Language Disorders in Children

Fundamental Concepts of Assessment and Intervention

Joan N. Kaderavek
University of Toledo

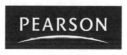

Boston   Columbus   Indianapolis   New York   San Francisco   Upper Saddle River
Amsterdam   Cape Town   Dubai   London   Madrid   Milan   Munich   Paris   Montreal   Toronto
Delhi   Mexico City   São Paulo   Sydney   Hong Kong   Seoul   Singapore   Taipei   Tokyo

Vice President and Editor in Chief:
  Jeffery W. Johnston
Executive Editor and Publisher:
  Stephen D. Dragin
Editorial Assistant: Anne Whittaker
Vice President, Director of Marketing:
  Quinn Perkson
Senior Marketing Manager: Christopher
  D. Barry
Senior Managing Editor: Pamela D. Bennett
Senior Project Manager: Linda Hillis Bayma

Senior Operations Supervisor:
  Matthew Ottenweller
Senior Art Director: Diane Lorenzo
Cover Designer: Kellyn E. Donnelly
Cover Art: SuperStock
Full-Service Project Management: Thistle
  Hill Publishing Services, LLC
Composition: Integra Software Services
Printer/Binder: Courier Stoughton, Inc.
Cover Printer: Courier Stoughton, Inc.
Text Font: Sabon

Credits and acknowledgments borrowed from other sources and reproduced, with permission, in this textbook appear on appropriate page within text.

Every effort has been made to provide accurate and current Internet information in this book. However, the Internet and information posted on it are constantly changing, so it is inevitable that some of the Internet addresses listed in this textbook will change.

Copyright © 2011 Pearson Education, Inc., Upper Saddle River, New Jersey 07458. All rights reserved. Manufactured in the United States of America. This publication is protected by Copyright, and permission should be obtained from the publisher prior to any prohibited reproduction, storage in a retrieval system, or transmission in any form or by any means, electronic, mechanical, photocopying, recording, or likewise. To obtain permission(s) to use material from this work, please submit a written request to Pearson Education, Inc., Permissions Department, 501 Boylston Street, Suite 900, Boston, MA 02116, fax: (617) 671-2290, email: permissionsus@pearson.com.

Library of Congress Cataloging-in-Publication Data

Kaderavek, Joan N.
  Language disorders in children : fundamental concepts of assessment and intervention/
Joan N. Kaderavek.
    p. cm.
  Includes bibliographical references and index.
  ISBN-13: 978-0-13-157492-2 (pbk.)
  ISBN-10: 0-13-157492-2 (pbk.)
  1. Language disorders in children.   2. Communicative disorders in children.   I. Title.
RJ496.L35K34 2011
618.92'85—dc22

                                                           2009049520

10 9 8 7 6 5 4 3 2 1

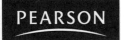

www.pearsonhighered.com

ISBN 13: 978-0-13-157492-2
ISBN 10:   0-13-157492-2

With love and gratitude to my husband, Dave

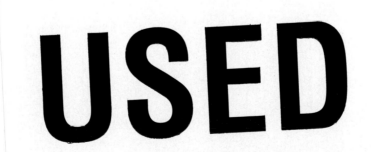

USED

Preface

This book considers issues of assessment and intervention for children with language impairments. It is written for undergraduate students who are just beginning to think about how to work with young children and school-age students who are language impaired. The assumption is that the student who uses this book will have already completed a course on normal language development.

I have developed the principles used in this book over a number of years of teaching undergraduate speech-language pathology (SLP) and special education students. Many undergraduate books provide an overview of terminology and describe a broad range of assessment and intervention approaches. As a teacher, I discovered a problem with this approach. The books (and the way I was teaching—primarily with lectures) promoted a passive learning mode. The undergraduates successfully passed tests; but these "good students" were not prepared to begin the analytic thought and problem solving that I expected (and they needed) in graduate-level training. I decided the problem was not with the students, but with the way I was teaching! My efforts to become a better teacher are reflected in the first overarching theme of this book.

THEMES OF THIS TEXT

Instead of expecting students to memorize terms and answer short-answer questions (e.g., *List three communication characteristics associated with autism spectrum disorders*), I began to train students to "think like a clinician." I began to emphasize decision-making processes used by highly skilled SLPs and educators. I realized that students did not need to be exposed to "everything." I could, however, motivate students to think deeply, ask questions, and solve problems.

I realized many students need to "talk through" problems and processes. If I described the problem (and the solution), students nodded wisely and wrote down what I said. When I asked if anyone had any questions, no hands were raised. In contrast, when I asked the students to explain what they had just learned, students could not verbalize the point that seemed so straightforward just a moment before. Clearly, I needed to do more.

I began to teach differently. I started each day with a mini-lecture; I tried to keep it under half an hour. Following the introduction of content, I assigned students to work in small groups. I varied the activities. I found this approach worked very well in face-to-face classes and also worked very well when I taught the course via distance learning. Rather than having the students demonstrate knowledge only with objective tests, I set up weekly activities during class time. I asked students in the distance learning class to complete the activities individually, with a partner, or a small group (depending on the weekly project). I began to include activities such as the following:

- I presented the students with a decision tree and asked them to put descriptive words at each decision point capturing expected communication behaviors they might see. Students explained the decision tree to a partner. I provide decision trees throughout this book.

- I provided simplified versions of assessment tools (trying to capture the essential elements of the decision-making process) and asked students to view videotapes and classify behaviors using the provided assessment tool. I realized that students' administration might not be highly accurate! However, I emphasized that students needed to verbalize "why" they choose to classify behaviors in a particular way—critical thinking was the goal. I provide simplified versions of assessment tools in this book.

- I encouraged students to "put words into their own mouths" by using role-playing activities. For example, I asked students to role-play an explanation of an intervention approach presenting to a "teacher" or "parent." In a distance-learning course I asked students to write out a script. Information that seemed easy to students during a lecture suddenly presented challenges when students were asked to teach someone else! I include many suggestions for role-playing in the chapter activities.

- I iteratively circled back to major points; I asked students to continually explain how fundamental principles applied to the topic under discussion. Instead of merely teaching theoretical perspectives during the first week of the course, I asked students to apply theory in response to all issues of assessment and intervention. As an example, in a discussion of intellectual disability, I might say *"Work with the person next to you and write down how social interaction theory, behaviorism, and systems theory might apply to our work with an individual with an intellectual impairment."* As I walked around the classroom, students asked many questions and actively engaged in solving the problem. I mirror this technique in many of the Focus boxes and In-Class Activities in each chapter. I also iteratively present information on language theory, form/content/use, and typical development throughout this book and link theoretical information to assessment and intervention decision making.

- I developed a numbered system for talking about language subdomains. Previously I had typically presented the concepts of *form, content,* and *use* in the parallel form (as it was taught to me). However, I was frustrated that during case example problem-solving activities, students didn't know where to start—they appeared to randomly focus on a domain (e.g., syntax for a child who was at the beginning language learning stage). I wanted students to move sequentially through a thought process that first considered an individual's beginning pragmatic skills, then single word and word combinations, then syntax, and so forth. The subdomain numbering (introduced in Chapter 1) provided a scaffold for this problem-solving task.

- I began talking to students about connections when I introduced new topics. I linked new information to previous information and also discussed how the information might apply more broadly across disorder types. I used the educational principle of helping students move from the known to the unknown. I mirror this approach in this book by including a section called *Connections* in many of the chapters. The Connections sections are linkages to previously learned concepts (e.g., applying the form/content/use model to children with autism spectrum disorders) or include a discussion of information that can be applied broadly across disorder types (e.g., counseling families).

• Finally, and most importantly, I begin to explicitly teach "meta" problem-solving skills. I tried to always explain why an SLP or educator might choose one approach over another or clarify the underlying analytic process fundamental to the task. I gave examples, and then asked students to discuss possible solutions to the problem *and* provide a rationale for their decision. I told students: *"Right now it is not important if you are wrong or right with your clinical decisions; I might make a different clinical decision than you. But what I want from you right now is to give me a reason (base it on language theory or research evidence or family concerns) to support your decision. That is your task at this early stage in professional training."* With this approach, students started to take chances and hypothesize about a particular assessment or intervention strategy for a specific child. At the end of the discussion, I typically shared my thoughts and explained why I might make a different clinical decision. But, before giving my opinion, I wanted students to begin to make decisions about intervention approaches that might work, based on their current knowledge. Throughout this book, I provide examples, case studies, and ideas for class discussion to stimulate this process. Chapter 3, the chapter on clinical decision making, grew out of my efforts to teach "meta" processes.

In sum, I began to be a better and more effective teacher for undergraduate students. This book is the result. My hope is that this approach will help other instructors actively engage students and help students become active learners.

A second overarching theme of this book is to represent current issues central to speech-language pathology and special education. This includes discussions of evidence-based practice (EBP), Response to Intervention, classroom-based assessment and intervention, connections between oral language and literacy learning, and multicultural issues. To this end, I give specific attention to each issue in one section of the book, but come back to each topic in other chapters. My intent is not to be redundant, but to make it clear that certain topics affect broad aspects of service delivery and decision making. My emphasis on EBP is also represented in my decision to only present two or three intervention approaches for each of the disorder groups. Rather than present a full range of possible intervention approaches (without a detailed discussion), I wanted to discuss relevant research for select exemplary approaches and explain how they represent "levels of evidence" within EBP.

I used to wait until graduate-level training to expose students to primary research. I now believe, with the emphasis on EBP, that students need exposure to primary research as the beginning training level. I hope instructors will supplement my discussions of intervention by providing examples of primary intervention research. Students need to begin to evaluate the quality of primary research. I supply a description of the elements of high-quality research studies in Chapter 4.

I have enjoyed my years as a practicing SLP and I am committed to teaching students to think like a clinician. My greatest hope is that this book helps that occur.

ACKNOWLEDGMENTS

My acknowledgement section is short, but my gratitude, affection, and the learning prompted by these four remarkable colleagues is limitless. Each is a talented professional colleague and steadfast friend. *Thank you* to (alphabetically) Laurie Dinnebeil, Aileen Hunt, Laura Justice, and Lori Pakulski.

Thank you to my husband, Dave (who helped prepare the permission requests for this book), to my children (Megan Kaderavek Tsai and Brian Kaderavek), and to my sisters (Lynn Nybell and Susan Nybell) who have listened to me talk endlessly about "the book!" You kept me going.

And, Mom (Elizabeth Gotter Odgen), I know you are watching all of this and thinking it is great fun!

I would like to thank the following people who reviewed the text and provided feedback: Eileen Abrahamsen, Old Dominion University; Linda K. Crowe, Kansas State University; Ellen Meyer Gregg, University of Northern Colorado; William O. Haynes, Auburn University; Henriette Langdon, San José State University; Peter Paul, The Ohio State University; Elaine Silliman, University of South Florida; and Nora Swenson, Valdosta State University.

Joan N. Kaderavek

Brief Contents

CHAPTER *1*   Language Theory and Language Development   1

CHAPTER *2*   Assessment of Language Disorders   44

CHAPTER *3*   Decision Making in Assessment and Intervention   97

CHAPTER *4*   Principles of Intervention   133

CHAPTER *5*   Children with Specific Language Impairment   175

CHAPTER *6*   Children with Hearing Loss   210
               Lori A. Pakulski

CHAPTER *7*   Children with Intellectual Disability   244

CHAPTER *8*   Children with Autism Spectrum Disorders   277

CHAPTER *9*   Early Literacy, Reading, and Writing for School-Age
               Children   305

CHAPTER *10*   Augmentative and Alternative Communication (AAC) and
               Individuals with Complex Communication Needs   356
               Julia M. King

CHAPTER *11*   Multicultural Issues   383
               Stephanie M. Curenton

APPENDIX *A*   *A Tutorial: The Meaning of Standard Scores*   413

APPENDIX *B*   *Language Sample Analysis Worksheet*   418

APPENDIX *C*   *Report Writing*   419

Glossary   425

References   439

Index   471

Contents

CHAPTER 1   *Language Theory and Language Development*   *1*

Definitions and Background Information: Language Disorders   2

The Speech Chain   3

Theoretical Approaches to Language and the Implications for Assessment and Intervention   6

Behaviorism Theory   *8*

Cognitive Theory   *9*

Nativist Theory   *13*

Neurobiological Research and Neural Maturation   *15*

Social Interaction Theory and Sociocultural Principles of Language Development   *19*

Information Processing/Connectionism   *21*

Systems/Ecological Approach   *23*

The Domains of Language: Form, Content, and Use and Five Communication Subdomains   24

Subdomain 1: Early Pragmatic Skills   28

Joint Visual Attention   *28*

Development of Early Pragmatic Functions   *29*

Early Discourse Skills Within Communication Subdomain 1   *30*

Clinical Implications for Communication Subdomain 1   *30*

Subdomain 2: Vocabulary Development   31

Clinical Implications for Communication Subdomain 2   *32*

Subdomain 3: Multiple Word Combinations   34

Clinical Implications for Communication Subdomain 3   *35*

Subdomain 4: Morphosyntax Development   36

Clinical Implications for Communication Subdomain 4   *38*

Subdomain 5: Advanced Pragmatic and Discourse Development   38

Clinical Implications for Communication Subdomain 5   *39*

Summary   *40*

Discussion and In-Class Activities   *42*

Case Study   *42*

CHAPTER 2   Assessment of Language Disorders   44

Assessment Tools   45
  Defining Norm-Referenced, Criterion-Referenced, and Dynamic Assessment   45
  Advantages and Disadvantages of Assessment Tools   47
  Psychometric Features of Assessment   48

Assessment Process   74
  Screening   74
  Diagnosis and Identifying Potential Intervention Targets   75
  Synthesizing Assessment Results, Counseling Families, and Writing Reports   89

Summary   93
Discussion and In-Class Activities   94
Case Study   95

**CHAPTER 3   Decision Making in Assessment and
Intervention   97**

A Model of Decision Making   98
  Critical-Thinking Parameters   99
  Questioning as a Tool for Critical Thinking   101
  Decision Trees as a Tool for Critical Thinking   103

Decision Making: Assessment   104
  Response to Intervention   107
  Prevention   111
  Case Example: Decision Making During Assessment   112

Decision Making: Intervention   113
  *Goals of Intervention: Infants, Toddlers, Preschoolers,
  and School-Age Students   114*
  *Critical-Thinking Questions During Intervention: Considering Underlying
  Language Theory   114*
  Public Policy (IDEA) and Decision Making   115
  Student Motivation and Decision Making   118
  Backward Design   118
  Case Example: Decision Making in Intervention   119

Decision Making: Environment   120
  Routines-Based Interviews   120
  Classroom Contexts for Remediation   123
  Case Example: Decision Making and Environment   125

Decision Making: Progress Monitoring and Dismissal   125
  Progress Monitoring   126

Dismissal from Therapy   *128*

Case Example: Decision Making in Progress Monitoring   *128*

Summary   *130*

Discussion and In-Class Activities   *131*

Case Studies   *132*

CHAPTER 4 Principles of Intervention   **133**

The Intervention Toolbox Part I: Theories, Domains, and Evaluation of Intervention Research   134

Intervention Techniques and Their Relationship to Language Theory   *134*

Intervention Techniques in Relation to Language Form, Content, and Use   *147*

Evaluating Evidence-Based Intervention Strategies   *153*

The Intervention Toolbox Part II: Structuring and Implementing Treatment   158

Structuring Intervention   *158*

Implementing Effective Interventions   *164*

Summary   *171*

Discussion and In-Class Activities   *173*

Case Study   *174*

CHAPTER 5 Children with Specific Language Impairment   **175**

Definition, Prevalence, Causation, and Major Characteristics   176

Definition   *176*

Prevalence and Causation   *176*

Major Characteristics   *177*

Associated Problems   *182*

Connections   184

Children's Social Communication   *184*

Peer-Mediated Intervention Approaches   *186*

Assessment   187

Parent-Child Interaction Assessments   *188*

Curriculum-Based Language Assessment   *192*

Intervention   193

Intervention Approach: Enhanced Milieu Teaching (EMT)   *194*

Intervention Approach: Conversational Recast Training (CRT)   *200*

Intervention Approach: Sentence Combining   *204*

Summary   *207*

Discussion and In-Class Activities   *208*

Case Study   *209*

CHAPTER **6**   Children with Hearing Loss   210

Lori A. Pakulski

Description of the Disorder   211
   Prevalence   211
   Types of Hearing Loss   211
   Variations in HL by Race/Ethnicity   212
   Degree of Hearing Loss   212
   Auditory Perceptual Problems   213

Causation, Risk Factors, and Communication Impairments   215

Factors Influencing Outcomes for Children with Hearing Loss   216
   Early Detection   216
   Neuroplasticity   217
   Choosing a Communication Modality   218
   Family Involvement in the Remediation Process   225

Connections   226
   Counseling Parents of Children with Special Needs   226
   The Grief Process   228
   Family Role in Intervention   229

Assessment and Progress Monitoring   230
   Assessment Tools   230

Intervention   235
   Learning to Listen   235
   Language Experience Books   237

Summary   240

Discussion and In-Class Activities   241

Case Study   242

CHAPTER 7   Children with Intellectual Disability   244

Description, Prevalence, Causation, and Major Characteristics   245
   Description of ID and the Ecological Model   245
   Prevalence   248
   Causation and Risk   248
   Characteristics of ID and the Implications for Remediation   252

Connections   258
   Language Delay Versus Language Disorder   258
   Form, Content, and Use Within Subtypes of ID   259

Assessment   262

Limitations of Norm-Referenced Assessments for
Individuals with ID   263

Functional Assessment   263

Achieving Communication Independence: A Comprehensive
Guide to Assessment and Intervention   264

Intervention   266

Intervention Approach: Functional Communication
Approach   266

Intervention Approach: IT's Fun Program   271

Summary   273

Discussion and In-Class Activities   274

Case Study   275

CHAPTER *8*   *Children with Autism Spectrum Disorders*   277

Description of the Disorder   278

Characteristic Deficits of ASD   278

Five Disorder Types Within the Autism Spectrum   281

Prevalence of Autism and Co-Occurrence
of Other Disorders   284

Causation/Risk Factors   285

Neurophysiologic and Neurochemical Investigations   285

Genetic Investigations   285

Environmental Factors   286

Connections   286

Developmental Issues   286

Family Involvement   287

Assessment and Progress Monitoring: Autism   288

Identifying Children with Potential ASD: Screening   288

Assessment of Verbal and Nonverbal
Communication Functions   291

Ongoing Progress Monitoring   294

Intervention   295

Intervention Approach: Applied Behavioral Analysis (ABA)   296

Intervention Approach: SCERTS   298

Summary   302

Discussion and In-Class Activities   303

Case Study   304

CHAPTER Early Literacy, Reading, and Writing for School-Age Children   305

The Role of the Speech-Language Pathologist in Reading and Writing   306

Emergent Literacy   308

Prevention of Reading Disability in Young Children at Risk for Reading Failure   308

Primary Targets of Emergent Literacy Prevention Programs   309

Assessment of Children's Early Literacy Skills   314

Early Literacy Interventions: The Embedded-Explicit Approach   317

Cultural Considerations in Emergent Literacy Development   322

School-Age Children with Language Impairment   323

School-Age Students: Phonological Awareness   324

School-Age Students: Narratives   328

School-Age Students: Spelling   331

School-Age Students: Reading Comprehension   336

School-Age Students: Writing   339

Working with Teachers   340

Cultural Considerations in Reading and Writing Development for School-Age Children   340

Reading and Writing Interventions for Students with Significant Levels of Impairment   342

The I-to-I Model: Overview   342

I-to-I Model: Level I   343

I-to-I Model: Level II   344

I-to-I Model: Level III   344

I-to-I Model: Level IV   345

I-to-I Model: Level V   345

Intervention for Students with Reading and Writing Disability: Evidence-Based Practices   346

Explicit Phonological Awareness Intervention   346

Writing Lab Approach   348

Summary   352

Discussion and In-Class Activities   353

Case Study   355

CHAPTER *10* Augmentative and Alternative Communication (AAC) and Individuals with Complex Communication Needs 356

Julia M. King

Background and Description 357
The AAC System 357
Multi-Modal Communication 358

The AAC System Components: What Is AAC? 358
AAC Symbols 358
The AAC Aid 359
AAC Strategies 359
AAC Techniques 363
AAC Selection Set 363
What Is Not AAC? 365

Assessment 366
Symbol Assessment 370
Feature Match 371

Intervention 372
The System for Augmenting Language (SAL) 372
Visual Scene Displays (VSDs) 373
Picture Exchange Communication System (PECS) 376

Summary 377
Discussion and In-Class Activities 378
Resources 379
Case Study 380

CHAPTER *11* Multicultural Issues 383

Stephanie M. Curenton

Ethnicity and Culture 385
Relationship Between Ethnicity and Culture 386
Working with Diverse Populations 386
Multicultural Challenges 386

Description of Diverse Populations 389

Issues to Consider When Working with Ethnically Diverse Populations 391
Acculturation 393

Individualism Versus Collectivism   394
Bilingualism   396
Dialects   397
Connections   400
Assessment of Ethnic Minority Children   401
Assessing a Child in His or Her Native Language   401
Pragmatic Differences   403
Intervention   403
Consideration #1: Consider the Role of Nuclear and Extended Family in Family Interventions   404
Consideration #2: Consider the Family Values About Child Communication Norms   405
Avoiding Cultural Conflicts During Intervention   405
Micro- and Macro-Levels of Intervention   407
Summary   409
Discussion and In-Class Activities   410
Case Study   411

APPENDIX A   A Tutorial: The Meaning of Standard Scores   413

APPENDIX B   Language Sample Analysis Worksheet   418

APPENDIX C   Report Writing   419

Glossary   425

References   439

Index   471

CHAPTER *1*

Language Theory and Language Development

Chapter Overview Questions

1. What are the differences between a language disorder, a language difference, and a language delay?
2. What are the three levels of communication described within the speech chain? Which level is the focus of this book?
3. What are the seven different theories influencing language development as described in this chapter?
4. How does each theory influence intervention approaches?
5. What are five different communication subdomains? What is the most important communication characteristic associated with each subdomain?
6. How do practitioners use information regarding the subdomains to guide clinical interventions?

Welcome to this book about language disorders. The language disorders course in which you are now enrolled is probably your first course focusing on children with communication deficits. Up to this point, your training has concentrated on communication development in children who are developing typically. It is an exciting professional turning point when you begin to consider how to guide assessment and interventions for individuals with language disorders.

This book's goal is to help you think like a practitioner. I focus on underlying theories and fundamental principles guiding clinical decision making. The ability to synthesize information, weigh scientific evidence, and see connections between basic principles will prepare you to work with children who have language impairments.

One book on language disorders cannot teach you everything you need to know to be a successful speech-language pathologist (SLP) or special educator. This book does not try to teach you everything! Instead, I have chosen to (a) emphasize basic principles and then (b) discuss selected assessment and intervention protocols as illustrative examples. I believe at this early point in your professional training it is better to provide more extensive information and examples for some exemplary assessment and intervention approaches (and clarify why they are exemplary) in contrast to briefly describing many different approaches.

To help you become a decision maker, I include many examples, case studies, and opportunities for you to practice problem solving. By working through the examples, you will learn important analytic processes. In this chapter, I (a) review basic definitions and background on language and language disorders, (b) review a basic model of communication (i.e., the speech chain model), (c) review theories of language development highlighting the clinical implications of each theory, (d) discuss the concepts of language form, content, and use, and (e) explain how form, content, and use can be subdivided into five communication subdomains.

Definitions and Background Information: Language Disorders

There are differences between the terms *language, speech,* and *communication.* **Language** is a complex and dynamic system of conventional symbols used for thought and expression. Language can be expressed orally, through writing or pictured symbols, or manually (e.g., sign language).

Speech is not the same thing as language. While language involves a symbol system, **speech** is the articulation and the rate (i.e., fluency) of speech sounds and quality of an individual's voice. **Communication,** in contrast, includes symbolic *and* nonsymbolic information (i.e., facial expressions, body language, gestures, etc.). As an example, if I frown and cross my arms, although I am not using symbolic communication, I am communicating! A communication disorder may be evident in the process of hearing, language, speech, or in a combination of all three processes.

In U.S. schools, children with speech and language disorders (as a specific diagnostic category) make up 1.79% of the total school population. Additionally, there are other subgroups of children who are not counted in the 1.79% who also have language disorders. Practitioners serve children who have hearing loss (.11% of schoolchildren), multiple disabilities (.2%), intellectual disabilities (1.81%), and learning disabilities (4.14%; IDEA, 1997). Each of these subgroups demonstrates language impairments.

A **language disorder** is impaired comprehension and/or use of spoken, written, and/or other symbol systems. A language disorder can represent a deficit in receptive language, expressive language, or a combined expressive-receptive deficit. **Receptive language** refers to an individual's ability to understand and process language; **expressive language** refers to an individual's ability to express and communicate meaning with language. Typically, an individual's receptive language abilities are better than his or her expressive language abilities.

Sometimes a young child (2 to 3 years old) who exhibits a developmental lag in language is called **language delayed** or a **late talker.** This terminology is used because experts state that a language disorder cannot be reliably diagnosed in young children in the absence of a primary disorder (e.g., cognitive impairment, autism; Bishop, Price, Dale, & Plomin, 2003; Rescorla, 2009).

An individual with a language disorder is different from someone with a language difference. **Language difference** results from a variation of a symbol system used by a group of individuals that reflects and is determined by shared regional, social, or cultural/ethnic factors. It is essential that professionals distinguish between aspects of language production representing dialectal patterns (i.e., language difference) as compared to true disorders in speech and language (ASHA, 2003). For example, a teacher may say to her students, "*I've got y'all's assignments here.*" This is a form of dialect associated with the southern United States; although it may be an unfamiliar expression to some U.S. speakers, it does not represent a language disorder. Information regarding language difference associated with dialect use is presented throughout this book.

As a final important point, I want to underscore that much of what you will learn about language disorders applies across disability categories. Rather than focusing on a child's diagnostic category (e.g., autism, specific learning disability), skilled practitioners use a descriptive-developmental framework to guide intervention. A **descriptive-developmental approach** focuses on a student's language development and function in a variety of natural contexts (Zipoli & Kennedy, 2005). A practitioner who uses a descriptive-developmental approach works to understand the individual's communication strengths and limitations rather than focusing on his or her diagnostic label. This is a particularly important point because I have organized subsequent chapters in this book by disability category. There is, for example, a chapter on autism, a chapter on intellectual disability, and so forth. I organize chapters by disability categories because—in my teaching experience— beginning practitioners learn most easily with this organizational strategy. However, to counterbalance my organizational strategy, I continually clarify descriptive and developmental similarities between disability groups and highlight connections between intervention approaches across disability types. Read more about categorical versus descriptive approaches in Focus 1.1.

The Speech Chain

The **speech chain model** is a basic model of communication used to explain the processes of communication from the speaker's production of words, through transmission of sound, to the listener's perception of what has been said (Denes & Pinson, 2001). I present this model to point out how language fits into an individual's communication system. The speech chain model is visually presented in Figure 1.1.

FOCUS 1.1 *Learning More*

The categorical model organizes language disorders on the basis of an individual's syndromes of behavior; it is fundamentally a medical model (Paul, 2007). Its advantages are that it (a) is easily understandable, (b) often is necessary to qualify a child for educational services, and (c) provides a basic explanation of how a particular child may be different from other children. The limitations of the categorical model are the following:

- There is not always a cause-effect relationship between an individual's diagnosis and the language impairment. Does a hearing loss mean that a child will automatically have a language delay? (You will read more about this in Chapter 6.)

- Children with different diagnostic labels may be quite similar. A child with a pragmatic disorder may be classified as having autism, intellectual impairment, or specific language impairment.
- Children's degree of involvement may vary dramatically within a diagnostic category. For example, a child with autism may be very mildly impaired; the diagnostic label may unfairly prejudice teachers or communication partners with regard to his or her abilities.
- Knowing a child's diagnostic classification may not be very helpful in planning an intervention program. SLPs instead use a decision-making process based on an individual's communication strengths and limitations.

The first point I want to emphasize is that the speech chain model reminds us that language has both a receptive and expressive component. The speaker/listener role is visually represented in Figure 1.1 with the left-to-right nature of the diagram. A good communicator speaks *and* listens. Within a conversation a person alternates between listening (using receptive language) and speaking (using expressive language). A competent communicator effortlessly comprehends the listener and produces meaningful language output. Remember that language output can be represented by spoken language, writing, or manual communication (i.e., sign language).

The second point about the speech chain is that the communication system requires a number of mechanisms to occur. Acoustic information must be transferred (Level 1 in Figure 1.1) motor activity must take place (Level 2), and the brain is activated at Level 3 to create meaningful symbolic (i.e., linguistic) information. All three levels of the system must be operating effectively for communication to occur. I elaborate on each of the three levels below.

Level 1 represents the acoustic level of communicative function: the external or environmental system. This level describes how physical energy is transferred between communication partners. In its simplistic form, Level 1 represents the molecular vibration forming sound waves and transferring physical energy from the speaker to the listener. It is very likely you studied the external physical component of communication in a course called Speech Science or Physics of Sound.

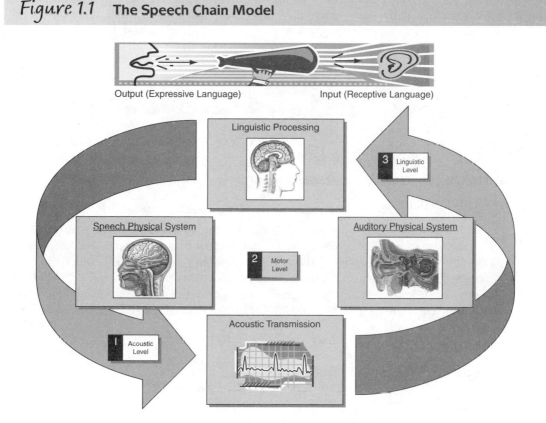

Figure 1.1 **The Speech Chain Model**

Level 2 represents the internal physical/motor system required for communication. In the listener, the physical system consists of the hearing mechanism and the transfer of neural messages to the brain's language center. In the speaker, Level 2 represents the speech system including respiration, articulation, and phonation. The physical speech systems must be coordinated to produce intelligible speech. It is likely that you studied aspects of Level 2 motor communication in a course called Anatomy and Physiology. You will learn about disorders occurring in the speech system in coursework covering articulation disorders, motor-speech disorders, and voice disorders. You will learn more about Level 2 (i.e., physical) hearing problems in your audiology coursework.

Level 3 of the speech chain model represents the linguistic component of communication. Level 3, the linguistic component, is the focus of this book. The linguistic level is the ability of the listener to receive incoming Level 2 energy (i.e., neural signals) and turn the physical energy into meaningful information via receptive language. The speaker creates meaningful linguistic information at Level 3.

The speech chain model emphasizes the complexity of the communication system and helps you integrate what you are learning in this course with other coursework. As you progress through your professional training program, continue to frame new knowledge within this basic model of communication functioning.

Let's now move beyond the speech chain model and consider the three fundamental language domains of form, content, and use.

Theoretical Approaches to Language and the Implications for Assessment and Intervention

To become an effective linguistic communicator, a speaker must master three language areas: the *form* of the message, the *content* of the message, and the message *use* or function. Language form includes phonology, morphology, and syntax (i.e., the structure of language). Language content consists of semantics (i.e., meaning of language); language function consists of pragmatics (i.e., how language is used within social contexts). See Table 1.1 for formal definitions and examples of each of these terms.

Table 1.1 Language Definitions

Form

Morphology is the system that governs the structure of words and the construction of word forms.

> Example: At age 13 months a child says "*Two birdie!*," but by 24 months says "*Two birdies!*" The child has learned to add the *s* morpheme to indicate a plural form.

Syntax is the system governing the order and combination of words to form sentences, and the relationships among the elements within a sentence.

> Example: At age 24 months, the child asks a question by saying "*Doggie outside?*" With this utterance, the child omits the copula verb *is* needed for a question form; this is a typical error at 24 months. However, by 36 months the child says, "*Is the dog outside?*" In the second instance, the child demonstrates understanding of English word order by placing the copula verb *is* at the beginning of the sentence demonstrating the use of interrogative reversal syntax form.

Phonology is the sound system of a language and the rules that govern the sound combinations. To learn more about phonological disorders go to the ASHA website: www.asha.org/public/speech/disorders/ChildSandL.htm

Content

Semantics is the system that governs the meanings of words and sentences.

> Example: At age 11 months, the child calls out "*da-da*" whenever she sees a male. But, by 15 months, she only calls "*da-da*" or "*daddy*" for her father; she says "*man*" for unfamiliar men. In the first example, the child overgeneralizes the meaning of *daddy,* using it to refer to any male figure. This is a common early semantic pattern. As semantic knowledge develops, the child learns the meaning of the word *daddy* and only uses this word for her father.

Use

Pragmatics is the system that combines the above language components in functional and socially appropriate communication.

> Example: A child tugs on his father's pants and points to the TV. This is an example of a nonverbal request.

Source: Information from *Definitions of Communication Disorders and Variations [Relevant Paper],* 1993, American Speech-Language-Hearing Association (ASHA). Available from www.asha.org/policy.

Given the complex communication system described in the speech chain model, it is amazing to conceive how a young child becomes a proficient language learner in a relatively short span of time. This process is remarkable because there are significant challenges confronting the language learner. Tomasello and Bates (2001) summarize the fundamental challenges facing the language learner:

- There are challenges related to speech perception and production. The language learner must make sense of the continuous sequence of spoken sounds and segment the speech stream into meaningful units. The motor system must be intact so the speaker can reproduce the sounds that are heard.
- There is the challenge of communicating meaning. The language learner must learn to use language to direct the attention of others.
- There is a challenge associated with mastering grammar and using language creatively. The language learner must learn to combine words into novel utterances using correct syntax and morphological structure.

Given this list of challenges, it is hardly surprising that there are a number of language theories to explain the language-learning process. At the mention of language theories, I hope you are not groaning inwardly! An important component of this book focuses on explaining how language theories are important principles used to identify children's language challenges and develop intervention programs. I will be referring back to language theory throughout this book when I discuss intervention options for children with communication impairments.

It is important to recognize that any one theory cannot explain the complex process of communication, but each theory makes a contribution towards understanding how language develops and how intervention helps children who struggle to communicate. Below I present information on seven theories of language development: behaviorism, cognitive theory, nativist theory, neural maturation, social interaction theory, information-processing theory (i.e., connectionism), and systems/ecological approach. I highlight clinical implications for each theory.

BEHAVIORISM THEORY

Behaviorism is a theory suggesting that learning occurs when an environmental stimulus triggers a response or behavior. Behavioral principles are used to reward children with the goal of increasing the frequency of positive behaviors and decreasing or altering negative behaviors. B.F. Skinner (1957) is the individual most closely associated with behaviorism principles.

Skinner proposed that language, like other behavior, is produced because caregivers selectively reinforce words. For example, the parent says the word "*cracker,*" and the child responds by saying "*ka-ka.*" The parent says, "*Yes, this is a cracker!*" and gives the child a cracker. The reinforcement is the parents' positive response and the cracker.

The word *ka-ka* gradually is shaped to match the adult production of the word. **Shaping** occurs when an individual is expected to produce closer approximations to the behavioral target prior to reinforcement. In this example, the parent eventually expects the child to say "*cracker*" before providing the desired item.

A number of important concepts used in speech-language pathology and special education are based on behaviorism theory:

- *Reinforcement:* Reinforcing a child's behavior makes it more likely that the behavior will occur in the future. **Positive reinforcement** is a stimulus increasing the frequency of a particular behavior using pleasant rewards. In contrast, **negative reinforcement** is unpleasant to the child. An example of negative reinforcement is when an adult frowns, nags, or makes disapproving comments to a child and continues to do so until the unwanted behavior ends. The child stops the unwanted behavior (presumably producing a more desirable behavior) to avoid the negative stimuli. Reinforcement can be social ("high-fives," smiles, encouragement, or praise), activities (participating in a pizza party following successful completion of therapy activities), or material (allowing the child to have favorite foods or earn points for toys).
- *Extinction:* Extinction is based on the behavioral principle that when a child's response is not reinforced, the ignored behavior will decrease or disappear. An example of extinction is ignoring a child's negative behavior.
- *Antecedent:* An antecedent event is a stimulus that precedes a behavior. The child's behavior (with reinforcement) can be linked to the antecedent event. For example, the child sees the cookie (the antecedent event) and the child says, "*Want cookie!*"

- *Punishment:* Punishment is a negative response that the child views as undesirable; punishment follows a behavior that the adult wishes to eliminate. Punishment makes it less likely that the negative behavior will occur; an example of punishment is placing a child in a "time-out chair" following the child's misbehavior.
- *Chaining:* **Behavioral chaining** occurs when an activity requires a number of linked steps; a complex behavioral sequence is broken down into smaller units so the child can be trained to complete a multistep task. For example, if a child is being trained to wash his hands, he is first taught to turn on the water, then to use soap and engage in hand washing, then taught to turn off the water, and then to dry his hands. Individual components are rewarded in successive steps.

Clinical Implications of Behaviorism Theory.　Behaviorism has influenced educational practice in many ways. First, drill-and-practice activities within intervention sessions are based on behaviorism (Fey, 1986). The goal in drill-and-practice sessions is to stimulate many child behaviors that can be shaped and rewarded by the interventionist. Drill-and-practice also tends to focus on discrete, isolated aspects of language with the idea that small skills are sequentially linked in a step-by-step approach to form more complex communication behaviors. The step-by-step principle underlies many intervention programs for children with more significant levels of disability (e.g., cognitive impairments, autism [Pelios, MacDuff, & Axelrod, 2003]).

Second, behaviorism principles underlie the practitioner's focus on observable and measurable behaviors. Behaviorism demands that a child's responses are documented and that change in language performance is demonstrated by ongoing progress monitoring. The skilled practitioner documents a child's performance and progress toward achieving long-term goals.

All language theories have limitations and strengths in explaining language learning. The limitation of behaviorism is that it is not a comprehensive theory; it does not explain how an individual produces complex and novel behaviors. For example, children produce utterances they have not heard without reinforcement; behaviorism does not explain this phenomenon. However, behavioral theory helps explain how children learn discrete behaviors. As a result, the application of behaviorist principles is useful within certain intervention programs.

COGNITIVE THEORY

Cognitive theory is based on the numerous writings of Jean Piaget (e.g., Piaget, 1952). Piaget examined children's logical reasoning abilities (i.e., problem solving) and proposed a sequence of progressively more sophisticated cognitive skills, from primitive thinking (at the beginning of the sensorimotor stage) to advanced cognitive ability (in the formal operations stage). Characteristics of Piaget's four stages of cognitive development are summarized in Table 1.2.

The interpretation of cognitive theory proposes that specific cognitive achievements are fundamental to linguistic development. Linkages exist between children's

Table 1.2   **Piaget's Cognitive Stages**

Age	Stage	Characteristics
Birth to 2 years	Sensorimotor	Begins with reflexive and motor learning. Progresses rapidly, learning object permanence, means-end, etc.
2 to 7 years	Preoperational	Most rapid stage of language learning. Child learns to solve physical problems.
7 to 11 years	Concrete operations	Child learns to categorize and organize information; begins to be a logical thinker.
11 to 15 years	Formal operations	Learns to be an abstract thinker, tests mental hypotheses.

motor ability, play behavior, and language development. Figure 1.2 illustrates a child at play who is developing her problem-solving skills.

The parallel development of motor, play, and language milestones is summarized in Table 1.3. Practitioners use Piagetian principles to evaluate cognitive skills

Figure 1.2   **An Infant's Exploration of Her Physical Environment Facilitates Cognitive Development**

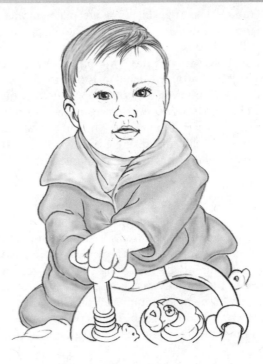

Table 1.3 **Linkages Between Piaget's Sensorimotor Substages and Motor/ Cognitive, Play, and Communication Behaviors**

Substage (age)	Motor/ Cognitive	Interactions and Imitation	Play	Communication
I Reflexive (Birth-1 month)		• Interactions are caregiver initiated		
II Primary circular (1–4 months)		• Child repeats own behaviors	• Grasping, looking at object	• Cries, laughs, coos
III Secondary circular (4–8 months)	• Behaves as if he or she is cause of all actions (early causality)	• Imitates behaviors that he or she has produced before • Child begins to initiate interactions	• Begins to interact with people with gestures and vocalizations	• Babbles (child actively interacts) • Beginnings of semantic understanding (6–8 months)
IV Causality (8–12 months)	• Looks for object if sees it being hidden (object permanence) • Knows other people can cause activities (more developed causality) • Evidence of planning of intentional behaviors (means-end)	• Imitates behaviors not produced before		• Links gestures and vocalization • Expansion of semantic function
V Tertiary circular (12–18 months)			• Figures out how to make toys work (cause and effect)	• First meaningful words
VI Representational thought (18–24 months)		• Imitates actions that has stored mentally	• Progresses to symbolic play	• Multiple-word utterances

Source: Adapted from *Born to Talk: An Introduction to Speech and Language Development* (p. 5), by L. M. Hulit and M. R. Howard, 2006, Boston: Pearson Education. Adapted with permission.

needed for language development and often observe children's play behavior with a Piagetian perspective. A detailed description of a play-focused observational proto-col is provided in Chapter 5. The following important concepts are based on Piaget's cognitive theory:

- **Schema:** A schema is a concept, mental category, or cognitive structure; children form many different schemata as they interact with their environments. (**Schemata** is the plural form of *schema*.)
- **Assimilation:** A child evidences assimilation when he takes in new information and incorporates it into his existing schemata. When a child sees an unfamiliar animal (e.g., a camel) and says, "*horse,*" he is evidencing assimilation.
- **Accommodation:** A child evidences accommodation when he adjusts his schemata resulting from new information. In the former example, the child eventually accommodates new information and uses the word "*camel.*"
- **Equilibrium:** Piaget believed that children attempt to find a balance between assimilating new information into old schemata, and developing new schemata through accommodation. This balance is called equilibrium.
- **Disequilibrium:** As the child recognizes that two schemata are contradictory, disequilibrium occurs. Reorganization to higher levels of thinking is motivated by this disequilibrium. Disequilibrium was evidenced in the above example when the child recognized that the word "*horse*" failed to capture the camel's unique characteristics.
- **Symbolic play:** Symbolic play is evidenced when the child uses one object to represent another. For example, a child might tie a towel around his neck and say the towel is a cape and he is Superman.
- **Object permanence:** The child evidences object permanence during the sensori-motor stage of development when he realizes that an object exists even when it cannot be seen. Very young children cannot understand that objects continue to exist even when they can't be seen or felt. As an example, prior to achieving object permanence, a child will quickly lose interest in (and not search for) a hidden toy.
- **Object constancy:** Object constancy is another concept of the sensorimotor stage; the child learns that he is viewing the same object regardless of distance, light, or different viewing angle.
- **Means-end:** Means-end behavior is evidenced when the child demonstrates intentionality; it occurs when the child identifies a problem and makes a plan to solve the problem. An example of means-end behavior is when a child pushes a button or pulls a string to make a toy move. A child calling out "*Mama!*" and waiting for his mother to appear also demonstrates means-end behavior.

Practice your clinical problem-solving skills by considering the information in Focus 1.2. What Piagetian concepts are the children demonstrating in each example?

FOCUS 1.2 *Clinical Skill Building*

Use what you know about Piaget's sensorimotor stages. What cognitive process (or processes) is each child demonstrating?

- Child pulls off his sock; he gleefully throws it on the ground then looks down to see where it has fallen.

- Child pulls a toy toward herself using a string tied to the toy.
- Child waves good-bye as he leaves his father; his father is waving and saying *"bye-bye!"*
- The child's mother walks around a corner and the child immediately starts to cry.

Clinical Implications of Cognitive Theory.   Practitioners observe children's play behaviors to gauge children's general cognitive ability and level of representational thought. I provide an example of this decision-making process in Figure 1.3. Representational thought is the child's ability to represent one object with another. An example of high-level symbolic play (the first step in Figure 1.3) is a child who pretends to cook dinner, sets the table, places dolls and stuffed animals around the table, and pretends to serve dinner. Practitioners look for evidence of representational thought to gauge a child's readiness for symbolic language.

The limitation of Piagetian theory is the proposal that (a) children move through discrete and qualitatively different stages of development and (b) they work through the stages sequentially. A child at the sensorimotor stage is thought to problem-solve using qualitatively different strategies as compared to a child at a later stage of development. However, children do not always follow this linear and step-by-step developmental progression. Sometimes children solve surprisingly difficult problems (i.e., problems seemingly beyond their cognitive stage) within certain contexts and with the right support. On the other hand, the strength of Piagetian theory is that it helps practitioners understand how children use physical exploration to increase their problem-solving abilities.

NATIVIST THEORY

Nativist theory (sometimes called psycholinguistic language theory) is connected to the writings of Noam Chomsky (1965, 1990a, 1990b). Chomsky proposed that children have an innate (i.e., inborn) ability to learn language; this biological brain mechanism is called the Language Acquisition Device (LAD). Nativist theory de-emphasizes the contribution of the child's environment; it proposes that children need only minimal language exposure to prime the LAD. Nativist theory examines similarities in cross-cultural examples of children's early sentence construction: Similarities support the idea of innate linguistic rules (i.e., linguistic universals). For example, children across cultures demonstrate parallel language abilities at similar developmental periods. Further, very different languages (e.g., American Sign

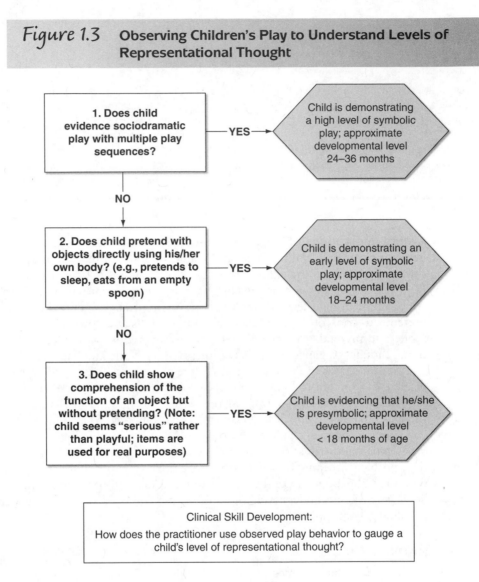

Figure 1.3   Observing Children's Play to Understand Levels of Representational Thought

1. Does child evidence sociodramatic play with multiple play sequences?

— YES → Child is demonstrating a high level of symbolic play; approximate developmental level 24–36 months

NO ↓

2. Does child pretend with objects directly using his/her own body? (e.g., pretends to sleep, eats from an empty spoon)

— YES → Child is demonstrating an early level of symbolic play; approximate developmental level 18–24 months

NO ↓

3. Does child show comprehension of the function of an object but without pretending? (Note: child seems "serious" rather than playful; items are used for real purposes)

— YES → Child is evidencing that he/she is presymbolic; approximate developmental level < 18 months of age

Clinical Skill Development:

How does the practitioner use observed play behavior to gauge a child's level of representational thought?

Language) use complex rules using many similar processes. Nativist concepts include the following:

- **Surface structure:** Surface structure is the actual sentence the speaker produces ("*The dog is petted by the child*").
- **Deep structure:** Deep structure is the underlying meaning of the sentence the speaker wants to produce ("*The child pets the dog*"). (This sentence and the sentence above mean the same thing; they have the same deep structure.)

- **Phrase structure grammar:** Phrase structure grammar describes the basic structure of a sentence regardless of the language being spoken.
- **Transformational grammar:** Transformational rules are specific to each language. For example, in English, when I ask a question, I use the interrogative reversal syntax construction (*"Am I late?"*). In an interrogative reversal, the auxiliary verb is placed at the beginning of the sentence. In other languages, the question-formation rule is different. Transformational grammar emphasizes the use of syntactic structures rather than semantics or pragmatics.

Clinical Implications of Nativist Theory. The nativist position has influenced professional recognition of the biological base for language learning, although it is now recognized that it may not be as specific as the LAD. For example, a linguist, Derek Bickerton (1990), studied the formation of Creole language in tropical colonies. Escaped slaves, living together but originally from different language groups, were forced to communicate in a restricted common form of language known as a pidgin (i.e., a very basic combination of words). The slaves were adults well beyond the period of typical language acquisition; accordingly, the language was rudimentary. However, the children of the slaves, as native speakers, developed the pigdin into a full language called Creole. Creole languages have morphemes and grammatical structure. The nativist theory helps explain this innate human ability to develop sophisticated language systems (Botwinik-Rotem & Friedmann, 2009). Nativist theory also has fostered an exploration of cross cultural language.

A limitation of Chomsky's work is that it was created at a theoretical level; it was not based on listening to what children do when they learn language. It also does not take children's environments into account and does not consider the influence of children's caregivers on language learning. A final limitation is that it focuses primarily on syntax learning instead of considering language form, content, and use.

The nature versus nurture debate in language considers the foundation of language learning. It asks the question: Is language learning based on a child's innate language ability (i.e., nativism) or nurture (i.e., the environment)? As you realize by now, language learning requires both nature *and* nurture. Even though both are required, the nativist position is helpful in this debate because it extends and clarifies the amazing language-learning ability (and drive to communicate) demonstrated by typically developing children.

NEUROBIOLOGICAL RESEARCH AND NEURAL MATURATION

Neurobiological research and **neural maturation** is not a theory of language development but rather a growing area of science explaining the relationship between language and brain development in young children. It is now well proven that maturation changes in the brain occur in overlapping stages and that successive changes in brain structure facilitate behavioral "bursts" of competency. The relationship between brain development and communication development is demonstrated in a number of recent research studies (Cheour et al., 2004; Hahne, Eckstein &

Friederici, 2004; Imada et al., 2006; Mills, Plunkett, Prat, & Schafer, 2005; Oberecker, Friedrich, & Friederici, 2005; Rivera-Gaxiola, Klarman, Garcia-Sierra, & Kuhl, 2005; Silva-Pereyra, Rivera-Gaxiola, & Kuhl, 2005). A diagram of the relationship between brain development and speech-language development is shown in Table 1.4.

The most recent research indicates that the relationship between brain development and behavior is not one way, but rather bidirectional (Clancy & Finlay, 2001). Specifically, not only does brain development facilitate language performance, but also a child's learning facilitates changes in brain regions devoted to a specific task. The brain is composed of highly integrated neural circuits (i.e., connections between brain cells). A child's environmental experiences build simple neural circuits; repeated and increasingly complex activities develop more advanced brain circuitry. The brain is, in a sense, "plastic." The term *plasticity* refers to the capacity of the brain to change (National Scientific Council on the Developing Child [NSCDC], 2007).

Table 1.4   **Communication Behaviors and Brain Development**

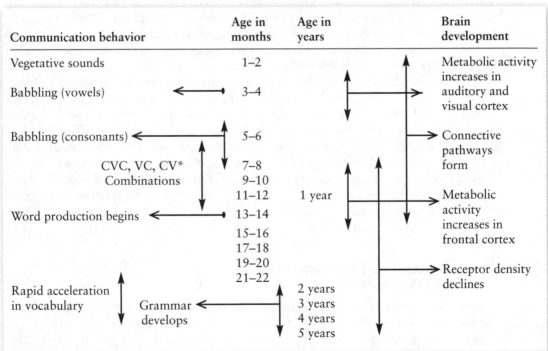

Communication behavior	Age in months	Age in years	Brain development
Vegetative sounds	1–2		Metabolic activity increases in auditory and visual cortex
Babbling (vowels)	3–4		
Babbling (consonants)	5–6		Connective pathways form
CVC, VC, CV* Combinations	7–8		
	9–10		
	11–12	1 year	Metabolic activity increases in frontal cortex
Word production begins	13–14		
	15–16		
	17–18		
	19–20		Receptor density declines
	21–22		
Rapid acceleration in vocabulary	Grammar develops	2 years	
		3 years	
		4 years	
		5 years	

*CVC = Consonant-Vowel-Consonant, VC = Vowel-Consonant, CV = Consonant-Vowel (These combinations are more "wordlike" than previous babbling sounds.)

Research on neural maturation also documents that as individuals mature, the brain becomes less capable of reorganizing and adapting to new environmental input: Brain plasticity decreases with age. Once a circuit is "wired," it becomes increasingly difficult to modify the neural activation patterns (NSCDC, 2007). This research highlights the need for very early intervention for children with developmental delays and sensory impairment.

Since the 1980s, technological advantages have dramatically altered the ability to understand the brain–language relationship. Technologies include electroencephalography (EEG), event-related potentials (ERPs), magnetoencephalography (MEG), magnetic resonance imaging (MRI), functional magnetic resonance imaging (fMRI), and near-infrared spectroscopy (NIRS). Figure 1.4 demonstrates how some of this technology is used with infants and young children.

The most frequently used noninvasive technologies include MRI and fMRI. The refinement in technologies provides insight into a broad spectrum of neural correlates of language learning (Tropper & Schwartz, 2009). For example, data indicate that (a) at birth young infants exhibit a universal capacity to detect differences between phonetic contrasts used in the world's languages; (b) by the end of the first year, the infant brain is no longer universally prepared for all languages but instead primed to acquire the language(s) in the infant's environment; (c) infants with excellent phonetic skills advance toward more complex language learning more quickly; and (d) by one year of age infants do not accept mispronunciations of common words, demonstrating that their representations of these words are well-specified after the first year (Kuhl & Rivera-Gaxiola, 2008).

Clinical Implications of Neurobiological Research.   Recent neural development research has altered decision making for some intervention programs. The basic principles of neuroscience indicate that early intervention produces more favorable outcomes than remediation later in life. As an example, experts now propose that children with hearing loss need early and intense auditory stimulation to build neural circuits for sound perception (Gordon, Papsin, & Harrison, 2003; Sharma, 2007; Sharma et al., 2004). In your professional career, neuroimaging technology will be an important contributor to the field of communication sciences. This research has the potential to answer important questions (Kuhl & Rivera-Gaxiola, 2008):

- How does social interaction affect the brain's ability to learn language?
- How is language mapped in the bilingual brain? Does experience with two or more languages early in development affect the brain's underlying processing?
- How do developmental disabilities such as autism and specific language impairment affect the brain's processing of speech and language?
- Which mechanisms underlie the critical period for second language acquisition? Why are adults unable to learn as well as young children? Can techniques be developed to help adults learn a second language?

A limitation of neurobiological research is that, at present, the technologies have only limited application for intervention. Eventually, however, neuroimaging may be used to document the effectiveness of a particular intervention approach.

Figure 1.4 Methods of Noninvasive Neuroimaging Used to Investigate Brain–Language Relationships

Neuroscience techniques used with infants

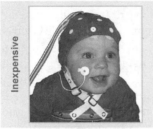

Inexpensive

EEG/ERP: Electrical potential changes
- Excellent temporal resolution
- Studies cover the life span
- Sensitive to movement
- Noiseless

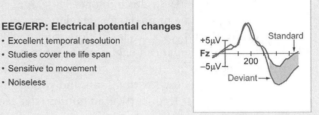

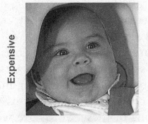

Expensive

MEG: Magnetic field changes
- Excellent temporal and spatial resolution
- Studies on adults and young children
- Head tracking for movement calibration
- Noiseless

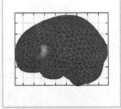

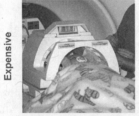

Expensive

fMRI: Hemodynamic changes
- Excellent spatial resolution
- Studies on adults and a few on infants
- Extremely sensitive to movement
- Noise protectors needed

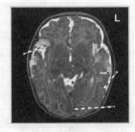

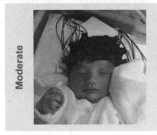

Moderate

NIRS: Hemodynamic changes
- Good spatial resolution
- Studies on infants in the first 2 years
- Sensitive to movement
- Noiseless

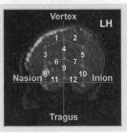

Kuhl P, Rivera-Gaxiola M. 2008.
Annu. Rev. Neurosci. 31:511–34.

Source: Reprinted, with permission, from the *Annual Review of Neuroscience*, Volume 31 © 2008 by Annual Reviews. www.annualreviews.org.

SOCIAL INTERACTION THEORY AND SOCIOCULTURAL PRINCIPLES OF LANGUAGE DEVELOPMENT

Two different (but related) theories are summarized in this section: social interaction language acquisition theory and Vygotsky's theory, sometimes referred to as sociocultural theory.

Social Interaction Theory.   Social interaction theory is based on the principle that communication interaction plays a central role in children's acquisition of language. The effects of social interaction on child language development have been demonstrated in the unfortunate situation where children have been denied access to human interaction due to severe neglect or abuse. In this situation, children fail to acquire normal language skills (Fromkin, Krashen, Curtiss, Rigler, & Rigler, 1974). Research shows that children's language development is strongly tied to children's appreciation of others' communicative intentions, their sensitivity to joint visual attention, and their desire to imitate others' behaviors and speech (Kuhl, 2004). The following concepts are based on social interaction theory:

- **Infant-directed talk:** Infant-directed talk (also called **motherese** [Baldwin & Meyer, 2007]) describes the characteristics of child-directed communication that enhance an infant's ability to learn language. Characteristics of infant-directed talk include the use of content words (i.e., nouns, verbs) in isolation, placement of content words at the ends of sentences ("*A doggie, see the doggie?*"), increased pitch on content words, and talking about objects and events in the "here and now." It has been theorized that these facilitating characteristics help infants extract the important information and make linkages between speech and objects or events.
- **Coordinating attention:** Adults follow an infant's focus of attention and match their communication to the child's eye gaze. Also, in Western cultures, adults try to direct infants' attention to a specific objects by pointing or showing (Baldwin & Meyer, 2007).
- **Parent-child communication routines:** Adults structure infant play routines in systematic patterns sometimes called scripts. **Scripts** involve predictable patterns of action facilitating infant participation. The interaction familiarity allows the child to anticipate his or her role in the interaction, building pragmatic communication skills (Baldwin & Meyer, 2007; Bruner, 1981). Examples include "*How big is baby? SO big!*" (the child is encouraged to lift his or her arms overhead); "*Peek-a-boo!*" (the child anticipates the "*boo!*" by laughing; eventually the child initiates hiding); repeated book-reading routines (parent repeats familiar vocabulary or prompts actions); waving "*bye-bye.*"

Vygotsky's Sociocultural Theory.   Vygotsky's (1962, 1978) theories build on the social interaction models that are described above. Vygotsky elaborated on the social interaction models by including cognitive development *and* language development in his theoretical position. Like Piaget, Vygotsky believed that children construct their own knowledge. However, whereas Piaget believed that cognitive development occurs primarily through children's interaction with physical objects, Vygotsky believed that cognitive development is socially mediated. That is to say, a child's interactions with others influence his or her cognitive understandings (Bodrova & Leong, 2007).

Vygotsky proposed that initially a child and a more capable partner (an adult or older child) solve problems together, but eventually the child internalizes the process and is able to carry out the function independently (Benigno & Ellis, 2004). There has been an explosion of research exploring Vygotskian principles in recent years (Winsler, 2003).

Vygotsky also asserted that language plays a critical role in shaping learning and thought. For example, he proposed that **private speech** plays a role in cognitive development. Private speech occurs when children speak aloud as they are engaged in play. Vygotsky's view was that private speech is a step that allows children to internalize important concepts. Other concepts based on Vygotsky's theories include the following:

- **Zone of proximal development (ZPD):** The ZPD is the competence that a child demonstrates with minimal assistance. The ZPD is the area between the zone of competence (what a child can do independently) and the zone of incompetence (what a child is unable to do, even with assistance [Baroody, Lai, & Mix, 2006]). Vygotsky proposed that teaching children within the ZPD (at the point where children can *just* perform the task with some assistance) is the key to maximizing child learning. Using the ZPD principle has prompted practitioners to introduce tasks to young children even though they are difficult (Kaderavek & Justice, 2004). For example, preschool children are engaged in early literacy activities with adult support. You will learn more about this concept in Chapter 10.
- **Scaffolding:** Scaffolding refers to the adult support that allows the child to engage in a challenging activity. Scaffolding techniques can include simplifying the task, providing directions and clarifying the task, reducing the child's frustration, modeling the correct response, and motivating and soliciting the child's task engagement. When used effectively, scaffolding is faded from levels of high support to minimal levels of guidance.
- **Mediation:** The term *mediation* is related to scaffolding. In scaffolding, the focus is on the adult's manipulation of the task to increase the learner's success. In mediation, the goal is to provide the learner with insights in order to teach the learner "how to learn." During a mediated learning task, the student is encouraged to accept responsibility so that he or she can function more independently. When mediating a task, the practitioner might say, *"Tell me the steps you are going to follow to finish this project."* The practitioner's goal is to increase the student's awareness of the steps required for task completion.

Clinical Implications of Social Interaction Theories.   SLPs and special educators base many of their assessment and intervention decisions on social interaction theories. Social interaction and sociocultural theories have encouraged practitioners to incorporate children's caregivers into intervention programs and to work with children in their homes and classrooms to build social interactions.

Social interactionists such as Jerome Bruner (1982) suggest the language behavior of adults when talking to children is specially adapted to support the acquisition process. Consequently, parents of children with language delay are taught to use strategies to enhance language input. I will be describing strategies to enhance children's language input in Chapter 5.

Other recent research supports the social interaction theory by demonstrating that increased maternal responsiveness facilitates greater growth in infants' social, emotional, communicative, and cognitive competence (Landry, Smith, & Swank, 2006). Accordingly, practitioners carefully observe and document caregiver interaction patterns in children with language deficits and delays.

The limitation of social interaction theories is that, taken on their own, they do not explain everything about language development. For example, in some cultures caregivers do not use infant-directed speech, yet children still develop language (Heath, 1983). Again we are reminded that one language theory, by itself, is not sufficient to explain the complex behavior of language development.

INFORMATION PROCESSING/CONNECTIONISM

Information-processing theories, also called **connectionism,** were initially called **parallel-distributed processing** (PDP) models. PDP models are used to simulate normal and impaired language development; the models are similar to computer software. PDP reflects a network in which neurons communicate in succession like a chain reaction (i.e., the serial model) or in a pattern where neurons fire along parallel routes (i.e., parallel processing). Serial and parallel processing also can be combined in what are known as hybrid models.

An important characteristic of information-processing models refers to **resource allocation:** the way in which energy is distributed in the system. The efficiency of the entire system depends on how many units are operating at one time; processing within one part of the system may be limited by demands on parallel processing units.

The model is complex and is represented by processing units, activation vectors (i.e., the connection between one unit and another), patterns of connectivity among units (i.e., the influence of one unit on another unit), rules that represent the initial pathways of activation, and learning rules describing how pathways are altered based on experience (e.g., change of weightings). The principle of weighting is used to explain how some connections are more easily initiated as compared to others.

Thinking of the brain as a computer highlights several important facts (Elman, 2001). First, an individual's cognitive ability to process information is completed by a large number of very simple processing elements. Each element (i.e., a clump of neurons in the brain called a node) responds to input from other nodes and either excites or inhibits connecting nodes. Second, a node's activation potential can change; a node may be particularly sensitive under some conditions but insensitive to activation under other conditions. Finally, output generated by the system relates to the connection patterns between the nodes (i.e., resource allocation). The weighting principle results in some patterns of connection occurring more frequently than others.

Here is an example of how connectionism is used to understand learning behavior associated with reading development. Weighting suggests that at the beginning stages of decoding the connections between recognizing a letter shape and the phonological processor (i.e., knowing the sound that a letter makes) must be particularly strong; at later stages of reading proficiency a reader depends less on this connection and the weighting is reduced. **Decoding** refers to the various skills an individual uses to decipher and understand printed words. In this case, the child begins the decoding process by sounding out individual phonemes in an unfamiliar word; he or she then blends individual phonemes back together to form an understandable word.

The child's processing nodes are activated in a linked manner. Activated nodes include a visual-processing component (i.e., the orthographic processor that visually stores the shape of letters and words in the brain) and the phonological processor. The phonological-processing component allows the child to convert the letter combination into a sound; if the child sees the word *ship,* the phonological processor associates the *sh* letter combination to the "sh" sound. Together the orthographic and phonological processors connect to a semantic node that allows the child to determine the word's meaning. This interconnected linkage of different processing components explains how children require both visual letter recognition abilities and phonological-processing abilities to become fluent readers. The information-processing model also explains how weighting at initial stages of reading highly favors phonological awareness but is reduced in skilled readers; readers at later stages of development focus more on comprehending word meaning (see Chapter 9 for more about reading development).

Clinical Implications of Information Processing Theories.   Research has demonstrated that weaker phonological processing connections are a likely cause of reading disability (Harm & Seidenberg, 1999). This information prompts practitioners to focus on building linkages between letter names and letter sounds in intervention programs for struggling readers. You will learn more about phonological awareness (PA) intervention approaches in Chapter 9. PA interventions often use information-processing models as a foundational theory (e.g., Gillon, 2004).

Also, the information-processing model offers a framework to explain individual processing challenges. Research has examined how simulated impairments in the information-processing model mimic errors noted in individuals with reading impairments (Harm & Seidenberg, 1999; Joanisse, 2009). The information-processing model also considers how cognitive-processing components—attention, memory, and transfer of information—affect the communication skills of individuals with intellectual disability (see Chapter 7).

A limitation of the information-processing model is that it is seen as being reductionist. In other words, it attempts to describe language processing in terms of neurons firing and communication between nodes. The model's strength is its ability to help practitioners understand how a weakness in a particular aspect of language functioning may result in language impairment.

SYSTEMS/ECOLOGICAL APPROACH

The **ecological approach** (Bronfenbrenner, 1979; Schalock, Luckasson, & Shogren, 2007) and related approaches such as family systems theory (Bowen, 1978) have several important tenets. First, both approaches are based on the belief that an individual's family, community, and culture shape his or her functioning throughout the life span. Both models emphasize that human behavior and development must be viewed as occurring within complex systems. The ecological model proposes a series of related systems:

- Microsystem: An individual's family, caregivers, peer groups
- Mesosystem: An individual's school, neighborhood, community organizations, workplace
- Macrosystem: Cultural contexts and legal policies influencing an individual's life

The model also emphasizes the interconnection and connectivity between systems: An individual's functioning must be analyzed as it is affected by varying levels.

Ecological approaches differ from traditional approaches, particularly in assumptions about what is normal and abnormal. Ecological approaches acknowledge a wide variation in individual, family, community, and cultural modes for dealing with challenges. Family and community support systems can contribute to an individual's dysfunction or promote an individual's self-reliance and growth. As a result, ecological approaches consider the impact of an individual's communication impairment in relation to the functioning and relationships within the family and community. Intervention focuses on strengthening supports and minimizing barriers within the ecological system.

Clinical Implications of Ecological Approaches.   The systems/ecological approach builds on an individual's family and community support. It proposes that behavior and learning is the result of dynamic interactions between the person and his physical and social environments. Furthermore, modifying any aspect of a person's physical or social environment will change some aspect of the person's behavior.

The systems/ecological approach tends to focus on functional or life-skill goals linking aspects of language use, form, and function and is particularly useful for older students or adults with cognitive impairments. As an example, a systems/ecological communication goal might be stated as "John will use socially appropriate language (*"Hi,"* *"How are you doing?"* *"See you later!"*) when he greets and leaves his communication partners at his workplace." The social/ecological system is discussed in more detail in Chapter 7 when I talk about interventions for individuals with cognitive impairments.

The Domains of Language: Form, Content, and Use and Five Communication Subdomains

Lois Bloom and Margaret Lahey (1978) developed the form-content-use language model and demonstrated how the three language areas intersect during communication (see Figure 1.5). The interlocking circles in the diagram are a reminder that (a) vocabulary (i.e., semantics) is used to produce (b) sentences involving the use of syntax structure and morphology, and that sentences are meaningless without (c) proficiency in language use. Lahey (1988) proposed that language disorders are caused when there is a disruption in language form, content, or use or a combination of disordered components. The form-content-use model is used widely in the communication disorders literature.

The interlocking circles (i.e., Venn diagram) representing form, content, and use remind us that the three domains are interdependent and that an effective communicator demonstrates proficiency in all three domains. However, now that you appreciate the interrelated nature of form, content, and use, let's discuss an elaborated model of early language development.

Figure 1.5   Form, Content, and Use Diagram

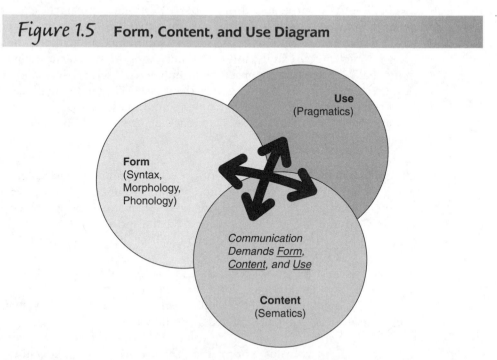

Source: Adapted from *Language Disorders and Language Development,* by M. Lahey, 1988, New York: Merrill/Macmillan. Adapted with permission.

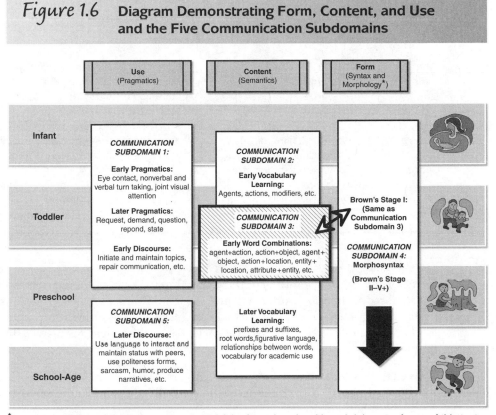

Figure 1.6   Diagram Demonstrating Form, Content, and Use and the Five Communication Subdomains

*Phonology also is an important component of the form domain, although it is not a focus of this text.

Figure 1.6 presents form, content, and use in parallel boxes aligned in relation to four age groups: infancy, toddler, preschool, and school-age students. Form, content, and use are represented by the left to right columns in Figure 1.6; the age groups are shown from top to bottom. Form, content, and use are subdivided into five communication skill subdomains: early pragmatics, vocabulary, early word combinations, morphosyntax, and discourse. Practice your clinical decision making skills regarding form, content, and use by reading and thinking about the information in Focus 1.3.

The five subdomains are presented in the following pages in this order: (1) early pragmatics, (2) vocabulary, (3) early word combinations, (4) morphosyntax, and (5) discourse. This order is different than the way the subdomains are typically discussed. This order parallels the thinking process of the skilled practitioner. When a skilled practitioner observes an individual's communication, he or she mentally "checks off" specific language abilities that are (or are not) observed. The process

FOCUS 1.3 *Clinical Skill Building*

Consider the following case examples and decide if the deficits reflect form, content, or use. Remember that sometimes a deficit impacts more than one domain.

- A fourth-grade student is having difficulty comprehending his reading especially in science and geography. He is very social and gets along well with his peers.
- A sixth-grade student who has been diagnosed with a learning disability does not appear to understand when other students are using sarcasm; he takes their statements literally. This situation is causing problems at school.
- A 2-year-old has 50+ words but almost all of the words are nouns. He is not combining words into two-word combinations.
- An eighth-grade student is getting poor grades in writing composition. His teacher says his writing is "immature" and that he does not write with enough complexity.

is not hit-or-miss; on the contrary, the important communication behaviors are identified, deliberately observed, and sequentially documented. To train students to use this process, I ask students to consider each subdomain one step at a time. During a child language observation, I ask each student to answer the following questions:

- Do you see the early pragmatic skills associated with Subdomain 1?
- Do you see the beginning use of vocabulary in the young speaker associated with Subdomain 2?
- Do you see the word combinations expected in Subdomain 3?
- Is the student developing the advanced vocabulary expected at later stages of Subdomain 3?
- Do you see the morphosyntax features associated with Subdomain 4?
- Do you see the sophisticated discourse skills typically seen within Subdomain 5?

When the student answers each question, he or she focuses attention on the sequential process of communication development. Through this step-by-step process, students' critical thinking skills become more deliberate and focused. I hope this overview is helpful as you read about each of the communication subdomains. As you read about each of the communication subdomains, merge this model with all of your prior knowledge of language development.

The subdomains also should be connected with your understanding of Brown's stages of language development. Roger Brown (1973) traced children's syntax acquisition by considering children's mean length of utterance (MLU; i.e., average sentence length) and documenting the morphemes occurring at varying levels of MLU. Brown's Stage I is demonstrated in children between 12 and 26 months of age; it describes children prior to their use of morphemes. In contrast, Brown's

Stages II–V+ describe children with MLUs of 2–4+ words/utterance. Brown's Stages II–VI occur in children developing typically between the ages of 27 and 46 months (2 to 4 years of age).

At Brown's Stages II–V+, children demonstrate an increasing use of morphological forms. I will be describing children's morphosyntax development in the section describing Communication Subdomain 4. More background on Roger Brown and his stages of language acquisition will be provided in Focus 1.4. An overview of Brown's stages of syntax development and his morphological features associated with each stage is demonstrated in Table 1.5.

Following the discussion of each communication subdomain, the implications of the subdomain skills in relation to assessment and intervention are briefly discussed. I will refer back to the five communication subdomains in upcoming chapters.

FOCUS 1.4 *Learning More*

In 1962, Roger Brown and his associates at Harvard began a long-term study of syntax and morphological development. They followed the language development of three children they called "Adam," "Eve," and "Sarah." Researchers observed and transcribed the children's speech every week for a period of one year (for Eve) to five years (Adam and Sarah). Observations lasted from 30 minutes to over 2 hours. Brown partitioned the children's increasingly longer utterances into five stages according to the children's mean length of utterance.

Brown noted that during Stage II, the children's utterances typically become longer than two words and other linguistic forms (morphemes) emerged. Brown intensively analyzed 14 of the morphemes; he suggested the morphemes emerge in a specific sequence in most children. The morphemes included (in order of appearance in children's speech): (1) the present progressive *ing* inflection on verbs, (2) *and* (3) the locative prepositions *in* and *on* (these come in at the same time), (4) the plural *s* inflection on nouns, (5) past irregular verbal inflections like *did, went,* and *came* (Brown looked at a large set of irregular past tense verbs), (6) the possessive *'s* inflection on nouns, (7) the uncontractible copula *be* (In sentences like "*Here I am*" and "*There it is*" the copula cannot be contracted), (8) the definite and indefinite articles *a* and *the,* (9) the past regular *ed* inflection on verbs, (10) the third person, present tense regular verb inflection *s* ("*I talk*" and "*You talk*" but "*He talks*"), (11) the third person, present tense irregular verb inflections *does, doesn't,* and *has,* (12) the uncontractible auxiliary *be* (The past tense form cannot be contracted; we must say "*He was going*"), (13) the contractible copula ("*It's red*"), and (14) the contractible auxiliary *be* (*He's going*").

Source: From Segal, E. F. (1975). Psycholinguistics discovers the operant: A review of Roger Brown's "A first language: The early stages." *Journal of the Experimental Analysis of Behavior, 23,* 149–158.

Table 1.5   **Brown's Stages of Language Development**

Age/Brown's stage	Morphemes	Examples
18–24 months/ *Stage I MLU 1.0–2.0*	Semantic combinations: Two-word utterances	See Communication Subdomain 3 (morphological development has not yet emerged)
24–30 months/ *Stage II MLU 2.0–2.5*	*ing* verbs prepositions (in, on) plural *s*	*"Boy run<u>ning</u>."* *"<u>On</u> box."* *"See two kitti<u>es</u>."*
30–36 months/ *Stage III MLU 2.5–3.0*	Irregular past tense verbs Possessive *'s*	*"I went home."* *"That Daddy's car!"*
36–42 months/ *Stage IV MLU 3.0–3.75*	Uncontractible copula Articles (*a, the*) Regular past tense Regular 3rd person verbs	*"He <u>is</u>."* *"<u>The</u> toy broke."* *"Grandpa cook<u>ed</u> dinner."* *"She <u>likes</u> it."*
42–60 months/ *Stage V–V+ MLU 3.75–4+*	Irregular 3rd person verbs Uncontractible auxiliary Contractible auxiliary Contractible copula	*"The dog <u>has</u> a bone."* *"<u>Is</u> he going?"* *"Kitt<u>y's</u> eating."* *"He's little."*

Subdomain 1: Early Pragmatic Skills

Communication Subdomain 1 begins at birth and is observed in children's prelinguistic communication. Figure 1.7 is a visual graphic for Communication Subdomain 1. At the earliest stages, children make sounds, movements, gestures, and give visual attention without communication intention. However, communication partners attribute meaning to these actions, with the result that children developing typically eventually produce these same behaviors with communication intent. Children are thought to have **communication intent** when they exhibit a collection of behaviors including (a) producing gestures, vocalization, and/or eye contact to direct the attention or actions of a communication partner, (b) exhibiting joint visual attention, (c) waiting after a communication attempt (i.e., expecting the partner to respond), or (d) persisting in a communication attempt that is not understood. The frequency and rate of early intentional communication behaviors are associated with more advanced language during the child's later years (Calandrella & Wilcox, 2000).

JOINT VISUAL ATTENTION

Joint visual attention (JVA) is a particularly important early communication skill. The child demonstrates the ability to respond to JVA when he follows the visual direction of an adult's gaze (i.e., looks where the adult is looking). The child initiates JVA when he points or shows an object with the intention of drawing his partner's

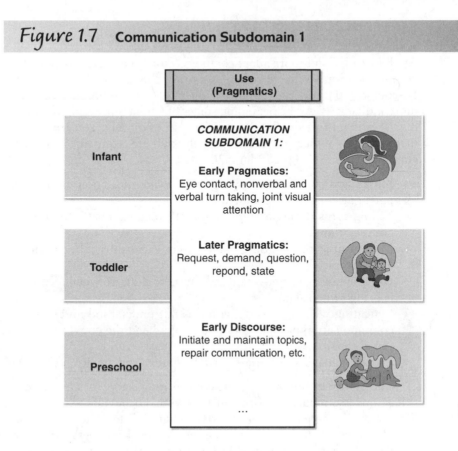

Figure 1.7 **Communication Subdomain 1**

Use (Pragmatics)

Infant

Toddler

Preschool

COMMUNICATION SUBDOMAIN 1:

Early Pragmatics:
Eye contact, nonverbal and verbal turn taking, joint visual attention

Later Pragmatics:
Request, demand, question, repond, state

Early Discourse:
Initiate and maintain topics, repair communication, etc.

...

attention to the object or event. JVC is one of the first interactive communication acts. Children reliably produce JVA between 10 and 12 months of age. It is important to remember there will be cultural variation with respect to children's use of eye gaze along with differences in other aspects of early pragmatic function resulting from cultural communication patterns (Ochs & Schieffelin, 2001).

DEVELOPMENT OF EARLY PRAGMATIC FUNCTIONS

Between 8 and 15 months, children begin to demonstrate a range of pragmatic functions. These functions include requesting objects or activities, refusing, and commenting. Between 16 and 23 months, new pragmatic functions are added, including requesting information, answering questions, and acknowledging a response (Chapman, 2000). It is important to remember that children's pragmatic functions can be demonstrated using varying communication means. For example, a child can demonstrate a request by pointing, gesturing, using a word + gesture, or producing one- or two-word utterances ("*Want cookie*"). In all cases, the child is producing a request, although the way he or she is requesting varies from nonlinguistic to linguistic.

EARLY DISCOURSE SKILLS WITHIN COMMUNICATION SUBDOMAIN 1

As children become more adept communicators, they begin to actively participate in communication exchanges demonstrating the skills associated with **discourse**. Discourse is the connected and contingent flow of communication between two or more individuals. At the beginning stages of Communication Subdomain 1, a child's conversational turns will be nonverbal (e.g., pointing, gesturing). Discourse skills include the following conversational rules that are required to complete a successful communication (Hedge & Maul, 2006):

- Initiating a conversation rather than always depending on the communication partner to initiate a new topic
- Taking turns during a conversational exchange rather than monopolizing the conversation
- Maintaining the ongoing topic of conversation rather than making overly abrupt topic changes
- Using language or nonverbal indicators to indicate when a conversational topic is being switched
- Indicating when the conversation is not understood and/or sensing when the communication partner does not comprehend the conversation (i.e., conversational repair)
- Using language appropriate for the context and situation (i.e., code switching)

The ability to use and request conversational repair is an important discourse skill. **Conversational repair strategies** are verbal behaviors exhibited by a speaker or listener during a communication breakdown. A listener uses conversational repair to indicate he or she has not understood the speaker's message. A repair can be as simple as "*What?*" or indicated by a more formal request "*I don't understand what you just said.*" A speaker uses conversational repair when he or she realizes there has been a communication breakdown. Preschoolers use an early level of communication repair when they repeat their message verbatim. More sophisticated conversational repairs are evidenced when the speaker restates or elaborates the utterance.

The term **code switching** refers to an individual's ability to alternate between formal and informal language in conversations. It also to refers to an individual's ability to vary between dialectal language patterns and General American English. (I describe dialectal variations and code switching in detail in Chapter 11.) A child demonstrates conversational code switching when he or she uses one questioning style with a peer ("*Wanna go?*"), but switches to a formal questioning style when communicating to a teacher ("*May I please go to my locker right now?*"). Early discourse skills begin in preschool and continue to advance through the school-age years (see Subdomain 5).

CLINICAL IMPLICATIONS FOR COMMUNICATION SUBDOMAIN 1

The beginning pragmatic skills in Communication Subdomain 1 (i.e., joint visual attention, turn taking) underlie all later communication; children developing typically have pragmatic intent before they produce words (Chapman, 2000). This means that, as a skilled practitioner, you may focus on building pragmatic skills in older children with atypical communication. For example, if you are working with an older student with intellectual impairment who lacks joint attention, turn taking, and imitation, you would facilitate these basic pragmatic skills in your intervention program. Pragmatic interventions also include helping individuals with social communication deficits join in peer play or group interactions (Timler, Olswang, & Coggins, 2005).

A focus on underlying pragmatic abilities is generally the first aspect of communication that is "checked off" during the observational process. If the SLP or special educator identifies a weakness in the individual's ability to enter interactions, become a part of interactions, and stay in interactions, Communication Subdomain 1 becomes the focus of intervention (Fujiki & Brinton, 2009).

Subdomain 2: Vocabulary Development

The early stage of Communication Subdomain 2 (vocabulary development) overlaps with early pragmatic development. In fact, it is important to remember that all the stages within the form, content, and use domains co-occur and influence each other.

Vocabulary development begins towards the end of the first year of life and continues to develop throughout one's life. Vocabulary development "takes off" during the early preschool years and then experiences another surge during the school years when children develop advanced vocabulary associated with content areas (i.e., content words associated with social studies, science) and written language (see Chapters 5 and 9). Figure 1.8 is a visual presentation of Communication Subdomain 2.

A child's first words are typically produced between 10 and 16 months. First words usually describe:

- Appearance/disappearance/recurrence (*"more," "all gone," "hi," "bye-bye"*)
- Names of people, pets, and interesting objects (*"Mama," "Dada," "kitty," "light"*)
- Affective attitudes (*"hug," "no"*) (Chapman, 2000)

Fillmore (1968) proposed that children's semantic use of words precedes syntax and is guided by universal concepts. He named his theory *case grammar.*

Children's vocabulary development progresses quickly; by the time they are 2 years old, children typically produce 200 to 500 words and understand many more words than they produce (Fernald, Pinto, Swingley, Weinberg, & McRoberts, 2001). By 30 months, children's vocabulary consists of approximately 54% common nouns, 7% verbs, and 5% adjectives. Other categories include function words (*the, a, and, mine*) and sound effects (Caselli, Casadio, & Bates, 2001). Semantic deficits are characteristic of many language disorders, including developmental delay, autism spectrum disorder, hearing impairment, and specific language impairment. During the

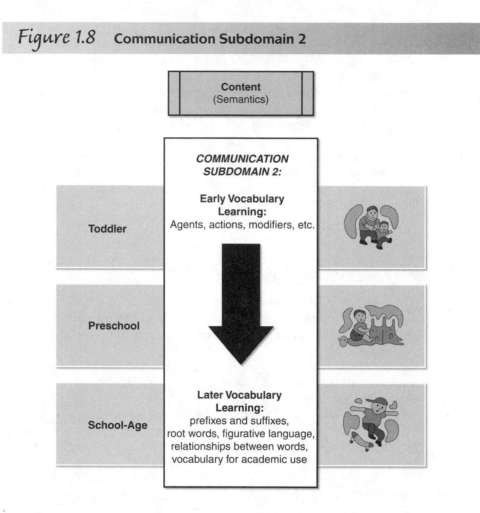

Figure 1.8   Communication Subdomain 2

Content
(Semantics)

Toddler

Preschool

School-Age

COMMUNICATION
SUBDOMAIN 2:

Early Vocabulary
Learning:
Agents, actions, modifiers, etc.

Later Vocabulary
Learning:
prefixes and suffixes,
root words, figurative language,
relationships between words,
vocabulary for academic use

school years, students with language-learning disabilities continue to demonstrate semantic problems. For example, students with language impairments have difficulty comprehending stories in both spoken or written form, have difficulty with figurative (i.e., nonliteral) language, and demonstrate problems with extended discourse (McGregor, 2009).

CLINICAL IMPLICATIONS FOR COMMUNICATION SUBDOMAIN 2

Practitioners continually evaluate whether vocabulary levels can support a child's communication and promote academic achievement. At early stages in vocabulary development, practitioners consider whether children's word usage reflects a variety of semantic categories. Many children with language impairments do not develop enough action words; this deficiency negatively impacts the formation of sentence production (Watkins & Rice, 1991). The interventionist may train caregivers to facilitate a variety of semantic forms.

Children's vocabulary use often varies in relation to their environmental experiences. Consider, for example, that first-graders from families with high socioeconomic levels know twice as many words as children from poor families (Hart & Risley, 1995). The interventionist takes this into account and works with some families to train them in book-reading strategies and implement other vocabulary-enhancing approaches (see Chapter 4).

Vocabulary continues to be a focus for school-age students. Since the average 17-year-old knows more than 60,000 words (Bloom, 2001), imagine the challenges for a student with language impairment who struggles to learn new vocabulary! Experts propose a number of best practices to help students become successful word learners (National Reading Panel, 2000; Nelson & Van Meter, 2006). Successful vocabulary interventions should (a) integrate new word meaning with familiar words; (b) provide repeated, meaningful, and contextual opportunities to learn new words; (c) provide explicit (i.e., teacher-directed, didactic) and implicit (i.e., naturalistic, exploratory) learning opportunities; (d) aim for fluent and automatic understanding and use of new words; and (e) teach students to be more independent word learners.

A concept associated with word learning is called syntactic bootstrapping. **Syntactic bootstrapping** occurs when a child is able to glean the meaning of a novel word from the surrounding function words. I provide more details and research regarding syntactic bootstrapping in Focus 1.5.

FOCUS 1.5 *Research*

Syntactic bootstrapping occurs when a child is able to glean the meaning of a novel word from the surrounding function words. For example, if I say, "*He saw a bleeper,*" you are likely to guess that the word *bleeper* is a noun because it followed the article *a*. Research has confirmed children's use of syntactic bootstrapping at a very young age. For example, Mintz and Gleitman (2002) showed that 36-month-old children identify a word as an adjective from its position in a sentence. In their experiment, a puppet described an object using a nonsense adjective. For example, "*Look at this stoof horsie! This horsie is very stoof.*" After presenting the training items, an experimenter showed the children two test objects side by side and asked, "*Look at these two things. Can you give the puppet the stoof one? Can you show the puppet which of these two things is stoof?*" The results indicated that preschoolers identified objects with shared descriptive characteristics (i.e., the same color or size) showing that preschoolers use syntax to make deductions about word characteristics. Syntactic bootstrapping helps children learn the meaning of new words.

Subdomain 3: Multiple Word Combinations

Once an individual produces approximately 50 individual words, word combinations begin to emerge. Figure 1.9 visually demonstrates the word combination stage I call Communication Subdomain 3. Early word use is not categorized by syntax terms such as "noun" or "verb." Consequently, Communication Subdomain 3 (early word combinations) and Communication Subdomain 4 (morphosyntax) are qualitatively different. I elaborate on what I mean by "qualitatively different" in the next two paragraphs.

Remember that Brown's stages of language acquisition are framed around syntax and morphological acquisition. Therefore, all of Communication Subdomain 1 (early pragmatics), early vocabulary learning (Communication Subdomain 2), and beginning word combinations (Communication Subdomain 3), all occur *before* a child demonstrates the use of syntax and morphology. I demonstrate this visually in Figure 1.10.

This concept can be confusing for the beginning practitioner. It is important to clear up any confusion, however, because (unfortunately) some interventionists focus on syntax and morphology too soon. So—at the risk of repeating myself—the foundational skills demonstrated within Communication Subdomain 1 (i.e., joint visual attention, turn taking, imitation, early pragmatic skills), the one-word productions uttered at the early stages of Communication Subdomain 2, and the semantic word combinations produced within Communication Subdomain 3 *precede* an individual's readiness for Communication Subdomain 4 (morphosyntax). During the first three subdomains, children are not using syntax and morphology. However, the communication skills characteristic of the first three subdomains are always noted; delayed or nonexistent skills within the first three subdomains are targeted for intervention.

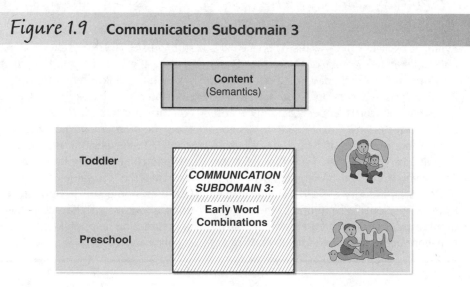

Figure 1.9   Communication Subdomain 3

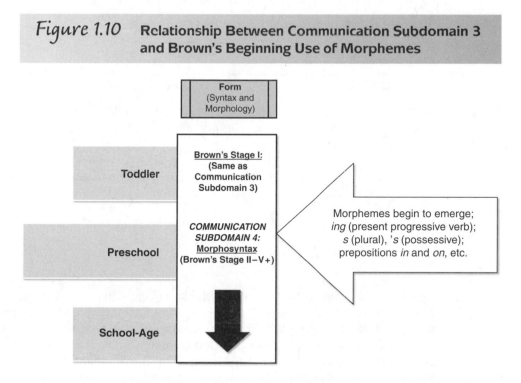

Figure 1.10 Relationship Between Communication Subdomain 3 and Brown's Beginning Use of Morphemes

So, to return to the issue of "qualitative difference," Communication Subdomain 3 is qualitatively different from Communication Subdomain 4 because, at this early word combination level, children are not governed by adult syntax rules and do not use morphological forms. Instead, during Communication Subdomain 3 children create combinations of words by naming objects or people of interest, stating the actions objects or people perform, describing the object's or person's characteristics, and describing who owns or possesses the object. Practitioners use semantic terms to describe these productions: agent (the "doer" of the action), object (the receiver of the action), action, location, possession, and object attribution.

Children's early word combinations must be judged within the contexts in which they occur. For example, a child might say "*Doggie house*" and mean "*The dog is in his doghouse*" or "*That is the dog's house*" or "*I want the dog to come in my house.*" Table 1.6 provides examples of early word combinations and demonstrates how the word combinations are described using semantic terminology.

CLINICAL IMPLICATIONS FOR COMMUNICATION SUBDOMAIN 3

Once a child is able to demonstrate Communication Subdomain 1 (early pragmatic skill) and has more than 50 single words (developed during early stage Communication Subdomain 2), practitioners target early word combinations (Communication

Table 1.6   **Examples of Two-Word Combinations**

Semantic combinations	Examples
Agent + action	*"car away," "kitty bye-bye"*
Action + object	*"kiss dolly," "need juice"*
Agent + object	*"kitty ball"*
Action + location	*"in box"*
Entity + location	*"Sam outside"*
Possessor + possession	*"my doll"*
Demonstrative + entity	*"that doggie"*
Attribute + entity	*"wet sock"*

Subdomain 3). Interventionists engage children in early play activities (e.g., building blocks, sociodramatic play with dolls, trucks) to facilitate multiple word combinations. A child's caregivers also are trained to facilitate these semantic combinations.

For older individuals with significant communication impairments, practitioners also may target Communication Subdomain 3. Communication may either be verbal or incorporate an augmentative or alternative form of communication (AAC). You will learn more about AAC in Chapter 10.

Subdomain 4: Morphosyntax Development

Communication Subdomain 4 coincides with Brown's stages of language acquisition II–V+. Now children's utterances begin to demonstrate characteristics of syntax and morphological development (i.e., language form). The emergence of syntax and morphemes occurs between 24 and 36 months for children developing typically. Examples of early developing morphological structures include the present progressive *ing* verb form and the initial occurrence of the plural *s*. (Review Table 1.5 for the list of Brown's morphemes.)

By age 5, children's sentences evidence complex syntax including the use of embedded phrases and clauses. Figure 1.11 is a visual presentation of Communication Subdomain 4.

I use the term **morphosyntax** to avoid wordiness throughout this book and because the lines between syntax and morphology are blurred (Leonard, 1998). For example, when a speaker asks the question *"Are you going to the party?"* she uses several morphemes (e.g., the auxiliary verb *are* and the *ing* verb). However, the speaker also uses syntax rules to sequence the morphemes into an interrogative reversal sentence. The term *morphosyntax* captures this combination of features. However, you should also keep in mind that the three components of language form (morphology, syntax, and phonology) have distinct properties that can independently

Figure 1.11   **Communication Subdomain 4**

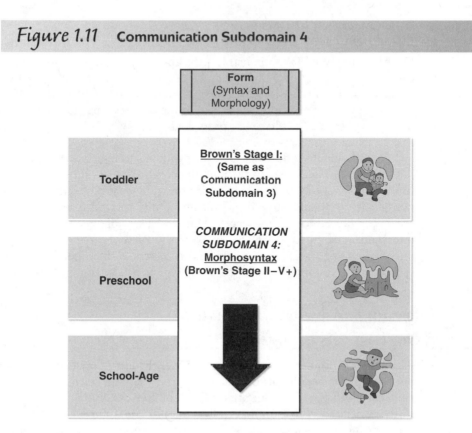

challenge children with language impairments. I describe particular morphological challenges of children with specific language impairments in Chapter 5.

Morphology by definition is the smallest unit of linguistic meaning. Some morphemes are considered to be free morphemes. Free morphemes can stand alone, as in the example of unmarked verbs (*walk, drive, go*) and in unmarked object names (*boy, tree,* and *street*). Bound morphemes carry meaning but must occur with a free morpheme. Bound morphemes include the plural *s* (*boys*), possessive *'s* (*girl's*), verb tenses (*walked*), and so forth.

An interesting feature of bound morphemes is their morphophonological features. **Morphophonology** refers to the phonological variations occurring with morpheme use. For example, when creating a plural form, speakers sometimes use an *es* and sometimes an *s* depending on the final phoneme in the word. To illustrate, speakers produce the plural of *bus* with *es* (*buses*), but produce the plural of the word *hat* with *s* (*hats*). In a third version of plural form, speakers produce the plural of a word with a final /f/ (*leaf*) with *ves* (*leaves*).

Morphophonological variation also is demonstrated by different pronunciations of the past tense *ed* morpheme. Speakers produce a voiceless /t/ when the root verb ends with a voiceless phoneme (*pushed, walked, bounced*) but use a voiced /d/ when the root verb ends with a voiced phoneme (*played, carried, showed*).

CLINICAL IMPLICATIONS FOR COMMUNICATION SUBDOMAIN 4

Once an individual (a) demonstrates the ability to use foundational pragmatic functions (Communication Subdomain 1), and (b) produces multiword combinations using a variety of semantic categories (Communication Subdomain 3), practitioners typically evaluate a speaker's use of morphosyntax using the framework developed by Brown (1973). I describe the process used to complete a language analysis using Brown's stages in Chapter 2.

An individual's syntax competency continues to increase in sophistication during the school years. Consequently, practitioners focus on syntax skills in their interventions with school-age students who demonstrate weaknesses in this area. Often syntax deficits are demonstrated in students' ability to read difficult texts and write at the level required for school success. During the school-age years, syntax analysis and intervention often focus on the speaker's use of sentences with conjunctions (*and, but, then, or, because, after, unless*) and sentences with embedded clauses. I describe assessment and intervention of complex syntax production in Chapters 2, 5, and 9.

Subdomain 5: Advanced Pragmatic and Discourse Development

Although Communication Subdomain 5 is listed last in my ordering system, remember that all the aspects of form, content, and use have been developing side by side since the child began to communicate. In children developing typically, the discourse skills associated with Communication Subdomain 5 have evolved seamlessly from the early pragmatic/discourse skills associated with Communication Subdomain 1. Further, the older child's discourse skills require the vocabulary and syntax competency associated with the other subdomains. Remember that discourse is defined as the connected and contingent flow of language between two or more individuals. Vocabulary, morphological, and syntax skills are required to have a connected and contingent flow of information! A visual diagram of Communication Subdomain 5 is shown in Figure 1.12.

Between the ages of 3 and 7 children's developing pragmatic/discourse skills include the ability to use language to reason and to reflect on past experiences, predict events, express empathy, maintain status and interactions with peers, use and understand sarcasm and politeness forms, and code switch in order to adapt communication to the situation and listener (Chapman, 2000; Owens, 2007).

During the school years, students continue to increase the sophistication of discourse competencies. A successful learner develops communicative behaviors required for school success. High-level pragmatic/discourse skills are need to (a) gain access to social activities, (b) participate effectively in group learning activities (e.g., science experiments), (c) respond to others' comments by validating their opinions, (d) sustain cooperative group communication, (e) negotiate differences of opinion, (f) offer contradicting opinions with socially acceptable strategies, and (g) respond appropriately to teacher or peer feedback (Fujiki & Brinton, 2009).

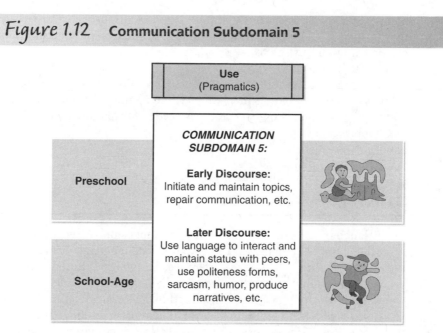

Figure 1.12 **Communication Subdomain 5**

Use
(Pragmatics)

COMMUNICATION SUBDOMAIN 5:

Early Discourse:
Initiate and maintain topics, repair communication, etc.

Later Discourse:
Use language to interact and maintain status with peers, use politeness forms, sarcasm, humor, produce narratives, etc.

Preschool

School-Age

Teacher-student communication is considered a form of discourse called classroom discourse. **Classroom discourse** generally is characterized by the teacher's initiation of a question, the teacher's evaluation of the student's verbal contribution, and the teacher's control of the conversational topic (Edwards & Mercer, 1987).

Students also have to learn to modify discourse styles for different situations. Some forms of discourse are called narratives. An **oral narrative** is a verbal retelling of past experiences or a telling of "what happened" (Ukrainetz, 2006). An individual's ability to produce narratives is associated with school success (Gillam & Johnston, 1992; Green, 2009). A different form of narrative is called an **expository narrative.** This is an informational genre; teachers ask for expository narratives when they ask students to describe a scientific experiment or summarize a historical event (*"Describe the events leading up to and causing the Civil War"*). Each discourse and narrative genre places unique demands on the language learner. I provide more information on narrative development and discourse interventions in Chapters 5 and 9.

CLINICAL IMPLICATIONS FOR COMMUNICATION SUBDOMAIN 5

Skilled practitioners track children's abilities to use vocabulary, produce sentences, and use advanced language within sophisticated discourse genres demonstrated in Communication Subdomain 5. SLPs and special educators recognize that very specific discourse demands are placed on students entering school; the challenges are even greater for children with language disorders (Peets, 2009). To obtain a complete picture of a student's discourse abilities, the practitioner must observe the student in the classroom, with peers, during production of narratives, and in response to a variety of stimuli and situational prompts (e.g., story retelling, expository narratives, group interactions).

The accurate assessment of discourse demands careful language analysis skills; I discuss discourse analysis in Chapter 2. Interventions focusing on peer interactions and the sophisticated language abilities needed for reading and writing are discussed in Chapters 5 and 9.

Summary

- A language disorder is impaired comprehension or use of spoken, written, or other symbol systems. An individual with a language disorder is different from someone with a language difference. Language difference is a variation of a symbol system used by a group of individuals that reflects and is determined by shared regional, social, or cultural/ethnic factors. Sometimes a young child (2 to 3 years old) who exhibits a developmental lag in language is called language delayed or a late talker; experts use this terminology because language impairment cannot be reliably diagnosed in young children in the absence of a primary disorder.
- Receptive and expressive language occurs at the linguistic level of the speech chain. Other communication processes that are within the motor/physical and the acoustic levels contribute to the communication system.
- Behaviorism suggests that learning occurs when an environmental stimulus triggers a response or behavior.
- Cognitive theory is based on the writings of Jean Piaget who proposed that children demonstrate a sequence of progressively more sophisticated cognitive abilities.
- Nativist theory proposes that children have an innate (i.e., inborn) ability to learn language; it is based on the writings of Noam Chomsky.
- Neural maturation is a growing area of science explaining the relationship between language and brain development.
- Social interaction theory is based on the principle that communication interactions play a central role in children's acquisition of language; this theory is often connected to the writings of Vygotsky.
- Information-processing theories historically have compared the brain to a computer, highlighting the interconnectivity of processing elements.
- The ecological approach and family systems theory are based on the belief that human behavior occurs within a complex system and an individual's family, community, and culture shape his or her functioning throughout the life span.

- Practitioners use behaviorism when they use reward systems to train behaviors.
- Practitioners observe children's play behaviors to informally gauge children's general cognitive ability and level of representational thought; this is an example of how cognitive theory has influenced clinical practice.
- The nativist position has influenced practitioners' recognition of the biological base for language learning.
- Recent neural maturation research has altered decision making for some intervention programs, suggesting that intervention should occur at very early ages.
- Social interaction theory has influenced many current therapies; practitioners use this theoretical approach to focus on enhancing interactions between communication partners.
- The information-processing model offers a framework to explain individual processing challenges; this theory explains how weaknesses in the processing system result in language deficits.
- The ecological/systems approach focuses on functional or life-skill goals; it is a particularly useful theoretical approach to guide interventions for older students or adults with cognitive impairments.
- Communication Subdomain 1 encompasses early pragmatic skills including joint visual attention, imitation, and turn taking.
- Vocabulary (Communication Subdomain 2) progresses from the early one-word level and continues to develop through adulthood.
- Once children have more than 50 words they typically begin to produce two-word combinations during the development of Communication Subdomain 3.
- Syntax and morphological development, often described in terms of Brown's stages of language development, are evidenced during Communication Subdomain 4.
- Children's discourse skills continue to develop in Communication Subdomain 5.
- Early pragmatic functioning (Communication Subdomain 1) is fundamental to all communication and may be the focus of intervention for individuals with severe social communication deficits.
- Practitioners may target teaching children a variety of semantic meanings at the one-word level and facilitate advanced vocabulary learning for children with vocabulary deficits (Communication Subdomain 2).
- Practitioners use language facilitation techniques and/or train caregivers to develop children's use of multiple-word utterances. Some children with severe disabilities may use augmentative or alternative forms of communication to communicate at this level (Communication Subdomain 3).
- If children are having difficulty with morphosyntax in Communication Subdomain 4, practitioners use language analysis to determine appropriate linguistic targets.
- Practitioners facilitate social use of communication to enhance the child's social and academic achievement; this is the focus of Communication Subdomain 5.

Discussion and In-Class Activities

1. In groups, give examples of communication behaviors in children's morphology, pragmatics, semantics, and syntax that will be demonstrated as the child matures.

2. In groups, brainstorm three activities that you could implement with an individual who demonstrated a deficit in each of the communication subdomains. Share your ideas in class. List the ideas and prioritize them. Why did you select some activities rather than others?

3. Following the activity above, try to identify the theoretical approach(es) supporting the particular activity that you see as best.

4. Explain the speech chain model to an individual who is not in your class. Draw a simple diagram to illustrate your explanation. Role-play this explanation in class.

5. Find a number of catalogs that contain intervention materials and assessments. In small groups, locate materials listed in the catalog that you believe are based on the following theoretical approaches: behaviorism, nativism (i.e., emphasis on morphosyntax analysis, transformational grammar), social interaction approaches, and cognitive approaches (i.e., sensorimotor emphasis). List or underline the words in the item description that support your conclusion. Share what you find with the entire class.

6. View video recordings of individuals with communication impairments. If you had to pick only one communication subdomain to target in intervention, which one would it be? Explain your answer.

Chapter 1 Case Study

Sachi is a 4-year-old female attending a preschool program; it is an inclusion program (i.e., some children are developing typically and others have developmental delays). Although Sachi has not been formally diagnosed, she demonstrates behaviors on the autism spectrum. She is not linguistic, does not socially interact with others, and does not initiate early pragmatic functions. She spends most of her time wandering around the classroom and carries a small battery-powered fan that she and turns off and on. As the assessor, you have identified goals in Communication Subdomain 1 as the most important communication targets. You have been working with Sachi in the classroom, incorporating her peers in turn-taking games like "marble raceway" (i.e., the children take turns dropping the marble into the spiral racetrack). Sachi is starting to respond to her name and make eye contact when it is her time to take a turn.

Sachi's parents are Japanese-American. They speak some English but to communicate effectively you must speak slowly and use simple vocabulary. Sachi's parents have scheduled a conference with you; they are concerned because you are not teaching Sachi "to talk." To explain your intervention goals you begin by showing video-recorded interactions of young children (toddler age). You turn off the volume, so that Sachi's parents will focus on the nonverbal signs of communication. You ask Sachi's parents to identify instances of nonverbal communication. With your help, they identify gestures, pointing, eye gaze, smiling, joint attention, and waiting behaviors. You emphasize the importance of these behaviors as a foundation for later communication.

Finally, you show a video recording of Sachi in her supported classroom interactions. You and Sachi's parents identify instances where Sachi is beginning to demonstrate early pragmatic communication. Together you and Sachi's parents begin to identify some activities at home to facilitate Sachi's early pragmatic skills.

Questions for Discussion

1. View videotapes of young children; watch while the volume is turned off. Locate instances of behaviors reflecting Communication Subdomain 1.
2. Role-play the interaction with Sachi's parents with other students in your class. Practice explaining your communication goals in simple terms. Draw a simple diagram to help Sachi's parents understand the need to begin with nonverbal pragmatic communication behaviors.

CHAPTER 2

Assessment of Language Disorders

Chapter Overview Questions

1. What are the characteristics, disadvantages, and advantages of norm-referenced and criterion-referenced assessment?

2. How do validity and reliability impact assessment tools? How are standard scores interpreted to identify students with language impairment?

3. How does the SLP or educator compute mean length of utterance? How does MLU differ from a T-unit analysis?

4. How does the assessor complete a microlevel analysis for a beginning language learner? For a higher-level language learner? What macrolevel analyses are completed for individuals with language impairment?

5. How does the assessor evaluate a child with regard to each of the communication subdomains? Describe an assessment protocol appropriate for Subdomains 1-5.

The information in the first chapter has prepared you to begin to think about the assessment process in ways that reflect your understanding of language theory, development, and the implications of the three language domains (form, content, and use). I organize this chapter in two major sections. First, I describe the tools of the assessment process. In the first section, I discuss how speech-language pathologists (SLPs) and educators use norm-referenced, criterion-referenced, and dynamic assessment to evaluate children's language abilities. I then describe psychometric characteristics of assessment (e.g., validity, reliability, standard scores). Language sample analysis (LSA) is a valuable criterion-referenced assessment protocol used to evaluate an individual's language production; I also describe LSA in the first section. In the second section, I describe the process of assessment: screening, assessment procedures, synthesizing assessment results, counseling families, and report writing.

Assessment Tools

DEFINING NORM-REFERENCED, CRITERION-REFERENCED, AND DYNAMIC ASSESSMENT

Norm-referenced assessments receive a great deal of attention. SLPs spend 21% of their time in evaluation and use norm-referenced assessments approximately 80% of the time to assess children's receptive and expressive language (Huang, Hopkins, & Nippold, 1997). Norm-referenced assessments are sometimes also called standardized tests or formal tests (Haynes & Pindzola, 2008). However, assessments that are not norm-referenced can be standardized, so I avoid using the term *standardized testing*.

The assessor uses **norm-referenced assessment** to compare an individual's abilities to those of his or her peers. A norm-referenced test provides a "snapshot" of a child's abilities at a point in time. A primary assumption of norm-referenced assessments is that children with language impairment will demonstrate below-average performance (Oetting & Hadley, 2009). Norm-referenced assessments are used to answer the clinical question: Does this child have a language impairment? Norm-referenced assessments have statistical properties that identify group differences (i.e., that allow the assessor to determine where the child is placed relative to his or her peer group). I discuss the psychometric properties of norm-referenced assessment in the subsection below.

Criterion-referenced assessments are test instruments in which the individual's performance is compared with a prespecified standard or a specific skill. Often the items in a criterion-referenced assessment are organized in a developmental sequence. Typically the assessor attempts to observe multiple examples of a skill within a particular domain. The number of items completed correctly reflects a student's mastery of the targeted skill. Criterion-referenced assessment answers the clinical question: How can this child perform on a particular communicative or academic task? Criterion-referenced tests are often clinician-developed. Like a norm-referenced test, a criterion-referenced assessment documents a student's abilities at a particular point in time. An example of a criterion-referenced assessment is shown in Figure 2.1. In this example, the criterion-referenced assessment is used to document a child's early print abilities, including the ability to recognize print in the environment and enjoy shared book reading. I discuss literacy development in detail in Chapter 9.

Both norm-referenced and criterion-referenced assessments are considered static assessments. As I mentioned above, both provide snapshots of an individual's performance at a particular point in time; they document a child's abilities and deficits. In contrast, dynamic assessment is considered a nonstatic assessment approach. **Dynamic assessment** is a method of conducting a language assessment identifying the

Figure 2.1 **Early Literacy Print Skills Checklist for 3- and 4-Year-Old Children**

Directions: Observe the child in an array of early literacy activities (for example, during shared-book storybook reading or whole-class writing and reading activities). Check each of the following that you observe.

1. Child recognizes that print runs from left to right.	
2. Child distinguishes scribbles ("writing") from pictures when drawing.	
3. Child knows that words are comprised of letters.	
4. Child uses a print vocabulary such as *word, read, write, letter.*	
5. Child responds to signs in the classroom.	
6. Child recognizes common logos, such as store names or a sports team.	
7. Child shows interest in what items say in the classroom.	
8. Child differentiates between pictures and print on posters and signs.	
9. Child asks for help to "read" signs and words in the environment.	
10. Child understands that print has a different function than pictures on signs.	
11. Child is interested in reading and sharing books.	
12. Child identifies the front and back of a book.	
13. Child holds book correctly (right side up, front side forward).	
14. Child can tell the title of a favorite book.	
15. Child turns pages from front to back when looking at book.	
16. Child knows that print tells the story.	

Source: From "Designing and Implementing an Early Literacy Screening Protocol: Suggestions for the Speech-Language Pathologist, by L. M. Justice, M. A. Invernizzi, and J. D. Meier, 2002, *Language, Speech, and Hearing Services in Schools, 33*, pp. 84–101. Used with permission.

skills that an individual possesses as well as his or her learning potential. Dynamic assessment has been described as being "fluid and responsive" (Lidz & Pena, 2009). In a dynamic assessment, the assessor demonstrates, and briefly practices, a language task with the child. During the practice session, the assessor observes the child's ability to modify his or her performance. Children who are developing typically usually make significant changes during the short-term teaching session. On the other hand, a child with language impairment often cannot change performance with a brief exposure to the task. Dynamic assessment answers the clinical question: Given exposure and opportunity, can this child perform a particular language or academic task? Dynamic assessment is particularly useful for a child from a culturally and linguistically diverse background because the assessor does not assume the child has prior knowledge of the communication task. Dynamic assessment allows the assessor to determine if the child has a language difference (i.e., dialect use, lack of exposure to specific vocabulary) or a language disorder. I discuss the dynamic assessment protocol in more detail in Chapter 11, "Multicultural Issues."

ADVANTAGES AND DISADVANTAGES OF ASSESSMENT TOOLS

There are many approaches to assessment; the professional recognizes the advantages and disadvantages of each assessment tool and uses the best tool to answer clinical questions. Typically, a combination of assessment procedures is used to (a) identify if the child does or does not have a language impairment (via norm-referenced assessment), (b) identify specific targets for intervention (via criterion-referenced assessments, language sample analysis, and developmental checklists), and/or (c) decide if the child has a language difference or a language disorder (via dynamic assessment).

Advantages and Disadvantages of Norm-Referenced Assessment.   Norm-referenced assessments have several advantages. Norm-referenced assessments are efficient to administer, and the guidelines for test administration are very clear. The psychometric properties of norm-referenced assessments allow the assessor to compute standard scores; this allows educators to qualify students for educational services (see section on computing standard scores in the subsection below). Norm-referenced assessment also is used at state and national levels to document school performance.

Norm-referenced assessment does, however, have disadvantages and weaknesses (Wiig & Secord, 2006). A primary disadvantage is norm-referenced assessments typically are administered individually in an unfamiliar context (e.g., the therapy room). Accordingly, a child's performance during a norm-referenced assessment may not capture his or her best performance. As you recall from Chapter 1, social interaction and systems theory suggests a child's performance should consider his or her everyday context. Norm-referenced assessments are less likely than criterion-referenced measures to document communication competency in daily living.

A second disadvantage is that norm-referenced assessment can overidentify children from minority cultures. Normative data (i.e., the data collected to compare children with their peer group) usually represent middle-income rather than low-income children, and often does not include adequate minority representation. As a result, some test norms prohibit fair comparison for children from minority cultures. Sometimes nonmajority children are identified with a language deficit when (in actuality) they have a language difference.

A third disadvantage is that norm-referenced tests often have only a few items to assess each language target. On a syntax test, for example, a particular verb form (e.g., *ed* [past tense]; *The dog bark<u>ed</u>*) may only be assessed one or two times. It is possible a student may use the past tense verb form correctly within conversation but miss the past tense verb during the test administration. In this case, the assessor may inaccurately identify past tense verbs as an intervention target. Due to the limited number of items per language task, norm-referenced tests should not be used to identify specific intervention targets; criterion-referenced assessments are the appropriate tool for this task.

Norm-referenced assessment also should not be used to document a student's progress in language intervention. Children may begin to use a language skill within familiar contexts but fail to use the developing skill in the more artificial norm-referenced assessment procedure. Norm-referenced tests are not designed to pick up subtle variations in skill.

In Chapter 1, I described five different communication subdomains. Norm-referenced tests are used most frequently when assessing Subdomains 2 (vocabulary; language content) and 4 (morphosyntax; language form). They are less helpful, and used less frequently, when assessing students who are significantly impaired (e.g., older students with difficulties in Subdomain 1 or 2) or for assessment of discourse function (Subdomain 5; language use). Some norm-referenced assessments assess an individual's ability across a variety of language domains. For example, the Clinical Evaluation of Language Function–Third Edition (CELF-3) is made up of a variety of subtests; different subtests evaluate different language domains (e.g., semantics, morphosyntax).

Advantages and Disadvantages of Criterion-Referenced Assessment. There are a number of advantages to criterion-referenced assessment, particularly in the area of intervention goal setting. SLPs and educators use criterion-referenced assessments to identify targets for intervention because enough items are chosen to meaningfully tap into an individual's skill level. The assessor chooses a criterion-referenced protocol to specifically address the student's communication weakness.

In contrast to norm-referenced assessments in which a student's performance is statistically compared to his or her peer group, during criterion-referenced assessment the assessor typically uses a raw score (i.e., number of correct responses) to summarize performance. The scoring simplicity is another advantage of criterion-referenced assessment. Criterion-referenced assessment is an appropriate tool to document a student's progress during intervention.

A disadvantage of criterion-referenced assessment is that the assessment protocol may not be well defined; this is in contrast to a norm-referenced test where the administration protocol must be followed exactly. The lack of defined protocol may result in some variation between assessors or between repeated administrations of the criterion-referenced assessment. The variation may result in reduced reliability of the assessment instrument (see subsection below on psychometric properties). Variability in test administration can be minimized by carefully describing the procedures used to collect data in a criterion-referenced protocol.

Criterion-referenced assessments are useful across all communication domains and subdomains. Some criterion-referenced protocols are used very frequently; a good example of this is the use of language sample analysis (see subsection below). I discuss other important criterion-referenced assessments, including play-based observation and curriculum-based language assessment, in Chapter 5, "Children with Specific Language Impairment."

PSYCHOMETRIC FEATURES OF ASSESSMENT

Assessment tools differ in their psychometric properties. As I mentioned previously, norm-referenced assessments use special statistical techniques in order to compare the performance of children with that of their peer group. On the other hand, criterion-referenced assessments are documented with raw scores. However, both norm-referenced and criterion-referenced assessments must meet basic standards of validity and reliability. I discuss validity and reliability next, then the specific statistical properties characteristic of norm-referenced assessment.

Validity.   Validity is the most important part of an assessment instrument (Lord & Corsello, 2005). A test has high **validity** if it measures what it says it measures. For example, if a student receives a lower-than-average score on a receptive language test, the SLP or educator expects the student to have difficulty following multipart directions and understanding complex sentences in his or her daily life. Obviously a norm-referenced test is not useful if the results do not reflect real life!

I discuss four types of validity: construct validity, content validity, criterion-related validity, and predictive validity. Typically, an instrument's validity and reliability are reported in the test's administration manual.

Construct validity refers to the underlying theory on which the instrument is based. In the first chapter of this book, I discuss fundamental theories of language development. In order for a language test to be useful, a logical theory must underlie the instrument's construction (Zeidner, 2001). As an example, imagine that I construct a test to document gender identity. I develop items asking questions such as *Would you rather repair a car motor or knit socks?* I decide that the answer *repair a car motor* will be recorded as a masculine response. If the individual chooses *knit socks,* the answer is assigned as a feminine response. "Wait a minute!" you respond. "Fixing cars or knitting socks has nothing to do with gender identity!" You point out my flawed thinking and suggest I read peer-reviewed literature on the topic. After educating myself, I admit that my test did not have construct validity, it did not reflect current understandings of gender identity. This example points out an important concept. Even if a test looks sophisticated, the underlying test construct can be flawed. The issue of construct validity underscores the need for professionals to understand the theory underlying clinical procedures.

Content validity is the degree to which test items represent a defined domain. To determine content validity, experts examine the test items and decide if there are enough items to represent the domain (i.e., area being examined), if the items logically link to the domain, and if the items appropriately assess the domain. For example, when an assessor measures receptive language, the test must be constructed so that the individual responds nonverbally. It would not make sense to ask the client to answer verbally—a verbal response taps into expressive language. So, receptive language tests have to allow pointing or nonverbal actions as a measure of comprehension.

Criterion-related validity considers the degree to which test results on one test align with another test measuring the same construct. Test developers report the statistical similarity between the tests in the test manual.

Predictive validity is similar to criterion-related validity. **Predictive validity** refers to how well a test score will predict a student's performance on a future criterion-referenced task. For example, will a test of syntax ability administered in first grade predict the writing complexity of a second-grader? Will students who scored well in first grade use more complex verbs, clauses, and descriptive language in third grade? This information allows the assessor to make important educational decisions from test results.

Reliability.   Reliability is the degree to which a test is free from errors of measurement across forms, raters, time, and within an instrument (APA, 1999). When an assessor tests or observes a child multiple times, scores reflecting the child's performance may not agree; this would suggest poor test reliability. The focus of reliability measures is to estimate the consistency of scores across repeated observations. Reliability data are reported as correlations; a correlation is a statistical measurement of score similarity. Two sets of scores that are perfectly correlated will have a correlation of 1.00. When making important educational decisions, a norm-referenced test should have a reliability of .90 or better (Webb, Shavelson, & Haertel, 2007). Table 2.1 lists a number of norm-referenced assessments often used to document an individual's expressive and receptive language abilities. Reliability is reported in the right-hand column next to each test.

Table 2.1   **Examples of Norm-Referenced Tests**

Test	Domain(s) assessed and description	Age group	Psychometric properties*
Examples of tests that evaluate a specific language domain			
Boehm Test of Basic Concepts–3rd Edition (Boehm, 2000)	Receptive language concepts; 50 basic concepts frequently occurring in kindergarten, first-, and second-grade curriculum. Spanish version available.	5–7:11 years	**RELIABILITY:** Test-retest reliability estimates ranged from .70 to .89 across forms and grades. Alternate form reliability, based on 216 first-graders, produced a reliability coefficient of .83. **VALIDITY:** Concurrent validity was based on comparisons with the Boehm-R, the Metropolitan Achievement Tests, the Metropolitan Readiness Test, and the Otis-Lennon School Ability Test, with correlations ranging from .48 to .96 depending on the comparison test.
Test of Pragmatic Language (TOPL) (Phelps-Terasaki & Phelps-Gunn, 1992)	TOPL evaluates six subcomponents of pragmatic language: physical setting, audience, topic, purpose (speech acts), visual-gestural cues, and abstraction. Student responds to a visual and verbal prompt illustrating a "dilemma."	5–13:11 years	**RELIABILITY:** Internal consistency and interscorer meet adequate standards. Interscorer reliability is excellent, but it was reported only between the two test authors. **VALIDITY:** Criterion-related validity of the TOPL is not well established. A coefficient of .82 between teacher ratings of pragmatic language and TOPL scores is reported, but the number of subjects in this study was small (n = 30).

Test	Domain(s) assessed and description	Age group	Psychometric properties*
Examples of tests that contain a variety of subtests assessing different language domains			
Clinical Evaluation of Language Fundamentals-Preschool 2 (CELF–Preschool 2; Wiig, Secord, & Semel, 2004)	Semantics (e.g., concepts, word classes, vocabulary), syntax (e.g., recalling sentences), morphology, preliteracy (e.g., phonological awareness), and pragmatics.	3–6 years	**RELIABILITY:** Reported test-retest corrected correlations for subtests by age ranged from a high of .94 for expressive vocabulary (ages 5 years to 5 years, 11 months) to a low of .75 for sentence structure (ages 6 years to 6 years, 11 months). Average internal consistency evidence was strong for the clinical groups with both overall test average alpha coefficient and split-half reliability coefficients at .90 or higher for most of the subtests. The test manual provides acceptable evidence for interrater reliability. **VALIDITY:** Evidence to support the validity of the CELF Preschool-2 is extensive and adequate.
Structured Photographic Expressive Language Test-3 (SPELT-3; Dawson, Eyer, & Stout, 2003)	Morphological use (e.g. preposition, plural, possessive noun and pronoun, present progressive, regular and irregular past, copula, and auxiliary verbs) and syntax skills (e.g., negative, conjoined sentence, *Wh* question, interrogative reversal, relative clause, and front embedded clause).	4–9:11 years	**RELIABILITY:** Test-retest reliability with a median interval of 11 days was .94. Interrater correlations ranged from .97 to .99. Internal consistency estimates on the standardization sample ranged from .76 to .92, with a median reliability estimate of .86. **VALIDITY:** Concurrent validity was established by using the Comprehensive Assessment of Spoken Language (CASL; Carrow-Woolfolk, 1999) as the criterion measure. The correlation between the two measures was .78, indicating substantial overlap between the measures.

(continued)

Table 2.1   **Examples of Norm-Referenced Tests (*Continued*)**

Test	Domain(s) assessed and description	Age group	Psychometric properties*
Clinical Evaluation of Language Fundamentals-4 (Semel, Wiig, & Secord, 2003)	Semantics, syntax, memory, pragmatics (provides checklist); Subtest scores can be combined to compute expressive and receptive language standard scores and compute language composite.	5–21 years	**RELIABILTY:** Test-retest reliability coefficients for each subtest and each age group range from poor (.60) to excellent (.90+). **VALIDITY:** The validity of use of the CELF-4 scores was assessed by correlating it with CELF-3 results for a clinical and a nonclinical group, and by conducting group studies with children diagnosed with language disorders. The correlations between CELF-3 and CELF-4 are moderate.
Test of Language Development Intermediate 3 (TOLD-I:3; Hammill & Newcomer, 2008)	Semantics (e.g., picture vocabulary, relational vocabulary, multiple meanings), morphology (e.g., choice between correct/incorrect sentences) and syntax (e.g., word ordering. Subtests can be combined to compute language composite.	8–17:11 years	**RELIABILITY:** Test-retest reliability coefficients ranged between .83 to .93 for the subtests and .94 and .96 for the composites. **VALIDITY:** The TOLD-I:3 composite scores were correlated with the Comprehensive Scales of Student Abilities (CSSA). Of the 25 coefficients, 17 were significant, indicating that the TOLD-I:3 was related to school achievement.

Examples of tests that evaluate reading, writing, or literacy-related skills

Test	Domain(s) assessed and description	Age group	Psychometric properties*
Test of Early Written Language-2 (TEWL-2; Hresko, Herron, & Peak, 1996)	Evaluates basic writing (e.g., spelling, capitalization, sentence construction) and conceptual writing (i.e., ability to construct a story to a picture prompt).	4-10:11 years	**RELIABILITY:** Both test forms were used in the determination of the test-retest reliabilities. Reliabilities ranged from .82 to .94 (M = .890). The range of coefficients for the interscorer reliabilities was between .92 and .99 (M = .952). **VALIDITY:** Current validity was considered by examining the relationship between the scores from the TEWL-2 and several other tests tapping similar abilities. The coefficients ranged from .24 to .90 (M = .490). Predictive validity was explored by comparing scores from the TEWL with later scores from the TEWL-2; correlations between the two tests were .69 and .62.

Test	Domain(s) assessed and description	Age group	Psychometric properties*
Lindamood Auditory Conceptualization Test-3rd Edition (LAC-3; Lindamood & Lindamood, 2004)	The LAC-3 measures an individual's ability to perceive and conceptualize speech sounds; the examiner asks the student to use colored blocks to represent changing syllable patterns.	5–18 years	**RELIABILITY:** Statistics indicate generally high overall reliability. **VALIDITY:** Evidence presented in the manual indicates that the LAC-3 has acceptable overall validity in terms of its content validity, criterion-related validity, and construct validity.
Test of Phonological Awareness-2nd Edition: PLUS (TOPA-2+; Torgensen & Bryant, 2004)	Phonological awareness (i.e., isolation of individual phonemes in spoken words and understanding the relationships between letters and phonemes)	5–8 years	**RELIABILITY:** Coefficient alpha values range from .80 to .90. Convincing evidence is presented that the TOPA-2+ has reasonable internal consistency and test-retest reliability. **VALIDITY:** Data show median correlation coefficients of .51 and .43 for phonological awareness and .40 and .54 for letter sounds with other similar subtests. Teacher ratings on the Learning Disabilities Diagnostic Inventory correlated the results with TOPA-2+ subscales. Overall, the associations found were moderate.
Test of Narrative Language (TNL; Gillam & Pearson, 2004)	Evaluates a child's ability to use episodic structure during narrative production; evaluates child's use of literate language features (e.g., temporal and causal adverbs, complex sentences).	5–11:11 years	**RELIABILITY:** Most coefficient alphas for the subtests and all items for the entire norm group, genders, and racial groups exceed the minimum criteria of .80. The test-retest reliability estimates are of concern. **VALIDITY:** Criterion-prediction validity included comparing the TNL and Spoken Language Quotient of the Test of Language Development-Primary: 3rd Edition (TOLD-P: 3) for 47 language-impaired children between the ages of 5 and 10 years. Their scores were similar.

*Reliability and validity data source: *The Seventeenth Mental Measurements Yearbook,* Buros Institute of Mental Measurements, 2007, Lincoln, NE: University of Nebraska Press.

When different assessors give the same test, a reliable test will give very similar results; this is called **interrater reliability.** A second type of reliability, called **test-retest reliability,** documents that a test given to the same individual on different occasions results in the same (or very similar) results. Although measures of reliability are not the only consideration when evaluating a test (and experts suggest reliability is not as important as test validity), it is one consideration in the responsible use and interpretation of tests (Webb, Shavelson, & Haertel, 2007).

Norm-referenced and criterion-referenced assessments vary in terms of their validity and reliability. It is generally accepted that criterion-referenced assessments are a more valid measure of performance since the child is provided multiple opportunities to respond and the assessment is generally based on real-life activities. Norm-referenced assessments, on the other hand, have detailed protocols to ensure consistent administration. The skilled assessor recognizes there is a tension between validity and reliability. Making a test more reliable tends to make a test less valid and vice versa; the goal is to use a variety of assessment procedures to account for this variation.

Psychometric Properties of Norm-Referenced Tests.   Norm-referenced assessments have special properties because the tests are designed, statistically analyzed, and revised so that the children's scores are distributed along a bell-shaped curve. The **normal distribution of scores** describes any behavior that clusters around the mean. For example, the mean height of a woman in the US is 5' 5". A certain proportion of women will be much taller and some much shorter, but the average woman will be somewhere around 5'5". Similarly, a well-designed norm-referenced test results in most children clustering around an average score; at the same time the test should discriminate between the average performer and those who are much better or much poorer performers on a particular task (Brown & Hudson, 2002).

When the assessor gives a norm-referenced test, he or she compares the individual's score to the normative sample and identifies if the individual is within normal limits (i.e., is within the expected range around the mean score). The ability to identify if an individual is below the normal performance range allows the assessor to identify children with language impairment. As a result, norm-referenced tests are an important part of the process used to qualify students for educational services.

One of the unique properties of norm-referenced assessments is that a child's raw score (i.e., the number of items completed correctly) is converted to a standard score. **Standard scores** are transformed scores measured in standard deviation units. For example, imagine that you test Mary, a 10-year-old female. Mary correctly answers 12 items on a norm-referenced test. Following the test, you check the test manual and find out that the mean score for 10-year-old females is a raw score of 12. (i.e., the average 10-year-old female typically gets 12 items correct on this test). In this case, the standard score is 100 (Note: for the purposes of this example, I am using the standard score of 100 to represent the mean). The transformed standard score of 100 indicates that Mary is performing within normal limits for her age (in fact, she is exactly at the mean for her age). The **mean** is the statistical average of all the scores in s sample.

If Mary misses many items (e.g., only selecting 6 correct answers), when you look up her raw score you see that she has a standard score of 70. A standard score of 70 indicates a very significant deficit. On the other hand, if Mary correctly selects many items (e.g., 20), you find her standard score is 125, indicating she is a higher-than-average performer.

Standard deviation describes the spread of scores around the mean. The average range around the mean is one standard deviation above and one standard deviation below (the middle part of the bell-shaped curve; see Figure 2.2). In a traditional standard score transformation, 100 represents the mean score and ±15 points above and below the mean is the range for the average performer (a standard score between 85 and 115). One standard deviation below the mean is 100 −15 resulting in a standard score of 85. One standard score above the mean is 100 +15 resulting in a standard score of 115. Typically, children who are performing at the lowest 10% of the population are considered to be language impaired; the lowest 10% represented in a normal distribution is represented by children who are 1.25 standard deviations below the mean (i.e., a standard score of 80 or lower).

Understanding the logic behind standard scores is very important: You will need to explain standard scores to other professionals and parents. At the end of the book (see Appendix A), I present a tutorial providing more detail about how standard scores are computed and how they represent a child's abilities. Focus 2.1 gives additional terms relevant to norm-referenced measurement.

Figure 2.2   **The Bell-Shaped Curve Representing Normal Distribution of Scores on Normative-Referenced Assessments**

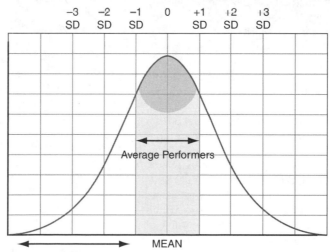

FOCUS 2.1 *Learning More*

Measurement Terminology and Explanations

There are a number of terms used in norm-referenced testing. The information below is summarized from Secord (1989) and Hegde and Maul (2006).

- *Age equivalent score:* The chronological age for which a raw score is the average score. Assessors are cautioned against using age equivalent scores because reporting that an older student (e.g., age 15 years) achieved an age equivalent of 8 years: 5 months is misleading. It is unlikely that a 15-year-old with a language delay communicates in ways that are equivalent to an 8-year-old student developing typically.
- *Basal:* The specific number of sequential items on a test or subtest that must be answered correctly before a student can continue taking the test. It is assumed that if the student answers three sequential items correctly (if the basal is set at 3), then prior items on the test or subtest would be answered correctly. By establishing a basal, the assessor avoids having to start at the lowest level for all students. Instead, students have varying "entry points" into the test items depending on chronological age or ability level.
- *Ceiling:* When the student misses a specific number of sequential items on a test, testing is discontinued. It is assumed that the student would miss test or subtest items beyond the ceiling.
- *Composite score:* A total score that consists of the sum or mean score on two or more subtests.
- *Percentile rank:* An indication of an individual's relative standing in terms of percentage; the percentage of people or scores that fall at or below a specific score. If an individual achieves a percentile rank of 60%, it means that 40% in the sample had higher scores.

- *Raw Score:* The actual score (number of items correct) on a test. The raw score is the number of items the student answers correctly between the basal and the ceiling items; the assessor then adds in the number of items below the basal (since he or she assumes that all items below the basal would have been answered correctly had they been administered).
- *Standard Error of Measure* (SEM): An estimate of the distribution of scores for any one person if he or she were repeatedly measured on the same test (assuming learning did not occur); a boundary of confidence that can be placed around a test score, calculated from the standard deviation and the reliability of the test. SEM is calculated because an individual's performance on a test will vary; there is no one "true" score. SEM is identified to represent the possible range of scores a student might achieve; determining SEM is particularly relevant for students who are near the boundaries for qualifying for services (e.g., at 1.5 standard deviations). A confidence band (adding or subtracting a certain number of points from the standard score) is used to calculate an individual's SEM. The test developer statistically computes the confidence band; the assessor looks up the SEM in the test manual. If the confidence band is ±3, and a student's standard score is 78, the student's true score could range from 75-81.
- *Stanine:* A standard score of with a mean of 5 and a standard deviation of 2.
- *T-Score:* A standard score with a mean of 50 and a standard deviation of 10.
- *Z-score:* A score calculated by obtaining the difference between the person's actual score and the mean of the normal distribution and dividing that value by the standard deviation; Z-scores are commonly used in educational research.

Language Sample Analysis.   Language sample analysis (LSA) is a criterion referenced task because the child's output is compared to developmental data. LSA evaluates an individual's spontaneous or self-generated speech in naturalistic contexts. Information from LSA provides information needed to develop intervention goals and has been proposed as the best means to identify children with language impairment. A high percentage (93%) of SLPs regularly use LSA as part of their assessment protocol; computation of the mean length of utterance (MLU) is the most frequently computed LSA procedure (Loeb, Kinsler, & Bookbinder, 2000). Experts consider LSA a more sensitive way to identify children with language impairments as compared to norm-referenced assessments. LSA often is used to confirm and elaborate on the information gained from norm-referenced testing.

LSA has both quantitative (i.e., numerical data) and qualitative (i.e., evaluation of morphosyntax complexity) components. The quantitative analysis answers the clinical question: Is the individual's length of utterance typical for his or her age? The quantitative protocol varies with regard to the child's length of utterance. For younger children (or beginning language learners), the assessor uses a quantitative protocol called mean length of utterance. For older students who speak in longer utterances (+4 words/utterance), the assessor often uses a quantitative analysis called T-unit analysis.

Following the quantitative analysis, the assessor completes a qualitative analysis of the language sample. In the qualitative analysis, the assessor evaluates the morphological complexity of the child's utterances (for beginning language learners) or evaluates sentence complexity (for later-language learners). The qualitative LSA answers clinical questions such as (a) What sentence constructions occur most frequently?, (b) Are there morphosyntax error patterns in the individual's utterances?, and (c) Does the student use appropriate levels of sentence complexity (e.g., embedded clauses, gerunds) for his or her age?

LSA is considered a formative assessment. **Formative assessment** is an evaluation of performance in a real-life context; formative assessment allows the assessor to gather information and make adjustments to assist student learning. In contrast, norm-referenced tests are considered summative assessments. **Summative assessments** typically are used to place a child in a particular category (e.g., language impaired versus non-impaired) or as accountability measures (e.g., state reading tests).

Quantitative Analysis in LSA: Beginning Language Learners.   The assessor completes four tasks in the first step of LSA. Remember that the clinical question for the first step of LSA is: Is the child's utterance length appropriate for his or her age? To begin to answer this question, the assessor first obtains a high-quality language sample. The specific steps to obtain a language sample are provided in Focus 2.2. In general, the assessor engages the student with open-ended questions and encourages the child to talk about pictures or describe an activity. It is best to obtain 50 to 100 child utterances.

Second, the assessor transcribes the sample (i.e., writes down what the assessor and the child say). After transcribing the sample, the assessor separates the child utterances into utterance segments. In young children, utterance segments are determined by

FOCUS 2.2 *Clinical Skill Building*

Obtaining a language sample

1. The child should be videotaped or audiotaped (or both). Have a familiar adult enter the room with the child.

2. For young children, provide toys that can be used to create a variety of activities such as eating utensils, dolls, a barn with appropriate animals, a gas station with cars and trucks, people figures, a schoolhouse and bus, a house with furniture, etc.

3. Have the preschooler play with toys while the examiner talks to the adult for approximately 5 minutes; then ask the adult to leave and play with the child for 15 minutes. The goal is to obtain 50 to 100 child utterances (100 utterances preferred).

4. Avoid questions that can be answered with one-word answers. Instead, manipulate the figures, comment on the actions, pause, and wait for the child to take a conversational turn.

5. After the play session, the familiar adult returns to the room and asks the child about the activities.

6. Older children do not need to be accompanied into the room. Students reluctant to talk can be engaged in age-appropriate activities: tiddlywinks, pick-up sticks, or balancing games (e.g., *Jenga*). Students can be engaged in conversation by asking them (a) to describe a favorite movie, (b) to describe the rules used to play a sport, or (c) questions such as "*Did your teacher/friend/brother/sister ever do anything that really bugged you? Tell me about it*" (Paul, 2007).

7. The assessor can repeat the child's utterances to aid transcription; this is done when the child is difficult to understand. Make sure that exact repetition occurs (e.g., if the child says "*I goed outside*" the assessor says "*I goed outside.*"

(a) voice inflection indicating the end of the utterance, (b) a pause of greater than 2 seconds, (c) inhalation, or (d) sentence structure indicating a "complete" thought (Eisenberg, Fersko, & Lundgren, 2001).

Third, the assessor counts the number of morphemes in the utterance sample. Recall that a morpheme can be a root word (i.e., an unmarked noun or verb) or a grammatical marker that communicates linguistic information (e.g., plural, possessive). Root words are called free morphemes; the grammatical marker is called a bound morpheme. Figure 2.3 provides a set of rules used to count morphemes within a child utterance. Unintelligible utterances are not counted.

Fourth, the assessor computes a child's mean length of utterance in morphemes (MLUm). I describe the procedure to complete MLU in the subsection below. It is important to note that assessors should be cautious when completing LSA for an individual who is culturally or linguistically different. For example, some children who are African American use African American English (AAE) some of the time. AAE is associated with differences in morphosyntax structure (e.g., *s* plural marker may be omitted ("*I have two book.*") or the auxiliary verb may be omitted ("*He walking.*"). Skilled assessors use variations of LSA so that an individual who uses AAE is not penalized for using AAE features. Learn more about alternative LSA procedures for children who use AAE in Focus 2.3.

Figure 2.3 **Language Analysis: Rules for Calculating the Mean Length of Utterance**

1. Start with the second page of the transcription unless the page involves a recitation of some kind. In the latter case, start with the first recitation-free stretch. Count the first 100 utterances satisfying rules 2 to 8.
2. Only fully transcribed utterances are used; none with blanks. Portions of utterances are entered in parentheses to indicate doubtful transcriptions.
3. Include all exact utterance repetitions. Stuttering includes repeated efforts at a single word; count the word once in the most complete form produced. In the few cases where a word is produced for emphasis (*no, no, no*), count each utterance.
4. Do not count such fillers as *mm* or *oh*, but do count *no, yeah,* and *hi*.
5. All compound words (two or more free morphemes), proper names, and ritualized reduplications count as single words. Examples: *birthday, rackety-boom, choo-choo, quack-quack, night-night, pocketbook, seesaw.* Justification is that there is no evidence that the constituent morphemes function as separate forms for the child.
6. Count as one morpheme all irregular pasts of the verb (*got, did, went, saw*). Justification is that there is no evidence that the child relates to the present form.
7. Count as one morpheme all diminutives (*doggie, mommy*) because children do not seem to use the suffix productively. Diminutives are the standard form used by children.
8. Count as separate morphemes all auxiliaries (*is, have, will, can, must, would*). Also all catenatives: *gonna, wanna, hafta*. These latter count as single morphemes rather than as *going to* or *want to* because evidence is that they function as one morpheme for the child. Count as separate morphemes all inflections; for example, possessive (*s*), plural (*s*), third person singular verb (*s*), regular past verb (*ed*), and present progressive verb (*ing*).

Source: Reprinted by permission of the publisher from A FIRST LANGUAGE: THE EARLY STAGES by Roger Brown, p. 54, Cambridge, Mass.: Harvard University Press. Copyright © 1973 by the President and Fellows of Harvard College.

Computing Mean Length of Utterance.   SLPs and educators establish a child's mean length of utterance to gauge a child's overall progress in developing mature speech (Rice, Redmond, & Hoffman, 2006). The MLU is completed by dividing the total number of morphemes by the number of utterances in the language sample. This gives the average, or mean, number of morphemes a child uses in his or her communication attempts.

As you recall from Chapter 1, Brown (1973) outlined stages of syntax development; each stage is associated with a chronological age and morpheme development. So, for example, let us consider a child, Johann, who is 36 months old. Given his chronological age, the assessor expects Johann to produce sentences between 2.5 and 3 words in length (Brown's Stage III). Further, if Johann's morphological development is within normal limits, the assessor expects Johann to produce specific morphological features associated with Brown's Stage III (i.e., irregular past tense

FOCUS 2.3 *Multicultural Issues*

Multicultural Issues In Language Analysis

- Many African Americans speak African American English (AAE) at least to some degree or some of the time. AAE is associated with differences in morphosyntax structure. For example, the *s* plural marker may be omitted ("*I have two book*") or the auxiliary verb may be omitted ("*He walking*").
- Since AAE linguistic structure varies from General American English, skilled assessors use different language analysis procedures so that children who use AAE are not penalized for using AAE features. Use of more sensitive language analysis procedures avoids a biased diagnosis of language impairment.
- To analyze language samples for students who use AAE, the assessor analyzes simple and complex C-units. A communication unit (C-unit) is an independent clause plus associated modifiers (Loban, 1976). In simple terms, this means the assessor separates the child utterance at the point when the child

uses a coordinating conjunction such as *and*. C-unit analysis also allows the assessor to count words such as *yes* or *uh-uh* when the child responds directly to the adult (these typically are omitted in MLU analysis).

- The assessor considers the frequency of production of C-units without complex syntax (simple C-units) as compared to complex C-units and computes a percentage of complex C-units. Examples of C-units with complex structure include (Craig & Washington, 1994) simple infinitives ("*They was tryin' to get in*"), noun phrase complements ("*I think this'll work*"), and gerunds ("*They saw splashing*").
- Children developing typically will demonstrate an increase in C-unit length and complexity (Craig & Washington, 2000).
- Read more about AAE language analysis in the following article:

  Craig, H. K., & Washington, J. A. (2000). The complex syntax skills of poor, urban, African American preschoolers at school entry. *Language, Speech, and Hearing Services in Schools, 25,* 181–190.

verbs [went, saw] and possessives). Johann also should produce grammar forms associated with earlier Brown's stages; in this case, the *ing* verb and plural forms (i.e., bound morphemes associated with Brown's Stage II).

The assessor also knows a child developing typically will make some morphosyntax errors; some grammar forms will be beyond the child's current level of ability. For example, a typically developing 36-month-old child may say, "*I cutting my paper.*" In this sentence, the child developing typically omits the auxiliary verb *am,* but uses the *ing* verb form. Auxiliary verb errors are expected because auxiliary verbs emerge during Brown's Stage V.

In the case of Johann, the assessor has to determine if Johann's errors reflect later-developing morphosyntax (Brown's Stages IV-V+) or if Johann is "behind" compared to a typically developing three-year-old. In summary, the assessor (a) considers Johann's MLU and morphosyntax skills, (b) considers the MLU and syntax and morphological skills produced by children developing typically, and then (c) compares Johann's actual performance to the predicted performance. This process is the first clinical decision of language sample analysis.

How does the assessor work through this clinical decision-making process? First, the assessor carefully considers Johann's language sample. If Johann's MLU is 2.5 to 3 morphemes per utterance and if Johann uses the morphological features associated with Brown's Stage III, the assessor concludes that Johann's language is within normal limits (given no other outstanding communication problems). Johann's length of utterance and his use of morphological features are appropriate for his chronological age. But what if Johann's MLU is less than expected for his chronological age? Let's consider the clinical decision-making process in more detail by considering three scenarios below. Figure 2.4 visually presents the clinical decisions representing different LSA scenarios.

In Scenario 1, the assessor determines the child has (a) an MLU consistent with expected chronological age norms and (b) nomorphosyntax errors (other than those considered to be beyond the child's developmental level). If the child was referred for assessment due to perceived communication impairments, the assessor completes other criterion-referenced and norm-referenced assessments to confirm or deny deficits in other communication domains (e.g., pragmatics, semantics). It may be that the child is not language delayed; on the other hand, the child may have communication problems that were not "picked up" in the language sample analysis.

In Scenario 2, the assessor notes the child's MLU is within normal limits, but also observes morphosyntax immaturity errors. Consider two utterances, both produced by a child who is 5 years old (i.e., 60 months).

- *Me no go outside mommy?*
- *I want to go outside.*

Both utterances are 5 morphemes in length. In the first case, however, the utterance is immature and ungrammatical. In the second case, the utterance contains an advanced syntax form (i.e., the infinitive verb *to go*). Children with the same MLU level can have very different qualitative differences in their utterance production (Eisenberg, Fersko, & Lundgren, 2001). In Scenario 2, the assessor documents the child's average-level MLU, but proceeds with a qualitative analysis of language form. I describe the qualitative analysis procedure in the subsection below.

In Scenario 3 (see Figure 2.4), the assessor observes reductions in the child's quantity and quality of language production. For example, in the case of Johann, imagine that his LSA revealed that he speaks in one- to two-word combinations. His MLU is 1.5. He produced the following utterances:

- *"Give it!"*
- *"Me"* (for *"mine"*)
- *"Look doggie!"*

The assessor determines that Johann is (a) below expected levels for MLU and (b) demonstrating immaturity in morphological development. In this example, Johann demonstrates both quantitative (i.e., MLU is below expected levels) and qualitative (i.e., morphosyntax is not age appropriate) differences. In both Scenarios 2 and 3, the assessor completes additional assessments to substantiate the child's difficulties in syntax and morphology and to identify other communication domains that are impaired.

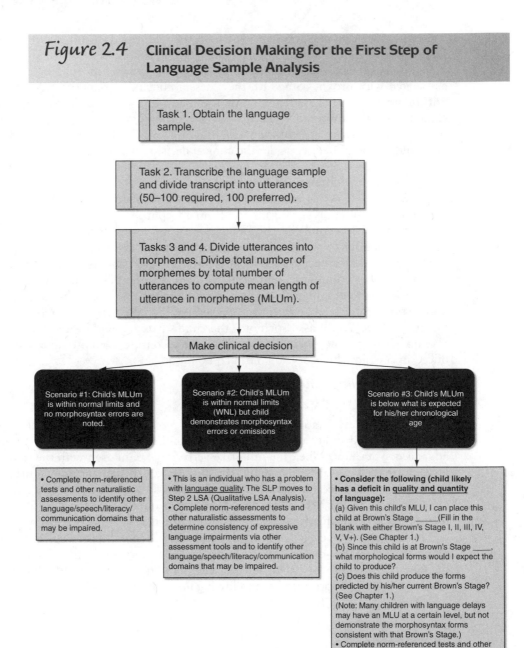

Figure 2.4 Clinical Decision Making for the First Step of Language Sample Analysis

Task 1. Obtain the language sample.

Task 2. Transcribe the language sample and divide transcript into utterances (50–100 required, 100 preferred).

Tasks 3 and 4. Divide utterances into morphemes. Divide total number of morphemes by total number of utterances to compute mean length of utterance in morphemes (MLUm).

Make clinical decision

Scenario #1: Child's MLUm is within normal limits and no morphosyntax errors are noted.

Scenario #2: Child's MLUm is within normal limits (WNL) but child demonstrates morphosyntax errors or omissions

Scenario #3: Child's MLUm is below what is expected for his/her chronological age

• Complete norm-referenced tests and other naturalistic assessments to identify other language/speech/literacy/ communication domains that may be impaired.

• This is an individual who has a problem with language quality. The SLP moves to Step 2 LSA (Qualitative LSA Analysis).
• Complete norm-referenced tests and other naturalistic assessments to determine consistency of expressive language impairments via other assessment tools and to identify other language/speech/literacy/communication domains that may be impaired.

• **Consider the following (child likely has a deficit in quality and quantity of language):**
(a) Given this child's MLU, I can place this child at Brown's Stage _____ (Fill in the blank with either Brown's Stage I, II, III, IV, V, V+). (See Chapter 1.)
(b) Since this child is at Brown's Stage _____, what morphological forms would I expect the child to produce?
(c) Does this child produce the forms predicted by his/her current Brown's Stage? (See Chapter 1.)
(Note: Many children with language delays may have an MLU at a certain level, but not demonstrate the morphosyntax forms consistent with that Brown's Stage.)
• Complete norm-referenced tests and other naturalistic assessments to determine consistency of expressive language impairments via other assessment tools and to identify other language/speech/literacy/ communication domains that may be impaired.

Number of Different Words.   The calculation of MLU is an important quantitative analysis of language form. Skilled assessors also complete a quantitative analysis of language content as part of the LSA procedure. Calculation of the **number of different words** (NDW) is a quantitative analysis of semantics (language content).

NDW is defined as the number of different words (sometimes called tokens) that occur in a 100-utterance language sample. NDW allows the assessor to determine if an individual does or does not demonstrate appropriate levels of vocabulary diversity. NDW should be used in combination with other measures of vocabulary. (I describe norm-referenced tests for vocabulary in subsections below.)

To compute NDW the assessor (a) collects a 100-utterance language sample (typically the same sample used for the MLU calculation), (b) counts the number of different words (a word used more than one time in the language sample is only counted the first time it is used), and (c) compares the student's NDW with normative data. If a root word occurs with different morphological endings (e.g., *walk, walks, walking*), only the first occurrence of the root word is counted. Children developing typically should have the following range of NDW (Dollagen et al., 1999; Leadholm and Miller, 1992):

- At 3 years: NDW between 100 and 164
- At 5 years: NDW between 156 and 206
- At 7 years: NDW between 173 and 212
- At 9 years: NDW between 183 and 235
- At 11 years: NDW between 191 and 267

There are other quantitative measures of lexical diversity in addition to NDW. These include the type-token ratio (TTR: number of different words divided by the total number of words in the language sample) and the number of total words (NTW). When calculating the NTW, every word produced by the child in the language sample is counted—even when the word is produced multiple times. NDW and NTW are better measures of lexical diversity than TTR (Watkins et al., 1995).

Quantitative Analysis in LSA: Later Language Learners.   In the preceding section, I described MLU as an appropriate quantitative technique for the beginning language learner who uses less than 5 words per utterance. Once a student begins to communicate in longer utterances, the assessor uses an alternative technique called T-unit analysis during the LSA process.

Completing a T-unit Analysis.   With school-age students, the assessor uses T-unit analysis to segment a student's utterances. A **T-unit** is one main clause with all the subordinate clauses and nonclausal phrases attached or embedded within the sentence (Paul, 2007). T-unit analysis is completed after a child is 42 months old or when his MLU is greater than 4.00. T-units are used because older children with language impairment often produce run on sentences linked with coordinating conjunctions.

Consider the following sentence: "*I went to the store, and I bought some bread, and I bought some candy, and I bought some pop.*" The individual's MLU equals

FOCUS 2.4 *Learning More*

A T-unit is one main clause including all the subordinate clauses and nonclausal phrases (Hunt, 1965; Paul, 2007). When a child uses long, run-on sentences consisting of many independent clauses connected with conjunctions *and, but,* or *so,* dividing the discourse into T-units avoids an inflated MLU (i.e., an MLU that is high, potentially indicating that the child had sophisticated verbal output, while in actuality his or her output was a series of linked simple sentences). Consider the following:

I went to the store and my mom had given me some money so I went and bought some

bread for her and I come back and gave her the bread and she said "OK, thanks, now you can go to the ball game."

The sentence above is one utterance. Consider the difference when the output is divided into T-units.

- *I went to the store*
- *(and) my mom had given me some money*
- *(so) I went and bought some bread for her*
- *(and) I come back and gave her the bread*
- *(and) she said "Ok, thanks, now you can go to the ball game.*

20 words; however, you can see that the sentence form is very simple, it represents a series of four simple sentences: *//I went to the store// (and) //I bought some bread// (and) //I bought some candy// (and) //I bought some pop//*. An MLU analysis would not be useful because the individual's output is beyond Brown's stages in terms of sentence length. An MLU analysis would not reliably identify language impairment. Instead the assessor must determine if the individual's sentence complexity is acceptable as compared to his or her peers and if sentence complexity is adequate for reading and writing.

T-unit analysis and LSA are important components of written language assessment for older students. Teachers and SLPs use LSA to analyze the writing samples of older students who struggle with reading and writing. I provide more information on reading and writing assessment and intervention in Chapter 9. I provide more details about T-unit analysis in Focus 2.4 in this chapter.

Qualitative Language Analysis.   As I described above, during the quantitative analysis, the assessor answers the question: Are the child's utterances an appropriate length? To answer this question, the assessor compares the child's production with that of an age-matched peer (e.g., a child of the same chronological age).

During the qualitative analysis, the assessor answers the question: Now that I have evaluated the child's length of utterance, what qualitative differences do I see in the child's language output? Individuals with language impairment typically exhibit both quantitative and qualitative language variations. I call the quantitative *and* qualitative analysis the "two-step process" of LSA. The two-step LSA process is visually demonstrated in Figure 2.5.

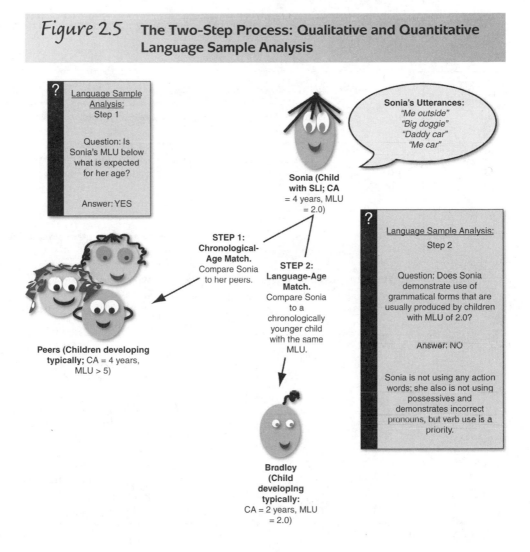

Figure 2.5   **The Two-Step Process: Qualitative and Quantitative Language Sample Analysis**

During the second step of LSA, the assessor compares the individual's language output with a language-age match. A **language-age match** is a chronologically younger individual with an equivalent MLU. So, for example, when evaluating a child with an MLU of 1.0 word per utterance, I compare his or her language output with the communication patterns of a child at Brown's Stage I.

Qualitative analysis is typically completed at both the micro- and macroanalysis level. **Microanalysis** considers each utterance as it stands alone. Microananalysis, for the beginning language learner, includes an analysis of the child's pragmatic abilities, semantic abilities, and morphosyntax skills at the utterance-by-utterance level. I provide a sample language analysis form in Table 2.2 to illustrate how the assessor documents microanalysis data for the beginning language learner. Microanalysis,

Table 2.2   **Utterance-Level Worksheet for Beginning Language Learners with MLU Between 1 and 3**

Child's Name: S.B.	Chronological Age: 3:8	**Language Sample Analysis (LSA) Step # 1 (Quantitative Analysis):** S.B.'s MLU is 3.0; he should be at an MLU +4 (Brown's Stage V considering his chronological age of 3 years, 8 months). However, his MLU is like that of a younger child.									
Examiner: J.K.	Date of sample: 2/7/09	**LSA Step #2 (Qualitative Analysis):** Since S.B.'s current MLU is 3.0 he should be producing morphemes consistent with Brown's Stage IV (i.e., morphemes such as articles, regular past tense, 3rd person regular verbs). However, S.B.'s morpheme use represents Brown's Stage I and II. Notes: S.B. demonstrates deficits in quantity (per MLU) and quality of syntax complexity.									
List Utterances Below:	(A) Pragmatic Functions (✔ Check one)							(B) Semantic Roles and Relations (Describe)	(C) Bound Morphemes and Brown's Stage Morpheme Typically Appears	# of morp.
	Requests	Declarations	Answer questions	Agree/disagree	Social speech	Imitation	Other	Examples: Agent Action Object Modifier Negation Agent + Action Action + Object Agent + Action Modifier + X Negation + X X + Location	Examples of bound morphemes: Present progressive (*ing*) Prepositions (*in, on*) Plural (*s*) Present tense aux. (*can, will*) Possessive (*'s*) Irregular past tense verb Articles (*a, the*) Copula and auxiliary "*BE*" Regular past tense verbs (*ed*) 3rd person singular verb (*s*)	
No go outside.				✔				Negation + action + location	0/1	3
Kitty drinking milk.		✔						Agent + action + object	Present prog./II	4
Mommy up!	✔							Agent + location	0/1	2

for later language learners, considers the individual's use of complex sentences at the utterance level.

   Macroanalysis considers the individual's ability to interact during a conversation; it considers his or her discourse skills. It moves beyond the utterance level to consider the individual's ability to initiate a topic, repair communication breakdowns, and use a back-and-forth conversational style. I discuss both micro- and macroanalysis qualitative procedures used in the second step of LSA in the section below.

Microanalyses for the Beginning Language Learner. The assessor evaluates the beginning language learner's pragmatic, semantic, and morphosyntax skills. During the qualitative analysis of pragmatic function, the assessor first considers the six early developing pragmatic categories: requesting, stating/commenting, protesting/denying, responding, socially interacting, and imitating (see Chapter 1 to review these terms). The assessor considers overall communication and determines whether or not the child with language impairment demonstrates a range of pragmatic function. If LSA reveals the child is not able to perform a pragmatic function (e.g., the child does not appear to use the pragmatic function of *request),* the assessor probes this communication skill. A **communication probe** is an interaction designed to elicit a specific child response. For example, to probe for *request,* the assessor may show a child a favorite toy or object and prompt a request. If the probe indicates the child is unable to produce a request, this skill is identified as a possible intervention goal.

Remember that language form, content, and use are never produced in isolation. A child with language impairment (LI) may appropriately produce a pragmatic function but demonstrate morphosyntax errors during the communication act. For example, a child with LI may demonstrate the pragmatic function *request* by saying, "*Outside now?*" The request is produced with rising intonation, instead of a grammatically correct sentence "*Can I go outside now?*" In this example, the assessor indicates the child produced a request in the pragmatic category (column A on the LSA form), but documents a morphosyntax error in column C in Table 2.2.

The six pragmatic categories in Table 2.2 (column A) describe pragmatic competency prior to 24 months. Between 24 and 36 months, children demonstrate increasingly sophisticated pragmatic functions including detailing, predicting, and requesting clarification. After age 3, children learn more sophisticated pragmatic functions including expressing feelings, giving reasons, and hypothesizing, and begin to maintain and elaborate on conversational topics (Carpenter & Strong, 1988; Owens, 2005). The assessor documents the use, or lack of use, of each pragmatic function in relation to the child's chronological age and level of language use.

Once the assessor considers pragmatic function for beginning language learners, he or she considers the semantic skills associated with Communication Subdomains 2 and 3 (see Chapter 1 for a review of communication subdomains).

At the earliest stage of language development (i.e., Brown's Stage I up to 24 months), children use word combinations to express a variety of meaning. For example, the utterance, "*Daddy car,*" could mean a possessive relationship, "*This is Daddy's car,*" a statement, "*Daddy is driving the car,*" or a request, "*Will Daddy take me in the car?*" Word combinations communicate a child's meaning unfettered by syntax and grammar constraints. As a result, during the second part of LSA (for the beginning language user) the assessor often completes a qualitative semantic analysis. In a semantic analysis the assessor documents a child's use of semantic combinations such as agent + object, action + object, agent + action, modifier + X, negation + X (X = any word, including a noun, an action word, or even a word like *more*).

Semantic combinations are building blocks for later-developing sentences. For example, I typically look for children at the two-word level to produce both agent + action ("*doggie eat*") and action + object ("*eat food*") combinations. Without the ability to produce such two-word combinations, children are likely to have difficulty producing the three-word agent + action + object combination, "*Doggie eat food.*" The agent + action + object semantic combination represents the noun + verb + noun structure required for more elaborate syntax and grammatical development. Table 1.6 (in Chapter 1) provided a description of all the semantic combinations for children at the early stages of language development.

Given that children with language impairment have a primary grammatical deficit, analysis of syntax and morphological ability is a critical component of LSA. Grammatical analysis considers a child's use of language form at Communication Subdomain 4.

During grammatical analysis, the assessor (a) describes the child's grammatical errors and (b) calculates the percentage correct use for grammatical errors. The assessor marks a grammatical form as an error if it is used incorrectly in an **obligatory context,** meaning that the conversation or situation calls for the use of a specific grammatical form. An error is counted if the child attempts to use the form but the grammatical feature is produced incorrectly (Fey, 1986). Consider the following example in which percentage correct use of the present progressive verb *ing* form is computed:

Utterance (from a 50-utterance sample)	Error*	Obligatory?
TEACHER: *What is the boy doing in this picture?*		
8) CHILD: *he <u>run</u>*.	1	Yes
9) CHILD: *I don't know what him <u>do</u>*.	1	Yes
TEACHER: *Tell me what you see happening at the circus.*		
45) CHILD: *That seal want to eat.*	0	No
46) *He <u>throw</u>* ball.*	1	Yes
47) *He <u>riding</u> bike with him hat on.*	0	Yes
48) *That elephant <u>stand</u>* up on him back legs.*	1	Yes
TOTALS	4	5

Number of errors divided by number of obligatory contexts
(4 ÷ 5 = .80) = 80% error in present progressive verb production

Note in utterance #45, an error was not identified in the use of present progressive verb tense. In this utterance, the child produced an error, but the sentence construction called for a third person regular verb (*wants*) rather than requiring a present progressive verb (*wanting*). The assessor must also consider that some morphosyntax features may represent cultural or linguistic differences and should not be counted as errors (see Focus 2.5).

FOCUS 2.5 *Multicultural Issues*

A morphological feature of African American English (AAE) includes use of subject and verb that differ in either number or person. For example, a speaker who uses AAE might say "*What do this mean?*" (Washington & Craig, 1994). What implications would AAE use have in the examples given in the text for calculating percentage of obligatory use (e.g., "*He throw ball*" and "*That elephant stand up on him back legs*")?

Microanalysis for the later-language learner. The qualitative morphosyntax analysis for beginning language learners is framed within Brown's stages II–V+. Once the language learner is beyond 4 words, the assessor begins to consider the use of complex language beyond Brown's stages. As I described above, the assessor segments language output for the older child into T-units.

Typically developing students (with an MLU of more than 5.0) produce sentences with embedded or conjoined clauses 20% of the time (Paul, 1981; Paul, 2007). In contrast, students with LI often produce few complex sentences. As a result, it is important to document an individual's use of complex sentences.

To determine the percentage of complexity, the assessor counts the number of T-units containing complex sentence construction and divides the number of complex T-units by the total number of T-units. If the percentage is below 20%, the assessor completes a more "fine grained" analysis by looking at specific types of sentence complexity and evaluates whether the student produces early or late complex sentence forms. Early forms of sentence complexity include simple infinitives ("*He likes to play baseball.*") and simple *wh* clauses ("*Why did he go?*"). Later forms of sentence complexity include relative clauses ("*That's the dress that I wore to the party.*") or gerunds ("*Swimming is a great sport.*"). I give examples of early and late sentence complexity in Table 2.3.

A child with an MLU between 3.0 and 4.0 (Brown's Stages IV and V) typically produces early sentence complexity; once a child produces an MLU between 4.0 and 5.0 (Brown's Stage V+ and beyond), later-developing complex sentence types emerge (Paul, 1981; Paul, 2007).

During intervention, the SLP or educator targets early-developing sentence complexity before targeting later-developing forms. Older children should be able to use complex sentence types during oral and written language production. I describe writing interventions for older students in Chapter 9.

Macroanalyses.   The analyses above describe microlevel analyses; microlevel analyses consider the communicator's pragmatic, semantic, and morphosyntax abilities at the utterance level. The assessor must also consider the communicator's

Table 2.3   **Early and Late Developing Complex Sentence Types**

Early Developing Complex Sentence Forms (MLU = 3–4) Examples

- Simple infinitive: The word *to* is used. However, the subject is deleted because it is the same as the main sentence. Does not include catenative forms of infinitive (*wanna, gonna,* etc.)
  - *She has to go.*
  - *The dog wants to run.*

- Full propositional complement: Cognitive verbs are used (*think, said, guess, know, wonder, hope*).
  - *She thought the room looked messy.*
  - *Guess how many I have.*

- Simple *wh*-clause: Includes a *wh*- conjunction: *what, where, when, why, who, how.* Does not include an infinitive *to.*
  - *Why did you say that?*
  - *See how he throws that ball?*

- Simple conjoining: Two clauses joined by a coordination conjunction (*and, but, so,* etc.) or subordinating (*because, after,* etc.).
  - *The boy likes to eat lunch early so that he avoids the crowd.*
  - *I ate dinner late and I'm tired.*

- Multiple embeddings: Sentences containing more than one embedded clause; may include a catenative.
  - *He's gonna have to go.*

- Embedded and conjoined: Sentence contains both an embedded and a conjoined clause.
  - *He's not really gonna buy it because he didn't wanna spend so much money.*

Late Developing Complex Sentence Forms (MLU = 4-5) Examples

- Infinitive clause with different subjects.
  - *He realized she wouldn't want to wait any longer.*
  - *The boat sailed next to the boy who wasn't able to swim.*

- Relative clauses: A subordinate clause that acts as an adjective; may or may not include *which* or *that.*
  - *That's the ice cream that I tasted.*
  - *The argument that they had was silly.*

- Gerunds: An *ing* form that is used as a noun.
  - *Reading is my favorite hobby.*
  - *She likes swimming in the outdoor pool.*

- *Wh-infinitives*: Use of *to*, along with *wh*-conjunctions.
  - *She doesn't know how to do it.*
  - *I thought you knew what to say.*

- Unmarked infinitives: *To* is not used; verbs include *make, help, watch,* or *let.*
  - *Make it go like this.*
  - *Let her play it.*

Source: From *Language Disorders from Infancy to Intervention* (3rd ed.), p. 486, by R. Paul, 2007, St. Louis, MO: Mosby. Copyright Elsevier (2007). Reproduced with permission.

abilities beyond the utterance level. Discourse-level analysis is a macroanalysis that considers an individual's language use (Subdomain 5). **Conversational discourse** is defined as the unstructured or unplanned spoken interactions that occur between two individuals.

At the discourse level, the assessor evaluates the child's ability to effectively convey information as a speaker and to adjust and respond to the listener. Consider the following two speakers who describe the same event.

Speaker 1:	Speaker 2:
• The little girl was on the way to school.	• She walked there.
• On the way, she saw a stray dog.	• And she saw it.
• So, she tried to catch it because she didn't want it to get hurt.	• She tried to catch it.
	• She didn't want it to get hurt.

As you can see from the two examples above, at an utterance level both speakers' utterances are grammatically correct. However, there are significant differences between the two speakers' communication abilities. We can understand the event described by Speaker 1, but we are confused by Speaker 2's version of the event. Macroanalysis reveals communication deficits not identified at the utterance level.

At the discourse level of analysis, the assessor considers a number of factors regarding an individual's conversational skill. For example, a skilled communicator provides sufficient information so the listener understands the speaker's intent. Consider Speaker 2 in the example just provided. If you were talking to Speaker 2, it would be unclear what had happened because the speaker does not provide enough decontextualized information. **Decontexualized information** is information able to be understood without environmental cues.

As another example of the need for decontextualization, imagine that you and I witness a car accident together and I say, "*Look at that! He crashed into her!*" In this instance, you understand exactly what I am saying because we shared the same visual cues and experience.

On the other hand, without a shared experience, the speaker must provide more information to the listener. If I walked up to you on the way to class and said, "*He crashed into her!*" you would be very confused. In the second conversation, in order to be an effective communicator, I must decontextualize the information. I might say, "*I saw a car accident. The driver of one car crashed into a girl who was driving a second car.*" I need to provide clear **referents** (specific nouns) to describe the people and objects (*the driver of one car* and *a girl . . . a second car*) rather than use ambiguous referents such as *that* and *her*. The ability to create clear linkages between new and old information (e.g., "*I saw a <u>man</u> driving a car; <u>he</u> crashed into another car*" [here the speaker uses the pronoun *he* to refer back to the "old" noun *a man*]) is called **referencing** (McCabe & Bliss, 2003; McCaleb & Prizant, 1985). The ability to decontextualize language is a very important skill for an effective speaker and writer. I discuss more about an older student's use of decontextualization in Chapter 9. The ability to decontextualize information begins in the late preschool years and continues to develop during the elementary- and middle-school years.

There are a number of other important macrolevel discourse skills assessed with children and older students. Important conversational discourse skills include:

- *Topic control:* Topic control is demonstrated when a speaker introduces a new topic. Children should initiate topics in addition to responding to other's topics. Effective speakers can discuss a variety of topics, rather than just one or two.
- *Topic maintenance:* Topic maintenance is demonstrated when a conversational turn connects to the previously introduced topic. An effective conversation has linked exchanges in which communication partners share information using topically linked exchanges. Children with LI are less proficient at introducing and maintaining new topics (Dollaghan & Miller, 1986). By the age of 3 years, children developing typically maintain a shared communication topic 50% of the time; by the age of 4, most children consistently maintain a conversation with a communication partner.
- *Conversational repair:* If one partner does not understand the other, or if the speaker senses the listener does not understand the communication, effective discourse partners repair the conversation either by paraphrasing, asking questions, or elaborating. By the age of 3, children developing typically begin to repair a communication breakdown when the listener says "*Huh?*" or "*What?*" The earliest form of conversational repair is repeating the utterance; as children mature they begin to rephrase their statement to increase listener comprehension.
- *Informativeness:* An effective communicator contributes new information during a conversational turn, rather than just repeating the same information. The communication should not be vague or confusing. Children developing typically begin to add information to a conversation at around age 3. Children need to be able to decontextualize the information so the listener understands the speaker's information.
- *Conjunctive cohesion:* Effective speakers use conjunctions to causally and temporally connect information during shared interactions. For example, in the utterance "*I want to go home and take a nap, because I didn't sleep last night*" I link information with the conjunction *because,* highlighting the causal link between the two ideas. Words such as *because, so, before, then,* and *next* make explicit connections between ideas and events. Children begin to use conjunctive cohesion typically between 3 and 4 years of age.

As you can see, there are many clinical considerations to be considered at a macroanalysis level. Figure 2.6 provides an example of a decision tree demonstrating how the assessor evaluates discourse skills. In addition to conversational discourse, individuals with LI often struggle with narrative and classroom-based discourse. I discuss other discourse forms in Chapter 9.

A final macrolevel analysis typically completed for older students is a mazing analysis. A **maze** is a disruption in speech that includes false starts, fillers, pauses of more than 2 or more seconds, revisions, and repetitions. The conversation of children

Figure 2.6 Decision Making at the Discourse Level

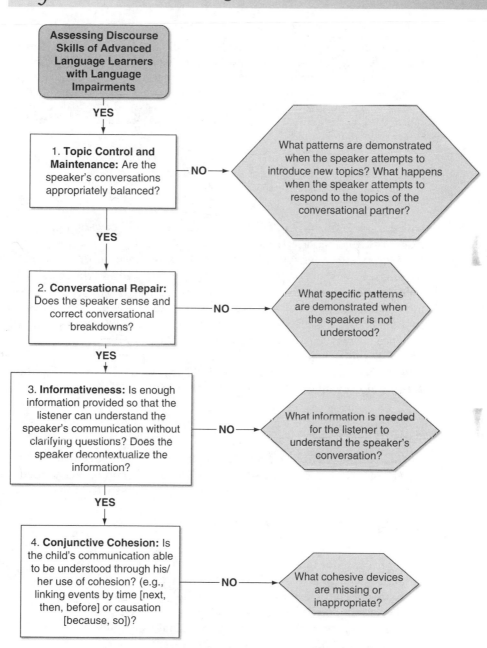

Source: From *Patterns of Narrative Discourse: A Multicultural, Life-Span Approach* (Table 1.1, Decision-Tree for Analysis of Higher-Level Language Skills, p. 19), by A. McCabe and L. S. Bliss, 2003, Boston: Allyn & Bacon. Reproduced by permission of Pearson Education, Inc.

Figure 2.7   Mazing Analysis

Consider the following discourse. The student is 14 years old.

I like video games, (you know, well) I like Mario (Mario) Brothers, there's a new one (that's called) that's called (uh [3 second pause]) new Super Mario Brothers. (Well, he runs around), (Mario [pause]) Mario runs around. And Luigi. You (try) try and get (her) the princess. Bowser, (Bowser, uh) he's the guy you fight. (Fire Mario), Fire Mario (throws) throws stuff. Like a turtle (uh a turtle). Mario (can) can get big. A shell . . . . . . (I like it, um) I like it. (My bro . . .) . . . my brother, (he's) good at Mario, too.

\# of mazed units ÷ # of total unmazed words = percent mazing
16 mazed units ÷ 57 unmazed words = 28%*
*>8% is considered excessive mazing

with LI is less fluent than children who are typically developing; consequently, students with LI demonstrate increased mazing behavior.

During maze analysis the assessor counts the number of speech disruptions (i.e., mazed units) as compared to fluently spoken words. Children developing typically produce less than six disruptions per 100-word speech sample; children who produce more than eight speech disruptions in a 100-word sample are considered to have significant difficulty (Dollaghan & Campbell, 1992; Miller, 1996). An example of mazing is a sentence such as "*He (um), (he's going), (I mean), (he) went, to the (um) (pause) car show.*" In this example there are a total of 12 words, with only 6 words fluently spoken. This sentence is recorded as containing 50% mazing (6/12 = 50%). Further examples of mazing, along with details for mazing analysis, are demonstrated in Figure 2.7.

Assessment Process

In this second section, I describe the process of assessment including screening, measuring skills and abilities, synthesis of results, counseling families, and report writing. An overview of the assessment process is visually presented in Figure 2.8.

SCREENING

Screening is the initial assessment process used to identify children or students who require formal evaluation. Failing a screening does not mean an individual has a language delay or disorder. A language delay or disorder is only identified after a full assessment. The assessor uses the screening process to separate children who clearly are developing typical language skills from children who need further assessment. Screening may be accomplished by using a published, norm-referenced test or informal checklist. Sometimes questionnaires are distributed to teachers or parents to identify children needing further evaluation; these also are considered screening measures. Some school districts have mandatory communication screening protocols completed for all children entering school (ASHA, 2000).

Figure 2.8   **Overview of the Assessment Process**

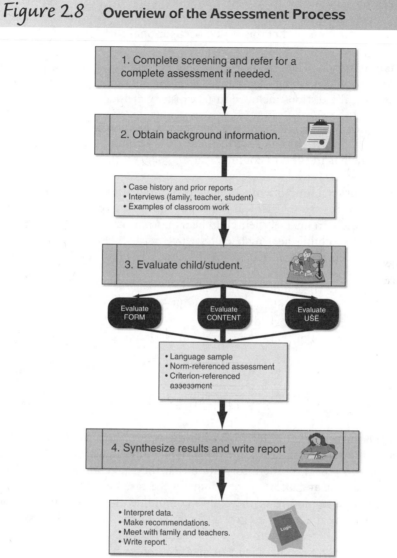

1. Complete screening and refer for a complete assessment if needed.

2. Obtain background information.

• Case history and prior reports
• Interviews (family, teacher, student)
• Examples of classroom work

3. Evaluate child/student.

Evaluate FORM   Evaluate CONTENT   Evaluate USE

• Language sample
• Norm-referenced assessment
• Criterion-referenced assessment

4. Synthesize results and write report

• Interpret data.
• Make recommendations.
• Meet with family and teachers.
• Write report.

DIAGNOSIS AND IDENTIFYING POTENTIAL INTERVENTION TARGETS

The skilled assessor begins the diagnostic process by evaluating the child's environment and considering how his communication disorder impacts the family. This process starts by reviewing case history information; typically the family sends this information prior to the diagnostic assessment. If the student is in school, the assessor interviews the classroom teacher. The assessor should observe classroom communication patterns and obtain examples of the student's written work. The assessor reviews all previous speech-language diagnostic reports in addition to reviewing information provided by other service providers (e.g., physicians, psychologists, physical therapists, and occupational therapists).

Case History.   The case history review begins by asking parents to supply written information describing their child's developmental, medical, and educational history. The critical questions included in case history include:

- When did the family first notice the child's speech-language impairment?
- How do the parents describe their child's communication at this time?
- How has the child's communication changed since the communication problem was observed?
- Do other family members have communication impairments? What are they?
- What illnesses or medical issues has the child experienced?
- Do the parents feel their child hears normally?
- Has the child's hearing been tested?
- How do the parents describe the child's overall development (physical, motor, self-help skills, eating)?
- What are the child's interests?
- How has the family tried to help the child's communication? What has worked? What has not worked?
- What kinds of therapy or other professional help has the family sought out for their child?
- How is their child performing in school? What (if any) are their educational concerns?
- What is the family's most important concern about their child's communication?

Family Interview.   After reviewing the written information that the family provides, the assessor follows up with a family interview. It is important not to ask the parents to repeat all the information that they have already provided as this duplicates the time and effort spent filling out the case history form. However, in order to obtain a clear picture of the child's communication, I summarize the information and then ask the family to give an example or elaborate their answer.

For instance, I might say, "*You indicated that Susan gestures and points to get her needs met at home. Can you give me two examples from the last week of what she 'asked for,' how she indicated what she wanted, and how you responded?*" Or, in order to clarify Susan's hearing ability, I might say, "*Describe for me what Susan does when the phone rings.*" By asking the family to provide examples, I finetune my plan for Susan's assessment. For example, if the family indicates that Susan does not look at others when they speak, I take additional time to assess Susan's pragmatic skills in a range of naturalistic interactions. If the parents indicate that Susan's sentences are too simple or too short, I will include several different procedures to assess Susan's morphosyntax skills. Finally, if the family indicates that Susan's written language is unsophisticated and lacks descriptive words, I will plan additional opportunities to assess semantic skills in Susan's oral language and written work.

Remember that family members do not always use the "right" words to describe a child's communication ability. For example, a parent may describe a child's difficulty as a "speech disorder" although technically the deficit is a language disorder. Also, sometimes parents make incorrect assumptions. I interviewed one parent who indicated her child understood many words because when the mother pointed to an item and asked, "*Is that a chair?*" her child would nod *yes*. The mother's description of her child's ability was not substantiated during the assessment; the child did not demonstrate any receptive comprehension of words during the diagnostic session (e.g., she could not point to the correct item when I said, "*Point to the doll.*")

In this example, the mother interpreted the child's nod as an indication of "knowing the word." However, as I'm sure you realize, nodding *yes* does not necessarily indicate word comprehension. It may not even indicate that the child understood the question! To obtain the needed information, I asked the mother for more examples and asked clarifying questions.

When parents lack understanding about their child's communication impairment, the professional provides more in-depth information. However, often all needed information cannot be provided during the initial interview. Instead, the professional knows the family will need more time and counseling to learn more about their child's communication disorder.

Basic Components of the Assessment.   Although this book focuses on language impairment, the professional must consider all aspects of communication during an assessment. Think back to the model of the speech chain presented in Chapter 1. In the speech chain model, I described the linkages between the motor system and the linguistic system. The motor system includes the mechanical aspects of hearing and the speech system. The linguistic system is the focus of this book; however, the assessor always remembers that the communication system includes both motor and linguistic components. Many children with LI have impairments in multiple communication components. Therefore, assessors consider all communication components during a diagnostic assessment. Not every area must be assessed with a norm-referenced test but the assessor formally or informally evaluates all communication components and describes the individual's abilities within the diagnostic report. In addition to the syntax, pragmatic/social, and semantic analyses that are the focus of this book, assessments during a speech-language diagnostic include the following:

- *Hearing screening*. Children who fail a hearing screening need to be referred for a complete audiological assessment. An illustration of a hearing screening is shown in Figure 2.9.
- *Speech-motor assessment*. The assessor evaluates the child's (a) facial symmetry, (b) structure and function of the lips, tongue, jaw, and velopharynx (i.e., the soft palate), and (c) the resonance, phonatory, and respiratory systems used for speech (Paul, 2007).
- *Speech/articulation assessment:* An articulation assessment evaluates the child's motor ability to produce phonemes. The assessor considers the child's sound production in isolation, syllables, words, sentences, and running speech. The

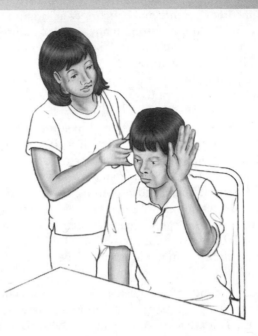

Figure 2.9   **Student Receives a Hearing Screening as Part of the Assessment Process**

norm-referenced Goldman-Fristoe Test of Articulation-Second Edition (Goldman & Fristoe, 2000) is a commonly used articulation test.

- *Phonological assessment and phonological awareness:* Phonological assessment, as discussed briefly in Chapter 1, considers the rules that govern the sound combinations in speech production. To uncover phonological processing disorders, the assessor looks for sound error patterns. Phonological processing disorders are considered a disorder of language form. An example of a test for phonological processing is the Hodson Assessment of Phonological Patterns-Third Edition (Hodson, 2004).
  - Phonological awareness (PA) is a receptive skill. PA refers to the ability to reflect on and manipulate phonemic segments of speech. PA development is highly correlated with early reading skill (see Chapter 9 for more about PA skills and literacy).
- *Assessment of cognitive ability:* The SLP or educator often documents early cognitive ability by observing child behaviors in play-based tasks (i.e., Piagetian framework for development; see Chapter 1) or by analyzing a child's drawing performance (Paul, 2007). For older children, the assessment sometimes includes a nonverbal IQ test such as the *Test of Nonverbal Intelligence* (Brown, Sherbenou, & Johnsen, 1997). (I describe criterion-referenced play-based assessment in Chapter 5).

- *Analysis of a child's rate and fluency of speech.* A child's fluency is typically evaluated informally during conversation. If a fluency disorder is present, a formal fluency assessment is completed.

Depending on the child's age and developmental level, different components of the assessment are emphasized. For example, a cognitive assessment is less appropriate for an older student when cognitive abilities have already been documented.

Identifying Potential Intervention Communication Targets: Communication Subdomains. During the assessment process, the professional considers the developmental sequence of language and considers the communication subdomains aligned with the individual's age and developmental level. The individual's performance within the five different subdomains helps the professional select intervention targets.

Subdomain 1. If the child, or older individual with significant communication impairment, is at the initial levels of communication, the assessment focuses on Subdomain 1: early pragmatic development. When focusing on early pragmatics, the assessor considers the individual's communication functions (e.g., asking, naming, requesting, negating) and evaluates whether the individual uses non-linguistic verbalizations (pointing, gesturing) or meaning-based symbols (words, signs, pictures) to communicate (i.e., the individual's communication means). A summary of Dore's (1975) and Halliday's (1975) pragmatic categories is provided in Table 2.4. The assessor evaluates an individual's pragmatic abilities as compared to the range of pragmatic functions shown in Table 2.4.

Subdomains 2 and 3. Subdomain 2 (vocabulary development) and Subdomain 3 (early word combinations) focus on semantic skills. Parent checklists, such as the MacArthur-Bates Communicative Developmental Inventories (Fenson et al., 2007) can be used to obtain norm-referenced data on children's semantic ability. A short-form version of the MacArthur-Bates (2000) is presented in Figure 2.10. In the MacArthur-Bates assessment, parents indicate the vocabulary items produced by their child (between the ages of 8 and 30 months); the number of words produced by an individual child is compared with normative data from other children the same age.

The assessor uses semantic-focused assessment data to determine the child's use of words and word combinations to communicate meaning. The professional combines information from a parent checklist (such as the MacArthur) with information obtained from a conversational language sample.

A few additional basic principles guide the assessment process for a child functioning within Subdomains 2 and 3 (Haynes & Pindzola, 2008):

- Determine if the child uses a wide range of semantic combinations or only a few. Remember at Brown's Stage 1 that children should be establishing a variety of semantic categories.

Table 2.4   **Pragmatic Categories for Young Children**

Halliday's* Communication Function (What is the child trying to accomplish?)	Dore's Primitive Speech Acts (What does the child do?)
Interacting Communication used to maintain contact with others	Labeling—identifies an object Answering—responds to a caregiver Calling—attempts to gain attention Repeating/Imitating
Regulatory Communication used to control others	Requesting an action Requesting an answer Calling Protesting—rejects an action or object
Personal Communication used to express emotions	Greeting—acknowledges a caregiver Practicing Calling Protesting
Heuristic Communication used to explore and categorize	Labeling Repeating/Imitating Practicing
Instrumental Communication used to satisfy wants/needs	Requesting an action Repeating/Imitating Calling Practicing
Imaginative Communication used during play	Labeling Calling Practicing Repeating/Imitating
Informative Communication used to share knowledge	Requesting Labeling Practicing

* Halliday (1975) and Dore (1974, 1975) categorized slightly different aspects of early pragmatic function. Halliday's pragmatic skills focus on what the child is trying to accomplish (i.e., What is the child's communication goal?) while Dore's categories focus on the child's communication functions at the one-word stage (i.e., What behaviors do we see the child attempting?). Both category systems are used to characterize early pragmatic skills.

- The child should have the lexicon (i.e., vocabulary) to describe his or her environment and communicate socially to achieve many different outcomes (e.g., greeting, negation, questioning, commenting, imaginative play).
- The child should be able to initiate communication and produce multiword combinations spontaneously (not only in imitation of an adult).
- As the child moves to Brown's Stages II and III, the assessor looks for beginning use of morphosyntax features in multiword combinations (e.g., plurals, past tense verbs).

Some children with language disorders continue to struggle to maintain vocabulary development as they enter school (Brackenbury & Pye, 2005). The reasons for vocabulary delay include difficulty with underlying vocabulary-learning processes such as (a) learning vocabulary through everyday interactions (particularly vocabulary that involves figurative speech), (b) storing the phonological information needed to produce words in short-term memory, (c) storing lexical items in long-term memory, and (d) expressively producing vocabulary. Figurative speech refers to nonliteral words or expressions such

---

Figure 2.10   **MacArthur Short Form: Level II (Form A)**

Vocabulary Checklist: Children understand many more words than they say. We are particularly interested in the words your child SAYS. Please mark the words you have heard your child use. If your child uses a different pronunciation of the word, mark it anyway.

BAA BAA	NECKLACE	PARTY	COLD
MEOW	SHOE	FRIEND	FAST
OUCH	SOCK	MOMMY	HAPPY
OH OH	CHIN	PERSON	HOT
WOOF WOOF	EAR	BYE	LAST
BEAR	HAND	HI	TINY
BIRD	LEG	NO	WET
CAT	BROOM	THANK YOU	AFTER
DUCK	COMB	SHOPPING	DAY
HORSE	MOP	CARRY	TONIGHT
AIRPLANE	PLATE	CHASE	OUR
BOAT	TRASH	DUMP	THEM
CAR	TRAY	FINISH	THIS
BALL	TOWEL	FIT	US
BOOK	BED	HUG	WHERE
GAME	BEDROOM	LIKE	BESIDE
APPLESAUCE	BENCH	LISTEN	DOWN
CANDY	OVEN	PRETEND	UNDER
COKE	STAIRS	RIP	ALL
CRACKER	FLAG	SHAKE	MUCH
JUICE	RAIN	TASTE	COULD
MEAT	STAR	GENTLE	NEED
MILD	SWING	THINK	WOULD
PEAS	SCHOOL	WISH	IF
HAT	SKY	ALL GONE	

Has your child begun to combine words yet, such as "*Nother cookie*" or "*Doggie bite*?"

❏ Not Yet   ❏ Sometimes   ❏ Often

Source: From "Short-Form Versions of the MacArthur Communicative Development Inventories," by L. Fenson, S. Pethick, C. Renda, J. L. Cox, P. S. Dale, and J. S. Reznick, 2000, *Applied Psycholinguistics, 21,* pp. 95–116. Copyright © 2000 Cambridge University Press. Used with permission.

Table 2.5   **Figurative Speech for Older School-Age Students**

Term	Definition	Example
Metaphor	An implied comparison between two unlike things. Metaphors carry meaning from one idea to another.	• Life is a journey. • I'm a night owl; you are an early bird.
Simile	A figure of speech that draws a comparison between two different words or concepts; usually contains the words *like* or *as*.	• Her heart soared like an eagle. • His headache pounded like a drum.
Proverb	A well-known saying that expresses a truth or offers advice.	• Penny wise and pound foolish • Practice makes perfect. • All's well that ends well. • Honesty is the best policy.
Idiom	An expression that cannot be understood from the combined meanings of the individual words; a colloquial expression	• Go the whole nine yards. • Come to grips with it. • Strikes a chord • Out on a limb • Not playing with a full deck • Taking the bait

as metaphors, idioms, and proverbs. For example, when I say, "*My friend flipped his wig*!" you know my friend was very upset; you do not literally believe that my friend's wig fell off! Nonliteral, figurative language can be challenging vocabulary learning for students with LI. I provide more examples of figurative speech in Table 2.5.

I mentioned above that children with LI have difficulty learning vocabulary because they may not easily learn new words in everyday interactions; this refers to a process called fast mapping. **Fast mapping** is a process in which young children learn a new word with only minimal exposure (Pence, Bojczyk, & Williams, 2007). For instance, young children developing typically hear a word only a few times and then, remarkably, are observed to produce the word spontaneously. Learn more about the research exploring the process of fast mapping in Focus 2.6.

The assessment process of semantic skills assesses a child's receptive and expressive vocabulary. **Receptive vocabulary** refers to the words the child understands, both in spoken and written form, while **expressive vocabulary** refers to the words a child produces. To test receptive vocabulary, the assessor says a word and asks the child to point to a picture representing the word spoken. In an expressive vocabulary test, the assessor shows a picture and asks the child to name the pictured word. Typically, a child comprehends many more words than he is able to produce expressively (Bates, Dale, & Thal, 1995). A description of some commonly used vocabulary tests is provided in Table 2.6.

Subdomain 4:   As the child's sentence length increases the assessor begins to consider the language features associated with Subdomain 4 (morphosyntax development). In Subdomain 4, an individual developing typically demonstrates the

FOCUS 2.6 *Research*

Fast mapping is a process in which young children learn a new word with only minimal exposure (Pence, Bojczyk, & Williams, 2007). It is proposed that children, when asked to identify an unfamiliar object, form a tentative hypothesis leading to a partial construction of word meaning. Over time, with repeated exposure, the meaning of the word is clarified. For example, imagine that a child is helping his mother in the kitchen and she says, "*Give me the whisk.*" Because the child recognizes the spoon, knife, and spatula, but does not recognize the fourth item on the counter (the whisk), he hands her the whisk. The child assumes that the novel word is the unfamiliar item. Fast mapping helps explain how children learn so many vocabulary words in such a short time. However, fast mapping is only a step in true vocabulary development since research demonstrates that words must be integrated into a child's lexicon before word meaning is retained (Alt & Plante, 2006).

Children use other linguistic cues to assist in fast mapping; the effects of linguistic features on children's fast mapping abilities are tested in research studies. To avoid the effect of previous exposure to the words, the examiner often uses nonsense words. For example, imagine that you are testing the effects of a child's knowledge of syntax. You ask the child, "*Show me the blick.*" If the child has syntax knowledge, he is likely to point to an object (i.e., a noun) rather than an action word (i.e., a verb). On the other hand, if you ask, "*Show me, 'She is <u>blicking</u>',*" the child with syntax knowledge is likely to pick an action picture (i.e., a verb).

Children with language impairment (LI) have reduced fast mapping ability; they need more exposures to a word to complete a fast mapping task. Research suggests that reduced fast mapping is part of the reason that young children with LI have more difficulty learning new vocabulary items (Alt & Plante, 2006). Researchers continue to investigate how different linguistic information is used to assist (or limit) fast mapping abilities.

---

maturing use of adultlike syntax and learns to combine root words with plural and possessive forms. A **root word** is the fundamental or unmarked part of a word (e.g., *look, walk, boy*).

The assessor incorporates a variety of norm-referenced and criterion-referenced tools (such as language sample analysis) into the morphosyntax assessment. Morphosyntax tasks can take several forms:

- Receptive morphosyntax tasks
  - In order to determine if the student understands the meaning of a morpheme the assessor shows several pictures and asks, "*Show me the <u>boys</u> are running. Now, show me the <u>boy</u> is running.*" A student who understands the use of the plural *s* points to a picture of several boys in response to the first sentence, and points to a picture of one boy in response to the second sentence.
  - In order to assess the student's understanding of correct sentence structure (i.e., syntax), the assessor tells the student, "*The boy is pushed by the baby.*" The assessor shows several pictures; in one picture, the boy is pushing the baby, in the other picture, the baby is pushing the boy.

Table 2.6   **Examples of Norm-Referenced Vocabulary Tests**

Test	Description	Age Norms	Psychometric Properties*
Expressive One-Word Picture Vocabulary Test-2000 Edition (EOWPVT; Gardner & Brownell, 2000)	Expressive single-word vocabulary. The student is asked to label the word when the examiner points to the picture. Spanish version available.	2.0–18:11 years	**RELIABILITY:** In terms of reliability, coefficient alpha was computed to assess homogeneity of test items. The median coefficient was .96 with a range of .93 to .98. Split-half coefficients reflected a median of .98. These coefficients speak well with regard to the internal consistency of this instrument. **VALIDITY:** For content validity, the EOWPVT was correlated with 12 other vocabulary measures. Correlations are not overly high (median: .79).
Peabody Picture Vocabulary Test-4 (PPVT-4; Dunn & Dunn, 2006)	Receptive, single-word vocabulary; the student points to one named picture when shown four pictures. Spanish version available.	2.6–adult	**RELIABILITY:** Internal consistency alpha: .92 to .98 (median: .95). Split-half: .86 to .97 (median: .94). Alternate-form .88 to .96 (median: .94). Test-retest .91 to .94 (median: .92). **VALIDITY:** The PPVT-3 had an average correlation of .69 with the OWLS Listening Comprehension Scale and .74 with the OWLS Oral Expression Scale. Its correlations with measures of verbal ability are: .91 (WISC-III VIQ), .89 (KAIT Crystallized IQ), and .81 (K-BIT Vocabulary).

Test	Description	Age Norms	Psychometric Properties*
Receptive One-Word Picture Vocabulary Test-2000 Edition (ROWPVT Gardner & Brownell, 2000)	Receptive, single-word vocabulary; the student points to one named picture when shown four pictures. Spanish version available.	2.11–12 years	**RELIABILITY:** Interrater reliability was evaluated by examining the consistency with which examiners are able to follow the scoring procedure after the test has been administered. The results of the analysis showed 100% agreement; however, the sample size was relatively small (N = 30). Test-retest correlations ranged from .78 to .93 with a coefficient of .84 for the entire sample (the average test-retest interval was 20 days), indicating that the ROWPVT has temporal stability characteristics. **VALIDITY:** The ROWPVT did very well when compared to standard measures such as the PPVT-4 with a coefficient of .64 and the Wechsler Intelligence Scale for Children-Third Edition (WISC-III) Vocabulary with a coefficient of .93. The manual also presents the relationship between the ROWPVT and other broad-based tests of language. Again, the corrected correlations ranged from .45 to .92 with a median of .76. The evidence presented in the manual demonstrated strong support for the overall validity of the ROWPVT scores.

(*continued*)

Table 2.6   **Examples of Norm-Referenced Vocabulary Tests (*Continued*)**

Test	Description	Age Norms	Psychometric Properties*
Comprehensive Receptive and Expressive Vocabulary Test-Second Edition (CREVT-2; Wallace & Hammill, 2002)	Expressive single-word vocabulary. The student is asked to label the word when the examiner points to the picture and define the word.	4.0–89:11 years	**RELIABILITY:** Test-retest reliability was .90. Two measures of alternate form reliability were calculated with averaged subtest reliability coefficients ranging from .88 to .95. Total test reliability coefficients were acceptable for making educational decisions regardless of the measure of reliability. **VALIDITY:** The total test scores on the CREVT-2 correlate highly with the total test scores of two comprehensive language abilities tests, the Clinical Evaluation of Language Fundamentals-Revised (CELF-R) and the Test of Language Development-2 Primary (TOLD-2:P). Correlations are lower for three tests of spoken vocabulary, ranging from .39 to .75.
The WORD Test-2-Elementary (Bowers, Huisingh, Barrett, LoGiudice, & Orman, 2004)	Semantic concepts. Subtests include associations, synonyms, semantic absurdities, antonyms, definitions, and multiple definitions.	7–11 years	**RELIABILITY:** The lowest test-retest reliability coefficient is .37 in the Flexible Word Use task for the 11 years to 11 years, 5 months age group. The manual explains that several reliability indexes may be low because of the restricted scoring range of the group. The 97.8% of agreement in scoring six protocols among nine SLPs does not

Test	Description	Age Norms	Psychometric Properties*
			provide convincing evidence of high interscorer reliability. **VALIDITY:** A major problem with this test is the lack of validity evidence.

*Reliability and validity data source: *The Seventeenth Mental Measurements Yearbook,* Buros Institute of Mental Measurements, 2007, Lincoln, NE: University of Nebraska Press.

- The assessor reads a short paragraph and asks the student comprehension questions about the story.
- Expressive morphosyntax tasks
  - The assessor shows a picture and asks the student to complete the sentence. *"This is David. Whose book is it? It is _____ (his)."* The student demonstrates use of possessive pronouns by completing the sentence with the word *his*.
  - The assessor provides a picture and a word (e.g., *although*). The assessor asks the student to make up a sentence about the picture using the target word.
  - The assessor produces a sentence and asks the student to repeat the sentence. For example, *"Was the boy followed by the girl?"* The assessor notes any errors in morphsyntax during the student's sentence imitation.

As you review the assessment procedures in the examples above, remember different test procedures place varying demands on an individual's syntax, morphology, semantic, and phonological abilities. For example, a sentence imitation task taps into an individual's short-term memory; difficulty with an imitative task may be a result of a short-term memory problem rather than a morphosyntax deficit.

The test directions and even the scoring system can alter the student's ability to perform. Specifically, on some tests, approximations of the correct response receive some point value (e.g., a point value of 0 [incorrect], 1 [partially correct], or 2 [completely correct]). On other tests, responses are marked as either correct (e.g., a value of 1) or incorrect (e.g., a value of 0). It has been suggested that assessors should carefully examine individual items to determine the task requirement or even take the test themselves to appreciate task demands (Sabers, 1996).

Subdomain 5. As I discussed in the section on macroanalysis, the assessor must consider a child's ability to initiate and maintain conversational discourse (Subdomain 5). Advanced pragmatic use also consists of observing a student's use and comprehension of slang, sarcasm, and politeness forms. These subtle language functions become increasingly important in school-age students. A list of pragmatic skills relevant for school-age students is provided in Table 2.7.

Table 2.7   Pragmatic Skills for School-Age Students

Social/Pragmatic skill	Difficulties that might be demonstrated by a school-age student with pragmatic weaknesses
The student should be able to note the current social situation in which the communication interaction is occurring, including the nonverbal cues.	• Student attempts to enter a conversation where the communication partners are clearly engaged in a private conversation. • Student has difficulty telling when others are teasing or are being sarcastic.
The student should be able to engage in mutually pleasant conversations with others.	• Student talks about a topic that is not interesting to the communication partner. • Student interrupts others. • Student does not link questions or comments to the communication partner's topic. • The student's conversation is disjointed and/or the student does not link his spoken ideas together in ways that promote comprehension.
The student should be able to repair a conversation when others do not understand.	• Student does not note communication partner's nonverbal behaviors that indicate lack of communication. • When the student repairs (attempts to clarify) his message, he repeats himself. The student does not rephrase his communication to increase comprehension. • The student does not adjust his conversation tone (i.e., code-switching) when he speaks to varying audiences. For example, the student uses slang or overly casual language when talking to teachers.
The student should follow the implicit rules of a conversational interaction.	• The student stands too close to others when talking. • The student uses inappropriate volume (too loud, too soft). • The student asks too many personal questions. • The student does not raise his or her hand before speaking in a classroom.

SLPs and educators use varying assessment instruments to assess an individual's function in Subdomain 5. It is important to remember that, regardless of the type of assessment used, educators are under increasing pressure to demonstrate the practical benefit of assessment for improving a child's pragmatic communication at home, preschool, or within elementary and secondary classrooms (Zeidner, 2001).

SYNTHESIZING ASSESSMENT RESULTS, COUNSELING FAMILIES, AND WRITING REPORTS

After the assessment protocols are completed, the assessor synthesizes the information that has been gathered. This information includes (a) case history information and information from prior educational or professional tests and reports, (b) interview with family, teachers, and student (if appropriate), (c) observation of client in conversation with family and peers, (d) criterion-referenced assessment, and (e) norm-referenced assessment. In this process, the SLP or educator answers the following questions:

- Does the child have language impairment?
- What language domains are impaired (form, content, use)?
- Does the child demonstrate consistency of ability across testing procedures?
- What are the child's strengths and weaknesses in communicating?
- What are the most important communication behaviors that limit the child's everyday functioning?

The first challenge is for the assessor to identify information overlap from the tests, interviews, and observations. The SLP or educator seeks to confirm the communication problem across measures or tests.

The second challenge is to summarize the information in a meaningful way so that family members understand their child's communication issues. I have found the form-content-use model is a helpful way to communicate information to parents and teachers. I am careful, however, to avoid using jargon and unfamiliar terms. For example, my explanation may go something like this:

> As you described when you came in this morning, Kylee seems behind in her ability to use words and sentences. I completed some different assessments today to check on Kylee's communication. The information you gave me was very helpful. I also want to tell you how much I enjoyed interacting with Kylee today—she really enjoyed playing with the housekeeping center!
>
> First, I completed some assessments of Kylee's ability to communicate her needs. We played together and I looked at her ability to let me know when she needed a toy, wanted help with something, or wanted to let me know that she didn't like the toy I gave her. I was happy to see that she is very able to communicate what she wants, but as you noted, she doesn't do it with words. Instead, she used pointing and sounds to indicate her ideas. Although she isn't using words to communicate, I was happy to note that she is able to get her needs met

nonverbally. This is a very good sign, because sometimes children do not seem to understand that they can communicate with others—even nonverbally—to get their needs met.

Next, I looked at the number of words that Kylee understands and uses. I compared the number of words that she understands to the words she is able to produce verbally. To check her understanding of words, I used an assessment in which I showed Kylee four pictures. After showing her the pictures, I said one of the words and then I asked Kylee to point to the correct word. Kylee's understanding of vocabulary words was somewhat behind what we would expect for her age. In our play interactions, I also saw that she is able to follow very simple one-step instructions, such as *"Show me the book."* But, she has some difficulty with more complex directions such as, *"Put the ball under the table."* Taken together, the results showed me that Kylee's ability to understand what others say is slightly below what is expected for her age.

Finally, I completed some observations and some formal tests during which I looked at the number of words that Kylee can produce. I would expect at her age that Kylee should have between 50 and 100 words and that she would be beginning to make some word combinations like *"Me go bye-bye"* and *"Baby sleeping."* But, as you have noticed, Kylee has only one or two words and is not combining words together. Her difficulty in using words to express her ideas demonstrates a moderate level of delay. Do you have any questions about anything I've said so far?

Take a close look at the information I provided to Kylee's parents. In the first paragraph, I summarized the information that her parents provided in the initial interview. Parents are the experts about their child's communication and I acknowledged this contribution. I also provided feedback on Kylee's behavior during the assessment. I know that parents are typically very anxious about their child's abilities. I used this opportunity to build the ongoing relationship I will need to establish an effective intervention program.

In the second paragraph, I began by describing Kylee's pragmatic skills (i.e., language use). Notice that I did not use the word *pragmatics,* but I described Kylee's ability to use language to request, negate, and question. I also highlighted the importance of pragmatic skills.

In the third paragraph, I described semantics (i.e., language form). I framed this discussion by talking about Kylee's understanding of words (i.e., receptive language). If you read this paragraph carefully, you noticed that I discussed both a norm-referenced test (i.e., the test during which I asked Kylee to point to pictures) and an observational, play-based task in which I asked Kylee to follow directions. This is an example of how I used multiple data sources to understand Kylee's abilities.

Also in the third paragraph, note that during this first explanation of results, I did not provide Kylee's parents with Kylee's standard score on the receptive vocabulary test. I typically give this information to the parents in another discussion; I often discuss test scores when I present the final written report. Many parents are overwhelmed by too much technical information at one time.

In the fourth paragraph, I discussed Kylee's expressive language ability. First, I framed the findings by describing the MLU that Kylee should be using. Then, I described Kylee's verbal output in relation to developmental norms. Can you determine (a) what Brown's stage Kylee should be at from my description and (b) her actual level of performance? If you can do this critical-thinking task, you understand how language sample analysis is used to gauge language development. Finally, at the end of my discussion, I paused and took time to answer questions.

In my discussion of Kylee's results, I used the terms, *slightly below* and *moderately delayed*. The use of the terms *mild, moderate,* and *severe* should always be used carefully. However, with this caution in mind, I typically think about a standard score between 1.25 and 1.5 standard deviations as being a mild level of impairment (these are below the 10th percentile) and scores between 1.5 and 2.0 standard deviations as a moderate level of impairment. A standard score at or below 2 standard deviations (2nd percentile of performance) is typically considered a severe impairment. Standard scores are always interpreted in conjunction with observation and criterion-referenced measures.

Clinical Report Writing.   The final challenge in the assessment process is to write the assessment report in a way that clearly summarizes the findings. In Appendix C, I provide a sample of an assessment report and explain the rationale for individual sections and writing style. There is not one right way to write a report other than the report must be accurate, concise, and link the various assessment protocols together in a logical way. However, I ask beginning students to use a report style that is consistent with the form-content-use language model. I do this because often beginning students administer tests but cannot explain what language domains (form, content, use) are being evaluated. This is particularly relevant when interpreting norm-referenced tests (e.g., the CELF-3) where different subtests within the test evaluate different language domains—one subtest evaluating syntax, another evaluating semantics, etc. Whereas the skilled assessor determines what domain is assessed within each subtest, the beginning student sometimes reports test scores without understanding the implications of the subtest score. However, if the report is divided into sections on form, content, and use, the assessor must consider each language domain individually and link information from norm-referenced tests and criterion-referenced assessments.

The skilled assessor also considers the difficulty level of the subtest task. For example, a syntax subtest might ask the student to repeat a sentence (a relatively easy syntax task). Alternately, in another syntax subtest, the student may be provided with three words and asked to construct a novel sentence (a more difficult syntax task). The assessor looks at an individual's varying ability across subtests and provides an explanation.

Beyond the above-mentioned suggestions, there are general professional writing guidelines used when writing a report. In Table 2.8, I describe writing guidelines and present examples of writing styles to use and avoid.

Table 2.8 **Guidelines for Report Writing**

Guideline	Like this:	Not like this:	Why?
• Use clear, short sentences. • Use specific language rather than ambiguous terms.	Mary has significant difficulty in the classroom following two- and three-step directions.	Following observations, it was revealed[1] that Mary is not functioning up to the norm for her level. She acts confused periodically[2] in the classroom.	[1] An expression like *it is revealed* adds words, but does not add writing clarity. [2] Expressions like *up to the norm* and *confused periodically* are ambiguous; they cannot be measured.
• Use non-technical language, or explain terms. • Do not use an abbreviation unless it is defined.	The examiner assessed Sonia's ability to point to words when they were named. This is a measure of receptive vocabulary. The Peabody Picture Vocabulary Test-R (PPVT-R) standard score was within normal limits.	Semantic abilities were assessed using the PPVT-R.	Parents, teachers, and other professionals need to be able to understand the assessment results.
• Avoid colloquial expressions. • Use formal instead of casual word choices.	In a 30-minute period, John left his seat three times. His mother confirmed John's difficulty in attending to tasks at home.	John bounced off the walls[3] during the class; he had difficulty interacting with other kids. His mom[4] said that John is just like this at home.	[3] *Bounced off the walls* is a colloquial expression. [4] Use more formal word choices (e.g., *children, mother*) in written reports.
• Use active rather than passive sentences.	During an observation of a shared reading, Katrina's mother asked 5-6 questions on each page of the book.	A storybook reading was observed[5] by the examiner. During the observation, the examiner observed that there were numerous examples of direct questioning that were asked by Katrina's mother.[6]	[5] Avoid passive sentence construction such as *a storybook reading was observed.* [6] This sentence is not clearly constructed.
• Avoid qualifiers and noncommittal language. • Describe behavior rather than labeling the individual.	Thomas had difficulty with instructions containing the subordinate conjunctions *before* and *after.* (e.g., "*Before you touch the red square, touch the blue triangle.*") He refused to complete the subtest containing complex commands.	Thomas appeared to have some difficulty with more complex tasks and sometimes[7] struggled to follow directions. He appeared frustrated.[8]	[7] Eliminate noncommittal language. [8] This is a subjective labeling of the student's emotions.

Source: Based on information from "Documenting Cinical Service Delivery: Writing Style and Lexical Selection" by D. L. Wilkerson, 2000, *Contemporary Issues in Communication Science and Disorders* (27), pp. 6–13.

Summary

- Norm-referenced assessments have statistical properties that allow the assessor to compare the individual's performance to that of his or her chronological peer group. Norm-referenced assessments are typically used to determine if an individual does, or does not, have language impairment. Criterion-referenced assessments are used to document an individual's ability in a specific domain; the raw data are used to develop intervention plans and document behavior change. Validity and reliability must be considered when evaluating an assessment tool. Standard scores are transformed scores allowing an individual's performance to be compared with same-age peers on a bell-shaped curve.

- The assessor computes mean length of utterance (MLU) by dividing the total number of morphemes in a speech sample by the number of utterances; this provides an average for utterance length. The assessor can use MLU to quantitatively compare a child's length of utterances with developmental data from Brown's stages. A T-unit analysis is an analysis in which the assessor separates clauses by coordinating conjunctions; it is an analysis used with older school-age children. Microanalysis considers an individual's output utterance by utterance; microanalysis can include analysis of pragmatic function and semantic relationships for beginning language learners and morphosyntax features for later language learners. Macroanalysis considers an individual's ability to participate in conversation and includes discourse and mazing analyses.

- The professional develops an assessment plan that will evaluate the individual's (a) language use (e.g., How does the client communicate? Can he get his or her needs met? What is conversation like when communicating with this individual?), (b) language content (e.g., What words does the individual know and use? Is the individual's semantic knowledge adequate for school success?), and (c) language form (e.g., What morphosyntax features does the individual understand and use? Do morphosyntax weaknesses negatively impact academic performance?)

- Assessment priorities change depending on the relevant communication subdomain. In Subdomain 1 (early pragmatic), the assessor often uses criterion-referenced assessments and parent surveys to understand the individual's use of pragmatic communication behaviors. When considering Subdomains 2 and 3 (word learning and early word combinations), the assessor uses a semantic focus to document the individual's lexicon and the semantic combinations used when combining words. Norm-referenced, criterion referenced, and observational assessments are all used for individuals at Subdomains 2 and 3. When assessing Subdomain 4 (morphosyntax), the assessor typically uses a combination of language sample analyses, along with norm-referenced and criterion-referenced assessment. When assessing Subdomain 5, the assessor completes a discourse analysis and considers advanced pragmatic skills.

- In addition to evaluating an individual's language abilities, the assessor considers all aspects of the communication system during a speech-language assessment.

This includes hearing ability, speech motor ability, cognitive ability, fluency and rate of speech, sound production, awareness of phonemes, and voice quality.

- The assessor evaluates case history data, interviews family members and teachers, evaluates the child or student using a variety of assessment tools, synthesizes test results, and writes a clinical report to complete the assessment process.

Discussion and In-Class Activities

1. Divide into groups with other students in your class. Look over a brief outline of a child with a language disorder given to you by your instructor (e.g., Child 1, who is 8 years old, is having difficulty in school learning to read and write; Child 2, who is 5 years old but can only speak with a few word combinations (i.e., child has a severe disability), Child 3, who is 3 years old, has a slight language delay and is making morphosyntax errors). Together with students in your group, brainstorm activities, observations, interviews, and criterion-referenced assessments that could be used with each case to obtain background information and conduct the assessment. Who should be interviewed before the assessment, and what questions will you ask? What points should be included in the final interview with parents and teachers? What information needs to be obtained during classroom observations?

2. Your instructor will provide a videotape observation of a young child in play with another child or an adult. Use the Language Sample Worksheet (see Appendix B) to document observed behaviors. Did the child you observed demonstrate a sufficient range (given his or her age) of pragmatic function? Could the context or environment be altered to promote a greater variety of pragmatic behaviors? How did the child try to communicate (communication means)? Did he or she use gestures, sounds, words, or word combinations?

3. Your instructor will show you a video of the administration of a norm-referenced test; score at least part of the test using score sheets provided to you. Your instructor may choose to give you score sheets already scored for the target child. After completing the scoring process (with your instructor's guidance), refer to the normative data table from the test manual. Find the page in the manual with standard scores for the target child's chronological age). Use the manual and your test data to (a) compute the raw score, (b) transform the raw score into a standard score, and (c) identify the confidence intervals. Following this exercise, you and your classmates can work together to role-play an interview with a parent in which the assessor explains the student's performance on the norm-referenced test.

4. Your instructor will provide you with a brief example of a child language transcript. Compute the child's MLU and NDW. Answer the following questions: (a) What Brown's stage should the child be at given his or her chronological age? (b) Is the child's MLU consistent with this stage? (c) If not, what Brown's stage is the child at? (d) Is this child within normal limits for sentence length and vocabulary variety?

5. Pick a norm-referenced test (you may be able to choose one from the university speech-language clinic). In an oral or written presentation, provide information about the assessment's (a) reliability data, (b) validity data, (c) purpose (Does it test form, content, use?), and (d) tasks used to assess different domains.
6. Your instructor will provide you with examples of good, average, and poorly written assessment reports. Edit the reports either individually or in a group with your classmates. Why did you change certain components of each report? Compare your changes with those of the other students. Following your edits, role-play how an SLP might interpret the assessment results to parents.

Chapter 2 Case Study

A student, Michael, is in the 4th grade and is 10 years, 3 months old. He speaks slowly, but sound production and syntax are correct. He is performing at just below average levels academically. He does not appear distracted but has difficulty following instructions in the classroom.

The assessor administered two norm-referenced tests, the Peabody Picture Vocabulary Test (PPVT; a receptive vocabulary test) and the Clinical Evaluation of Language Function-3 (CELF-3).

Michael received the following standard scores (SS):

TEST/Subtest	SS (M = 100)	SS (M = 10)
PPVT	87	
CELF-3		
Concepts and Directions		6
Word Classes		9
Semantic Relationships		7
RECEPTIVE CELF-3 SCORE	84	
Formulated Sentences		13
Recalling Sentences		8
Sentence Assembly		5
EXPRESSIVE LANGUAGE SCORE	92	

Overall, Michael's normative assessment data indicated that his receptive-expressive language and vocabulary knowledge were generally within normal limits, but he demonstrated significant levels of difficulty with sentence assembly. The assessor noted that Michael had difficulty organizing the sentences into more than one sentence type (a requirement of this sentence assembly subtest).

The assessor evaluated some of Michael's written work. Michael's written work was grammatically accurate, but he used simple rather than complex sentence constructions. His story writing was "flat," lacking descriptive language or temporal or clausal connections.

Questions for Discussion

1. Explain why Michael could score reasonably well on most of the CELF-3 and PPVT, but have the described difficulties in the classroom.
2. Describe a criterion-referenced task that you might use to further evaluate Michael's abilities.
3. Find a copy of the PPVT and the CELF-3; look at the different tasks that are used to assess each language domain. Which tasks are easier? Which are more difficult?
4. Role-play an explanation to Michael's parents and teacher regarding Michael's assessment. Explain the results of his standardized scores.

Decision Making in Assessment and Intervention

Chapter Overview Questions

1. What are the three critical-thinking parameters? Give two examples of critical-thinking questions reflecting each parameter.
2. How does the practitioner use decision trees to increase understanding of clinical decision making? Draw a simple decision tree.
3. How is the response to intervention model (RTI) different from a more traditional model of assessment? Give three examples of

critical-thinking questions reflecting the RTI model.
4. What changes in public policy have influenced decision making for students with language impairment?
5. What are some examples of questions used to elicit information from a family during a routines-based interview?
6. How is progress monitoring impacted by IDEA? What role does it play in implementation of the RTI model?

As a speech-language pathologist (SLP) or special educator, you will be making daily decisions directly impacting the lives of children and families. Read the following case examples and consider the decisions you might be called on to make in the following situations:

1. Tanzia is 7 and is significantly impaired. She communicates in simple sentences and her verbal productions are often off topic. Last year, her teacher worked on increasing Tanzia's sentence length and complexity. This year, Tanzia has been assigned to you.
2. Mrs. Shultz is a preschool teacher in your school; she teaches in an inclusive classroom. Six children in her classroom have special needs and six

children are developing typically. Mrs. Shultz used to be a first-grade teacher. When you observe her classroom, you find the children spend a lot of time completing worksheets at a table. Mrs. Shultz is very worried about the need for her students to identify all the alphabet letters and write their names. You want to help the children learn these concepts but also want to promote a more active learning style.

3. Jahara is 16 and has a cognitive impairment. In the past year, her intervention has focused on improving her syntax (e.g., correct use of pronouns) and working on correct articulation of the /r/ and /l/ sounds. You are meeting with Jahara and her family and need to develop her intervention goals for the upcoming school year.

4. Thomas is 8 and is struggling in school. His sentences often contain morphosyntax errors including errors with verb forms and subordinating conjunctions (i.e., *because, so, if*). Errors are demonstrated in his spoken and written language. You will be working to develop a progress-monitoring protocol for his Individualized Education Program (IEP).

This chapter will highlight strategies you can use to make important clinical decisions in situations like the case examples described above.

A Model of Decision Making

The world you will be entering as a professional is very different from the professional world I entered over 30 years ago. When I began my training in the 1970s, undergraduate education focused on teaching vocabulary terms and the facts and figures connected to language disorders. We did not have the Internet, so teachers focused on providing terminology and basic knowledge fundamental to the field.

As students in the new millennium, you have grown up accessing facts at the click of a mouse. The quantity of easily available information changes how young professionals should be trained. Now, rather than presenting only the facts, training must focus on helping students synthesize and evaluate available information. Young professionals must learn how to use theory and data to make clinical decisions. This chapter focuses on that important challenge: learning to become an effective clinical decision maker, someone who has moved beyond simply knowing the basic facts. An effective clinical decision maker:

- Knows how to choose among a wealth of information and is able to select credible information.
- Is able to understand and explain to parents and teachers—who also have access to a great deal of information—(a) the theories that underlie specific approaches and (b) the pros and cons associated with various intervention approaches.
- Understands how to weigh research evidence to choose approaches that demonstrate strong efficacy, evidence, and efficiency. **Efficacy** is measured by studies that determine the extent to which a specific intervention, procedure, or service

produces a beneficial result under ideal conditions (for example, in a very controlled clinical study when it is administered by highly trained interventionists). **Effectiveness** is determined in studies examining the extent to which a specific intervention results in positive outcome when it is used in routine practice (e.g., in a school setting administered by regular SLPs). **Efficiency** is a priority when funding sources are limited; the decision maker must consider the most efficient means to rehabilitate an individual's communication disorder (Stout & Hayes, 2004).

- Understands the *why* and *how* associated with various intervention approaches. The skilled decision maker understands when to choose one approach over another, sets specific and targeted goals supported by research evidence, and documents change in an individual's communication behaviors.
- Is sensitive to a multicultural environment, because increasingly SLPs and educators are providing services for children and families with a variety of life experiences and cultural practices.
- Develops a professional approach that welcomes innovation and change. The skilled decision maker recognizes that continual professional training is required to keep abreast of what works as demonstrated by high-quality research.

This chapter is designed to help you begin to develop important decision-making skills. I set you on the course to becoming a skilled decision maker by (a) presenting a series of three critical-thinking parameters, (b) linking the critical-thinking parameters to questions you can use to implement high-level thinking skills, and (c) connecting the critical-thinking parameters to four components of clinical practice (i.e., assessment, intervention, the environment, and progress monitoring/dismissal). Throughout this chapter, I give examples and illustrate decision-making processes by providing case examples.

I have divided the important critical-thinking skills into three parameters: (1) accuracy and scope of information, (2) evaluating evidence, and (3) change and adaptability. These three parameters characterize important elements of thought demonstrated in higher-order decision making. See Figure 3.1 for a graphic presentation of the three parameters.

Below I briefly describe each of the three critical-thinking parameters. These parameters are adapted from the work of Paul and Elder (2008).

CRITICAL-THINKING PARAMETERS

The first critical-thinking parameter is *accuracy and scope of information*. Accuracy prompts the decision maker to gather supporting evidence to identify the communication problem and make conclusions. A communication problem cannot be remediated until it is objectively described. The decision maker uses both objective and subjective data to accurately document a communication disorder; **objective data** are based on observable phenomena (e.g., ratings scales, behavioral/classroom observations, test scores). **Subjective data** represent an individual's opinion. A family's belief about their child's communication disorder is subjective; but it is information that must be included as part of the decision-making process. Accuracy also is an essential

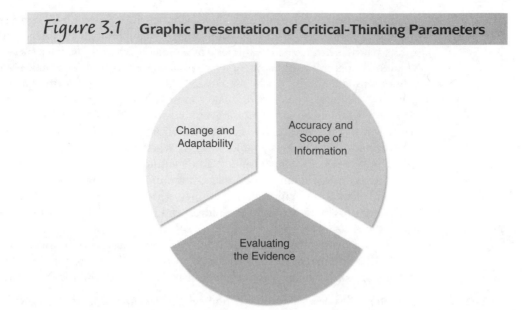

Figure 3.1   Graphic Presentation of Critical-Thinking Parameters

Change and Adaptability

Accuracy and Scope of Information

Evaluating the Evidence

feature of intervention; the practitioner makes recommendations based on child data, carefully documents intervention outcomes in high-quality reports, and accurately documents a child's progress.

The data must be accurate, but the decision maker also must take care to gather enough pertinent information to reach a meaningful conclusion. In Chapter 2, I discussed issues of reliability and validity. Accuracy is most similar to reliability—the decision maker wants to accurately capture and describe the individual's communication behavior. But, as you recall, validity is even more important than reliability! In order for clinical conclusions to be valid, the decision maker must gather sufficient scope of information to document the individual's communication skills in real-life settings. For example, the decision maker considers the scope of information by asking the family *"Can you give me an example or illustration of that behavior?"* or *"Could you elaborate on that point?"* during the assessment interview. Scope of information also provides the rationale for completing classroom observations and working closely with classroom teachers.

The second critical-thinking parameter is *evaluating evidence*. This second parameter underlies the need for practitioners to know and understand how to use scientific evidence to identify high-quality assessment tools and intervention programs. In Chapter 2, I presented information about adequate correlation levels to document reliability levels in assessment tools. This information helped you consider the evidence supporting the use of particular assessment tools.

Practitioners also evaluate evidence when they choose an intervention program. Decision makers use external evidence (e.g. research studies) as well as internal evidence to choose between varying intervention approaches. Internal evidence includes individual family and child characteristics and the practitioner's knowledge of theory and development. For example, the decision maker considers internal evidence when he or she determines if a proposed intervention is responsive to the client's cultural and family background. If it is not responsive, the practitioner acquires more evidence to clarify the individual's unique circumstances.

The practitioner also uses a thorough knowledge of language theory and development as internal evidence to support specific clinical practices. Throughout this book, I provide numerous examples and developmental frameworks to build your ability to use internal evidence.

The third decision-making parameter is *change and adaptability*. The skilled practitioner learns to consistently note and document change in an individual's communication abilities. Communication interventions must make a real difference in the life of the individual. The skilled practitioner also notes if the intervention is motivating for a particular individual; if not, the intervention should be modified to increase motivation.

Adaptability also requires that the practitioner is personally open to change. A skilled practitioner stays open-minded with regard to intervention approaches and new evidence. It is easy to fall into intervention habits and use the same or similar approaches for different children with dissimilar communication challenges. The professional should beware of entering a clinical comfort zone; it is easy to use a familiar approach. Skilled professionals continually seek out new information to determine if another approach may be more helpful.

In summary, a skilled decision maker uses critical-thinking skills to (a) gather relevant and sufficient information to aid the decision-making process, (b) compare decisions via internal and external evidence, (c) consider multicultural influences on communication behavior, (d) observe and document change in communication behavior, and (e) flexibly adapt interventions to promote effective outcomes.

QUESTIONING AS A TOOL FOR CRITICAL THINKING

We are all familiar—through Court TV or television dramas—with the proceedings of the courtroom. The prosecuting attorney faces the witness and asks a number of focused questions. The assumption is that questioning reveals information that allows the jury to reach a verdict. The process of asking and answering questions is central to this process. Focused questioning allows facts to be less distorted, clarifies confusing issues, and guides thoughtful reasoning (Browne & Keeley, 2007; Paul & Elder, 2008; Phillips & Duke, 2001).

As a developing critical thinker, you must learn to ask, and answer, critical-thinking questions. At first, you will need to deliberately ask yourself questions and write down your answers. As you become a skilled decision maker, the question asking and answering process will become automatic and internalized. Asking and answering questions will guide you to become reflective, increase thinking clarity, and help you achieve important critical-thinking skills.

Examples of the critical-thinking questions you will learn to use are provided in Table 3.1. You should notice that the questions are aligned along the three critical-thinking parameters (accuracy and scope of information, evaluating evidence, change and adaptability). Although you might not ask yourself every question with

Table 3.1 Critical-Thinking Parameters, Questions, and Aspects of Clinical Practice

Critical-thinking parameters	Critical-thinking questions	Assessment, intervention, environment, progress monitoring
Accuracy and scope of information	1. Has screening indicated that this child needs more in-depth assessment?	Assessment
	2. Do I have enough details about the language disorder to understand the issues?	Assessment, intervention, environment
	3. Are there multicultural issues that may impact this language disorder that I need to consider?	Assessment, intervention, environment, progress monitoring
	4. Do I know what language domains are impacted?	Assessment, intervention, environment
	5. Can I clearly explain the relevant issues facing this individual?	Assessment, intervention, environment, progress monitoring
	6. Have I considered this student's language disorder from all relevant points of view (e.g., family, teacher, employer, student)?	Assessment, intervention, environment, progress monitoring
	7. Have I gathered data from several sources to verify my information (norm-referenced tests, criterion-referenced protocols, environmental scans)?	Assessment, intervention, environment, progress monitoring
Evaluating the evidence	1. Does the assessment protocol and intervention approach I have selected have evidence to support its use?	Assessment, intervention
	2. Does all of the information I have about this individual make sense together?	Assessment, intervention, environment
	3. Are my decisions on intervention and dismissal based on student outcome data?	Intervention, progress monitoring
	4. Have I established a data monitoring system that allows me to track student progress?	Progress monitoring
Change and adaptability	1. Do I need to look at this communication problem from a different perspective?	Assessment, intervention, environment, progress monitoring
	2. Will the intervention be motivating to the student? If not, how can I change it?	Assessment, intervention, environment

Critical-thinking parameters	Critical-thinking questions	Assessment, intervention, environment, progress monitoring
	3. Will the intervention target behaviors making a real difference in the student's life?	Intervention, environment
	4. Am I providing intervention within an environment (i.e., family routines, classroom) that is likely to promote change?	Intervention, environment
	5. Am I providing the intervention that is best for the client or does my intervention reflect what is convenient for my schedule and me?	Intervention, environment
	6. Have I continued to learn and grow as a professional? What have I learned to do differently or better in the past year?	Assessment, intervention, environment, progress monitoring

every student, you should consider each of the three parameters during the clinical decision-making process. This list does not include all of the possible questions that could be asked; it is only a beginning to help you get started.

Not only are the questions in Table 3.1 aligned with the three critical-thinking parameters (the column on the left in Table 3.1), I also aligned questions in relation to important aspects of clinical practice: assessment, intervention, environment, and progress monitoring. The rest of this chapter is organized around these four important aspects of clinical practice.

DECISION TREES AS A TOOL FOR CRITICAL THINKING

A **decision tree** is a graphic example of the alternatives in the decision-making process. I incorporate a number of decision trees throughout this book to efficiently help you become a skilled decision maker. A decision tree allows you to see the thought process that underlies the decision-making process. A very simple illustration of a decision tree is illustrated in Figure 3.2; it is an illustration of my thought process at the age of 18 when I was deciding on a major as an undergraduate student. I considered different occupations, and chose speech-language pathology. The decision tree illustrates how I chose among the varying alternatives.

I include decision trees and graphic illustrations of critical-thinking processes throughout this book; I include these features to help you understand underlying decision-making processes. Take time to consider the decision trees included in this book. Use the decision trees to address the provided case examples. Just as one needs practice to become a skilled athlete, you must practice decision-making skills to become proficient.

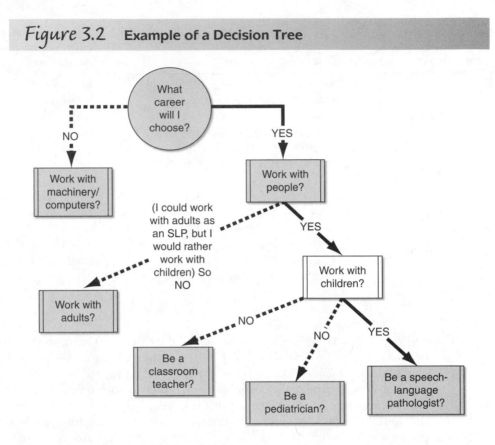

Figure 3.2   **Example of a Decision Tree**

When an SLP student or student teacher is assigned his or her first clinical experience, the student often looks at the supervisor in horror and says *"But what should I DO?"* Although the student has learned a great deal of information prior to the first clinical assignment, he or she often fails to master critical-thinking skills. Do not let this happen to you! Start now to develop the critical-thinking skills you will use throughout your professional career.

In the sections below, I describe critical-thinking skills as they relate to four aspects of clinical practice: assessment, intervention, environment, and progress monitoring. I explain how critical-thinking questions are used to fine-tune the decision-making process. I illustrate critical-thinking questions and how they relate to the four aspects of clinical and educational practice in Figure 3.3.

Decision Making: Assessment

As you recall from Chapter 2, assessment is used to (a) describe a child's communicative functioning, (b) determine what domains or communication functions should be targeted during intervention, and (c) determine a child's eligibility for special educational

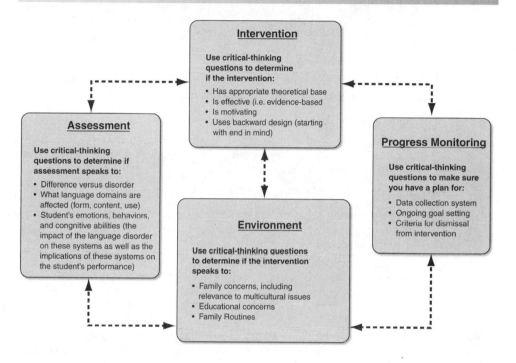

Figure 3.3   **Critical-Thinking Questions as They Relate to Assessment, Intervention, Environment, and Progress Monitoring**

or rehabilitative service (Paul, 2007). In the clinical decision model, the practitioner begins this process by asking some of the following questions:

- What aspects of language should be evaluated for this student (e.g., form, content, use)?
- Have I used a variety of clinical measures to describe the student's language disorder (e.g., norm-referenced and criterion-referenced tools)?
- Does this student require a referral?

The examples listed above are some of the questions to consider during the assessment process. I highlight additional points with regard to the critical-thinking parameter of *accuracy and scope of information* in the section below.

The need for *accuracy* significantly impacts the assessment process. You learned a great deal about assessment in Chapter 2. Now, expand your ability to use this knowledge by looking at Table 3.2 and consider how you might use questions to guide your assessment with (a) a toddler who is not interacting socially with his communication partners, (b) a preschool child who is not speaking in word combinations, (c) an older school-age student who is having difficulty following the teacher's instructions.

Table 3.2   **Critical-Thinking Questions Related to Aspects of Communication or Related Skills**

Prelinguistic

* Does the child or student have the basic principles of communication (i.e., imitation, joint attention) underlying social interactions (first evidenced at nonverbal level)?

Cognitive

* Does the child or student demonstrate the cognitive skills (i.e., means-end, object permanence, cause and effect) that impact language development?

Pragmatic (early skills)

* Does the child or student have early communication behaviors (e.g., turn taking, range of pragmatic acts [requesting, commenting, protesting]) needed for social interaction (verbal or nonverbal)?

Lexical

* Is the beginning language learner combining words into two- and three-word combinations using a variety of semantic combinations (i.e., agent + action, action + object, agent + object)?
* Are there vocabulary items or concepts that would significantly improve communication or make clear impact in his or her academic setting or workplace? Does the student have the needed vocabulary to be successful academically?

Morphosyntax

* Are there morphosyntax features that, if targeted, would improve social communication and/or academic achievement? Does the student have appropriate levels of syntax complexity for his age/grade?

Pragmatic (discourse)

* Does the student have good ability to introduce topics, maintain a topic, switch topics appropriately, and ask questions in ways that promote social interaction?
* Can the student make conversational repairs?

Literacy

* Are early literacy skills being targeted in ways that engage young children in active learning?
* Are there reading and writing skills for the older student that, if facilitated, would improve communication, academic skills, work skills, or quality of life?
* Are there learning strategies that an older student can learn that will help him or her be more successful in the classroom?
* Can the student tell and/or write a narrative? Is the student motivated to work on narrative production?

Assessment also requires the practitioner consider the *scope of information;* an important decision is to consider whether the child's language behaviors reflect a **language difference** versus a **language disorder.** A language difference reflects a cultural or regional pattern. The practitioner's task is to separate children who have a language difference from children with a true language disorder. In using your critical-thinking ability, you may need to move beyond only considering the formal definition of a language disorder (i.e., a language disorder is the impaired comprehension and/or use of spoken, written, and/or other symbol systems; ASHA, 1993). In order to determine if you are observing a true language disorder you need to ask:

- Does this student score significantly lower than average on standardized testing and/or naturalistic testing <u>and</u> is the student perceived as having a communication disorder by his or her significant communication partners?

If you can answer yes to both parts of the question, you are likely to have identified a language disorder instead of a language difference (Paul, 2007). Use the Internet site described in Focus 3.1 to learn more about language differences and multicultural language. I highlight additional information with regard to multicultural issues throughout this book. It is a very important aspect of your clinical training.

Scope of information also implies that you have considered the breadth of behaviors that may be affected by the student's disability. Ask yourself about the student's cognitive and perceptual skills, coping behaviors, social interactions, and academic skills. Consider if any related domains are impacted by the communication impairment and if so, will your proposed intervention accommodate the student's associated deficits? If not, take the time to complete more observations and conduct more interviews with the student, teachers, or family members during the assessment process. What do the stakeholders feel are the student's most significant communication issues? To determine if you have met this critical-thinking threshold, you can ask yourself, Has my assessment evaluated the student's most critical communication challenges as perceived by those closest to him or her?

RESPONSE TO INTERVENTION

You will be making assessment decisions in a constantly evolving professional world. As an example, in 2004 a new educational model was proposed, the **response to intervention (RTI) model** (also referred to as the **responsiveness to intervention**

FOCUS 3.1 *Multicultural Issues*

You can access more information about the multicultural knowledge and skill requirements outlined by the American Speech-Language Hearing Association at www.asha.org/docs/html/KS2004-00215.html

model). The RTI model begins with a different set of assumptions as compared to the more traditional assessment model described in Chapter 2.

As you recall, in Chapter 2 I introduced the concept of static versus dynamic assessment. Static assessment provides a snapshot of an individual's abilities at a particular moment in time. Dynamic assessments, on the other hand, identify an individual's learning potential. The RTI model is a form of dynamic assessment. Consider the differences between clinical questions using the two models. In a traditional model of assessment, the practitioner poses the following questions:

- Does this student's standard score on a norm-referenced test fall significantly below that expected for his or her age?
- Is the child's mean length of utterance below what is expected as compared to children who are the same chronological age?
- Does the student produce utterances with sufficient levels of complexity?
- Do the student's everyday communication abilities appear to be different from other students his or her age?

In contrast, in the RTI model, the practitioner begins with a different set of critical questions. The practitioner asks:

- Has this student had previous exposure to the concepts or skills required for a particular task?
- Has this student been provided with evidence-based (i.e., scientifically proven) instructional methods in his or her classroom?

With the RTI-framed clinical questions, the practitioner considers that a child's poor performance on a language/literacy task may be due to the student's (a) lack of experience with the task or (b) lack of evidence-based instruction (i.e., instruction was not based on scientific research).

As an example, many preschoolers have few opportunities to practice rhyming words (e.g., *"What word rhymes with hat?"*). In a preschool-level screening test, a child without sufficient rhyming experience may perform very poorly when asked to rhyme. In the RTI model, the practitioner makes certain that every child has many learning opportunities to rhyme before assuming that there is a "rhyming deficit."

The need to focus on rhyming ability in young children is based on scientific research. Consequently, classroom-based opportunities for rhyming must be provided to all children during their preschool years. In the RTI model, exposure to key language and literacy targets within the general education classroom is called Tier 1 intervention. Tier 1 intervention is typically provided by the general education teacher and involves the use of instructional methods with good efficacy, effectiveness, and efficiency. The assumption is that a child should not be identified as being impaired until he or she has many opportunities to learn important language/literacy skills at the classroom level.

RTI applies to preschool children (as in the rhyming example above) and also older school-age students. In elementary school, practitioners do not wait until a student is diagnosed as learning disabled prior to initiating scientifically based educational interventions. With the RTI model, all students receive high-quality evidence-based educational instruction in the classroom. Reading instruction has been a significant focus in the RTI model. Scientifically based reading instruction for school-age students includes a focus on phonological awareness skills, reading comprehension, and reading fluency. I describe the important components of scientifically based reading research in more detail in Chapter 9.

In summary, the RTI model is based on the principles that (a) there are specific instructional practices (identified in scientific research) linked to academic success that should guide instruction for all children, (b) it is easier and better to prevent academic failure in contrast to waiting until a child experiences academic failure, (c) all children should receive Tier 1 instruction at the classroom level, and (d) most children will learn with high-quality Tier 1 instruction.

However, some children—even with high-quality classroom instruction—will fall behind. A second important component of RTI is that children who do not develop at the Tier 1 level are provided more intensive instruction at the Tier 2 level. Tier 2 instruction is typically provided several times a week in small groups; an SLP, teacher, teacher assistant, or tutor provides the instruction (Ehren, Montgomery, Rudebusch, & Whitmire, 2006; Haager, Klingner, & Vaughn, 2007).

In the RTI model, children's skill development is used as an indicator for more intense levels of instruction. Therefore, a child failing to progress with high-quality classroom instruction alone will be moved to Tier 2 where they will receive more explicit and intense exposure to the targeted skill. Explicit instruction is more adult-directed and provides more opportunities for focused skill repetition. For example, a Tier 2 intervention for preschoolers may focus on a particular skill, such as alphabet letter recognition. For example, during a Tier 2 small-group intervention, the adult may read a storybook and provide multiple opportunities for children to look for, point to, and name letters during the shared book reading.

Some children may continue to struggle, even with Tier 2 small-group intervention. A student who does not show adequate skill development in Tier 2 is referred for Tier 3 instruction. Children referred for Tier 3 instruction (i.e., highly specialized and focused intervention) often include students with more severe levels of disability (i.e., children with cognitive impairments, children with significant language disabilities). An example of a Tier 3 approach for an older school-age student may include training the student to use specific strategies prior to reading to improve his or her comprehension. The student may be trained to list specific key words to look for during the reading process. At the Tier 3 level, the practitioner helps the student implement the comprehension strategy during classroom reading assignments and monitors the student's successful use of the new strategy. Figure 3.4 shows the relationship between Tiers 1, 2, and 3.

To reiterate the fundamental principle of RTI, a student's response to instruction is used as the criteria for placement in Tier 1, 2, or 3. If a student improves after Tier 2 or Tier 3 intervention, he or she moves back down to the Tier 1 level. This approach varies from a discrepancy criterion model. Prior to implementation of the response to intervention (RTI) model, the **discrepancy criterion model** was used to qualify children as having a learning disability. The discrepancy model required that a child demonstrate a significant difference between IQ (i.e., overall cognitive ability) and school achievement in order to qualify for educational services. Use of the discrepancy model often resulted in delaying intervention until the student's achievement had fallen significantly below his or her peers.

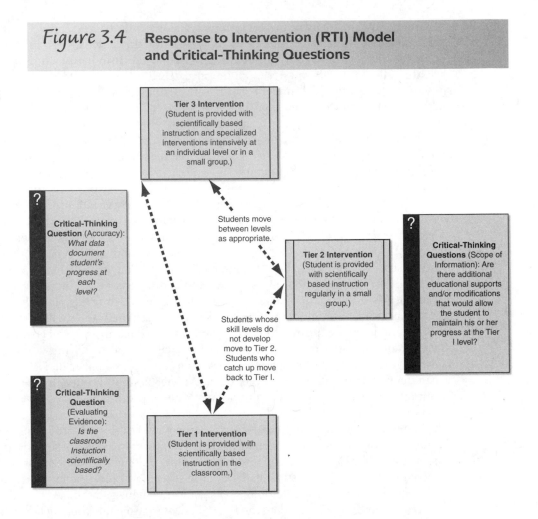

Figure 3.4 **Response to Intervention (RTI) Model and Critical-Thinking Questions**

Tier 3 Intervention
(Student is provided with scientifically based instruction and specialized interventions intensively at an individual level or in a small group.)

? **Critical-Thinking Question** (Accuracy): *What data document student's progress at each level?*

Students move between levels as appropriate.

Tier 2 Intervention
(Student is provided with scientifically based instruction regularly in a small group.)

? **Critical-Thinking Questions** (Scope of Information): Are there additional educational supports and/or modifications that would allow the student to maintain his or her progress at the Tier I level?

Students whose skill levels do not develop move to Tier 2. Students who catch up move back to Tier I.

? **Critical-Thinking Question** (Evaluating Evidence): *Is the classroom Instuction scientifically based?*

Tier 1 Intervention
(Student is provided with scientifically based instruction in the classroom.)

Educationally, there are clear limitations for the discrepancy criterion model. Once a child has fallen behind in school, it is difficult to help a child catch up. The common pattern of reading failure typifies this problem. The child who struggles to read reads less often, and often dislikes reading. With less practice, the struggling reader has less exposure to new vocabulary causing the poor reader to fall farther behind. Skilled readers, in contrast, enjoy reading, tackle increasingly difficult texts, and become more and more proficient (Torgesen et al., 2001). To counteract the downward spiral of reading disability, the RTI model advocates high-quality instruction for children at the classroom level, with immediate and increasingly intensive levels of instruction for students who do not catch up. More intense intervention begins as soon as a lack of progress is noted; the child does not have to qualify for special education before receiving additional help. Consequently, RTI is viewed as a preventative approach to academic failure.

PREVENTION

Prevention is an important concept for SLPs and special educators. Prevention also is a fundamental concept embedded within the RTI model. A **preventative approach** provides instruction, or modifies an individual's environment, before a deficit is observed. Preventative approaches reduce the likelihood that a deficit will occur. When SLP was a new profession, in the 1940's, practitioners focused on identifying and treating children with already-existing communication disorders. However, in recent years, the profession has expanded to include a focus on the prevention of communication disorders and academic failure. There are a number of important skills related to prevention; to prevent communication disorder, SLPs and special educators should (ASHA, 1991):

- Use prevention terminology appropriately (see Focus 3.2 for definitions).
- Understand conditions that place individuals at risk for various communication disorders.

FOCUS 3.2 *Learning More*

Terminology for Prevention of Communication Disorders

Effective prevention of language disorders requires the appropriate use of prevention terminology. Below I provide prevention definitions and explain how these terms are applied throughout this text. For more information about prevention in speech-language pathology, access the Internet at www.asha.org/docs/html/RP1991_00211.html

- *At risk:* The potential to develop a disorder based on specific biological, environmental, or behavioral factors. In Chapters 6 and 9, I will discuss risk factors associated with hearing loss and autism.
- *Disability:* An individual's reduced ability to meet the needs of daily living; determined by the severity of the impairment, the person's lifestyle, or the extent to which the individual can compensate. In this text, I discuss how an individual's ecological system can alter an individual's level of disability (see Chapter 8).
- *Handicap:* The social disadvantage that an individual experiences because of an impairment and resulting disability. The degree of handicap depends in part on the attitudes and

biases of those with the disability or those who interact with the individual. For example, I will discuss in Chapter 6 that some deaf adults do not view their hearing loss as a handicap.

- *Impairment:* Any loss or abnormality of psychological, physiological, or anatomical structure or function. In this text you will learn about a number of impairments, including specific language impairments (Chapter 7) and cognitive impairments (Chapter 8).
- *Primary prevention:* The elimination of the onset and development of a communication disorder by altering susceptibility or environment for susceptible persons. Use of Tier 1 instruction in the response to intervention model is an example of primary prevention.
- *Secondary prevention:* The early detection and treatment of communication disorders. Early detection and treatment may lead to the elimination of the disorder or the retardation of the disorder's progress, preventing further complications. Screening is an example of secondary prevention.
- *Tertiary prevention:* The reduction of a disability by attempting to restore effective functioning. I will present a number of intervention approaches in this text as examples of tertiary prevention.

- Understand factors, either biological or environmental, that cause communication disabilities.
- Understand practices and educational strategies that enhance children's communication abilities.
- Identify and intervene as early as possible to prevent serious communication handicaps.

In this book, you begin to learn about prevention approaches by reading about (a) the conditions that place students at risk for language disorders, (b) risk factors for language impairments, (c) effective practices for preventing communication disorders, and (d) intervention approaches appropriate for very young children. Your knowledge in these areas will continue to develop throughout your professional career. As an SLP or special educator, you will ask yourself critical-thinking questions to determine if you (or your school or organization) are implementing an effective prevention program. Critical-thinking questions may include the following:

- Do we have a screening program to identify children at earlier ages?
- Do we provide information to community members or school personnel to help parents and teachers recognize language disorders at an early age?
- Do we provide intervention with very young children, if appropriate?

CASE EXAMPLE: DECISION MAKING DURING ASSESSMENT

Review Case Example 1 at the beginning of this chapter. Tanzia is 7 years old and has a significant impairment that prevents her from interacting socially with her peers. She avoids interactions, does not initiate communication with other adults or children, and plays by herself; she often demonstrates repetitive activities (e.g., spinning a top). She speaks in simple two- to three-word sentences but her sentences often do not relate to the ongoing activity. Before completing an assessment, you ask yourself the critical-thinking question:

- What domains of communication (i.e., form, content, use) are most impaired for Tanzia?

Before you read further, reflect on what you have already learned and try to think of the answer.

After thinking about Tanzia's communication problems, I hope you considered the communication subdomains and remembered that Subdomain 1 (social interaction) is the foundational skill underlying advanced language learning. It is likely you determined that Tanzia has difficulty with this underlying social interaction skill since she has problems in requesting, responding, turn taking, and (perhaps) even eye contact.

Now, let's continue with this critical-thinking exercise. Ask yourself a second question:

- What assessments should I use to understand Tanzia's communication challenges?

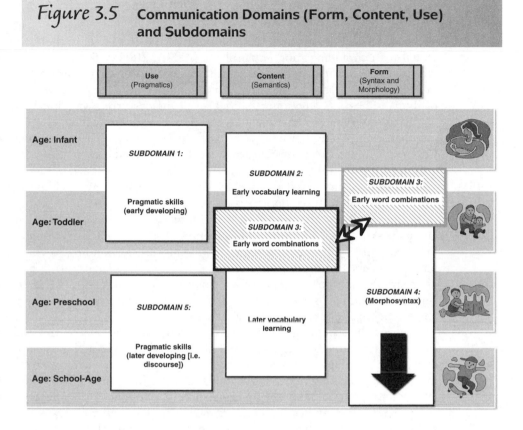

Figure 3.5 **Communication Domains (Form, Content, Use) and Subdomains**

And finally, ask:

- Am I more likely to use norm-referenced or criterion-referenced assessments as part of the assessment protocol?

At this point in your professional training, I do not expect you to name specific tests. Instead, I want you to describe several tests or procedures appropriate for a student like Tanzia. Refer to Figure 3.5 to review the communication subdomains to help you respond to this case example.

Decision Making: Intervention

In this section on decision making and intervention, I outline the general goals of intervention with respect to varying age groups; I then describe how critical-thinking questions help the skilled practitioner relate language theory to language intervention. In the second and third subsections, I describe how public policies and issues of motivation influence decision making.

GOALS OF INTERVENTION: INFANTS, TODDLERS, PRESCHOOLERS, AND SCHOOL-AGE STUDENTS

The goals of speech-language intervention change with respect to the age of the individual with communication impairments (ASHA, 2004a). For infants and toddlers who are at risk for communication impairment, the practitioner concentrates on increasing the caregivers' sensitivity to the infant's needs and teaches caregivers to facilitate preverbal communication (i.e., eye contact, turn taking, imitation).

Early intervention also includes teaching caregivers to facilitate early speech (i.e., babbling, word approximations) and the communication skills associated with Communication Subdomains 2 (early words) and 3 (word combinations). Social interaction, play, and emergent literacy skills (e.g., engaging in joint action routines; interactions using toys and books) also are included as intervention targets at the earliest ages.

Intervention for preschoolers continues to focus on social interaction, play, and early literacy. Now, the practitioner also targets increasing sophisticated receptive language skills (e.g., attention and listening skills; vocabulary development; following directions; understanding sentences and stories; responding to communicative intent of peers and adult partners) and expressive language skills (e.g., using age-appropriate phonology and articulation skills; using a variety of words; formulating simple and complex sentences; telling simple oral narratives; expressing a variety of communicative functions; engaging with peers).

During the school-age years, intervention includes a focus on the student's educational curriculum, future vocational needs, and peer interaction. The practitioner considers the student's knowledge and use of language for listening, speaking, reading, writing, and thinking. Interventions often include an emphasis on phonology and print symbols, complex syntax structures, advanced vocabulary, discourse structures for comprehending and organizing spoken and written texts, pragmatic skills for communicating appropriately in varied situations, and metacognitive and self-regulatory strategies for handling complex language, literacy, and academic demands (ASHA, 2004a).

In summary, the goals of communication intervention at any age include (a) facilitating communication development, (b) changing or eliminating an individual's underlying communication problem, (c) changing specific aspects of the individual's communication function by teaching specific skills, or (d) teaching compensatory techniques to improve the individual's communication functioning (Olswang & Bain, 1991). Throughout the intervention, the skilled practitioner asks the critical-thinking question:

- Is this individual's intervention focusing on goals that reflect abilities consistent with age and communicative needs?

CRITICAL-THINKING QUESTIONS DURING INTERVENTION: CONSIDERING UNDERLYING LANGUAGE THEORY

One important question regarding intervention is motivated by the critical-thinking parameter *evaluating the evidence*. As I described at the beginning of this chapter, evaluating assessment and intervention approaches requires both external and internal evidence. In the next chapter (Chapter 4), I discuss how to evaluate external evidence. Weighing the scientific evidence supporting (or not supporting) a particular approach is an essential component of evidence-based practice. To begin this process, let's consider how a practitioner evaluates an intervention's internal evidence using a critical-thinking question like this one:

- What theoretical approach is represented by the intervention I have chosen?

Different professionals have very different theoretical approaches to language intervention. In Chapter 1, I discussed a number of language theories, including behaviorism, nativism, neural maturation, social interaction, information processing, and the systems-ecological approach. Different intervention approaches draw from different theoretical positions.

As an example, consider possible intervention choices for a student who has difficulties with vocabulary and grammar. If an SLP or special educator believes that social interaction theory is fundamental to language development, the practitioner is likely to use theme-based materials to engage the student in meaningful conversations during intervention. It is unlikely that the practitioner would attempt to remediate the targeted syntax skills by using worksheets or rote drills. On the other hand, a practitioner who believed in behaviorism might use highly controlled interactions and focus on reinforcing specific student responses with a skills-based approach (Ukraintez, 2005).

There are differences of opinion regarding appropriate interventions for children with different communication disorders. For example, some experts propose that interventions based on behaviorism are most appropriate for young children with autism. Other experts argue that children with autism should participate in interventions based on social interaction theory. Some practitioners use a combination of methods (Solomon, Necheles, Ferch, & Bruckman, 2007). When you weigh the appropriateness (or inappropriateness) of a particular intervention, you will first want to consider the following questions:

- Does the intervention I am proposing fit with my beliefs about language development?
- Do parents and teachers understand the underlying principles that frame this intervention?

Your ability to answer these critical-thinking questions will demonstrate the critical-thinking parameter of *evaluating evidence*.

PUBLIC POLICY (IDEA) AND DECISION MAKING

Public policy has increasingly impacted educational interventions in recent years. A landmark federal policy is the **Individuals with Disabilities Education Act** (IDEA); this policy was reauthorized in 2004 and took effect in October 2006. IDEA 2004 ensures that all eligible children with disabilities have a right to a free, appropriate public education (FAPE) in the least restrictive environment (LRE), and that the rights of children and parents are protected. IDEA mandates that schools provide special education for children from birth through age 21 and ensures the effectiveness of these services.

The term *least restrictive environment* is a fundamental concept under IDEA 2004. LRE policy mandates that a child with special educational must receive services within the general education classroom to the greatest degree possible. That is to say, a child with language impairment should only receive services outside the classroom when classroom-based intervention is not in the child's best interests.

Students with disabilities in the following areas are eligible for services under IDEA: hearing impairment, deafness, speech or language impairments, mental retardation, visual impairments, blindness, serious emotional disturbance, orthopedic impairments, autism, traumatic brain injury, other health impairments, specific learning disabilities, deaf-blindness, and multiple disabilities.

Part C of IDEA guarantees services for infants and toddlers (to age 2 years) with disabilities; it is a federal grant program that helps states provide early intervention services for children and families. In order for a state to participate in the program, it must ensure that early intervention will be available to every eligible child and his or her family. Children served under Part C of IDEA have developmental delay in domains including cognitive development, physical development (including vision and hearing), communication development, social or emotional development, and adaptive development (i.e., difficulty performing activities needed for daily living).

For school-age children, IDEA regulations specify that academic failure is not a requirement for receiving special education and related services (i.e., the student does not have to demonstrate a discrepancy between IQ and achievement). Assessment should be broad based and consider educational performance across school environments (i.e., classroom discussions, peer interactions, extracurricular).

Identification of a disability that impairs a student's academic performance results in the development of an **Individualized Education Program** (IEP). An IEP is a plan outlining special education and related services specifically designed to meet the unique educational needs of a student with a disability. Every child who receives special education and related services under IDEA must have an IEP. The IEP has two general purposes: (1) to set reasonable learning goals for the child, and (2) to state the services that the school will provide for the child. Parents, general education teachers, school administration, and members of the special education team (including the SLP) all participate and agree to the final plan during the IEP process.

Critical-thinking questions considered during the IEP process include:

- To the maximum extent possible, does this IEP guarantee that the student with a disability is educated with children who are nondisabled?
- For students who cannot be educated solely in the general education classroom, is there a continuum of alternative placements (i.e., from less restrictive [as in receiving supplementary services part of the day] to more restrictive [as in a self-contained classroom for children with disabilities])?

Two final concepts are motivated by IDEA and the critical-thinking questions listed above: inclusion and differential instruction. The first term, inclusion, requires children to be educated in the least restrictive environment. Inclusion means that children with disabilities are educated in the same context as nondisabled peers. Inclusion is different from **mainstreaming,** which is when students with disabilities spend a portion of their school day in the general education program and a portion in a separate special education program. The term *inclusion* is the preferred term; professionals avoid the use of the older term, *mainstreaming* (Idol, 2006).

Research demonstrates children in inclusive preschool classrooms have improved developmental abilities, auditory comprehension, expressive language, and social skills when compared to their language-delayed peers in segregated classes (Rafferty, Piscitelli, & Boettcher, 2003). Inclusive education also benefits older school-age students. Idol (2006) studied elementary and secondary schools and reported that inclusion benefited students with special educational needs. Further, data demonstrated that inclusion did not negatively impact educational outcomes for students developing typically—-this is a concern voiced by critics of IDEA.

The second term is *differentiated instruction.* When children are in inclusive classrooms, teachers must use **differentiated instruction** to determine what children will learn, how they will learn it, and how students can express what they have learned (Tomlinson, 2003). Differentiated instruction may include altering the content of what is taught, altering how the content is taught, or altering a student's curriculum goal (i.e., reducing task demands). Differentiated instruction increases the likelihood that each student will learn as much as possible, as efficiently as possible. For example, when altering content, the practitioner may decide to reduce the number of pages a student is required to read to complete an assignment. If the practitioner decides to alter how the student is instructed, the student may be provided simultaneous auditory and written instruction instead of auditory-only instruction.

Critical-thinking questions motivated by the principle of differentiated instruction include:

- Will this student benefit if he or she is taught to use a self-management skill (i.e., checking work, planning prior to beginning the task) to facilitate the curriculum goal?
- Will this student benefit by being trained to use reflective questions prior to and during the curriculum task?
- Would simplifying the task (e.g., reducing the number of spelling words for a spelling assignment) be an appropriate curriculum modification?
- Should this student focus on a foundational communication goal during a higher-level classroom activity (e.g., the student [who has a significant language impairment] practices initiating conversation during a small-group science activity)?

The skilled SLP or special educator helps teachers develop a range of differentiated instructional strategies. By using differentiated instruction, children with special educational needs remain in inclusive classrooms but receive the specialized intervention required by their IEP.

STUDENT MOTIVATION AND DECISION MAKING

When you are a skilled practitioner working with a student with communication impairment, you are likely to ask the question:

- Is this intervention motivating for the student?

A student's level of motivation profoundly impacts academic achievement (McTigue, Beckman, & Kaderavek, 2007). Students who are motivated to learn will spend more time on the task and will seek out opportunities to practice the targeted skill (Lepola, Salonen, & Vauras, 2000). Moreover, students who exhibit high task motivation internalize the targeted skills resulting in more permanent behavior change (Edmunds & Bauserman, 2006). The issue of student motivation is prompted by the critical-thinking parameter *change and adaptability*. If a student is not motivated during intervention, the practitioner must flexibly adapt the intervention to improve motivation and improve the student's opportunity for a good outcome.

Increasingly, trends in special education emphasize choosing interventions to impact an individual's daily activities and classroom achievement (Whitmire, 2002). This movement has stemmed from IDEA requirements, along with current research demonstrating the relationships between language skills and academic ability (Catts & Kahmi, 2005). Student motivation is enhanced when the practitioner emphasizes the positive effects of the intervention in everyday events. As an example, imagine that you are working with a high-functioning student with social communication impairment who has difficulty with peer interactions. As a skilled practitioner, you explain and give examples to the student to demonstrate how improved discourse skills will positively affect peer relationships. Your goal is to enhance the student's understanding of how the targeted skills will be used in daily life to increase motivation and use of the intervention strategies.

BACKWARD DESIGN

Considering the parameter, *change and adaptation,* motivates the practitioner to focus on communication behaviors most likely to impact an individual's everyday interactions. One way to achieve this goal is to begin intervention with the end in mind (Ehren, 2007). This approach is called backward design. **Backward design** advocates that the practitioner first consider the desired results for a particular student. Then, after clearly outlining the ultimate goal, the practitioner identifies interventions needed to equip students to achieve the goal (Wiggins & McTighe, 1998). Using backward design prompts several critical-thinking questions, such as:

- What does the student need to understand?
- What does the student need to do that he or she cannot do now?
- What interventions and approaches will promote understanding, interest, and competency in the targeted area?

The issue of backward design is relevant whether the individual is a preschooler, a school-age child, or an older student preparing for a career. The skilled SLP or special educator continually considers the individual's environment by asking the overarching question: Will this intervention make a real difference in the individual's daily life?

CASE EXAMPLE: DECISION MAKING IN INTERVENTION

Consider the case of Mrs. Shultz, the preschool teacher (Case Example 2 at the beginning of this chapter). You are concerned about what you see in the classroom because you are thinking about the critical-thinking parameter of *evaluating evidence*. You are aware that having preschoolers sit for extended periods doing worksheets is not a recommended educational practice. You know the importance of early literacy skill building, but ask yourself the following question:

- What language theory should guide early language/literacy intervention for preschool children?

Your knowledge of language theory prompts you to reflect on social interaction theory; social interaction theory suggests that young children learn best when they are actively engaged with others. Because of your training, you know that young children need to explore and "think, do, and talk" to learn early literacy skills.

Reflect on how you might share your critical-thinking questions with Mrs. Shultz. Do you have any suggestions for changing how preschoolers could learn alphabet letters or name-writing within a preschool classroom with a more active learning approach? (You will learn more about how to foster early literacy skills in Chapter 9.) Use the example questions in Table 3.2 to guide your critical thinking. An example of a preschool literacy activity incorporated within an engaging art activity is illustrated in Figure 3.6.

Figure 3.6 **Children Incorporate Emergent Writing into an Engaging Art Activity**

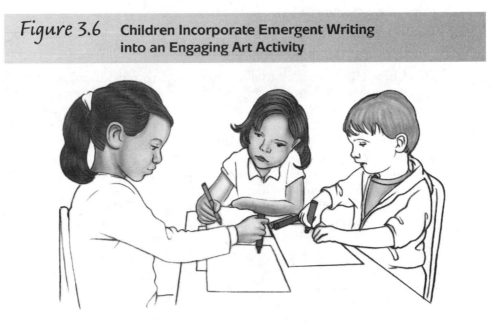

Decision Making: Environment

Undoubtedly, a child's environment makes a difference in language development. A child's exposure to high-quality language at home results in significantly higher child language output and vocabulary development (Hart & Risley, 1995). In the preschool environment, rich and frequent high-level teacher language results in improved academic gains for children (Wasik, Bond, & Hindman, 2006). Peers also influence language development; preschoolers in classrooms with higher peer language levels demonstrate improved receptive and expressive language development (Mashburn, Justice, Downer, & Pianta, 2009). During the school years, opportunities for peer socialization and interaction with a caring, supportive adult promote positive language outcomes for students with language impairment (Gillam et al., 2008). Finally, children who come from culturally or linguistically different homes are likely to have differences in language use. A skilled practitioner considers the impact of environment and considers *scope of information.* Questions include:

- Have I considered the communication impairment from the perspective of the child and/or the child's family?
- Am I considering all communications environments and environmental influences on language development?
- Do I understand the family discourse patterns between adults and children (and children with other children) for individuals from a specific culture?

In this subsection, I highlight two issues to help you more carefully consider communication environments: routines-based interviewing and classroom contexts for language learning. I will discuss more about the impact of culture on language learning in Chapter 11.

ROUTINES-BASED INTERVIEWS

In Chapter 1, you were introduced to the social-ecological approach, also referred to as family systems theory. This approach recognizes that children are part of a multilayered system. Family systems may be very nurturing or may be dysfunctional. Some teachers may be highly sensitive to the needs of a particular child. In contrast, other teachers may need a great deal of support to provide individualized instruction. When using an ecological approach, and in order to demonstrate the critical-thinking parameter *accuracy and scope of information,* skilled practitioners often use a routines-based interview (McWilliam & Clingenpeel, 2003).

The practitioner uses the **routines-based interview** (RBI) to pose questions to family members to (a) assess a child's developmental and communication status, (b) gain information about day-to-day life, and (c) tune in to a family's feelings about their child. The goal is to gather a sense of the family's most important concerns in order to prioritize intervention goals. The word **routine** is used to describe times of day and/or familiar activities such as eating, bathing, bedtime, hanging out, going to the store, and traveling in the car.

An introductory question to initiate the routines-based interview often starts with the question:

- What does a typical day look like for your family?

This question is used to determine those routines that are most important for the family. The interviewer also asks:

- What activities does your family enjoy for fun?
- What does your family do on holidays?
- What do you do on weekends?

After identifying four to six of the most important routines, the interviewer then asks the following questions about each of the important routines:

- What does everyone do during this routine?
- What does your child do?
- Is the child highly engaged (e.g., eager, high attention) or poorly engaged (e.g., "wandering," low attention) to the routine? (See Focus 3.3 for more information on engagement.)
- What does the child do independently as part of this routine?
- How does the child communicate during this routine?
- How satisfied are you with your child's interaction and participation during this routine?

Gathering routines-based information helps the practitioner target meaningful outcomes that build on a family's strengths. For example, imagine that you have a child, Tabitha, on your caseload. Tabitha is 14 and is hearing impaired; she wears hearing aids and communicates verbally, although her language is delayed. She is struggling in school and her reading skills are below average. After interviewing the family, you find that after dinner is a time when family members typically spend time together. You ask if reading chapter books (e.g., the *Harry Potter* series) together with Tabitha would be an enjoyable shared family event. The parents are enthusiastic about taking turns reading aloud. At first, Tabitha is reluctant, but eventually is willing to read aloud with her parents' support. Eventually, she rereads the books independently because she is familiar with the vocabulary. In this example, you used the routines-based interview to integrate a language/literacy goal into a family's daily schedule.

Routines-based questions also are used to target the most important opportunities for intervention during child care. Frequently occurring child care routines include entering the classroom at the beginning of the day, free play, center time, meal time, nap time, outdoor play, transitions (e.g., moving from one activity to another), and going to the bathroom. The practitioner asks the child care provider routines-based questions (e.g., *What does the child do when it is time to change activities?*) and uses classroom observations to clarify the child's participation and engagement during the child care routines (McWilliam, Scarborough, & Kim, 2003). Using routines-based interviewing focuses the practitioner on the parameter *accuracy and scope of information.*

During routines-based interviewing, the practitioner also considers the critical-thinking parameter *change and adaptability*. This parameter reminds the practitioner to consider issues of child motivation; motivation in young children is sometimes called **engagement.** Engagement refers to a child's duration and complexity of play and quality of interaction with others.

When young children exhibit positive engagement in classroom routines and activities (i.e., when they are highly focused, cooperative, self-directed), students learn more. Further, classrooms where more children are engaged more of the time promote positive academic achievement (Powell, Burchinal, File, & Kontos, 2008). Consequently, skilled SLPs and educators evaluate child engagement levels to monitor classroom environments and facilitate change if engagement is not high.

Child engagement levels vary from high to low and are typically ranked on a 4-point rating scale. A hierarchy of the levels of engagement and the scoring system used to rate child engagement levels is detailed in Focus 3.3. A child can be highly

FOCUS 3.3 *Clinical Skill Building*

McWilliam and de Kruif (1998) developed a hierarchy to code preschool children's level of engagement during classroom routines (e.g, circle time, center activity, mealtimes). The following scale has been adapted (McWilliam & de Kruif, 1998; McWilliam, Scarborough, Kim, 2003).

Child Level of Engagement

4. *High engagement:* (a) Child demonstrates problem solving and challenge, often indicated by a failed first attempt. The child either changes strategies or uses the same strategy again to solve the problem or reach a goal. (b) Child uses language, pretend play, drawings, etc. that allow him or her to reflect on the past, talk about the future, and construct new forms of expression through combinations of different symbols and signs.
3. *Moderate-high engagement:* (a) Child manipulates objects to create, make, or build something. He or she puts objects together in some type of spatial form, but not just handling an

object or banging blocks together; the child includes some indication of intentionality. (b) The child demonstrates differentiated behavior that demonstrates adaptation to environmental demands and expectations. This level includes active interaction with the environment, including typical play.
2. *Moderate-low engagement:* Child demonstrates attention to the activity by looking at an object or person(s); attention must be sustained for at least three seconds. The child evidences engagement at this level when he or she is observed to demonstrate a serious facial expression and a quieting of motor activity.
1. *Low engagement:* (a) Child demonstrates undifferentiated behavior; he or she interacts with the environment without differentiating behavior (i.e., performs low-level actions in repetitive manner). (b) Child demonstrates non-engaged behavior; e.g., staring blankly, wandering aimlessly, crying, whining, aggressive or destructive acts, rule-breaking behavior (i.e., throwing or kicking toys).

engaged in some activities (e.g., free play) but demonstrate low engagement during more structured activities. The practitioner uses engagement ratings to help the teacher modify instructional practices to increase the child's engagement across the school day. Combining family and child care provider information, in addition to using direct observation of child levels of engagement, demonstrates the practitioner's commitment to critical-thinking parameters.

CLASSROOM CONTEXTS FOR REMEDIATION

Considering *scope of information* motivates the practitioner to consider the location of school-based interventions. In **pullout models** of service delivery, the special educator or SLP works with an individual or a small group of children in an area outside of the classroom (McGinty & Justice, 2006). In contrast, when a practitioner provides intervention using a **classroom-based approach** to service delivery, he or she works with a student in the classroom. In a classroom-based approach, the curriculum materials or ongoing classroom activities typically are the stimulus for communication. Language intervention is embedded within the child's familiar activities and incorporates the child's teachers and peers.

Pullout intervention and classroom-based intervention represent two different service delivery models. A **service delivery model** refers to an intervention protocol aimed at achieving a particular educational goal. The service delivery model includes the personnel, materials, specific intervention procedure, the schedule for provision of services, settings in which intervention services will be delivered, and the direct or indirect roles of the practitioner as he or she provides language intervention to students with language impairments (Cirrin & Penner, 1995).

Despite IDEA's focus on classroom-based interventions as the optimal model of service delivery, most practitioners continue to provide school-based services using a pullout model of therapy. Unfortunately, the frequent use of pullout intervention occurs even though research and best practice supports the use of classroom-based intervention (ASHA, 2002).

There are several reasons for the limited use of classroom-based approaches with school-age students. First, many school-based SLPs have high caseloads; a high caseload reduces planning time and limits the time needed to complete paperwork and collaborate with teachers (Chiang & Rylance, 2000). Second, many SLPs currently working in schools were not trained to use curriculum-based assessment and intervention. Despite the challenges, the American Speech-Language-Hearing Association continues to advocate the use of classroom-based intervention approaches with school-age students (ASHA, 2002).

Young children also benefit from a classroom-based model of service delivery. Inclusive, classroom-based service delivery is advantageous for young children with language disorders because the practitioner can focus on enhancing the preschooler's communication within classroom routines. During conversational routines, the child practices his new communication behaviors with his typical peers (Wilcox, Kouri, & Caswell, 1991).

Direct versus Indirect Classroom-Based Intervention.   The classroom-based service delivery model can be implemented in several ways; the approaches are typically categorized into indirect and direct approaches (McGinty & Justice, 2006). In the **indirect service classroom-based approach,** the SLP or special educator serves as a consultant to the general education teacher. The practitioner provides expert guidance so that the teacher can adjust instructional methods to meet a child's special needs. In the **direct service classroom-based approach,** the practitioner (a) collaborates with the teacher using a team-teaching method or (b) the teacher and SLP take turns providing specific lessons to the entire class (McGinty & Justice, 2006; Meyer, 1997). Often practitioners use a combination of direct and indirect methods as part of the classroom-based approach.

Skilled practitioners ask themselves critical-thinking questions to evaluate their level of classroom-based service delivery approaches. Questions include:

- Am I serving as a "coach" to the teacher?
- If not, how I can I increase my support to facilitate differentiated instruction for the child with language impairment?

The implementation of classroom-based approaches requires that the practitioner coach other adults (Dinnebeil, Pretti-Frontczak, & McInerney, 2008). Coaching helps the classroom teacher acquire intervention skills to help children meet IEP goals and objectives.

When the practitioner coaches another adult, he or she (a) models specific strategies that can be used in the classroom to increase communication, (b) demonstrates how the approach can be implemented in the classroom, (c) observes the teacher using the strategy, and (d) provides feedback and reinforcement to the teacher in his or her implementation of the targeted strategy (Showers & Joyce, 1996). The goal of high-quality classroom intervention is to help teachers embed differentiated instruction throughout the school day in keeping with the child's level of ability. For example, the classroom teacher is trained to prompt question-asking during snack time or naming during outdoor play. An embedded intervention for an older student may include reminding a student to use a series of prompts (posted on the student's desk) to organize a writing assignment.

Embedded learning opportunities take place as part of children's contextualized interactions as they occur in the classroom. In an embedded approach, the adult is seen as a facilitator of a child's communication (Justice & Kaderavek, 2004). When teachers—supported by the SLP or special educator—provide instruction across classroom activities and routines, children have learning opportunities that match everyday communication demands. This match facilitates generalization. **Generalization** refers to the ability of an individual to take a learned skill and apply it in a novel situation (Kahmi, 1988). Embedded instruction also insures that instruction is provided when children are highly involved in an interesting activity; this increases children's engagement and motivation.

The concepts of embedded learning and classroom-based instruction lead the practitioner to consider the positive effects of distributed practice. **Distributed practice** refers to providing children with opportunities to practice a skill frequently throughout the day. Distributed practice contrasts with **massed practice** where skill training is massed into less-frequent and longer sessions. Experts suggest that distributed practice promotes learning (Cepeda, Pashler, Vul, Wixted, & Rohrer, 2006).

CASE EXAMPLE: DECISION MAKING AND ENVIRONMENT

In Case Example 3, you are meeting Jahara and her family for a family interview. You remember to consider issues related to accuracy and scope of information (i.e., having enough information to help make decisions) and change and adaptability (i.e., making a real difference in an individual's life). You decide to use the principle of backward design to focus on the family's perceptions for Jahara's ultimate communication goals. You also want to carefully consider Jahara's communication environments. You ask the family the following question:

- What are your hopes and wishes for Jahara in the next 5 to 10 years?

You discover that Jahara will be entering a vocational training program and she hopes to work in a hospital. She will be trained to work in the hospital laundry. This is likely to be her long-term employment setting. With more questioning and assessment, you find that Jahara communicates in simple sentences but is understandable about 50% of the time to unfamiliar listeners (i.e., her speech is poorly articulated and she often mumbles). Jahara is motivated and excited to begin her job training.

Now, after learning this information, ask yourself some critical-thinking questions. Look back at Table 3.1 for possible questions. What language domains do you feel should be targeted in intervention? How does Jahara's future work environment and motivation to succeed affect her intervention program? Use this opportunity to improve your critical decision-making skills.

Decision Making: Progress Monitoring and Dismissal

The skilled practitioner maintains data to continuously monitor the changes in a child's language abilities. Data document specific child outcomes and also reflect the type and frequency of intervention. Both IDEA policy and the response to intervention model require frequent progress monitoring and the use of child response data to make educational decisions (Ehren, Montgomery, Rudebusch, & Whitmire, 2006). Progress monitoring reflects the critical-thinking parameters of *evaluating evidence* and *accuracy and scope of information.*

Deciding when a child or student should be dismissed from treatment is one of the most important decisions in the clinical process. The American Speech-Language Association and IDEA both provide guidelines for dismissal. I discuss these guidelines later in the chapter.

PROGRESS MONITORING

Progress monitoring provides data about the student's communication progress during intervention and guides decisions and programmatic changes (ASHA, 2006). In the RTI model, the SLP or special educator uses progress monitoring to document a student's status in response to evidence-based instruction within the classroom (i.e., Tier 1 level of intervention). The practitioner considers the following question at Tier 1:

- Is there a progress-monitoring system in place to document the student's change as a result of classroom evidence-based instruction?

If the student does not progress, or falls behind expected levels of performance, the progress-monitoring system triggers movement to Tier 2 or 3 where the student receives more frequent, intense, and specialized intervention.

If a student is placed on an Individualized Education Program (IEP), progress monitoring continues to play an important role. IDEA 2004 requires that parents receive regular reports on the student's progress toward annual goals. Progress is measured by comparing changes in a student's speech-language skills to established performance baselines, including curriculum-based language assessments and classroom observations (ASHA, 2004a).

Additional critical-thinking questions that the practitioner may ask include:

- Do I have a progress-monitoring system allowing me to document the student's progress across time?
- Have I shared the progress data with the student (if appropriate) and the student's teachers and parents?
- Is the progress-monitoring system efficient and effective?

There are several methods of data collection appropriate for progress-monitoring systems; they are discussed next.

Data Collection.   Data collection procedures (a) allow the practitioner to track a student's progress from one session to another, (b) document the effectiveness of the intervention approach, and (c) maximize the effectiveness of the intervention (Paul & Cascella, 2006). The practitioner uses record forms and documentation procedures consistent with the underlying theory guiding the intervention. For example, data keeping in an intervention based on a behavioral approach is likely to reflect a student's correct or incorrect attempt when performing a targeted skill. Counting the number of correct attempts reflects quantitative data. **Quantitative data** are numbers expressing quantity, amount, or range of a targeted behavior.

In contrast, a social interaction or systems-based intervention is likely to result in the practitioner using qualitative data to document progress. **Qualitative data** are words or labels describing observed attributes or properties. Qualitative data can be organized into categories and assigned a number. However, with qualitative data the numbers do not have value by themselves; rather, they represent descriptive attributes. A rubric is a commonly used data system for qualitative behavior documentation. A **rubric** is a set of criteria and standards used to assess an individual's performance on a specific task. You can see an example of a rubric used to document a student's ability to tell a story in Table 3.3. In this example, the practitioner rates the storyteller on a

Table 3.3 **Rubric for Evaluating Storytelling**

Category	Ratings (1–4)			
	4	3	2	1
Characters	The main characters are named and clearly described (through words and/or actions). The audience knows and can describe what the characters look like and how they typically behave.	The main characters are named and described (through words and/or actions). The audience has a fairly good idea of what the characters look like.	The main characters are named. The audience knows very little about the main characters.	It is hard to tell who the main characters are.
Pacing	The story is told slowly where the storyteller wants to create suspense and told quickly when there is a lot of action.	The storyteller usually paces the story well, but one or two parts seem to drag or to be rushed.	The storyteller tries to pace the story, but the story seems to drag or be rushed in several places.	The storyteller tells everything at one pace. Does not change the pace to match the story.
Knows the story	The storyteller knows the story well and has obviously practiced telling the story several times. There is no need for notes and the speaker speaks with confidence.	The storyteller knows the story pretty well and has practiced telling the story once or twice. May need notes once or twice, but the speaker is relatively confident.	The storyteller knows some of the story, but did not appear to have practiced. May need notes 3–4 times, and the speaker appears ill-at-ease.	The storyteller could not tell the story without using notes.
Audience contact	Storyteller looks at and tells the story to all members of the audience.	Storyteller looks at and tells the story to a few people in the audience.	Storyteller looks at and tells the story to 1-2 people in the audience.	Storyteller does not look at or try to involve the audience.

Source: RubiStar, 2000–2009. Copyright ALTEC at the University of Kansas. Development of this educational resource was supported, in part, by the U.S. Department of Education award # R302A000015 to ALTEC (Advanced Learning Technologies in Education Consortia) at the University of Kansas. Reprinted with permission.

series of four components of good story telling (e.g., introducing characters, familiarity with the story, pacing, and audience contact). The storyteller is rated on each component with a rating varying from either 4 (very good demonstration of the skill) down to a level of 1 (very poor demonstration of the skill). Chapter 4 provides more details on data-keeping systems.

DISMISSAL FROM THERAPY

A practitioner uses critical-thinking skills to determine when an individual should be dismissed from language intervention. Careful progress monitoring allows dismissal from therapy to be tied to student outcomes and achievement. Experts suggest that the SLP or special educator use the following factors to determine a school-age student's continued eligibility for intervention (Steppling, Quattlebaum, & Brady, 2007):

- Student's age
- Rate of student progress as documented by progress monitoring
- Student's motivation

The practitioner also considers ASHA standards when making decisions about dismissal from intervention. ASHA standards indicate dismissal is appropriate when an individual's communication disorder (a) no longer negatively affects health status or social, emotional, or vocational performance, (b) there is no longer any measurable progress, (c) the individual's goal and objectives have been met, or (d) the individual has obtained the desired level of enhanced communication (ASHA, 2004b). A decision tree illustrating the dismissal decision-making process is presented in Figure 3.7.

Once a student is dismissed from direct therapy, indirect support in the student's classroom may be a viable option. IDEA also has criteria governing dismissal from speech-language school-based services. Under IDEA, dismissal occurs when a student's speech-language impairment no longer negatively affects educational performance.

CASE EXAMPLE: DECISION MAKING IN PROGRESS MONITORING

In Case Example 4, at the beginning of this chapter, you were asked to develop a progress-monitoring tool to document Thomas's morphosyntax skills. Thomas demonstrates frequent errors with verb forms and subordinating conjunctions. You consider issues related to *accuracy* (i.e., keeping accurate data) and *change and adaptability* (i.e., documenting real-life changes) and ask the following critical-thinking questions:

- What method of progress monitoring will best document changes in Thomas's morphosyntax?
- How can I gather data to help Thomas, Thomas's parents, and his teacher see changes in morphosyntax during everyday speaking and writing tasks?

In order to document change in verb forms, you decide to incorporate both quantitative and qualitative data-keeping systems. To keep quantitative data, you decide to have Thomas describe an event for 2 minutes and count the number of correct and

Figure 3.7 **Dismissal Decision Tree**

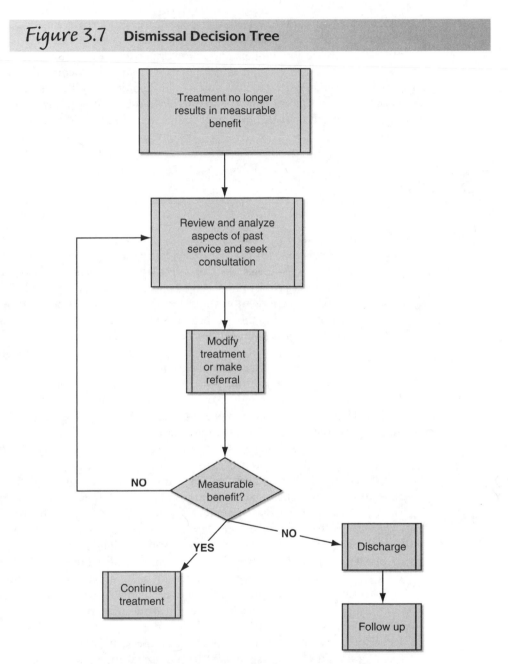

Source: Reprinted with permission from Admission/discharge criteria in speech-language pathology [Guidelines]. Available from www.asha.org/policy. Copyright 2004 by American Speech-Language-Hearing Association. All rights reserved.

incorrect verb forms. As a qualitative procedure, you create a rubric to evaluate changes in the quality of Thomas's written work.

As a clinical skill-building exercise, develop a rubric to capture qualitative differences in Thomas's use of verb forms during his writing assignments. After you develop a rubric for verb use, write out how you would quantitatively and qualitatively evaluate Thomas's use of subordinating conjunctions. Your ability to develop appropriate progress-monitoring tools demonstrates your developing critical-thinking skills.

Summary

- The critical-thinking parameters outlined in this chapter include (a) accuracy and scope of information, (b) evaluating evidence, and (c) change and adaptability. *Accuracy* prompts the decision maker to gather supporting evidence to identify the communication problem and make conclusions; *scope of information* creates critical-thinking questions to motivate careful documentation of an individual's communication reflecting the breadth of communication skills needed in multiple settings and considers cultural differences. *Evaluating evidence* demands that the practitioners evaluate internal and external evidence supporting assessment tools and intervention protocols. The final parameter, *change and adaptability,* demands critical-thinking questions to make sure that the practitioner looks for real change in real-life settings for individuals with communication impairments, assesses student motivation, and is open to professional development and personal change.
- A decision tree is a graphic example of the alternatives in the decision-making process. A decision tree helps the practitioner see the thought process that underlies decision-making process.
- Different approaches and procedures influence decision making. An important new approach is called response to intervention (RTI). In RTI, intervention is based on scientific, research-based evidence using a tiered approach. Intervention is organized with three tiers of intervention. Tier 1 (classroom-based intervention on a daily basis) is provided to all children. For those children who do not improve in response to Tier 1, Tier 2 (small-group or individualized intervention) is provided on a regular, weekly basis. Tier 3 intervention, consisting of intense, individualized intervention, is provided for children who do not progress with Tier 2 intervention. RTI is a preventative approach in that it provides scientifically based intervention for all children at the Tier 1 level to reduce the occurrence of later academic problems. In RTI, a child's ability to respond to intervention indicates whether a child does, or does not, have a significant level of impairment. In traditional assessment, test scores and observational data are used to document the presence of a disability.
- The Individuals with Disabilities Education Act (IDEA) is a law ensuring services to children with disabilities throughout the nation. IDEA governs how states and public agencies provide early intervention, special education, and related services to eligible infants, toddlers, children, and youth with disabilities. IDEA has

prompted SLPs and special educators to provide classroom-based intervention in inclusive classrooms and train teachers to provide differentiated instruction to students with special educational needs.

- When making decisions about the student's environment, the SLP can use the routines-based interview (RBI) to pose questions to family members. RBI is used to (a) assess a child's developmental and communication status, (b) gain information about day-to-day life and family routines, and (c) tune in to a family's feelings about their child. A family routine includes familiar activities such as eating, bathing, bedtime, hanging out, going to the store, or traveling in the car.

- Progress monitoring results in data about the student's communication progress during intervention and guides decisions and programmatic changes. Progress monitoring assists the SLP to develop goals, monitor progress, and formulate dismissal criteria. Progress monitoring is needed in the response to intervention model to move students between the three tiers of intervention; it is a requirement under IDEA policy.

Discussion and In-Class Activities

1. Alone, or in a small group, develop critical-thinking questions to guide assessment and intervention for an individual at Communication Subdomains 1, 2, 3, 4, and 5. As an elaboration to this activity, write critical-thinking questions for an individual with language challenges in the subdomain who is (a) a preschooler and (b) an older school-age student. Note how the questions change in relation to the child's age and environmental expectations (i.e., classroom, vocational, peer).

2. Go to the Internet and research information on the response to intervention model. Two good sites include:

   - www.rti4success.org/
   - www.asha.org/slp/schools/prof-consult/RtoI.htm

   Prepare a brief report of additional information on RTI beyond what is presented in this chapter.

3. Go to the Internet and research information on IDEA. Two good sites include:

   - http://idea.ed.gov/
   - www.asha.org/advocacy/federal/idea/default.htm

   Prepare a brief report of additional information on IDEA beyond what is presented in this chapter.

4. Read more about embedded learning in preschool classrooms and develop embedded learning activities to engage young learners in early literacy learning:

   - Justice, L. M., & Kaderavek, J. N. (2004). Embedded-explicit emergent literacy intervention I: Background and description of approach. *Language, Speech, and Hearing Services in Schools, 35*. 201–211.

- Kaderavek, J. N., & Justice, L. M. (2004). Embedded-explicit emergent literacy intervention II: Goal selection and implementation in the early childhood classroom. *Language, Speech, and Hearing Services in Schools, 35.* 212–228.

5. Develop a rubric to document (a) a preschooler's topic initiation and maintenance in the preschool classroom, (b) the quality of an oral presentation in front of the class for a fourth-grade student, or (c) social interaction for an older school-age student with peers. An Internet resource is http://rubistar.4teachers.org/index.php

Chapter 3 Case Studies

1. Cameron is 4 years old and has autism. His parents ask you if they should enroll him in an intensive behavioral communication intervention. Cameron will be receiving one-on-one intervention learning (at the initial level) to point to pictures and follow one-step commands. He will receive 3 to 4 hours of intervention per day. Describe some of the points you want to consider when you talk to them. Base your discussion on internal evidence. In other words, give them background on the different theoretical approaches that can be used with children with autism (i.e., behavioral versus social interaction theory).
   a. List some critical-thinking questions that help you clarify this situation.
   b. Research information about interventions for children with autism at www.autismspeaks.org.
   c. Role-play a conversation in which you explain the theories that underlie each approach to Cameron's parents.
2. Alana is 3 years old and is in a preschool classroom. She has a language delay; she communicates with one-word utterances. Describe some classroom routines that may be appropriate opportunities to facilitate Alana's verbal communication.

Principles of Intervention

Chapter Overview Questions

1. What does the interventionist consider when choosing stimuli to use in intervention? What techniques are used to elicit responses? What factors influence reinforcement?

2. Describe five different language facilitation techniques. How are they related to social interaction theory? How are they used within language intervention sessions?

3. How does the interventionist use the assertive-responsive scheme and the continuum of naturalness for intervention planning?

4. What are intervention techniques related to issues of a child's language form, content, and use? Give examples.

5. What differentiates Level I, Level II, Level III, and Level IV research in evidence-based practice (EBP)? How does an interventionist use EBP to guide intervention?

6. What are the basic components of an intervention goal?

7. What are two different techniques for maintaining intervention data?

In this chapter, and throughout this book, my goal is to provide you with a toolbox of theoretical principles, developmental guidelines, and underlying state-of-the-art practices to guide your clinical work as a speech-language pathologist (SLP) or language specialist. This chapter focuses on tools and techniques you will use during language intervention. To this end, I first review basic elements in the section below called The Intervention Toolbox: Part I. This section provides information with regard to (a) specific intervention techniques and linkages between techniques and underlying theories, (b) intervention techniques as they relate to the language domains of form, content, and use, and (c) a discussion of the influence of evidence-based practice (EBP) on decision making in language intervention. In the section called The Intervention Toolbox: Part II, I provide information on structuring and implementing intervention.

The Intervention Toolbox Part I: Theories, Domains, and Evaluation of Intervention Research

INTERVENTION TECHNIQUES AND THEIR RELATIONSHIP TO LANGUAGE THEORY

A skilled professional incorporates EBP to make intervention decisions. I describe below how professionals evaluate scientific evidence to identify high-quality interventions. Scientific evidence is called **external evidence;** it documents the successful or unsuccessful implementation of a particular approach within published research (Dollagen, 2007).

Professionals also consider **internal evidence** as part of EBP. Internal evidence includes (a) client and clinician issues and (b) considering why a particular approach might be expected to work. The *why* is answered by understanding the theory underlying a proposed intervention (Ratner, 2006). Review Chapter 3 for clinical questions related to evaluating internal evidence. In the section below, I highlight connections between frequently used intervention techniques and theoretical perspectives.

Intervention Techniques: Influences from Behavioral Theory.   In Chapter 1, I discussed several concepts based on behavioral theory: reinforcement, behavioral extinction, punishment, and chaining. In the section below, I highlight additional intervention concepts related to behavioral theory. Specifically I discuss information to guide (a) selection of stimuli used to elicit target behaviors, (b) techniques to elicit communication, and (c) reinforcement used during interventions.

Choosing Stimuli for Intervention.   In keeping with the behavioral model, the professional carefully considers and defines aspects of the intervention eliciting the target behavior. Stimuli are either nonlinguistic or linguistic. Examples of nonlinguistic stimuli include showing a picture to elicit naming, making eye contact, or touching the child to prompt a pointing response. Linguistic events include calling the child's name, asking a *wh*-question, or initiating a conversation.

Choosing the right stimulus type and context is an important component of effective interventions. For example, young children learn more easily when they are engaged with an activity (McWilliam & Casey, 2007). Consequently, it makes sense to use objects as compared to pictures when teaching words to very young children or children with significant levels of delay. Object use also allows the object name (e.g., *ball*) to be paired with actions (e.g., *throw, catch, roll)*. When a child is learning to use verbs and prepositions (e.g., *in, on, under*), the ongoing activity makes word meaning more transparent (Gentner, 2006).

Interventionists often use pictures to elicit language when they work with older children. Usually, by age 2, children developing typically can learn new vocabulary by looking at pictures and transferring newly learned vocabulary to the real world (Ganea, Bloom-Pickard, & DeLoache, 2008). For children at early levels of language learning, realistic photographs promote more word learning as compared to illustrations (Ganea et al., 2008). Shared storybook reading is a frequently used and effective stimulus for language intervention; the book's illustrations connect children to the written text. Importantly, incorporating storybook reading into interventions not only facilitates a child's vocabulary, morphological, and syntax abilities, but also fosters children's emergent literacy skills (Kaderavek & Justice, 2002).

SLPs and educators increasingly use computers to deliver stimuli during language interventions. However, skilled professionals carefully consider EBP when choosing a computer-based intervention. In a recent study, researchers compared computer-based morphosyntax interventions with comparable SLP-administered interventions. Specifically, adult-delivered intervention using imitation, modeling, and elicited production was more effective with a group of school-aged students compared to a computer-delivered approach (Cirrin & Gillam, 2008). In another example, Bishop, Adams, and Rosen (2006) reported that computerized intervention treatments using slowed speech or modified speech input did not produce better results than regular school services.

Although computers do not replace adult-provided intervention, professionals use computers effectively in specific contexts. Cochran and Masterson (1995) suggested that computer games provide an engaging topic of conversation for many school-age students. Some computer programs allow the user to create and illustrate stories, create a greeting card, or use problem-solving strategies (e.g., SimCity). In this case, software programs serve as a context for discourse between the adult and individual with language impairment. The computer stimuli function much like the board games or arts-and-crafts activities used traditionally in language interventions (Paul, 2007). I provide examples of computer software programs used in language intervention in Table 4.1.

Computers also provide practice opportunities for school-age students who struggle to develop topics for papers, organize writing assignments, or edit and revise written work. In this case, adults train students to use brainstorming software (such as Inspiration) to improve prewriting skills and word processing programs to facilitate editing and writing revisions.

Eliciting Responses.   SLPs and educators use a variety of intervention techniques to elicit children's responses. I discuss the following terms and concepts: prompting, shaping, and modifying contexts.

Prompts are instructions or stimuli used to ensure a child responds correctly. Generally, the adult uses combinations of multiple prompts at early stages of learning and then reduces the number of prompts as the child develops skill. As an example, imagine you are the interventionist responsible for the communication program for a 3-year-old minimally verbal child, Isaac. Isaac uses some gestures and a few words to communicate in his preschool class. After "morning circle," the children typically

Table 4.1   Examples of Software Programs Used in Language Intervention

Software	Description
Tiger's Tale (Laureate Learning Systems)	Children talk for an animated character who has "lost his voice." Voices are recorded to create a movie; students watch their movies and hear themselves speaking.
Itchy's Alphabet (ABB Creations Ltd.)	A phonics program designed to teach children alphabet skills; focuses on letter sounds and lowercase letter formations.
Preschool Playtime Volumes 1 & 2 (Say It Right™)	Children view videos in which they see children taking turns, sharing, requesting, cooperating, and shifting activities through real-life social situations like a day at the park or going on a play date. The child is asked to identify, produce, and explain social situations.
Exploring Verbs (Laureate Learning Systems)	Provides stimuli to elicit 50 early developing verbs; students select verbs while computer illustrates the actions.
Irregular Verb Videos (Say It Right™)	Students view video clips and see an action; they are prompted to use the correct verb form. Recording function allows children to hear their own voice using the correct verb tense.

request to move to a preferred activity (e.g., art table, dramatic play, sand table, book center). Along with Isaac's preschool teacher, you develop a sequence of prompts to facilitate Isaac's verbal productions. First, the teacher shows Isaac a series of pictures visually demonstrating activity choices (pictures = prompt #1); the teacher then asks, "*What do you want to do today, Isaac?*" (teacher request = prompt #2). If Isaac does not respond, the teacher touches Isaac's arm and says, "*Show me what you want to do today*" (tactile = prompt # 3). If needed, the teacher uses a hand-over-hand method to help Isaac point to his favorite activity—the sand table (physical support = prompt #4). The teacher then says, "*Isaac, say 'sand table'*" (imitation = prompt #5). Gradually, Isaac learns to respond to the teacher's question, "*What do you want to do today?*" without the use of additional prompts.

Shaping is used to teach increasingly complex behaviors. When using **shaping,** the language trainer facilitates easy, small steps, gradually approximating the goal behavior. Consider the following example: the interventionist is training a nonverbal child to pair motor actions with verbalizations. Specifically, the professional decides to train the word *in* paired with an action (e.g., dropping blocks into a coffee can). At the beginning of the shaping procedure, the adult models and rewards the client as he imitates the motor act of dropping a block into the can. As this behavior emerges, the adult pairs a sound, *uh!,* along with dropping the blocks. Now, the adult shapes the child's behavior by only providing reinforcement when a sound and action are produced together. Eventually, the adult uses the word *in* as she drops the block. Once again she uses shaping; she now reinforces the child only when an approximation of the word *in* is paired with the motor action. Eventually the word and action are transferred to other similar motor activities (e.g., putting trash into a trash can, loading laundry into a basket).

Rewarding Communication Responses.   As I discussed in Chapter 1, reinforcement increases the probability a behavior will occur. There are many decisions to consider regarding how to implement reinforcement during intervention. Professionals choose the most appropriate reinforcement for an individual and modify the reinforcement schedule to facilitate generalization of new behaviors.

When considering reinforcement, professionals prefer to use social reinforcement in contrast to primary reinforcement (e.g., food). Social reinforcement is preferred because it is always available and because responsiveness to social cues is "programmed into our species" and serves as a powerful tool for changing behavior within a social context (Baum, 2005). Just as adults view a smiling baby as highly reinforcing and a crying baby as highly aversive, children have a predisposition to respond to the positive or negative social responses of others. Social reinforcement includes smiling, nonverbal responses, "high fives," or positive sounds and verbalizations (e.g., *Oh! Yea! Good job!* Baum, 2005). When food is used as reinforcement (e.g., for a child with very significant disabilities), the goal is to use it only at the initial stages of intervention, to pair food with social reinforcement, and to fade food reinforcement as quickly as possible (Owens, 2009).

Several intervention techniques are important when an interventionist considers how to generalize a new behavior into other communication contexts. **Fading** is a technique in which adult prompting is reduced with the goal of spontaneous occurrence of child behaviors in daily interactions. Generally at initial stages of intervention, target behaviors are elicited with strong modeling, cuing, and prompting. Eventually, the intensity of the elicitation behaviors is faded. Fading is a part of intervention at all levels, at the initial stages of teaching a behavior through the final stages of generalization. In fact, an interventionist's overall goal is to "fade out of the picture." The real goal of language intervention is to help the child to produce the appropriate communication behavior with complete independence.

Part of fading from the picture is fostering a child's ability to produce the target behavior with less externally provided reinforcement. At first the adult provides frequent reinforcement and feedback; ultimately the goal of intervention is for new behaviors to be used and reinforced via everyday social interactions (Fernald, 2008). At the initial stages of intervention, the adult often uses continuous reinforcement. **Continuous reinforcement** means every correct response is followed by an event increasing the probability the response will be repeated. Once the behavior is established, the adult reinforces the target behavior intermittently. In **intermittent reinforcement,** sometimes called **partial reinforcement,** only some correct responses are followed by the reinforcing event.

Other kinds of feedback also are important. For example, feedback can be used to improve a child's awareness of the targeted behaviors. Consider the following feedback during an intervention session. The intervention goal is to facilitate auxiliary verbs (e.g., *is* and *are*) within a noun phrase + verb phrase sentence. The interventionist chooses this goal because the child omits auxiliary verbs; he says, *"The dog barking outside"* instead of *"The dog is barking outside."* The child also does not use auxiliary verbs when asking questions; he says, *"Dog barking?"* instead of using an interrogative reversal, *"Is the dog barking?"*). The adult and child are playing with a farm set.

> **Adult:** *"The pig <u>is eating</u> his dinner. <u>Is</u> the pig <u>eating</u> his dinner? Yes, the pig <u>is eating</u> his food!"* (SLP makes eating noises.)
>
> **Child:** *"Pig is eating!"*
>
> **Adult:** *"Yes, the pig is eating! I liked how you used the special <u>is</u> word. You said, 'The pig <u>is</u> eating!'"*

In this example, the adult provides feedback increasing the child's awareness of the goal behavior. Explicit feedback is designed to highlight the specific behavior needed to correctly complete the task. Explicit feedback increases the likelihood a target behavior will occur; this is true whether the professional is training parents (e.g., *"When you were talking to Samuel you slowed down your speech rate, this is very helpful!"*), or when interacting with the child directly (Speights Roberts, Tingstrom, Olmi, & Bellipanni, 2008).

In the example above, the adult used another effective therapeutic method, **sentence recasts.** Sentence recasts are similar to expansions (definition provided below), except in sentence recasts the language facilitator changes the sentence modality (e.g., changes the sentence from a statement to a question). In this example, the adult produced the auxiliary verb during a statement (*"The pig is eating"*) and also produced the sentence as an interrogative reversal (*"Is the pig eating?"*).

Intervention Techniques: Influences from Social Interaction Theory.   Social interaction provides the context for, and has the potential to, effect developmental change in children (Schneider & Watkins, 1996). Vygotsky (1978, 1987) maintained that initially a learner completes a task with the support of a more skilled participant, but with repeated opportunities, the learner internalizes underlying concepts and learns to perform the task independently. The social interaction perspective motivates the practitioner to promote children's communication attempts within positive and socially relevant interactions. The practitioner builds on a child's communication bids using modeling and by indicating that the child's efforts are important and accepted (Prizant, Wetherby, & Rydell, 2000).

Below I describe techniques used to facilitate children's language learning within the powerful context of adult–child interactions. Parents and teachers also use these language facilitation techniques when they interact with language learners.

Language Facilitation Techniques.   A child with language impairment (LI) is less likely to engage in conversation than children developing typically (Westby, 2008). Children with LI have reduced vocabulary and are less skilled at producing word combinations to express their experiences. Once they begin to use word combinations, children with LI typically have unsophisticated morphology and syntax. In order to facilitate children's communication output, adults use a variety of strategies

Figure 4.1 Language Modeling Can Consist of Expanding or Extending a Child's Utterance

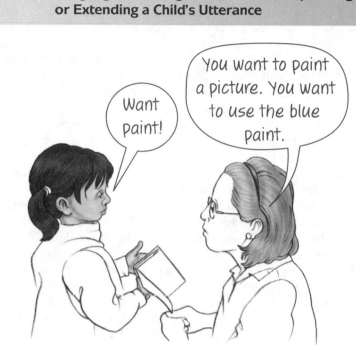

to encourage children to say more (i.e., increase the frequency of talk, vocabulary richness, and sentence length) and to elaborate their output (i.e., increase morphosyntax complexity). Techniques discussed below include self talk, parallel talk, modeling, expansions, extensions, and buildups and breakdowns. Figure 4.1 demonstrates a teacher using modeling techniques.

Self talk is language in which the adult describes what he is thinking, feeling, or seeing (Van Riper, 1978). Self talk statements typically begin with *I*. For example, playing with a dollhouse the adult might say, "*I'm putting the baby to sleep. Night-night baby. I'm rocking the baby. Rock, rock!*" The adult uses words to link the ongoing experience with interesting words, phrases, and sentences. Self talk is a particularly helpful technique for children who are reluctant to talk; it is most effective when the adult observes what the child is doing and then performs similar actions with similar materials (Fey, 1986).

Parallel talk differs from self talk in that the adult uses language to describe what the child is thinking, feeling, and doing. As in self talk, the adult does not require the child to respond; instead the adult provides "play-by-play" descriptive language connected to the child's actions.

Both self talk and parallel talk are consistent with language modeling. **Modeling** describes a technique in which the adult talks and the child listens (Fey, 1986; Miller & Yoder, 1972). Modeling is an opportunity for the child to deduce linguistic structures because the communication partner provides multiple examples of the language target.

During self talk and parallel talk the adult typically uses simplified language; sentences have less vocabulary variation, are shorter, have less complex syntax, and are semantically redundant. For example, the adult uses redundancy when he says, "*I see a doggie. The doggie is big! He is barking! The big doggie is barking at the cat!*" This simplification draws upon Vygotsky's principle of operating in a child's zone of proximal development (van Kleeck et al., 2009).

Children are most likely to talk when they are highly engaged (McWilliam, Scarborough, & Kim, 2003). Parallel talk is likely to be effective because the adult's communication is based on the child's interests, level of engagement in the ongoing activity, and focus of attention. In early stages of language development, children also are more likely to talk about their own actions as compared to talking about what others are doing. Consequently, parallel talk stimulates a child's independent utterances (Fey, 1986). Adults subsequently build on children's independent utterances through elaboration and expansion (elaboration and expansion are defined below).

There is controversy regarding the level of simplification adults should use in their utterances to young children and children with language delays (van Kleeck et al., 2009). For example, with a child who is very language delayed or very young, the adult may say, "*doggie walk*" instead of "*The dog is walking.*" This sentence construction pattern is similar to children's early word combinations sometimes called telegraphic speech. **Telegraphic speech** typically includes only content words, such as nouns, verbs, and a few adjectives/adverbs with few or no function words (e.g., auxiliary verbs, articles, conjunctions, and prepositions) or morphemes (e.g., present progressive "*-ing,* plural *s,* past tense *ed*). Function words and morphemes are not needed to communicate the meaning of a sentence. Examples of telegraphic speech include word combinations such as "*Mommy fix*" or "*put table*" (Brown, 1973). The adult uses telegraphic speech in the following example (Hancock and Kaiser, 2006):

Child: (points to cookie)
Adult: "*Say, 'want cookie.' *"
Child: "*Cookie.*"
Adult: "*Want cookie.*"

As a counter example, consider the following interaction where the adult uses short utterances but includes function words and consequently avoids telegraphic speech (van Kleeck et al., 2009):

Child: "*Truck.*"
Adult: "*Say, 'push the truck.' *"
Child: "*Push truck.*"
Adult: "*I'll push the truck. Now, you push the truck!*"

Many experts suggest telegraphic speech should never be used; in contrast some language specialists argue telegraphic speech is appropriate for children with a mean length of utterance less than 2.0 and appropriate within language interaction programs (Kaiser & Trent, 2007). However, all experts agree that adults should avoid using decidedly nongrammatical sentences, such as asking a child, "*What doing?*" (in contrast to using the correct form, "*What are you doing?*"), and agree that adults should not use telegraphic speech in everyday conversations with children.

A child is not required to talk during self talk and parallel talk; however, the adult's use of self talk and parallel talk encourages the child's spontaneous communication. The adult subsequently builds on the child's spontaneous communication by using **language expansions** and **language extensions.** In an expansion, the adult repeats the child's verbalization but adds morphemes or words to make the sentence an acceptable adult sentence (Paul, 2007; Vigil, Hodges, & Klee, 2005). An example of an expansion follows:

> *Child:* "*Daddy go outside?*"
>
> *Adult:* "*Yes, Daddy went outside!*"

An extension is very similar to an expansion, but during an extension the adult adds additional information related to the ongoing event. For example:

> *Child:* "*Baby night-night*"
>
> *Adult:* "*The baby is going night-night. The baby is tired. Night-night, baby.*"

To summarize, expansions are elaborations of a child utterance in which the adult fills in missing grammar; an extension is produced when grammatical forms as well as semantic information are added.

Researchers have documented the use of expansions between parents and children developing typically; parents expand about 30% of the utterances of their 18-month to 3-year-old children. Children developing typically imitate 10 to 24% of the parents' expansions (Goldstein, 1984).

A technique called buildups and breakdowns is another powerful language facilitating technique. The **buildup/breakdown technique** was proposed in the early 1960s. It is designed to deconstruct a sentence into its separate components (e.g., noun phrase, verb phrase, prepositional phrase, adverb and adjective clauses; Weir, 1962). Buildups and breakdowns are observed in conversations between parents and young children. Parents say a sentence, repeat smaller segments of the sentence, and then finally repeat the entire sentence. Buildups and breakdowns are associated with positive language growth in young children developing typically (Cross, 1978). Here is an example of a buildup/breakdown. In this example, the adult and child are playing with building blocks:

> *Child:* "*House.*"
>
> *Adult:* "*I'm building a tall house with my blocks. A tall house! Building a tall house. I'm building. I'm building a tall house. I'm building a tall house with my blocks.*"
>
> *Child:* "*Build house.*"

Expansions, extensions, and buildups and breakdowns are all highly contingent on the child's behavior. **Contingency** refers to how closely the language facilitator's communication relates to the child's output. All four techniques start with the child's communication and then modify the child's output to correspond to the adult language form. The frequency of contingent language during adult–child interactions positively predicts child language development (Hoff, 2006).

Assertive-Responsive Communication Scheme.   Fey (1986) proposed a scheme in alignment with the social interaction approach; he proposed the interventionist should observe an individual's **conversational assertiveness** and **conversational responsiveness.** An assertive communicator initiates a conversational turn. A responsive communicator responds to others' communication attempts. An effective communicator is both assertive and responsive. However, individuals vary along a continuum of assertiveness and responsiveness. Fey (1986) named this the assertiveness-responsiveness scheme; the assertiveness-responsiveness scheme profiles an individual according to levels of social participation. A visual representation of the scheme is shown in Figure 4.2. Consider the following example as an illustration of the scheme.

Imagine you are at a party and you introduce yourself to the people around you. First, you begin a conversation with a woman who is extremely talkative. You have difficulty fitting in a comment. When you do make a statement, she ignores your comment. She continues to talk about her own ideas and thoughts without

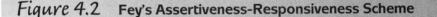

Figure 4.2   **Fey's Assertiveness-Responsiveness Scheme**

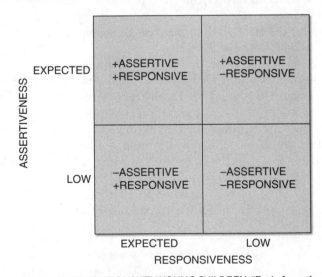

Source: Fey, LANGUAGE INTERVENTION WITH YOUNG CHILDREN, "Fey's Assertiveness-Responsiveness Scheme," p. 70, © 1986 Pearson Education, Inc. Reproduced by permission of Pearson Education, Inc.

fostering the expected back-and-forth flow of conversation. In the assertiveness-responsiveness scheme this individual is classified as highly assertive and minimally responsive (+ assertive; − responsive).

You seek out another conversation partner. Your second conversation is completely different. Now you are talking to a man who answers your questions, but does not elaborate on his ideas and does not bring up new topics. You feel frustrated because you are doing all the conversational "work" and your communication partner is passive during the interaction. In the assertiveness-responsiveness scheme this individual is classified as an unassertive but responsive communicator (− assertive, + responsive).

The examples above are exaggerations; however, I imagine you have experienced a version of the events I have described. In contrast to the two examples above, an effective communicator achieves a balance between assertiveness (i.e., able to initiate a topic as needed, makes statements or comments) and responsiveness (i.e., responding to what other people say). An individual who is + assertive and + responsive generates the expected back-and-forth conversational pattern.

As Figure 4.2 demonstrates, there are four communication types in the scheme. Beyond the three types discussed above (+ assertive, − responsive; − assertive, + responsive; + assertive, + responsive), there is a − assertive, − responsive classification. In this case, the individual does not initiate or respond to other's communication. This communication type describes an individual with a severe disability.

The assertiveness-responsiveness scheme is helpful when the interventionist considers the aspects of communication to be targeted within an individual's intervention program. Remember, the effective communicator (+ assertive, + responsive) produces a range of assertive communication acts and also responds well to others' conversational attempts. Assertive conversational acts include asking for information from others, requesting actions or objects, making comments and statements, joking, and teasing.

A variety of communication behaviors are classified as responsive communication. Responsive communication acts include responding to others' requests for action or objects and acknowledging others' comments. A list of assertive and responsive communication acts is shown in Table 4.2.

An SLP or educator provides intervention for children who vary along the continuum of assertive and responsive communication. For example, as a language facilitator you may work with an individual who is highly verbal but has difficulty responding contingently to others' conversational attempts. In this case the communication profile is classified as + assertive, − responsive.

The intervention focuses on improving the individual's communication responsiveness. An example goal for a + assertive, − responsive student is *Elissa will respond contingently to a conversational partner's comments at least three times within a 3-minute conversation.* Elissa's intervention program includes (a) practicing responsive communication behaviors using prompts (prompts include a written set of directions to serve as a reminder of the conversational rules and an adult hand gesture to signal the responsive act; prompts are faded), (b) videotaping and analyzing videotapes of conversations (Elissa participates in analyzing her conversational skills), and (c) practicing the responsive communications skills with peers in the classroom setting.

Table 4.2 Examples of Assertive and Responsive Communication Acts

Assertive Acts

- Requests for information
  - *"Why you going?"*
  - *"Where my Mommy?"*
  - *"You want you Mommy?"*
  - *"Wanna go outside?"*
  - *"It's nice, isn't it?"*
- Requests for action
  - *"Gimme that!"*
  - *"Push the chair in."*
  - *"You say it."*
- Requests for clarification
  - *"What?"*
  - *"No?"*
  - *"Excuse me?"*
- Requests for attention
  - *"Look at this!"*
  - *"See this?"*
  - *"Mommy!"*
- Comments, statements, and disagreement
  - *"This is the biggest one."*
  - *"They hanged up."*
  - *"That's my dog, Jackie."*
  - *"Do it this way."*
  - *"You have to push it."*
  - *"That's not mine."*
  - *"No."*
  - *"I'm not telling you."*
- Discourse-level assertive conversational acts
  - Initiating a new topic
  - Extending a topic (adding new information)

Responsive Acts

- Responses to requests for information
- Responses to requests for action
- Responses to requests for clarification
- Responses to requests for attention
- Responses to comments and statements and disagreement
  - *"Sure."*
  - *"I know."*
  - *"Yeah."*
  - *"Right."*
- Discourse-level responsive conversational acts
  - Maintaining topic (does not add information)

Source: Adapted from Fey, LANGUAGE INTERVENTION WITH YOUNG CHILDREN, Table 5-1 "Examples of Assertive and Responsive Communication Acts," pp. 72–73, © 1986 Pearson Education, Inc. Reproduced by permission of Pearson Education, Inc.

In contrast to the example demonstrated with Elissa, you may work with a student who is − assertive, + responsive. Imagine in this case, the student is having difficulty in the classroom because he fails to initiate comments to peers, does not request objects or actions when needed, and fails to ask for clarification when he is confused. You and the student's teacher design the following goal: *Daniel will use assertive communication acts at least three times during classroom small-group science activities.* Daniel practices completing assertive communication with you during role-playing simulations.

Prior to each small-group science activity, Daniel and his teacher write out three assertive communication acts (i.e., comments, statements, or requests). The first several times Daniel tries his assertive acts, you visit the classroom and help with the science activity. You cue and support Daniel's use of assertive communication acts; gradually Daniel's teacher provides the needed level of support. Eventually, Daniel practices embedding assertive conversational acts into other classroom activities.

Note in the above examples, I did not mention the students' diagnoses. One of the compelling features of the assertiveness-responsiveness scheme is that it is not organized around an individual's diagnostic label (e.g., autism, cognitive disability, hearing impairment). Instead, the assertiveness-responsiveness scheme focuses on an individual's quality of participation during social discourse. The interventionist uses this scheme to make sure there is a focus on how the individual interacts with others in daily life. The assertiveness-responsiveness scheme is a valuable tool for your intervention toolbox as it can be used to plan intervention approaches for children with varying disabilities.

Intervention Techniques: Influences from Cognitive Theory.   As you learned in Chapter 1, cognitive theories include the concepts proposed by Piaget. Cognitive theories focus on individuals' mental processes including perception, memory, and problem solving. The influence of cognitive theories on language intervention is profound, ranging from facilitating early learning strategies to enhancing sophisticated processes associated with high-level cognition.

Imitation and Practice.   The most fundamental cognitive processes are facilitated through imitation and practice. **Imitation** occurs when one communication partner copies another's actions or sounds. Imitation often is used as a first step in teaching a specific language target. Providing a gesture, sound, word, phrase, or sentence for imitation allows the child to have more opportunities to talk and provides more opportunities for pragmatic, phonological, semantic, and morphosyntax practice (Paul, 2007). Adults also reciprocate by imitating children's behaviors and communication attempts. Young children increase vocalization and communication attempts when adults imitate child utterances or motor acts (e.g., waving "bye-bye" back to a child). Imitation can be used to foster back-and-forth conversational turns within interactions (MacDonald, 2004).

Children must practice language to become proficient communicators. **Practice** is defined as the repetition of a task to gain proficiency; practice fosters cognitive development. To understand the importance of practice in language learning, think of the skills needed to become a skilled dancer.

Learning to dance is a good analogy for language learning (Moerk, 2004). Dance is based on basic stepping patterns that are likely to be innate. Dance occurs within all world cultures in different forms and is a learned social skill. To become a skilled dancer, an individual learns different dance components from different sources; individual components of dance must be separated and then recombined into new combinations. Much of this learning is internalized unconsciously. Dance is primarily taught through modeling and imitation, but it can also be taught didactically (e.g., through formalized and explicit instruction). The individual internalizes concepts to become proficient. Practice is essential.

As a language facilitator, you will facilitate multiple opportunities for individuals to practice their communication skills just as a dancer must practice dance steps. During intervention, skilled practitioners monitor the frequency of adult talk in relation to the amount of child talk. The practitioner waits for the child to respond. Children with communication disorders often need more time to compose their ideas and more opportunities for practice.

Direct questions (questions requiring only a brief answer) are avoided. Instead, modeling procedures and open-ended comments (e.g., "*What's happening now?*") are preferable because they provide increased opportunity for practice. To facilitate even more practice, practitioners work closely with teachers and family members so children can practice communicating more often. When intervention goals are highlighted throughout the day, the individual has more opportunities for practice.

Metacognition.   Practitioners foster high-level cognitive skills when they facilitate a student's metacognition and metalinguistic skills. **Metacognition** refers to the conscious recognition and application of abstract concepts. The student learns to "think about thinking." **Metalinguistics** refers to a student's ability to focus on and talk about language (Westby, 1998). A student uses metacognitive tasks to (a) consider how to approach a learning task, (b) when he monitors his comprehension during reading, or (c) when he evaluates his progress in an academic task. A number of intervention strategies build meta-awareness (Margolis & McCabe, 2006). To facilitate metaskills, a language facilitator can:

- *Describe* the learning strategy so the student internalizes the skill. For example, if the practitioner is teaching strategies to improve reading comprehension, he or she first describes the underlying process (e.g., "*I will outline at least five important paragraphs in each science chapter and ask myself questions about it, so I can understand the material.*")
- *Model* the strategy for the student. In this example, the practitioner shows the student how he or she selects the important items from the text.
- *Rehearse* the strategy with the student both verbally and in guided practice. The practitioner breaks the task into separate steps; together the practitioner and student take sections of the step and practice the task.

- *Discuss* how the student can use the strategy in a variety of situations. The practitioner plans time for the student to use the strategy during class.
- *Teach the student to monitor* his use of the strategy. In the example above, the practitioner and student make a check sheet with basic *wh* questions (e.g., *What is the primary point of the text? What facts support the primary point?*). The student learns to use the check sheet to monitor his comprehension.
- *Teach struggling learners to reinforce* themselves when they correctly use the strategy. In this example, the practitioner and student have fun looking in a mirror and saying "*I am doing great; I used questions today after I read my science assignment!*"
- "*Provide task-specific feedback* (e.g., "*You made an excellent topic sentence for each section of your outline.*"). Specific feedback, in contrast to general feedback (e.g., "*Good job!*"), promotes meta-awareness.

There is an increasing emphasis on enhancing metaskills as students move past the early primary school years into middle school. The assumption is that early leaning focuses on skill acquisition, but older students should focus on applying effective strategies to guide thinking and language use (Law, Campbell, Roulstone, Adams, & Boyle, 2008).

INTERVENTION TECHNIQUES IN RELATION TO LANGUAGE FORM, CONTENT, AND USE

In the section above, I described intervention techniques associated with theories of language development. I suggested that language theory helps the professional answer why a particular technique is chosen for intervention. Language intervention techniques also can be organized in relation to the language domains of form, content, and use. Form, content, and use guide the professional to think about what aspects of communication should be targeted for intervention. Interventionists use different language intervention strategies based on an individual's impairment within pragmatic, semantic, or morphosyntax domains. Basing a child's intervention on his or her abilities in form, content, and use is preferred to designing an intervention based on a child's diagnosis (Nelson, 1998).

Intervention: Pragmatics Domain.   Interventions focusing on pragmatics often are used with individuals who are at an early developing level of communication functioning. Early developing pragmatics skills include turn taking, requesting, and responding to others' communication attempts (See Chapter 1; Subdomain 1). For children who have impairments across multiple domains (i.e., difficulties with pragmatics, semantics, and morphosyntax), family members typically identify the pragmatic impairment as the highest priority (Nelson, 1998).

Communication includes learning to enter into the interactions of others. For children with significant pragmatic difficulties, the practitioner focuses on facilitating a child's turn-taking abilities, encouraging the child to initiate interactions, and increasing the amount of time the child stays in interactions with others. Practitioners use facilitative techniques during their interactions with young children and also train parents to use the techniques at home (Kaiser & Hancock, 2003). Techniques include the following:

- *Be responsive* to child verbal behaviors. Meaningful, related responses encourage child communication.
- *Give a limited number of instructions.* Giving instructions only for important behaviors increases child compliance and increases child communication.
- *Create a balanced interaction.* Encourage child-initiated utterances and limit utterances so that the child has time to contribute to the conversation. Wait for the child to take a conversational turn and indicate nonverbally and with eye contact that you expect the child to communicate.
- *Expand and extend* the child's utterances; keep language modeling related to the ongoing activity.
- *Follow the child's lead in the interaction;* watch what the child is interested in doing and make his or her actions and comments the focus of the conversation. The idea is to be a language responder, rather than a leader, teacher, or questioner (Weitzman & Greenberg, 2002).
- *Make the interaction affectively more positive.* Praise the child often; limit the number of negative responses or comments. Children's language is enhanced when they interact with positive and warm caretakers who are responsive to the child's needs and interests (Chapman, 2000).

Intervention: Morphology and Syntax Domains.   Once a child demonstrates social engagement (Communication Subdomain 1), demonstrates concepts and vocabulary associated with everyday activities (Communication Subdomain 2), and begins to regularly produce word combinations demonstrating simple sentence structure (Communication Subdomain 3) it is appropriate to begin interventions focusing on the morphosyntax concepts associated with Communication Subdomain 4. Interventionists target morphosyntax skills using the developmental sequence of children developing typically. Four morphosyntax intervention strategies are highlighted next: (a) establishing discourse contexts to elicit specific morphosyntax targets, (b) increasing the "detectibility" of targeted morphosyntax features, (c) identifying errors and absent grammatical features, and (d) choosing intermediate language targets.

The first strategy underscores the need to establish an appropriate discourse context to elicit specific morphosyntax features. As an example, the third person singular verb (verb + *s*) is used in its simple present only in state verbs such as *knows, goes, needs, wants, loves,* or *uses.* **State verbs** describe a person's state of being in contrast to describing an action. The use of third person with state verbs does <u>not</u> imply that the condition (or state of being) has lasted over a long period of time. For example, I can say, "*She needs a glass of water.*" This statement does not indicate that she has needed water for a long period of time, but rather she needs water at this moment.

In contrast, when third person is used with action verbs (*drives, cooks, watches*) it is implied that the action occurs every day or over a long period of time. So, for example, if I see a girl studying in the library, I say, "*She is studying.*" If I know she goes to the library regularly, I say, "*She studies at the library.*" In the latter case, with the action verb "*studying,*" I changed the verb to third person regular (i.e., *studies*) to indicate that the action happens regularly.

Skilled practitioners are careful to set up discourse contexts that require the targeted form when establishing a morphosyntax intervention. In the above example, the adult must create an appropriate context to elicit a third person action verb by demonstrating that the action occurs frequently or consistently (Oetting & Hadley, 2009). For example, the child and adult could create a play routine with a toy school bus and comment, "*The boy rides to school every day.*" Conversely, the adult avoids asking the child to use a third person verb in an inappropriate discourse context.

A second strategy underscores the need to make targeted morphosyntax features easily detectible. Children are more likely to attend to new morphosyntax features if they are embedded within sentences containing familiar vocabulary and include familiar tasks (i.e., functions).

Accordingly, if an interventionist is teaching present progressive verb use *is + ing,* the form is first embedded into a sentence with simple vocabulary (e.g., "*The girl is riding a bike.*"). The interventionist realizes complexity is increased with unfamiliar vocabulary, (e.g., "*The veterinarian is examining the dog.*").

Similarly, interventionists teach new forms within familiar functions (Slobin, 1973). For example, children learn to produce statements (e.g., "*That is mother's purse.*") before question forms ("*Is that mother's purse?*"). Consequently, teaching the possessive morpheme (*'s*) is facilitated when it is produced in a statement rather than a question. Skilled practitioners realize that form, content, and use are interconnected. At the initial stage of learning, when form (i.e., morphosyntax) is the intervention target, content and use should be familiar. Learn more about the relationship between form, content, and use in Focus 4.1.

FOCUS 4.1 *Learning More*

In this chapter, I stated that when form is the intervention target, content and use should be familiar at initial learning stages. This statement was first expressed by Slobin (1973) in his adage, "New forms first express old functions and new functions are first expressed by old forms" (p. 184). In other words, children first learn new behavior (i.e., form, content) in a familiar context (i.e., function) and visa versa. So, for example, when children are learning to request an action, they are likely to use familiar words. They are unlikely to use new words (i.e., content) or new form (i.e., syntax) while practicing a new function.

- As an example, Mary (age 21 months), says, "*Hold you!*" which means "*Pick me up now!*" She has heard her parents say the familiar statement, "*Do you want me to hold you?*" so she uses part of the familiar form and content to produce a new function (Sara Jones, personal communication, January 23, 2009).
- A skilled professional considers Slobin's adage when developing an intervention program. If the goal is to have a child learn new words (i.e., content), ask him or her to produce new vocabulary within a familiar pragmatic task. Keep the syntax simple by embedding new vocabulary in simple sentences instead of complex sentences.
- Modify the pragmatic and syntax demands as the child's new vocabulary is established.
- Alternately, if the goal of intervention centers on teaching new syntax, the adult initially minimizes pragmatic and semantic demands of the task.

The third strategy suggests that interventionists must note the absence of particular morphosyntax forms, in addition to noting error patterns. I have observed that beginning students readily identify some morphosyntax deficits but have difficulty identifying other error patterns. For example, even beginning students cringe (along with the child's parents and teachers) when they hear "*Her do it*" or "*Me go outside now?*" Beginning students clearly identify the pronoun errors; in this example, the child's substitution of possessive or objective pronouns (*her* = possessive pronoun, *me* = objective pronoun) for subjective pronouns (e.g., *she, he, I*).

However, in addition to the pronoun errors, the child is failing to produce an important morphosyntax feature. Morphosyntax deficits also include the lack of grammatical features. Take a look at the example above, ignore the pronoun errors, and identify something the child is not producing. Did you notice the child is lacking auxiliary verbs? In both cases, the child omits the use of an auxiliary verb, "*Her <u>can</u> do it.*" and "*<u>Can</u> me go outside now?*" The verb *can* is a form of auxiliary verb called a modal verb (e.g., *can, do, will*). Children with language impairments frequently have difficulty with auxiliary verb form; they exhibit difficulty with modal verbs as well as auxiliary *be* verbs (e.g., *is, was, are*). Auxiliary verb deletion should be a focus of intervention because complex sentence construction requires auxiliary verb production (Justice, 2002). As a result, a skilled interventionist targets auxiliary verbs in addition to—or before—pronoun errors. The interventionist notes grammatical features that are *not* used, in addition to noting morphosyntax features used incorrectly.

The fourth strategy underscores the need to choose intermediate versus beginning-level morphosyntax targets. An **intermediate-level intervention goal** is a goal highlighting grammatical categories, operations, or processes (Fey, Long, & Finestack, 1993). For example, an intermediate pronoun intervention context for a child with subject pronoun errors potentially contrasts the use of subject pronouns with possessive pronouns "*This is <u>her</u> book. <u>She</u> is reading. Is <u>she</u> reading?" <u>She</u> is reading <u>her</u> book!*" The contrastive use of the subject and possessive pronouns is an intermediate target highlighting the relationship of pronouns to underlying sentence structure.

Along with intermediate pronoun intervention targets, the adult also demonstrated two different intermediate verb targets in the previous example. First, the adult contrasted auxiliary verbs in both the statement form and interrogative form. The statement form was produced as "*She is reading*" and the interrogative form was produced as "*Is she reading*?). Second, the adult contrasted two forms of the *be* verb; contrasting the copular *be* verb ("*This <u>is</u> her book*") with the auxiliary *be* verb ("*She is reading*"). Contrasting verb forms represents an intermediate goal as it highlights underlying verb-related operations. Note in the example above, I included both pronoun and two different verb form contrasts to demonstrate different intermediate-level morphosyntax goals. In actual practice, the practitioner carefully considers a child's ability level and typically focuses on only one structural contrast at a time. Practitioners often focus on early verb learning for children with language impairments; learn more about this in Focus 4.2.

FOCUS 4.2 *Learning More*

Why do children with language impairments have difficulty learning verbs?

- Verb use is connected to the subject and object of a sentence. This syntactic relationship impacts verb argument; verb argument refers to a phrase that appears in a syntactic relationship with the verb in a clause. In English, the two most important arguments are the subject and the direct object. The properties of verb argument result in verbs carrying more syntactic information than nouns.

- Correct verb use demands noun-verb agreement; there must be agreement in person. For example, I say "*She walks*" but I change the verb with a plural noun, "*They walk.*" I can say, "*I am a girl,*" but must change the copula verb with a third person singular pronoun as in "*She is a girl.*" The speaker must change the verb in relation to the subject; this makes verb learning more complex.

- Verbs also require varying relationship with direct objects. Consider the verb *smile* versus *move*. *Move* is a transitive verb, meaning

that it requires a direct object (e.g., "*John moves the car.*" *Smile,* in contrast, is an intransitive verb; it does not require a direct object (e.g. "*John smiles*"). Other verbs require a noun phrase + prepositional phrase sequence or a noun phrase + noun phrase sequence in the direct object position. The verb *give* is an example of such a verb. I can say, "*I give the present to the boy.*" or "*I give the boy a present.*" The speaker must know if a verb is transitive or intransitive; this also makes verb learning more complex.

- Accordingly, children must process more information to use verbs effectively. Research indicates that children with language impairment use fewer argument types in spontaneous speech as compared to children developing typically.

Source: Information from "Verb Argument Structure Weakness in Specific Language Impairment in Relation to Age and Utterance Length" by E. T. Thordardottir and S. E. Weismer, 2002, *Clinical Linguistics and Phonetics, 16,* pp. 233–250.

The practitioner chooses intermediate goals to foster systemwide change. An intermediate goal highlights the processes or operations behind a morphosyntax form and increases generalization. To further enhance generalization, the practitioner also embeds intervention targets into meaningful social contexts and includes multiple modalities (i.e., oral, writing, reading).

Intervention: Semantic Domain. Semantic deficits are an early sign of language impairment; young children with LI are typically delayed in their rate and quantity of word learning. Semantic deficits continue to limit academic performance in older students with LI (McGregor, 2009). As a consequence, practitioners target semantic skills (Communication Subdomains 2 and 3; see Chapter 1) for many children with language impairments.

When selecting semantic goals for young children, interventionists consider semantic transparency. **Semantic transparency** refers to words or phrases in which meaning is easily observed or intuited. For example, the verb *pour* (said as one pours water into a glass) is semantically transparent while the word *know* (e.g., "*I know I want water*") is less transparent. Children learn vocabulary more easily when the referent is connected to the label provided by the adult. In semantic interventions, the practitioner chooses words and manipulates the context to increase semantic transparency.

In order to learn new words, children with language impairments need more frequent exposure compared to children developing typically (Gray, 2004). To provide increased exposure to word meaning, the practitioner provides (a) repeated models of the new word within a play context, (b) prompts the child to produce the word, and (c) provides feedback on word accuracy. Adding semantic and phonological cues appears to enhance word learning for children with language impairments (Grey, 2005). Semantic cues include describing the physical characteristics, providing item function, or providing the word category (e.g., "*This is a muffler; it is something you wear; it's clothing.*") Phonological cues include emphasizing the initial sound or first syllable, clapping out syllables in the word, or providing a rhyming word (e.g. "*The word is* wheat; *it sounds like your brother's name, Pete!*").

At older ages, the practitioner works to increase the breadth (i.e., number of new words) and depth (i.e., nuanced vocabulary to express familiar concepts) in a student's semantic lexicon. McGregor (2009) indicates that the practitioner should work on:

- Idiomatic phrases (e.g., "*What does* flipping her lid *mean?*").
- More subtle vocabulary (e.g., *morose, depressed,* or *glum*) to replace a familiar word (e.g., *sad*).
- Alternative meanings to a familiar word (e.g., "*At night we can say it is dark. What do I mean when I say 'He has a dark personality'?*").
- Compound word construction (e.g., "*When we make a compound word, the describing word* [i.e., adjective] *goes first. We say blue + berry (not berry + blue) and mail + box (not box + mail).*"
- Prefixes (*readmit, bidirectional, autopilot, disappear*) and suffixes (*transition, presentable, nutritious*). **Prefixes** and **suffixes** are groups of letters attached to the beginning (prefix) or ending (suffix) of a word to form a new word; prefixes and suffixes sometimes change the grammatical function of the original word. (Learn more about prefixes and suffixes in Focus 4.3.)

In addition to the suggestions above, Beck and her colleagues (Beck & McKeown, 1985; Beck, McKeown, & Kucan, 2002) provide a helpful perspective for vocabulary intervention. They suggest a well-developed vocabulary consists of three tiers. Tier 1 words consist of basic vocabulary used on a daily basis (e.g., *climb, sofa, man, close*). Tier 1 words rarely require instructional attention for most school-age students.

Tier 2 words are used across domains by skilled speakers, writers, and readers. Tier 2 words occur within academic settings and in books but are difficult for students to learn in daily interactions. Consequently, Tier 2 words should be the focus of vocabulary intervention. Examples of Tier 2 words include *merchant, required, tend, maintain, identified, fortunate,* and *unscrupulous* (Beck et al., 2002).

FOCUS 4.3 *Learning More*

Prefixes and Suffixes

- Teaching students to find the base word along with the suffix and prefix is considered an intermediate-to-advanced word study strategy generally appropriate for children in third to fourth grades (Bear, Invernizzi, Templeton, & Johnston, 2007). Word study should relate to words children use while reading and writing.

- During word study, children learn to complete the following sequence when they come to an unfamiliar word while reading: (1) take off the prefix; (2) take off the suffix; (3) look at the base word to determine if it is familiar; (4) reassemble the word and make a hypothesis about word meaning; (5) try the hypothesized meaning in the sentence; (6) if the sentence does not make sense, look up the word in the dictionary; (7) record the word in a word study notebook.

- Suffixes and prefixes are learned in a developmental sequence.

- Early suffixes include identification of plural endings (*s* and *es*), suffixes related to size (*er, est*), compound words (*snowman, pancake*), and spelling rules such as changing the final *y* to *i* and adding *ed* or *s* (*cry-cries*). Simple prefixes include *un-, re-, sub-, in-*.

- Middle-level affixes include advanced rules that govern spelling, such as producing plurals by changing *y* to *i* (*babies* versus *toys*). Other middle-level suffixes include -*such, -ship, -ity, -ment,* and -*ic*. Middle-level prefixes include *dis-, mis-, pre-, pro-,* and *con-*.

- Late-developing word study focuses on teaching students to recognize common roots in English such as *port* (to carry; *portable, transport*), *duct* (to lead; *conduct, tear duct*), *spec* (to look at; *spectator, spectacles, inspect*).

In contrast, Tier 3 words are words related to a specific domain (e.g., science [acceleration, hibernation], occupation [lathe, stethoscope], social studies [peninsula, lava]). Beck argues that domain-specific words are used infrequently and are most appropriately learned when a specific need arises—such as when a learning unit is introduced in class.

The practitioner decides which words to target for vocabulary instruction by determining if the student has old, familiar words to describe the new Tier 2 word. So, for example, if the student knows the word *dishonest* or *cheating*, the practitioner may choose to teach the Tier 2 word, *unscrupulous*. A strategy to enhance student's vocabulary knowledge is described in Focus 4.4.

EVALUATING EVIDENCE-BASED INTERVENTION STRATEGIES

Evaluating research evidence is an important component of evidence-based practice (EBP); consideration of an intervention's documented effectiveness is an important component of the intervention process. In this section, I describe how professionals evaluate the quality and quantity of an intervention approach.

FOCUS 4.4 *Clinical Skill Building*

There are four guiding principles for vocabulary instruction. Effective instruction should help students (1) relate new vocabulary to background knowledge, (2) develop elaborated word knowledge, (3) become active participants in learning new words, and (4) develop strategies for learning new vocabulary (Nelson & Van Meter, 2007).

- A method called robust vocabulary instruction has been evaluated in research studies; it is an effective approach to helping students learn the meanings of words and improve reading comprehension (Beck & McKeown, 2007). With robust vocabulary instruction, students learn how a novel word is similar to, and different from, related concepts and how the word is used in a variety of situations.

Storybook reading is an effective context for robust vocabulary instruction. The language facilitator uses a storybook interaction to introduce new vocabulary, provide a child-friendly definition of the word, give an example of the word with a different sentence, and provide follow-up activities in which children choose between words, relate words to known concepts, and ask questions using the new words.

- This approach is effective with low income and middle class European-American children, but also is an effective and culturally sensitive strategy for improving vocabulary in African American students. Storybooks with cultural themes are used to connect the vocabulary to children's lives (Lovelace & Stewart, 2009).

EBP: Evaluating Research Quality.　A hierarchy of research quality is used to rank the scientific merit of a particular intervention; a summary of the guidelines is provided in Table 4.3. Quality ratings represent a continuum from Level I to Level IV. **Level I** evidence resulting from randomized experimental research is considered the best, or "gold standard" research design. Level I evidence also includes meta-analyses. A **meta-analysis** is a specialized form of systematic review in which the

Table 4.3　**Levels of Evidence for Scientific Studies**

Quality	Criteria
Level I	• Evidence from one well-conducted randomized clinical trial. • Systematic reviews or meta-analysis of high-quality randomized controlled trials.
Level II	• Similar findings demonstrated from nonrandomized experiments (with good experimental design) from several different researchers.
Level III	• Well-designed nonexperimental studies (i.e., correlational and case studies).
Level IV	• Expert committee report, consensus conference, clinical experience of respected authorities.

Source: Information from ASHA, www.asha.org/members/ebp/assessing.htm.

results from several studies are summarized using a statistical technique resulting in a single weighted estimate of their findings. **Level II research** reflects high quality, but nonrandomized, experiments. **Level III** evidence reflects well-designed nonexperimental studies and case studies. A nonexperimental design is typically a description of clinical results from one or a small group of students, without the use of a comparison treatment. **Level IV** represents experts' opinion.

Assigning a research study to one of four research levels reflects the scientific rigor of the study's methodology. Level I research reflects the most rigorous investigation standard because studies assigned to Level I (a) compare performance of two or more groups of students (i.e., control group design) and (b) randomly assign students to one group or the other. Sometimes in a control group design, two different interventions (also called treatments) are compared. For example, researchers compare results from the treatment group with results from the no-treatment group. In the no-treatment group, the students continue with their regular school or home activities but do not receive any special intervention. Although comparison between a treatment and no-treatment group is an acceptable design, a better research design compares two *different* treatments. In the treatment vs. no-treatment design, students in the treatment group may improve because they receive regular, positive interaction with an attentive adult; student gains may not be directly attributable to specific characteristics of the intervention. A comparison of two different interventions (in which both groups of children receive some kind of intervention) eliminates this problem.

Subject randomization also is a factor in Level I research. In a randomized research design, a group of students consent to participate in a study. Following consent, the students are randomly assigned to the treatment group or control group. Randomization adds certainty to the interpretation of results. If randomization is not used, there is a possibility for bias. For example, imagine I say, "*I would like you to participate in a study on the effects of exercise. You can choose to be in a group in which you will exercise four times a week, or you can choose to be in a group that exercises two times a week.*" In this situation, it is likely individuals with specific character traits (perhaps highly motivated individuals) will choose to be in the more frequent exercise group; less motivated individuals may choose the two-times-per-week group. Study results potentially represent variations in motivation levels rather than comparing exercise effects. Random assignment increases the validity of the experimental results.

Other factors contribute to the evaluation of research quality. An overall goal of high quality research is to (a) limit any extraneous factors potentially contaminating the results, (b) determine that participants in the group are similar except for treatment exposure, (c) document results with highly reliable and valid measures of performance, and (d) provide statistically significant and meaningful data (Gillam & Gillam, 2008). Each of these factors is described in more detail below.

One goal of high quality research is to document that reported effects are not contaminated by unintended variables. One factor causing contamination is research bias. Research bias occurs when an examiner unconsciously inflates a student's abilities because he or she knows the student participated in an intervention and "should" improve. Potential for research bias is reduced when blinding is used. **Blinding** means the individual who assesses the students is not the same individual who provides the intervention or directs the study. Without blinding, there is potential for contamination of outcome data.

Contamination also occurs when the individual providing the treatment fails to implement the treatment as planned. To counter this possibility, high-quality studies include measures of treatment fidelity. **Fidelity** refers to the degree to which the intervention is carried out as described. One way to document intervention fidelity is to videotape intervention sessions and count or code the interventionist's behaviors.

A second factor impacting research quality is documentation of group similarity prior to the intervention. As I have already pointed out, randomization makes it more likely that the groups do not differ. However, in communication disorders research, investigators must also demonstrate that subjects in treatment and control groups are relatively the same prior to the study. Without this assurance, it can be argued the participants' ability level or environmental circumstances influenced the results. For example, consider that I am completing a study and I find my control group students are significantly more impaired than my treatment group. My results are affected because I cannot be certain treatment-group improvement is due to intervention. Since the treatment group was (on average) less impaired, improvement may represent natural development and not represent change due to the intervention. To minimize this factor, researchers document participants' age, communication ability, socioeconomic status, classroom environment, intellectual ability, ethnicity, and so forth. Documentation and analysis clarifies group equivalency prior to the treatment implementation.

A third factor in research design relates to assessment. In Chapter 2, you learned the importance of using valid and reliable assessments in clinical practice; high quality research studies must also use standardized assessments or high-quality, criterion-referenced measures. Examples of standardized assessments are the Peabody Picture Vocabulary Test-4 (Dunn & Dunn, 2006) and the Clinical Evaluation of Language Fundamentals-Preschool 2 (Wiig, Secord, & Semel, 2004). Validity and reliability data for standardized tests are reported in a test's administration manual; the researcher includes these data in published research.

Criterion-referenced evaluation instruments used in Level I to III research also require documented reliability and validity. To demonstrate a criterion-referenced measure is high quality, the researcher clearly describes the behavioral parameters used to evaluate student behavior, uses an established protocol to administer the criterion-referenced measure, and documents the reliability of the measure's administration.

A final factor in research design is the requirement for data demonstrating that study results are significant as well as meaningful (Schuele & Justice, 2006). To determine significance, the (most basic) process is to compare mean performance between treatment and control groups. Significance tests reflect the probability that the reported outcome being due to chance, or random fluctuation, is adequately small (Silverman, 1998). When interpreting intervention research, statistical significance demonstrates the intervention made a real difference in student performance.

Although statistical significance is important, by itself it is not sufficient. It is possible for a study to produce statistical significance, but the degree of change may not be clinically meaningful. To overcome the limited interpretability of statistical significance, high-quality research studies report effect sizes. **Effect-size estimates** are numerical values designed to characterize results in functional and meaningful ways. Effect-size data indicate the magnitude of an effect in addition to estimates of probability (Schuele & Justice, 2006). Typically, effect-size estimates are interpreted with two processes. The first process uses a commonly accepted benchmark to differentiate small, medium, and large effect sizes (Cohen's *d*, .2 = small effect, .5 = medium effect, and .8 = large effect; Cohen, 1988). In a second process, the researcher compares his or her effect size to effect sizes achieved in similar studies.

Randomization and control-group design are important factors in quality leading to a Level I research rating. However, Level II, III, and IV studies also can be very high quality even though they are not randomized, control-group studies (Fey, 2006; Justice & Fey, 2004). High quality at Levels II to IV is documented with similar factors as described for Level I studies: careful description of subject characteristics, the use of valid and reliable measures to document change, minimizing contamination of results, and reporting outcome data to document significant and meaningful results.

EBP: Evaluating the Quantity of Data. When professionals use EBP decision making to guide intervention selection, they also consider the quantity of supporting evidence (ASHA, 2005; Justice, 2006). Interventions with a body of documentation have more evidence supporting their use. Many commonly used speech-language pathology interventions have not yet been evaluated by randomized, control-group treatment (RCT) design studies. In this case, the professional examines the body of evidence across all levels including nonrandomized research studies, case studies, and expert opinion.

Interventionists develop skills to assess research results and judge the accumulated body of research evaluating the proposed intervention. Increasingly there are Internet sites to provide summarized information about EBP. For example, the American Speech, Language, and Hearing Association (ASHA) maintains a Web site providing tutorials and working papers on EBP for ASHA members and student members (www.asha.org/members/ebp/). Also, professionals use searches to access peer-reviewed research such as the one available with Google Scholar (http://scholar.google.com/). In contrast to regular Google access (which typically does not represent peer-reviewed research), Google Scholar allows the professional to access peer-reviewed research (Nail-Chiwetalu & Ratner, 2006). As a student in the beginning level of training, you can start developing the needed skills by accessing the American Speech, Language and Hearing Association Web site (if you are a member of the National Student Speech, Language, and Hearing Association). The information in Table 4.4 provides a step-by-step process you can use to locate information on a particular topic.

Table 4.4   **Steps for Finding Peer-Reviewed Research Studies**

Step	Instructions
1.	As a member of the National Student Speech, Language, Hearing Association (NSSLHA), log on to the ASHA and NSSLHA Members Web page at www.asha.org and select "ASHA full-text journals" from the full menu on the far left-hand side of the screen.
2.	Select "Advanced Search" (this link is midway down the page under "Advanced Features"). This search allows you to access all ASHA journals and other peer-reviewed articles electronically.
3.	Type search terms (e.g., *preschool language intervention* or *focused stimulation*) in the text, title, or abstract box where it says "specify authors and keywords."
4.	Select either "all ASHA journals" or "search across multiple journals" at the bottom of the page. You will be able to access PDF versions of the relevant articles. If too many articles are identified, you can be more specific with search terms or request to see only recent articles (i.e., enter in dates under "limit results.")

Source: Information from "Teaching Graduate Students to Make Evidence-Based Decisions: Application of a Seven-Step Process Within an Authentic Learning Context," by S. L. Gillam and R. B. Gillam, 2008, *Topics in Language Disorders, 28,* pp. 212–228.

The Intervention Toolbox Part II: Structuring and Implementing Treatment

When planning an intervention approach, the interventionist makes a series of decisions in response to a student's specific needs. In the first section in this chapter, I described how language theory answers the question, *Why am I choosing this intervention?* A discussion of the language domains of form, content, and use in relation to language intervention. The interventionist considers an individual's abilities in the three language domains to answer the question, *What aspects of communication should be targeted in intervention?* The following section is designed to describe concepts and principles to answer *how.* The practitioner asks the question, *How do I structure and implement intervention to most effectively impact an individual's communication skills?* The information below helps answer this question.

STRUCTURING INTERVENTION

When making a decision about intervention structure, the practitioner considers how best to expose the child to the targeted language features and how to provide practice opportunities. The structure of the intervention varies in line with the overall therapeutic goal. If, on one hand, the goal is to teach specific linguistic structures, the session must provide frequent opportunities for exposure and practice. On the other hand, if the goal is to improve communicative patterns in everyday interactions, the intervention sessions are structured differently. Several concepts illuminate this process and are discussed below. The first concept centers on who leads the interaction; interactions can be classified as adult directed versus child directed. The second concept centers on the activities, location, and social aspects of an intervention. Fey's (1986) continuum of naturalness, which is discussed later in this chapter, provides a structure elaborating this concept.

Adult- versus Child-Directed Intervention.   The concept of adult- versus child-directed intervention describes who is "in charge" and what the intervention looks like. In **adult-directed intervention** the adult leads the interaction by (a) choosing the stimulus items; (b) regulating how the child will respond; (c) prompting particular responses through pointing, modeling, or the use of questions; and (d) providing direct feedback on the child's performance (e.g, "*Good talking!*"). One of the common features of the adult-directed approach is the three-part question sequence consisting of (1) an adult request to produce specific information, (2) child response, and (3) adult evaluative feedback (Kovarsky & Duchan, 1997). Adult-directed approaches tend to use many of the intervention strategies from behavioral-based intervention discussed previously in this chapter. I provide a treatment sequence illustrative of an adult-directed approach in Focus 4.5.

In contrast, during **child-directed intervention,** the adult follows the child's lead, responds contingently to the child's responses, and waits for the child to respond before initiating another conversational sequence. Social interaction is viewed as the reinforcing event in contrast to explicit reinforcement. Rather than taking on the

FOCUS 4.5 *Learning More*

An adult-directed intervention sequence has a typical question-statement-feeedback format. Below is an example:

Adult: "Joshua, I have different kinds of balls in this box. I am going to pull one out and throw it to you. Each time catch it and then tell me about the ball. Remember to use your descriptive words!"

Adult: "What kind of ball is this?"

Joshua: "It is a red ball."

Adult: "Yes, it is red. Is it big or little?"

Joshua: "It Is big."

Adult: "Try and put all your descriptive words together to make a big sentence."

Joshua: "This is a big, red ball".

Adult: "Good, you told me about the size and the color. You could have also told me about how it feels. Like this: 'This is a soft, bouncy ball.'"

Joshua: "This ball is soft and bouncy."

Adult: "Good try! Try it this way. This is a soft, bouncy ball."

Joshua: "This is a soft, bouncy ball."

Adult: "Good! That time you used your descriptive words before the word ball. You said, 'This is a soft, bouncy ball.' Let's try this next one. What about this ball?"

leader role, in child-directed intervention the adult modifies the situation's interactional and interpersonal characteristics to enhance the child's communication functioning (Kovarsky & Duchan, 1997). The approach reflects the modeling and balanced turn-taking strategies influenced by social interaction theory.

Fey (1986) proposed a third category, hybrid intervention, lying between adult- and child-directed approaches. In **hybrid intervention** the practitioner focuses on a small subset of language behaviors and focuses a great deal of attention on identified targets within the intervention session. However, rather than using the direct question sequence often seen in the adult-directed approach, the adult manipulates the context to entice the child to spontaneously use the targeted linguistic features. Often hybrid interventions use toys and play routines to create opportunities for practice. During the play routine, the practitioner uses specific modeling and responsive strategies to emphasize targeted features. An example of a technique consistent with the hybrid approach is sentence recasting. As I discussed earlier in this chapter, during sentence recasting the practitioner varies sentence structure in modeled sentences (i.e., interrogative vs. statement sentences) to increase the child's attention to the language target.

Focused stimulation is another approach considered to be a hybrid therapy. In **focused stimulation** a child is exposed to multiple examples of a linguistic target within a meaningful communication context. The practitioner does not require an imitative response but rather elicits spontaneous communication. Focused stimulation can be used to facilitate features within form, content, or use language domains (Leonard, 1981; Weismer & Robertson, 2006).

Empirical evidence supports the clinical use of focused stimulation for children who have language impairments, toddlers who are language delayed, and individuals with cognitive impairments. For example, a Level I research study demonstrated that focused stimulation intervention resulted in significant gains in toddlers' total number of words, number of different words, and mean length of utterance (Weismer & Robertson, 2006). Level II and III research also documents the effectiveness of this approach (e.g., Culatta & Horn, 1982; Wilcox, Kouri, & Caswell, 1991).

Developing a playlike, engaging context is an important component of focused stimulation. For example, imagine that the practitioner wants to teach a child to use auxiliary forms. The practitioner selects the modal auxiliary form *can* since modal verbs typically emerge earlier than *be* auxiliary verbs (Paul, 2007). In this interaction, the child and adult manipulate superhero action figures:

Adult: "Can *Superman fly? Yes, he* can *fly! Superman* can *fly. How about Aquaman? Can he fly?*"

Child: "*Aquaman no fly. Aquaman swim.*"

Adult: "*Oh, I see. Aquaman* can *swim. Superman* can *fly.*"

Adult: "*I wonder if Hulk* can *fly? What do you think?*"

Child: "*Hulk* can *fly!*"

Adult: "*Wow, I didn't know Hulk* can *fly! Show me again, how Hulk* can *fly!*"

Classic characteristics of focused stimulation are demonstrated in the previous example. The activity is carefully constructed so repeated exposure of the targeted form is modeled and produced. Play routines consist of dramatic play enactments (e.g., setting up a grocery store, getting ready for school) or manipulating toy figures and objects. Examples of play routines to elicit different form, function, and use targets are provided in Table 4.5.

Table 4.5 **Examples of Focused Stimulation Interventions for Form, Content, and Use**

Communication Domain	Focused Stimulation Activity
Form	• To increase the child's use of negation, the following activity is established: • The adult sets up a dollhouse with a man doll, cat, doll furniture, and car. The man is sleeping and the cat is under the bed. **Adult:** (Man wakes up). *"Where is that cat? He is <u>not</u> in the kitchen. He is <u>not</u> in the living room. Is he in the car? He is <u>not</u> in the car. I wonder where he is? Is he in the backyard?"* **Child:** *"No backyard."* **Adult:** *"He is <u>not</u> in the backyard!"*
Content	• To increase child's use of superordinate categorization, the following activity is established: • The adult shows the child a box containing doll furniture, doll clothes, and vehicles (cars, trucks, bus, taxi, bicycle). **Adult:** *"The box is a mess! We are going to organize this box into categories. Some of these objects are <u>furniture</u>, some of these objects are <u>clothing</u>, some of these objects are <u>transportation</u>."* (Adult lays out a picture of a house, a closet, and a garage). *"Let's figure out where these items should go."* **Child:** *"OK."* **Adult:** *"This is a hat. It's something you wear on your head. A hat is <u>clothing</u>. I can put it in the closet. We keep <u>clothing</u> in the closet. <u>Clothing</u> is stuff that we wear."* **Adult:** *"This is a bus. We ride on a bus. A bus is used for <u>transportation</u>. Where should we put the bus? OK, we can park the bus in the big garage. What kinds of things are we going to put in the garage?"* **Child:** *"Bus, car."* **Adult:** *"Yes, because a bus and a car are things we use for <u>transportation</u>, we use them to get places."*

(continued)

Table 4.5   **Examples of Focused Stimulation Interventions for Form, Content, and Use (*Continued*)**

Communication Domain	Focused Stimulation Activity
Use	• To increase child's use of the pragmatic function of *request*, the following activity is established: • The adult sets up a picnic using stuffed animals and plastic food. There are plates, cups, a pitcher for juice, etc. *Adult:* "*The bear says, 'I need a plate.' Can you give him a plate? Good. The cat says, 'I need a plate, please.' What does the dog say?*" *Child:* (does not answer, gives dog plate) *Adult:* "*Wait, before you give the dog a plate he has to ask. The dog says, 'I need a plate!'*" *Child:* "Need plate." *Adult:* "*Good, you made the dog ask for a plate! Let's see who wants some juice.*"

As discussed in the previous example, the practitioner does not demand that the child imitate a response but creates a context in which child productions are elicited. As the child's skill level improves, the practitioner decreases the number of focused models and increases opportunities for child responses.

The notion of adult- versus child-directed therapy, and the use of hybrid approaches, is a helpful concept for intervention planning. It is important to remember, however, an intervention does not have to be entirely one approach or another. Typically, practitioners use a combination of approaches within a therapy session. For example, a child might participate in an adult-directed warm up activity at the beginning of each therapy session, followed by a child-directed or hybrid approach during the rest of the therapy session. The duration and intensity of different approaches is varied in relation to the child's abilities, motivation level, and the intervention goal.

Continuum of Naturalness.   The degree to which an intervention session is adult versus child directed influences other aspects of the intervention. For example, interventions vary in terms of activities, location (i.e., physical context), and the number of participants (i.e., social context). Fey's (1986) **continuum of naturalness** is a helpful concept in describing these variations; the continuum of naturalness describes the degree to which an intervention session is very similar (or very dissimilar) to everyday interactions. The activities, location, and social context are variables contributing to an intervention's naturalness or unnaturalness. Figure 4.3 illustrates how activity, location, and social variables contribute to an interaction's naturalness rating.

First, intervention activities vary in the degree that they are natural versus unnatural. If the intervention activity is very structured and adult directed, it is

Figure 4.3 **Continuum of Naturalness**

		drill	organized games	daily activities
1.	Activity	0	+1	+2
2.	Physical Context	clinic 0	school +1	home +2
3.	Social Context	clinician 0	teacher +1	parents +2
4.	Overall Naturalness	low 0	+3	high +6

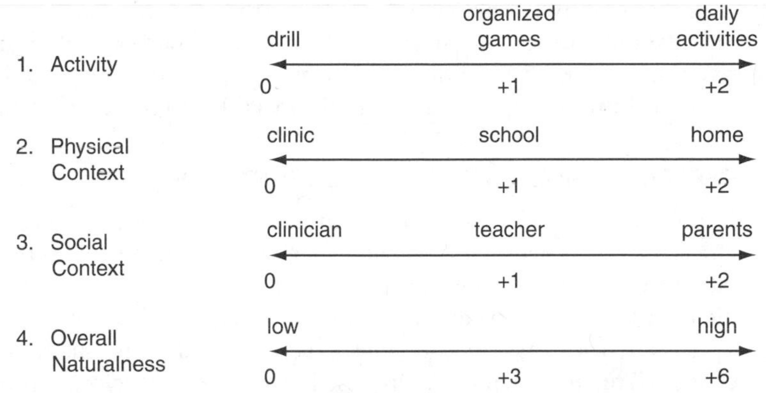

Source: Fey, LANGUAGE INTERVENTION WITH YOUNG CHILDREN, "Continuum of Naturalness," p.63, © 1986 Pearson Education, Inc. Reproduced by permission of Pearson Education, Inc.

considered unnatural on Fey's continuum. An example is drill, an activity often completed in response to pictures. **Drill** activities typically elicit a high number of child responses produced in response to adult questions. Drill play is somewhat more natural, but still highly structured. In **drill play,** an element of a play routine is used to increase motivation. Examples include mailing pictures into a mailbox (i.e., child produces the targeted form before mailing), selecting items to put into a toy box (e.g., child selects stickers, pictures, or miniature items), or playing a game in which multiple child productions are elicited.

Modeling and focused stimulation activities are considered a midpoint on Fey's continuum of naturalness; they are somewhat more natural as compared to drill and drill play. An example of a highly natural language intervention occurs when the practitioner creates opportunities for a child to communicate in the classroom or interacts with a child with toys following the child's lead.

The second variable influencing the continuum of naturalness refers to physical context. One-on-one interactions between the interventionist and child are highly unnatural while home-based and classroom-based interventions are more natural. In Chapter 3, I discussed the issue of classroom-based versus pullout models of intervention. The classroom-based model is more natural than the pullout model. An example of a midpoint along the physical context is when the interventionist works with a child one on one within the classroom environment (i.e., the adult works with the child at a separate table inside the classroom).

The final variable influencing the continuum of naturalness relates to social context. One-on-one, adult-child intervention is the least natural, while training parents to facilitate language targets at home is highly natural. The midpoint on the social interaction variable is demonstrated when the interventionist provides treatment in small groups or brings siblings or peers into the treatment session.

One caution in the use of Fey's continuum is the assumption that highly natural activities are always better than highly unnatural activities. Experts caution us against this thinking; highly natural activities are preferred *only* when they are effective. If two activities are equally effective, then the more natural activity is preferred. However, if the activity must be modified (i.e., made less natural) to increase effectiveness, the adult modifies the intervention accordingly. Gradually, as the child's skill level improves, the adult adjusts variables to increase naturalness (Fey, 1986).

IMPLEMENTING EFFECTIVE INTERVENTIONS

Making a measurable difference in an individual's everyday interactions is the heart of efficacious treatment. "It is the ultimate goal, indeed, the gold standard for impairment-based treatment" (Thompson, 2007, p. 5). In order to document changes made during intervention, the interventionist must write goals in which change can be described and measured, select appropriate goal attack strategies, and maintain data to document change. This information is discussed in the section below. I provide a decision tree illustrating the intervention process in Figure 4.4.

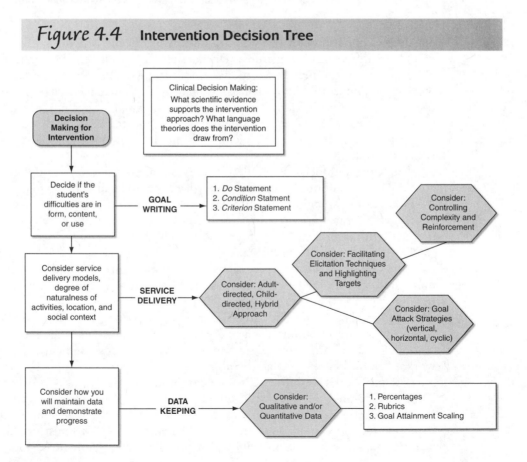

Figure 4.4   **Intervention Decision Tree**

Writing Intervention Goals.   When writing intervention goals the practitioner describes what the student's communication behavior will look like when the skill is mastered. A goal is made up of three components, the *do* statement, the *condition* statement, and the *criterion* statement (Roth & Paul, 2007). The *do* statement describes the behaviors the child will produce. It is important to write the goal with active, observable verbs such as *write, answer, state, imitate, respond,* or *produce.* In contrast, verbs such as *know, understand, realize, comprehend,* and *learn* cannot be measured. Some examples of active verbs in a *do* statement include

- John will <u>initiate</u> . . .
- Xavier will <u>express</u> . . .
- Sasha will <u>imitate</u> gestures . . .
- Kareem will <u>edit</u> his written work . . .

The second component of the behavioral goal describes the situation or conditions under which the behavior will occur. Remember that a communication goal describes target behaviors as they are produced at the initial learning stage (i.e., the child is provided strong support from an adult in a controlled interaction) to the final stage (i.e., the behavior is produced during natural, spontaneous interactions). Accordingly, the *condition* statement describes the stimuli, where the behavior will occur, and who will be there when the behavior occurs. *Condition* statements often include words such as *following, after, with, in response to, before,* and *during.*

- At the beginning stages of learning, the *condition* statement will indicate strong support and cuing. Examples include:
    . . . following an adult model
    . . . with picture cues
    . . . with a written reminder
- In contrast, the *condition* statement demonstrates the child's increasing independent production of the targeted skill at later stages:
    . . . before initiating a written assignment
    . . . in response to peers' questions
    . . . during interactive play routines in the classroom

The final component of the goal statement reflects the criteria determining goal achievement. The *criterion* statement can be measured qualitatively (e.g., with total correct or percentage data) or quantitatively (e.g., with a rubric or description of performance). Quantitative goals often include statements such as:

- . . . 8 out 10 times
- . . . with 90% accuracy
- . . . two times a day for two weeks
- . . . at least three times in a ten-minute conversation
- . . . less than three times during the twenty-minute therapy session

Typically, accuracy levels are set fairly high when they are expected to occur in an adult-directed and less naturalistic setting (i.e., 70–90% accuracy). At the final stages of intervention, when the child is expected to produce the behavior spontaneously, less stringent accuracy levels are expected (e.g., 50–70% accuracy; Paul, 2007).

A good goal allows the practitioner some flexibility (i.e., is not so specific that it completely limits the choice of therapeutic activity) but is descriptive enough that another professional could reproduce the activity and achieve similar results. An example of an overlimiting goal is, "When reading the story, *The Three Bears,* John will . . ." This goal limits the therapeutic activities and does not promote generalizability.

Selecting Goal Attack Strategies.   A goal attack strategy refers to the way in which multiple goals are approached or scheduled within an intervention session (Cirrin & Gillam, 2008). Three strategies have been identified: (a) a **vertical strategy** in which one goal at a time is targeted until a predetermined level of accuracy is achieved, (b) a **horizontal strategy** in which several goals are targeted within every session, and (c) a **cyclic strategy** in which several goals are targeted with a repeating sequence, each for a specified time period independent of accuracy (Cirrin & Gillam, 2008; Fey, 1986; Tyler, Lewis, Haskill, & Tolbert, 2003).

Each goal structuring method has advantages and disadvantages. Vertical structuring allows the practitioner to work on one goal at a time and the child achieves a high response rate for a single target in each session. The one-goal strategy may heighten the child's focus of attention on the targeted skill. However, vertical structuring may lead to a repetitious and potentially boring intervention.

In a horizontal structure, the practitioner presents two or more goals within the same intervention session. The goals may target related behaviors (e.g., use of *be* verb as a copula [*"The boy is a baseball player"*] with *be* verbs as an auxiliary [*"The boy is throwing the ball"*] or unrelated behaviors (e.g., a goal targeting syntax and a goal targeting semantics). New goals are added as the child reaches predetermined criteria on each goal. The amount of time to reach criteria will vary from goal to goal. One advantage of horizontal structuring is that the intervention session does not become as repetitive and the child is less likely to be bored.

Another advantage of horizontal structuring is that as a primary goal is achieved in a structured intervention context, the adult can relegate a primary goal to secondary status. The interventionist regularly monitors the student's use of secondary goals during natural, spontaneous speech. In this way, newly learned communication behaviors are generalized to everyday interactions. A disadvantage of horizontal structuring is that presenting multiple intervention targets may cause confusion for children who are easily distracted or more severely impaired.

In a cyclic goal attack strategy, the interventionist moves through a series of targeted goals using a predetermined schedule. For example, in the cycle approach Goal 1 is introduced during Week 1 and Goal 2 during Week 2. The interventionist then cycles back to Goal 1 on Week 3 and Goal 2 during Week 4. The cyclic approach has features of both vertical and horizontal attack strategies. When implementing the cyclic attack strategy, the practitioner introduces a different goal each week and then moves from one goal to the next regardless of the child's progress, or lack of progress, on a particular goal (Williams, 2000). Over time, as the cycle is repeated, the child increases competency on individual goals.

Consider the following example of an intervention program using the cycle approach. The interventionist develops three goals for a student who has deficits in three areas: (1) third person verb errors (example errors: *He* walk *to school, She* drive *the car*), (2) limited use of conjunctions, such as *so* and *but* (e.g., "*The man wants a new car,* <u>*but*</u> *he doesn't have enough money*"), and (3) poor comprehension of *why* questions. The interventionist writes a goal for each of the targets.

1. Macauley will produce third person regular verbs with 70% accuracy in focused stimulation activities in which third person verbs are contrasted with regular present progressive verbs. (Example: "*What is the girl doing? She is walking her dog. What* does *she like to do? She* likes *to walk her dog?* Does *she do it every day? Yes, she* walks *her dog every day.*"
2. Macauley will produce 4-6 sentences using coordinating conjunctions during a retelling of a familiar fairy tale with access to a written list of coordinating conjunctions.
3. Macauley will produce three different *why* questions and answer at least different three *why* questions during a shared book reading interaction using a first-grade level book.

The three goals are targeted on a rotating basis and the interventionist records the child's accuracy each session. If a goal reaches criteria, a new goal is brought into the cycle or the goal is modified to elicit more independent and complex productions. Goals that do not reach criteria continue to be targeted in the cycle. The child learns some skills in a period of a few weeks, while other skills take longer. The cyclic approach has been shown to be effective in teaching morphosyntax skills to preschoolers (Tyler et al., 2003) and in teaching phonological skills (Williams, 2000). A rationale for the cycle approach is that goal mastery is developmental and children require varying levels of exposure to meet criteria (i.e., some targets may be acquired with little stimulation while others take more time). The disadvantage is that generally professionals need more skill and experience to organize and maintain a cyclic intervention schedule.

Keeping Intervention Data.   An important outcome of EBP is the recognition that all intervention must be evidence based and there must always be data documenting changes in communication. Although the complex nature of communication means documentation takes organization and planning, it is possible. I tell beginning clinicians, "*Don't limit your intervention by choosing goal behaviors that are easy to document; instead decide what the child needs to practice or learn, and then figure out a way to document change of the needed skill.*" With that caution in mind, I present strategies for keeping data across the continuum of naturalness: (a) data collection during structured activities (e.g., drill, drill-play, hybrid) and (b) data collection during naturalistic activities. In all cases, the goal of data collection is to track the client's behavior from one session to another, document the efficacy of the intervention, and maximize the professional's effectiveness (Roth & Paul, 2007).

Data Collection During Structured Activities. Data collection in drill and drill-play activities is typically straightforward since the behaviors are adult-directed and highly controlled. The interventionist documents the type of child response (e.g., signed, gestured, verbal) and the degree or type of practitioner prompting. Typically, the practitioner compares a child's behaviors before, during, and after intervention. Sometimes a graph is used to document change; a **graph** is a visual representation of the occurrence of a behavior over time. The data obtained prior to intervention is called the **baseline.**

In the graph shown in Figure 4.5, the baseline of the child's productions of two-word combinations prior to intervention is documented on the first section of the graph on the *x*-axis (i.e. horizontal axis); the *x*-axis represents the session occurrence (i.e., Session 1, Session 2). The frequency of the child's spontaneous production of two-word combinations is represented by the *y*-axis (i.e., the vertical axis). During the intervention, the practitioner uses strong modeling techniques. The child's increasing production of two-word utterances is shown as higher data points on the *y*-axis.

As shown in Figure 4.5, the interventionist also documents the child's use of two-word phrases in a generalization probe. In the **generalization probe,** the practitioner does not use the strong modeling used during the intervention phase, but rather interacts in a typical back-and-forth interaction and documents the child's use of two-word phrases under more natural circumstances. In this case, the child demonstrates continued two-word productions, indicating he has generalized the behavior following the intervention phase.

As an alternative to graphing the results, sometimes the interventionist counts the occurrence of a behavior and represents it as a percentage. As an example, at the

Figure 4.5 **Graph of Intervention Data**

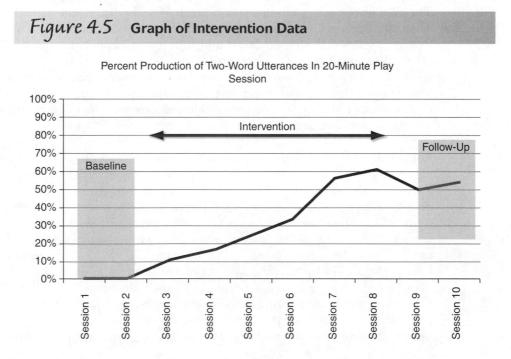

Percent Production of Two-Word Utterances In 20-Minute Play Session

baseline phase the professional reports: *Donald spontaneously produced 2% two-word utterances in a baseline probe during a 5-minute drill-play activity.* At the intervention and follow-up phases the professional documents changes in Donald's production levels with percentages. In order to compute a percentage, the practitioner counts all of Donald's verbal productions (one- and two-word productions) and then divides the number of two-word productions by the total number of utterances. Here is an example:

$$\frac{10\,(\text{two-word productions})}{30\,(\text{one-word and two-word productions})} = 10/30 = 33.3\%\ \text{two-word productions}$$

Practitioners often develop simple data sheets to record the child's productions as they occur during the intervention session. An example of a recording sheet is provided in Figure 4.6.

Figure 4.6 Data Recording Sheet

Student	Objectives:
1.	
2.	
3.	
4.	

Date	Attendance		Objective/Methods/Materials	Notes
	1			
	2			
	3			
	4			
Data Collection				
	1			
	2			
	3			
	4			
Data Collection				

Data Collection in Naturalistic Activities.   To collect data during naturalistic conditions, the interventionist can videotape interactions. Videotaping allows the practitioner to review an interaction and count behaviors or code the quality of a communication behavior. Alternately, the practitioner conducts direct observations. If, as an example, a student's communication goal is to increase assertive communication acts, the practitioner may observe the first ten minutes of the school day and document the student's use of topic initiations and social greetings in the classroom. Sometimes parents and teachers assist in collecting behavioral observations; they provide a summary of the number of times (or the duration of a behavior) as it occurred over a class period or conversation.

Rubrics are used to evaluate the qualitative nature of behaviors in naturalistic setting. The use of goal attainment scaling is a sophisticated use of a rubric. A **goal attainment scale** (GAS) is an individualized, criterion-referenced approach (Roach & Elliott, 2005). GAS allows the practitioner to document a student's baseline performance and numerically record behavioral changes. Steps in developing GAS include (1) selecting a target behavior, (2) describing the desired behavior or academic outcome in objective terms, and (3) developing three to five descriptions of the probable outcomes from least desirable to most desirable. By using numerical ratings for descriptive levels of functioning the practitioner documents student progress (Roach & Elliot, 2005).

To complete GAS, the practitioner includes a descriptive word or percentages indicating variation in the child's performance level ranging from a −2 to +2 level. For example, *Johanna never produces possessive pronouns correctly during a grade-level writing activity* is an example of a −2 level goal. In contrast, the goal *Johanna always uses possessive pronouns correctly in a grade-level writing task* represents a +2 level goal. Zero on GAS indicates the student's behavior is unchanged. In other words, zero reflects the student's baseline behavior.

Examples of descriptive vocabulary capturing the −2 to +2 variation include:

- *Frequency* (never—sometimes—very often—almost always—always)
- *Quality* (poor—fair—good—excellent)
- *Development* (not present—emerging—developing—accomplished—exceeding)
- *Usage* (unused—inappropriate use—appropriate use—exceptional use)
- *Timeliness* (late—on time—early)
- *Percent complete* (0%—25%—50%—75%—100%)
- *Accuracy* (totally incorrect—partially correct—totally correct)
- *Effort* (not attempted—minimal effort—acceptable effort—outstanding effort)
- *Amount of support needed* (totally dependent—extensive assistance—some assistance—limited assistance—independent)
- *Engagement* (none—limited—acceptable—exceptional)

Figure 4.7 documents a student's goal attainment scores over time. In this example, Brittany's initial production of past tense verbs in her written work was 25%. Interventions included one-on-one conversations discussing real-life events using past tense verbs (teacher uses a nonverbal signal to indicate past tense verb production), guided practice to help Brittany write sentences using past tense verbs, posting a

Figure 4.7 Goal Attainment Scale

Objective: Brittany correctly produces past tense verbs.

+2: Brittany uses past tense verbs correctly 70% of the time when writing about a past event in a written assignment of at least 20 sentences.

+1: Brittany uses past tense verbs correctly 31–69% of the time when writing about a past event in a written assignment of at least 20 sentences.

0: Brittany uses past tense verbs correctly 20–30% of the time when writing about a past event in a written assignment of at least 20 sentences.

−1: Brittany uses past tense verbs correctly 11–19% of the time when writing about a past event in a written assignment of at least 20 sentences.

−2: Brittany uses past tense verbs correctly less than 11% of the time when writing about a past event in a written assignment of at least 20 sentences.

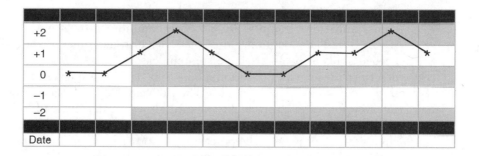

word list of regular and irregular past tense verbs near Brittany's desk, frequent checks of Brittany's independent work, and monitoring daily written assignments for past tense verb use. The target (+2) was written as: Brittany uses past tense verbs correctly 70% of the time when writing about a past event in a written assignment of at least 20 sentences. The teacher documented Brittany's use of past tense verbs for approximately 6 weeks. Examination of the GAS ratings demonstrated improvements on the target behavior on 60% of the assessment dates. The practitioner observed that Brittany's conversational use of past tense verbs also improved.

Summary

- Speech-language pathologists (SLPs) and educators consider a variety of issues with regard to intervention stimuli. Stimuli can either be nonlinguistic or linguistic and can be presented via pictures, objects, or computers. Prompts, shaping, and fading techniques are used in conjunction with stimuli to provide varying levels of support. Reinforcement can be primary (i.e., food) or social; reinforcement schedules are varied based on the child's needs and the behaviors being trained.

- Language facilitators use modeling techniques that are contingent on child interests and behaviors to facilitate children's language production. *Self talk* is language in which the adult describes what he is thinking, feeling, or seeing. In contrast, *parallel talk* is when the adult describes the child's actions. Both self talk and parallel talk facilitate child language output. Once a child produces a phrase or sentence, the adult uses *expansions* and *extensions* to modify a child's simple sentences into more sophisticated sentence constructions and to add related information. When using *sentence recasts* the adult changes the sentence modality to highlight specific linguistic features. In *focused stimulation* a child is exposed to multiple examples of a linguistic target within a meaningful communication context. Modeling techniques are based on social interaction theory. Social interaction theory maintains that children benefit from the support of a more skilled language user; with repeated supported exposure, children internalize underlying concepts and become independent language producers.

- The *assertiveness-responsiveness scheme* is a way for the interventionist to profile an individual's ability to initiate conversational turns and respond to others' communication attempts. An effective communicator is both assertive and responsive. The practitioner uses the scheme to determine if the child has the needed skills to be an effective communicator. The *continuum of naturalness* describes the activities, location, and social aspects of intervention. The practitioner considers these variables when developing an intervention program. Intervention varies from highly unnatural (e.g., adult directed, drill activities) versus highly natural (child directed, in the child's home or classroom, with the child's family or peers). The practitioner chooses between natural versus unnatural variables depending on the intervention goal and the child's abilities.

- Practitioners make intervention decisions based on a child's abilities with regard to form, content, and use. If a child has errors in form, the professional uses strategies to make certain the discourse facilitates the child's production of the required form, makes certain that targeted features are easily detected, notes a child's errors and absence of linguistic features, and chooses intermediate-level targets. Intervention related to content focuses on highlighting the semantic transparency of vocabulary and choosing Tier 2 level vocabulary with older children. Pragmatic intervention focuses on a child's ability to take conversational turns and initiate conversation. Pragmatic intervention with young children often includes parent training; parents learn to facilitate optimal parent-child conversations.

- A hierarchy of research quality is used to rank the scientific merit of a particular intervention with respect to evidence-based practice (EBP). Level I research, evidence resulting from randomized experimental research, is considered the best or "gold standard" research design. Level II research reflects high quality, but nonrandomized, experiments. Level III evidence represents well-designed nonexperimental studies; Level IV represents expert opinions. When using EBP to guide intervention, professionals consider internal evidence (i.e., client and clinician factors and theoretical support for an approach) and external evidence (i.e., research, case studies, and expert opinion).

- A goal is made up of three components, the *do* statement, the *condition* statement, and the *criterion* statement. The *do* statement describes the behaviors the child will produce. The *condition* statement describes the situation or conditions under which the behavior will occur; the *criterion* statement reflects how the goal will be measured.
- Data collection can be either qualitative or quantitative. Qualitative measures include rubrics, goal attainment scaling, or rating naturalistic interactions. Quantitative data are often computed with percentages or represented on graphs.

Discussion and In-Class Activities

1. In your small group, role-play intervention sessions for a 4-year-old child with (a) a pragmatic deficit, (b) a semantic deficit, and (c) a morphosyntax deficit. In each case, demonstrate the use of a variety of stimuli (i.e., pictures, objects, computers), reinforcement (i.e., primary, secondary), and varying use of prompts. Have students evaluate the different techniques and discuss the strengths and weakness of the demonstrated approaches.

2. Your instructor will show you videotapes of language intervention. After watching the session, identify the intervention goal, the prompts used by the adult, and the adult's evaluation of the child's responses. Discuss if you believe this was a successful session. Why or why not? What could have been changed to make the session more effective? As a second activity, develop a strategy for recording the child's behaviors. Watch the session a second time and record and evaluate the child's responses. Did everyone in the class evaluate the child's behaviors in the same way? How could the data collection procedure be modified to increase the reliability of the scoring method?

3. Brainstorm Tier 2 vocabulary that could be introduced to (a) a first grader who needs to use more interesting verbs, (b) a third grader who writes only sentences with Tier 1 vocabulary (e.g, "*The boy walks to his house*"), or (c) a fifth grader who is writing a report on Native Americans. Use a thesaurus or the Internet to develop a word list.

4. Pick one of the following topics and identify studies documenting the effectiveness of the approach. Determine if the study represents Level I, Level II, Level III, or Level IV scientific evidence. Topics include Fast ForWord, narrative intervention, print referencing, explicit phonological awareness intervention, milieu intervention, routine-based intervention, semantic mapping, Hanen Early Language Program, and self-regulated strategy development.

5. Write intervention goals for (a) a 3-year old child, (b) a 6-year-old child, and (c) a 12-year-old child. Make sure the goal contains a *do* statement, a *condition* statement, and a *criterion* statement. Indicate if the goal is focused on form, content, or use. Describe where the goal would be placed on the continuum of naturalness.

Chapter 4 Case Study

You are an SLP in a community speech-language hearing clinic. Your department supervisor assigns two new children to your caseload. You review their files; the first child, Cole, is 2 years, 6 months old, the second child, Maria, is 5.

Cole has no known developmental delays other than his language delay. His hearing is normal and his physical development is within normal limits. He appears to understand most of what is said to him but only uses a few words spontaneously (i.e., "*pizza*," "*no*"). During communication interactions he responds to what others say with physical actions and some word imitations but rarely initiates communication. Cole's parents are anxious to work with their son at home and want to be involved in the intervention program.

Maria is in kindergarten and is learning to read but is at the low end of academic performance as compared to other children her age. She is a personable child and makes friends easily. She produces a variety of grammar errors in her spoken language. Most noticeable are her incorrect use of prepositions (*on, under, in*) and her lack of possessive forms ("*Mother dress*" instead of "*Mother's dress*").

Questions for Discussion

1. Does Cole's primary language deficit represent form, content, or use? Does Maria's primary language deficit represent form, content, or use?

2. How would you describe Cole's and Maria's communication pattern using Fey's assertiveness-responsiveness scheme? How will you use this information to frame your overall intervention plans?

3. Using the continuum of naturalness, what kind of intervention will be most appropriate for Cole and Maria (i.e., child-directed, hybrid, adult-directed)? Provide a rationale for your answer.

4. What kinds of suggestions will you give to Cole's parents? Role-play your session in which you explain the language techniques you would like them to use.

5. Your department supervisor asks you to provide a rationale for your intervention plans for Cole and Maria. Explain your rationale; use one or more language theories (e.g., behaviorism, social interaction, cognitive theory) to support your intervention programs for Cole and Maria. Write language goals for Maria and Cole. How will you document change within their intervention programs?

Children with Specific Language Impairment

Chapter Overview Questions

1. What criteria are used to diagnose a child with specific language impairment (SLI)? How does SLI differ from the term *late talker*?
2. What is the primary language deficit of children with SLI? Give examples.
3. What are some intervention approaches used as part of social communication intervention?

4. How does language theory guide assessment? Explain two assessment protocols and describe their theoretical framework.
5. Describe three different intervention approaches appropriate for children with SLI. How do the interventions differ in theoretical stance and approach?

In this chapter, I present information about children who have **specific language impairment** (SLI). One of the most common reasons children are referred to the SLP is because of delayed expressive language development (Rescorla & Lee, 2000). Children with SLI have a language deficit, but without accompanying factors such as hearing loss, low intelligence scores, or neurological damage. While most children appear to learn language effortlessly, children who are SLI struggle to become effective language users.

This chapter is an important component of your clinical training. Many children—those with SLI and those with other diagnoses—have significant difficulties with syntax and morphological skills, as well as associated deficits in semantics and pragmatics. The information in this chapter will be widely applicable in your future clinical work.

Definition, Prevalence, Causation, and Major Characteristics

DEFINITION

Specific language impairment is a diagnosis based on **exclusionary criteria**. This means that other possible causes of language impairment must be eliminated as possible reasons for a child's language delay. The exclusionary characteristics of SLI include (a) a language test score -1.25 standard deviations or lower (corresponding to a standard score of 81 or lower on a test with a mean of 100), (b) nonverbal IQ of 85 or higher indicating that intellectual function is within normal limits, (c) normal hearing as determined by a hearing screening, (d) no oral structural or oral motor abnormalities, (e) no evidence of neurological disorder, and (f) within-normal social ability (i.e., the child is not on the autism spectrum). As you can see, many possible deficits must be excluded before a child is diagnosed as SLI. It is a clinical dilemma that some children do not meet all of the criteria for SLI but also do not fit into any other diagnostic category. Approximately 15% of children who are clinically considered to be SLI do not meet all the SLI criteria (Tomblin, 1996). However, since SLPs and special educators treat children and not disorder types, the lack of a clear diagnosis for a child's language disorder is not a significant clinical concern.

The *Diagnostic and Statistical Manual of Mental Disorders, Fourth Edition–Text Revision* (DSM-IV) (American Psychiatric Association [APA] 2000) lists three major subtypes of SLI; a major delay in receptive language, a major delay in expressive language, or a delay in both receptive and expressive language.

Some literature refers to a young child under the age of 4 with a language delay as a **late talker** rather than using the SLI classification. The term *late talker* is used because not all children with early language delay continue to have language impairment; in fact only 25–50% of children who are language delayed as toddlers go on to have long-term language impairments (Weiss, 2001). At present, there is a lack of agreement among professionals about when the term *late talker* should be used versus the term *SLI*. The fact that some late talkers catch up with their peers does not minimize the importance of early intervention for young children with language delay (Leonard, 1998).

PREVALENCE AND CAUSATION

The prevalence of SLI is 7% (Fox, Dodd, & Howard, 2002). There are discrepancies in the findings related to gender and SLI. While some experts report that SLI occurs more frequently in males than females, at a ratio of 3:1 (Leonard, 1998), other researchers have not found a greater occurrence in males (Tomblin et al., 1997).

In recent years, there has been a major breakthrough in genetic research: A gene locus has been identified in families with a history of severe speech and language impairments (Marcus & Fisher, 2003). This finding corroborates other literature indicating that a child with SLI is more likely to have a family member with language impairment as compared to a child who is not language impaired (Gopnick, 1990). Consequently, most experts now believe there is a genetic basis for SLI (Rice, 2000).

An extension of this genetic research includes studies determining how an inherited condition contributes to children's language-learning problems. Currently, two theories predominate (Leonard, Eyer, Bedore, & Grela, 1997). The first is called the **extended optional infinitive theory.** It proposes that young children with language impairment persist in using unmarked verbs (e.g., *walk* versus *walking, walks,* or *walked*) well beyond the point when children with normal language discontinue this pattern (Rice, Wexler, & Cleave, 1995). The second is called the **surface theory** proposing that morphemes' short duration and unstressed pronunciation contribute to learning difficulties for children with SLI (Leonard, McGregor, & Allen, 1992). In other words, morphological features are fleeting within spoken language and, as such, are difficult to comprehend. In the future, it is hoped that with gene identification and specific behavioral descriptions linked to inherited characteristics, practitioners will be able to implement highly targeted treatment approaches (Rice, 2000).

Along with genetic factors, a child's environment also affects language development. While it is true limited language stimulation negatively impacts children's language development, a lack of language stimulation is not typically the reason for most language impairments. Instead, experts believe that children with SLI require more intense and focused stimulation to become language proficient as compared with children who are developing typically.

Although the environment typically is not the cause of SLI, the practitioner knows that parent–child communication patterns should be monitored and sometimes modified to foster language. Communication is a two-way street; when a child fails to produce language, it is easy for parents to develop nonfacilitating communication patterns. For example, parents may be more conversationally directive with children who are language impaired. **Directive language** occurs when a parent requests that a child say or do something, or when the adult asks many questions (Pellegrini, McGillicuddy-DeLisi, Sigel, & Brody, 1986). The overuse of directive language is a concern because children with language impairments respond less positively to maternal use of commands and questions as compared to typical peers (Rabidoux & MacDonald, 2000; Rescorla & Fechnay, 1996).

In your work as an SLP or educator, you will determine if parents should modify their communication patterns as part of the overall intervention program. The play-based assessment, described below, is one approach often used to assess parent-child communication patterns. The enhanced milieu approach, also discussed below, is an intervention approach targeting parent-child interactions.

MAJOR CHARACTERISTICS

The morphosyntax features of language are the primary deficit for children with SLI. While children with SLI generally develop morphosyntax features in the same developmental sequence as their peers, they take longer to reach the same linguistic milestones (Tallal, 1988; Rescorla & Lee, 2000). Refer to Chapter 1 for a review of the terminology *syntax, morpheme,* and *morphosyntax.*

Specific morphemes are particularly problematic for children with SLI. Challenging morphemes include (a) verb forms (e.g., third person singular *s,* past tense *ed,* copula verbs [*is, are*], auxiliary verbs [*is, are, do, can*]), (b) articles (*a, the*), (c) possessive *'s,* and (d) pronouns (Rescola & Lee, 2000; Rice & Body, 1993). Table 5.1 provides an expanded list of morphosyntax features frequently delayed in children with SLI. As you can see from examining Table 5.1, research on morphosyntax primarily was completed during the 1970s and 1980s. Practitioners should remember that in some homes children do not hear or use General

Table 5.1 **Morphosyntax Deficits in Children with SLI**

Morphosyntax	Example of error	Citations
• *ing* (present progressive verb)[1]	*"Dog eat him food."* (The dog is ea*ting* his food.)	Albertini, 1980
• Plural */s/*[2]	*"Me got two cat."* (I have two cats.)[3]	Crystal, Fletcher, & Garman, 1989; Leonard, Bortolini, Caselli, McGregor, & Sabbadini, 1992
• *Wh* questions	*"What we can make?"* (What can we make?) *"What do you think what the boy broke?"* (What do you think the boy broke?)	Ingram, 1972a; Smith, 1992
• Prepositions *in* and *on*	*"Mommy put table, my book."* (Mommy put my book *on* the table.)	Albertini, 1980
• More likely to use demonstratives (*this, that, these, those*) without a paired noun	*"This mine!"* (*This book* is mine!)	Morehead & Ingram, 1973
• Pronoun usage, particularly the nominative (subject) case	*"Her sleeping."* (*She* is sleeping.) *"Me want it."* (*I* want it.)	Loeb & Leonard, 1988
• Difficulty using auxiliary verbs (e.g., *is, do, can*)	*"Sara do it!"* (Sara *can* do it!)	Hadley & Rice, 1996; Ingram, 1972b; Leonard, 1991; Rice, Wexler, & Cleave, 1995
• Difficulty with adverbials (omits adverbial in obligatory context)	*"We left."* (We left on Saturday.)	Wren, 1980
• Produce three-element noun phrases (determiner + adjective + noun) less frequently as compared to typically developing peers	*"The girl here. The girl big."* (The big girl is here.)	Gavin, Klee, & Membrino, 1993

Morphosyntax	Example of error	Citations
• Difficulty with copula *be* verb	*"Me Batman today!"* (I *am* Batman today!)	Cleave & Rice, 1995; Ingram, 1972b; Leonard et al., 1992
• Difficulty using articles (*a*, *the*)	*"Give me cookie, OK?"* (Give me *a* cookie, OK?)	Albertini, 1980; Lee, 1996; Leonard et al., 1992
• Pronoun case marking	*"Her do it." "That him bike."* (*She* can do it. That is *his* bike.)	Lee, 1996
• Possessive *'s*	*"That mommy coat."* (That is *Mommy's* coat.)	Albertini, 1980
• Regular past tense[1]	*"He push him."* (He *pushed* him.)	Loeb & Leonard, 1988; Rice et al., 1995
• Third person singular verbs[1]	*"Daddy fix cars."* (Daddy *fixes* cars.)	Gopnik, 1990; Leonard et al., 1992; Rice et al., 1995
• Difficulty with embedded clauses in *wh* questions	*"What do you think what Sara broke?"* (What do you think *that she broke?*)	Smith, 1992

[1] In general, children with SLI use more bare stem verbs (verbs without markings) as compared to typical peers; consequently they have difficulty with a variety of verb tense markers (Fletcher & Peters, 1984).

[2] This is controversial; some investigators have reported that plural forms are not deficient in children with SLI (Oetting & Rice, 1993; Rice & Oetting, 1993)

[3] Plural deletions with the use of numerical word (*two*) also can be a dialectal error, but in this example, it is meant to illustrate the omission of plural form.

American English dialect; dialects are characterized by distinct variations in morphosyntax structure. A child who is using his or her home dialect (and demonstrating the variations consistent with that dialect) should not be erroneously classified as SLI. Learn more about dialectal morphosyntax variations in Focus 5.1.

FOCUS 5.1 *Multicultural Issues*

A morphological feature of African American English (AAE) includes use of subject and verb that differ in either number or person. For example, a speaker who uses AAE might say *"What do this mean?"* (Washington & Craig, 1984). Another morphosyntax variation in AAE is nonobligatory use of the auxiliary *is* within the present progressive verb (*"He working"* instead of *"He is working"*). Skilled professionals consider a child's home dialect when determining his or her language abilities. Learn more about AAE in Chapter 11 and by checking out the information at this Web site: www.speechpathology.com/articles/article detail.asp?article id=287

As you might expect, when there is a primary deficit in morphosyntax, there is a trickle-down effect that impacts other aspects of language ability and academic functioning. This is certainly the case for children with SLI. For example, as children with SLI enter school, they have difficulty with the more sophisticated language needed for academics. Written language has more compound and complex sentences than spoken language. Children with SLI have difficulty with syntactically complex sentences and use embedded clauses less often than children who are developing typically (Gillam & Johnston, 1992). Figure 5.1 demonstrates how the morphosyntax of children with SLI lags behind that of their typical peers.

Semantic skills also are affected. Children with SLI have difficulty with vocabulary development. This pattern of slower vocabulary growth is seen in children at very young ages. Children with SLI often produce word combinations up to $3\frac{1}{2}$ years behind their peers and have difficulty learning to use verbs (Morehead & Ingram, 1973). Children with SLI use a smaller variety of verbs relying on a handful of high frequency verbs such as *want, get,* and *like*. Experts believe that the lexical problems of children with SLI relate to (a) the additional time needed for word retrieval, (b) decreased ability to expand new object names to objects in the same semantic category, and (c) the need to learn new words embedded within simple versus complex sentences (Ravid, Levie, & Avivi Ben-zvi, 2003).

The trickle-down effect also impacts pragmatic development in children who are SLI. For example, when communicating with adults, preschoolers with language impairment are less likely to initiate topics. Their conversational turns are more likely to merely acknowledge the communication partner's utterance instead of offering new information.

Pragmatic difficulties continue as children with SLI reach school age with resulting social communication problems. **Social communication problems** are limitations in an individual's social, cognitive, and language skills necessary for contextually appropriate, meaningful, and effective interpersonal communication (Adams, 2005).

As an example of social communication problems, older children with SLI have difficulty entering into peer-group conversations and struggle to make conversational repairs such as clarifying their communication when there is a conversational breakdown (Craig & Washington, 1993). Children with SLI have less opportunity to practice their communication skills because their typically developing peers tend to dominate shared interactions. Consequently, an unfortunate situation begins when children with poor language ability have reduced opportunity to practice and improve their communication performance. A negative cycle is created in which children with SLI fall farther and farther behind their peers in their social communication (Rice, Sell, & Hadley, 1991).

Other problems face children with SLI during their school years. For example, children with SLI are less adept telling an organized and elaborated narrative. A narrative is an oral or written monologue following formalized conventions; in simplest terms, a narrative is a story with a beginning, middle, and end. (I describe narrative assessment and intervention in more detail in Chapter 9.) The narratives of children with SLI contain fewer words and utterances and often lack a well-formed story

Figure 5.1 Comparison of Development of Children With and Without Specific Language Impairment

	Years																					
	2									3						4						5
										Months												
	18	20	22	24	26	28	30	32	34	36	38	40	42	44	46	48	50	52	54	56	58	60

Children developing typically (Typical age of development)

- 2-word phrases produced
- Plural /s/; auxiliary *be* emerges[1]
- *in/on, ing, 's* > 80%[5]
- MLU of 4.2[2]
- Mastery of copula and auxiliary *be* and auxiliary *do*[2]

Children who are SLI (Evidence of delayed production)

- 2-word phrases[4]
- MLU 2.6[2]
- Auxiliary *be* emerging for some children with SLI[1]
- Prepositions *in/on*
- 50% of children with SLI still having difficulty with copula and auxiliary *be* and *do* at 5–6 years[3]

[1] Hadley & Rice, 1996
[2] Roberts, Rescorla, & Borneman, 1994
[3] Rice & Wexler, 1995
[4] Trauner, Wulfeck, Tallal, & Hesselink, 2000
[5] Albertini, 1980

structure. Difficulty producing high-quality narratives affects children's social interactions and literacy development.

Research on the social challenges associated with SLI has influenced many professionals to include social and pragmatic interventions for children with language impairments. Early intervention can prevent a negative cycle of social and academic failure. A social peer-based approach to intervention is discussed in the *Connections* section below.

Children with SLI also have more frequent phonological impairments than their typically developing peers; about 40% of children with SLI have associated speech problems (Beitchman, Nair, Clegg, Ferguson, & Patel, 1986). The phonological differences emerge at an early age. For example, toddlers with SLI have smaller consonantal and vowel inventories and use a more restricted and less mature variety of syllable shapes as compared to their typically developing peers (Rescorla & Ratner, 1996). An example of a simple syllable shape is a consonant-vowel (CV) combination (e.g., *toe*); a more complex syllable pattern is a CCV (e.g., *play*) or a CVC (e.g., *hat*). Phonological and articulation deficits continue to be problematic during later years, resulting in reduced speech intelligibility.

ASSOCIATED PROBLEMS

Research demonstrates that children with SLI need more time to process information than children developing typically; this finding supports the claim that children with SLI have capacity limitations in their cognitive processing resources (Weismer & Thordardottir, 2002). The slower rate of processing results in reduced ability to rapidly name pictures and recognize words. The rate of **nonword repetition tasks** (i.e., repetition of nonsense words) also is reduced in children with SLI; the use of a nonword repetition task has been proposed as way to differentiate children with and without SLI (Weismer & Thordardottir, 2002).

Although the diagnosis of SLI excludes children with significant motor or neurological impairment, research has found evidence of neurological soft signs. **Neurological soft signs** are behaviors consistent with a neurological impairment; however, the brain scan of an individual with neurological soft signs does not show hard evidence of neurological damage. Neurological soft signs in children with SLI include higher incidence of difficulty with chewing, sucking, and drooling indicating potential oral-motor weakness (Whitehurst & Fischel, 1994); slight motor differences (i.e., children with SLI sometimes are reported as "clumsy" or "accident prone;" Tallal, Ross, & Curtiss, 1989); and a higher frequency of visual-motor integration problems (Beitchman et al., 1989).

A higher-than-expected proportion of children who are SLI are diagnosed with **attention-deficit/hyperactivity disorder (ADHD)**. In fact, 59% of children with significant levels of SLI also are diagnosed with ADHD (Beitchman, Hood, Rochon, & Peterson, 1989). Children with SLI with significant levels of receptive language impairment appear to be the most likely to exhibit behaviors of impulsivity, high activity, and distractibility associated with the ADHD diagnosis (Cantwell & Baker, 1987). Attention deficits likely contribute to language learning difficulties for many children with language impairment. Practitioners compensate for diminished attention capacity by providing repeated and focused stimulation of targeted linguistic structures and facilitating increasingly longer periods of sustained attention.

Approximately 80% of school-age children with SLI experience reading problems (Botting, Simkin, & Conti-Ramsden, 2006; Catts, Fey, Tomblin, & Zhang, 2002). It has been suggested that SLI and dyslexia are linked, with SLI forming a dyslexia subgroup. In this theory, children with SLI exhibit a more severe form of dyslexia in that they have phonological awareness difficulties associated with dyslexia in addition to morphosyntax problems (Bishop & Snowling, 2004). **Phonological awareness deficits** result in problems detecting, segmenting, and blending sounds in words, hindering children's **reading decoding** (e.g., sounding out and spelling words during reading and writing).

Writing, along with reading, poses challenges. Children with SLI demonstrate frequent grammatical errors in their writing and have difficulty with written verb morphology (Scott, 2002; Scott & Windsor, 2000). Complex sentence formation difficulty also affects writing performance. Children with SLI rarely write sentences with more than one subordinate clause. Spelling difficulties also are common and may be linked to underlying phonological, morphological, and semantic deficits (Apel, Masterson, & Niessen, 2004). Focus 5.2 gives more information about the support of reading development in school-age children. I discuss reading, writing, and spelling interventions for students with language impairments in Chapter 9.

FOCUS 5.2 *School-Age Children*

Reading demands coordinated use of high-level language skills. Children need a more sophisticated vocabulary and must be able to comprehend low-frequency syntax structures (e.g., passive sentences, embedded subordinate clauses, elaborated noun phrases) that more frequently occur in written language as compared to oral discourse (Wright & Newhoff, 2001). Other skills such as phonological awareness, print concepts, alphabetic knowledge, and spelling conventions also impact literacy development. In recent years, SLPs and educators have begun to directly support children's reading and writing development. During intervention with school-age children with SLI and associated reading and writing deficits, practitioners should do the following (American Speech-Language-Hearing Association, 2001):

- Integrate spoken and written language targets; students should alternate between reading, writing, and oral productions.
- Assist children in decoding/encoding and comprehending language at the sound, syllable, word, sentence, and discourse levels.
- Help children form associations between how groups of letters look, sound, and feel in the mouth, and link this awareness to word recognition and spelling skills.
- Develop children's meta-awareness of spoken and written language and facilitate students' use of computers and software to strategically support written language.

Connections

Children with SLI do not function socially like children with normal language development (Craig, 1993). Throughout this book, I describe how social interaction theory and the systems approach provide the theoretical base for many aspects of language intervention. Once again, these theories underscore the need to directly focus on the peer relationships of children with SLI. I describe peer-mediated intervention in this *Connections* section because peer-mediated social communication intervention is a form of intervention appropriate for students with a variety of disorders, such as students with intellectual disabilities or students who are on the autism spectrum (Goldstein, Schneider, & Thiemann, 2007).

CHILDREN'S SOCIAL COMMUNICATION

Peer-mediated treatment is a form of intervention focusing on a student's social communication. To facilitate social communication, practitioners follow one of three basic treatment paradigms (Hadley & Schuele, 1998). The first, **social intervention** with peers, involves identifying a social skill hierarchy, teaching the student with the communication disorder specific social skill strategies, and facilitating the student's use of social strategies with his or her peer group. The second paradigm is called **peer confederate training.** In confederate training, students with typical language are trained to use social strategies to encourage communication from students with communication disorders. The third paradigm, **sociodramatic script training,** involves engaging children in opportunities to role-play **social scripts** (Goldstein & Cisar, 1992). A social script is a repeated social interaction likely to occur in daily life; examples of social scripts include greeting, interactions over lunchtime or during recess, asking a friend to play, or joining in a group activity. During script training the adult uses role-play and cuing to familiarize the student with daily discourse routines. Below I describe two important social interactions for young children with communication impairments: peer entry and cooperative play. Following this information, I discuss issues of peer interaction for older students with communication impairments.

Peer Entry.   In order for a child to enter into a group-play situation, he or she must display a combination of verbal and nonverbal skills. Typically, children demonstrate 10 or more entry behaviors before being included in a group-play activity (Timler, Olswang, & Coggins, 2005b). Entry behaviors include low risk behaviors such as engaging in a similar activity as the other children in the group and high risk behaviors such as commenting on the activity or requesting to join the activity. It is interesting that positive comments about the activity have been identified as being a more successful means of gaining entry than asking to join the activity (Timler et al., 2005b). The hovering behavior often demonstrated by children with SLI is not a successful strategy; neither is directly demanding to be included, responding negatively to a peer's communication or activity, or ignoring others' comments and requests. Figure 5.2 is an example of a positive peer entry strategy.

Figure 5.2 **Child Entering Peer Group**

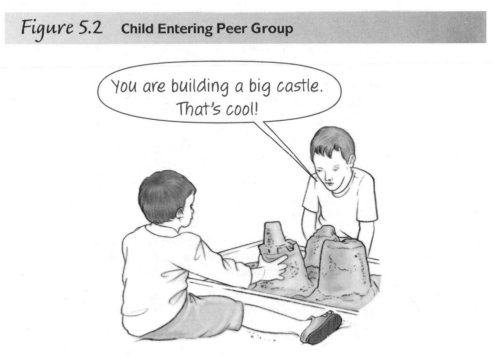

Cooperative Play. During cooperative play, children take on specific roles maintained with play organizer statements such as *"Let's say this house is on fire, and we'll both be firemen."* When there are disputes, effective communication strategies involve giving a reason for the problem (*"No, this is the house because, see, here's the roof."*), making a polite request, or suggesting a compromise. In order to be successful during cooperative play, children with SLI must be able to answer peer questions, acknowledge comments, ask for needed information, and comment about the activity.

Peer Interactions for School-Age Students. At older ages, students with language impairments continue to exhibit communication difficulties stemming from pragmatic deficits. Young adults with a history of SLI have few close friends and less-rewarding social relationships (Howlin, Mawhood, & Rutter, 2000). Students with a history of language impairment often have difficulty negotiating conflict and have lower social self-esteem as compared to their typical peers (Wadman, Durkin, & Conti-Ramsden, 2008). Consequently, practitioners continue to facilitate social communication skills for school-age children.

Before initiating a social communication intervention for an older child, the practitioner considers the student's environment by discussing patterns of social communication with the student's teachers, parents, siblings, and peers. Sometimes communication partners unconsciously develop nonfacilitative patterns of communication such as excessive direct questioning or answering questions for the student. The practitioner also talks directly to the student with language impairment about the need for social communication intervention. Teamwork makes it possible to alter the student's environment comprehensively. There is more likely to be a positive outcome when all team members realize changing social behavior is complex and social communication intervention demands significant time and effort (Brinton & Fujiki, 2005).

PEER-MEDIATED INTERVENTION APPROACHES

Intervention Strategies for Young Children.   When working with a young child with communication impairments the practitioner facilitates the child's assertive communication strategies while minimizing ineffective or disruptive strategies (Fujiki & Brinton, 2009). For example, a child with communication impairments may attempt to join a peer group by grabbing group members' toys or without making sufficient eye contact. The following example represents observational notes completed on a child with difficulty during social interaction:

> J outside; running circles around perimeter of the playground. Stops to go down the slide. Then runs to sand area and attempts to pour sand in a bucket with two other girls. Girls tell him to leave (J looks upset), begins to run around the playground again. (Timler, Olswang, & Coggins, 2005b, p. 171)

Timler et al. (2005b) identified intervention targets for children to facilitate (a) peer entry into groups and (b) cooperative play.

a. To facilitate peer entry, the practitioner teaches the child to:
   - Approach peers physically.
   - Watch what peers are doing and imitate the activity.
   - Make a positive statement about the group activity.
b. To improve cooperative play, the practitioner teaches the child to:
   - Establish eye contact.
   - Share play materials.
   - Take turns.
   - Make a play organizer statement, complement peers, request assistance, and offer assistance.
   - If a conflict arises, the child states a reason for the disagreement or suggests a compromise.
   - Answer when a peer asks a question, respond to peers' comments, and maintain the ongoing topic.

The behaviors listed above can be a starting point for identifying the social behaviors potentially limiting a child's peer interactions. Once deficits are identified, the adult continues the intervention by (a) teaching a specific social communication behavior, (b) practicing the behavior with the child in small-group activities, and (c) supporting the child as he or she begins to use the strategy independently.

Intervention Strategies for the School-Age Student.   Experts have proposed a number of intervention approaches to guide social communication interventions for school-age students (Adams, 2005; Timler, Olswang, & Coggins, 2005a). Techniques include increasing the student's ability to take another's perspective, practicing social routines, and understanding hidden meanings.

To facilitate the student's ability to take others' perspectives, the practitioner helps the student use and define emotion words to encourage understanding others' emotions. Some students with communication impairments need to be taught to evaluate a social situation from others' perspectives and to appropriately describe what others may be thinking or feeling.

For example, if you viewed two individuals engaged in a confidential discussion, it is unlikely you would attempt to enter the interaction. In contrast, a student with poor social communication skills may not consider others' nonverbal cues or emotions and attempt to join the discussion. In this case, the professional encourages the student to verbalize what others are thinking or feeling. Following role-playing social scenarios, the student with communication impairment practices answering questions such as, "*What was my friend thinking?*" "*How did my friend feel?*"

The practitioner also uses sociodramatic script training to improve school-age students' communication. The practitioner and student practice established social routines first during role-play and then in everyday situations. As the student gains competence, the practitioner establishes more flexibility by regularly adding small changes to the established routine.

A final intervention goal with older students is to help the student use and understand hidden meanings. Indirect communication is an example of a hidden meaning. For example, if you are at a party and you want to leave, you might say to your partner, "*Wow, it's getting late!*" You use an indirect statement as a subtle indicator that you want to leave the party. Indirect communication can be challenging for an individual with social communication impairments; he or she may not understand or act on the social implications of indirect statements.

Practitioners target indirect language by improving a student's meta-awareness of indirect communication. The practitioner and student view videotaped examples of indirect communication and discuss rules for deciphering hidden meanings. Practitioners sometimes use comic strips as a source of discussion. Students practice interpreting the hidden meanings of the comic strip; learning to explain "what makes it funny" helps the student understand implied meanings behind words.

Assessment

Assessment for the individual with specific language impairment typically includes an in-depth LSA and norm-referenced assessments such as the Preschool Language Scale, 4th edition (PLS-4; Zimmerman, Steiner, & Pond, 2002) or (for older school-age students) the Clinical Evaluation of Language Fundamentals-4 (Semel, Wiig, & Secord, 2003). More examples of norm-referenced assessments appropriate for students with SLI are provided in Chapter 2.

Criterion-referenced assessments also contribute important information with respect to deficits in language form, content, and use in everyday interactions. In this section, I discuss two different criterion-referenced assessment approaches: (a) parent-child toy play and book reading observational assessments and (b) curriculum-based language assessment.

Parent-child interaction assessment and curriculum-based language assessment are two forms of criterion-referenced assessment within an overarching category called naturalistic assessment. **Naturalistic assessment** provides multiple opportunities for an individual to perform skills across domains (i.e., social, cognitive, motor, communication). Naturalistic assessment can be a planned activity (as when the adult sets up toys and observes the child during play) but also includes observation of a child in his classroom or home. It is important to note that the naturalistic approaches described in this chapter also are appropriate for individuals with other types of communication disorders (e.g., children with hearing loss, children with intellectual disability, children on the autism spectrum). Learn more about naturalistic assessment by viewing the video clip at the Web site www.cde.state.co.us/media/resultsmatter/RMSeries/WhatIsAuthenticAssessment.asp.

PARENT–CHILD INTERACTION ASSESSMENTS

Throughout this book, I emphasize how language theory underlies clinical decisions. The relationship between clinical procedures and theory also plays a role in the assessment process. Language theory guides the assessment protocols used within the assessment battery.

Consider, for example, the professional who believes that social interaction theory plays a strong role in language acquisition. As you recall, social interaction theory is based on the theories of Lev Vygotsky. According to Vygotsky (1962), children's development results from social interactions with more capable peers. Within this perspective, as adults identify and interact within children's zone of proximal development, children's development is stimulated. Observations of parent-child book reading and toy play align with the social interaction approach.

To begin the parent-child observation, the assessor supplies appropriate books and toys and asks the child's parents to interact as typically as possible with their child. The assessor includes a variety of books (e.g., alphabet books, storybooks, simple books without text). The assessor also includes a variety of toys to prompt a range of play behavior; toys should include thematic toys (e.g., a farmyard, small "people" figures, vehicles, animals), toys for sociodramatic play (e.g., dishes, dish pan, sponge, baby doll, doll clothing), and toys stimulating motor play (e.g., stacking rings, mailbox with different-sized blocks to be inserted in "mail slots").

There are several advantages and disadvantages to parent-child interaction assessments (Losardo & Notari-Syverson, 2001). Advantages are that (a) young children are more likely to use complex language in child-initiated familiar routines, (b) children are more likely to interact in ways representing their true abilities, and (c) children are more likely to be highly engaged during play activities as compared to more formalized assessment procedures. Disadvantages include the fact that play-based assessments, like other naturalistic assessment protocols, require more planning and more expertise as compared to administration of norm-referenced assessment.

One area of expertise required to complete an effective observation is the assessor's ability to identify the parent's scaffolding strategies and to assess the effects of varying strategies on the child's communication. The term **scaffolding**, introduced in Chapter 1, refers to the graduated assistance provided to novice learners in order to help them achieve higher levels of conceptual and communicative competence. The assessor may use a criterion-referenced assessment tool to document observed parent scaffolding behaviors.

An example of a parent-child observational form used to document book-reading behaviors is shown in Table 5.2. The assessor notes parents' scaffolding strategies that are elaborative (i.e., expanding child utterances) or directive (i.e., asking the child to repeat words, or asking the child to "fill in the blank"; Crain-Thoreson, Dahlin, & Powell, 2001). When used most effectively, scaffolding is faded from levels of high

Table 5.2 **Parent Scaffolding Behaviors During Parent-Child Book Reading**

Child's name:
Book used:
Date:

Book type (alphabet, narrative, rhyming, etc.)

Scaffolding behaviors observed	Child response	Behavioral observations
1. Labeling and commenting	Positive/Negative	
2. Oral dialogue to explain/elaborate text	Positive/Negative	
3. Pauses	Positive/Negative	
4. Sentence recasting or language expansion (i.e., elaborative strategy)	Positive/Negative	
5. Simplified the book's text by simplifying syntax	Positive/Negative	
6. Tag questions (e.g., *"He's big, isn't he?"*)	Positive/Negative	
7. Direct questions (*"Where is the man going?"*) or asking the child to "fill in the blank" (i.e., *"The man is wearing a yellow ___"* (i.e., directive strategy)	Positive/Negative	
8. Follows the child's comment by making a linked comment	Positive/Negative	
9. Retells story by making up own words	Positive/Negative	
10. Other forms noted:	Positive/Negative	

Did the child evidence enjoyment of the book interaction?   YES   NO

Did particular parent scaffolding strategies work well to engage the child? List:

Did the child react negatively to particular scaffolding strategies? List:

If the child evidenced a lack of engagement or interest in the interaction, what scaffolding strategies might be most effective? List:

Further recommendations to improve the quality of book reading interactions: (book type, length of interaction, contextual demands, etc.)

Source: Adapted with permission from "Parent-Child Joint Book Reading: An Observational Protocol for Young Children," by J. N. Kaderavek and E. Sulzby, 1998, *American Journal of Speech-Language Pathology, 7,* pp. 33–47.

support (e.g., providing an imitative model; limiting the child to two choices) to minimal levels of guidance (e.g., asking open-ended questions).

While the assessor is noting parental scaffolding, the assessor also observes the child's responses to the adult's different conversational strategies. Variations in the child's communication and engagement suggest parent language approaches that should be facilitated or reduced. For example, if the child responds more when the parent follows the child's conversational lead—in contrast to the child's response to direct questions— parents can be coached to increase their use of the former conversational strategy.

The assessor also carefully considers the child's play behaviors during the observation. The assessor may choose to apply a Piagetian framework to the parent-child observation. A Piagetian-focused observation is likely to consider the child's ability to use means-end behavior, imitate motor behaviors, manipulate objects in functional ways, and use objects symbolically (see Chapter 1 to review the behaviors associated with Piaget's theories). The Piagetian perspective helps the assessor focus on behaviors associated with the child's level of cognitive development. An example of a criterion-referenced assessment documenting a child's use of sensorimotor, presymbolic, and symbolic play behaviors is shown in Table 5.3.

Table 5.3   Play and Language: Observation Checklist (9–24 months)

Play behaviors observed	Communication and language behaviors observed
9 to 12 months	
_____ Awareness that objects exist when not seen; finds toy hidden under scarf	_____ Sounds rather than language; may have words that are associated with actions
_____ Means-end behavior: crawls or walks to get what he/she wants; pulls string toys	Exhibits following communicative functions:
_____ Does not mouth or bang all toys – some used appropriately, manipulates objects	_____ Request _____ Command
13 to 17 months	
_____ Purposeful exploration of toys; discovers operation of toys through trial and error; uses variety of motoric schemas	_____ Context-dependent single words; for example, child may use the word *car* when riding in a car; words tend to come and go in child's vocabulary
_____ Hands toys to adult if unable to operate	Exhibits following communicative functions (linguistically or nonlinguistically):
	_____ Request _____ Protesting _____ Command _____ Interactional _____ Response _____ Personal _____ Greeting _____ Label

Play behaviors observed	Communication and language behaviors observed

17 to 19 months

_____ Beginning of pretending (early symbolic) play behaviors with himself/herself as agent (e.g., child pretends to go to sleep or pretends to drink from cup or eat from spoon)

_____ Beginning social play; child plays same or similar activity while engaging in social interaction with peer

_____ Uses most common objects and toys appropriately

_____ Tool use (uses stick to reach toy)

Beginning of true verbal communication. Words have following functional and semantic relations:

_____ Recurrence
_____ Agent
_____ Existence
_____ Object
_____ Nonexistence
_____ Action or state
_____ Rejection
_____ Location
_____ Denial

19 to 22 months

Symbolic play extends beyond the child's self:

_____ Plays with dolls; brushes doll's hair, feeds doll a bottle, or covers doll with blanket

_____ Child performs pretend activities on more than one person or object; for example, feeds self, a doll, mother, and another child

_____ Combines two toys in pretend play, for example, puts spoon in pan or pours from pot into cup

_____ Refers to objects and person not present

Beginning of word combinations with following semantic relations:

_____ Agent-action
_____ Action-locative
_____ Action-object
_____ Object-locative
_____ Agent-object
_____ Possessive
_____ Attributive (*many, dirty, big*)
_____ Dative (*that, this*)

24 months

_____ Represents daily experiences; plays house—is the mommy, daddy, or baby; objects used are realistic and close to life size; beginnings of make-believe play

_____ Completes short routines (e.g. puts food in pan, stirs, and eats; stacks and knocks down blocks; pours and dumps sand and water)

_____ Beginnings of cooperative social pretend play; child plays with others (but is not likely to use verbal communication while doing so)

_____ Uses earlier pragmatic functions and semantic relations in phrases and short sentences

Beginning use of morphological markers appear:

_____ Present progressive (*ing*) on verbs
_____ Plurals
_____ Possessives

Sources: Adapted with permission from "Assessment of Cognitive and Language Abilities Through Play," by C. E. Westby, 1980, *Language, Speech, and Hearing Services in Schools, 11*, pp. 154–168. Copyright 1980 by American Speech-Language-Hearing Association. All rights reserved.

Last, but not least, a parent-child observational assessment can be framed within a behaviorist perspective. A professional coming from a behaviorist position is likely to take note of slightly different aspects of a child's behavior. With this perspective, the assessor documents the occurrence of target behaviors and notes the antecedent events and reinforcements that precede and follow each behavior.

You may be thinking that all of this observation takes a very long time! In actuality, the professional moves back and forth between theoretical perspectives and identifies the most relevant aspects needed for each child. But, as I continue to emphasize throughout this book, the skilled professional understands the *why* that drives every clinical activity. Your understanding of the theoretical basis of varying protocols also helps you explain the assessment results to the child's parents and teachers.

CURRICULUM-BASED LANGUAGE ASSESSMENT

Curriculum-based language assessment is another naturalistic assessment process; the assessor considers the academic content and social interaction demands of the curriculum, assesses the language skills the student brings to the curriculum, determines the knowledge and language skills the student needs to succeed academically, and identifies instructional modifications to enhance the student's academic success (ASHA, 2001). Curriculum-based language assessment requires the assessor to (a) observe the child in the classroom, (b) identify (with the classroom teacher) aspects of the curriculum that are problematic, (c) consider aspects of the instruction (e.g., Are instructions provided verbally? In writing? What is the language complexity of the instructions?), (d) evaluate student work samples (e.g., written work is evaluated for error patterns), (e) evaluate textbooks and classroom materials to identify vocabulary and/or morphosyntax that is poorly comprehended by the student, and (f) identify strategies that the student can use to organize his or her work or improve performance (Deno, 1992). Learning to implement curriculum-based language assessment is a sophisticated skill that will be fine-tuned during your graduate training.

It is important for practitioners to use curriculum-based language assessment to develop effective interventions for school-age students. To be successful in the classroom, students must learn to identify the most important components for a specific academic task. Good students take this for granted, but it can be challenging for students with language impairments and learning deficits.

For example, imagine that you are conducting a classroom observation as part of your curriculum-based language assessment. You observe that, during a science unit, the teacher asks students to *"summarize what we have learned about butterflies and moths."* The students developing typically immediately begin listing the two categories and noting similarities and differences between the two species. However, the student with language impairment does not use this underlying strategy and his answer is disorganized and incomplete. The information you obtained during the assessment provides data documenting the need to improve the student's organizational strategies and semantic categorization skills.

In another example, you note that a student with language impairment is unable to produce a coherent response to a classroom story-writing assignment.

Her story has no clear plot, lacks descriptive words, and does not indicate cause and effect with conjunctions such as *because*. You note this difficulty, do some more assessment probes on the student's narrative abilities, and develop goals to target narrative production (see Chapter 9 for more information about narrative interventions).

In a final example, you may have a student complete a writing probe. A writing probe is an appropriate assessment protocol for a student whose written work consists of simple sentences, lacks descriptive words, and demonstrates poor punctuation and spelling. You supply a story starter (e.g., *One day I landed on a desert island and* . . . and ask the student to write for 10 minutes). At the end of the 10-minute period, you count the number of complex and compound sentences, evaluate the student's use of descriptive words, and count the number of punctuation and spelling errors. You target some or all of these areas in your intervention and periodically readminister the writing probe to assess progress.

As the examples above demonstrate, an advantage of curriculum-based language assessment is that the assessment procedure results in meaningful intervention goals. Another advantage is that curriculum-based language assessment requires close collaboration between the SLP and classroom teacher; professionals work together to identify areas of academic weakness and develop remediation strategies. This collaboration is likely to improve student outcomes. The disadvantages of curriculum-based language assessment mirror the challenges of other forms of naturalistic assessment. Curriculum-based language assessments are more time-consuming than, for example, norm-referenced assessments. Curriculum-based language assessment procedures also require professional expertise to evaluate curriculum materials and identify student weaknesses within the classroom.

Intervention

I present three interventions in this chapter on SLI: enhanced milieu intervention, sentence recast training, and sentence combining intervention. Milieu and sentence recast training are most appropriate for young children with language impairment while sentence combining (SC) intervention typically is implemented with students who are 5 to 12 years of age.

There are many different approaches that can be implemented for children with language impairments. I have chosen these three approaches for this chapter because they (a) are based on a clear theoretical position, (b) have results published in peer-referred journals, and (c) have data demonstrating efficacy. These three approaches are picked to illustrate variations in interventions for children with SLI; there are dozens of other viable approaches. If you are a member of the National Student Speech-Language-Hearing Association (NSSLHA), you can access the American Speech-Language-Hearing Association Web site to find additional intervention approaches for children with language impairments: www.asha.org/members/ebp/compendium/default

Remember that language interventions are not necessarily specific to a particular language diagnosis. Interventions designed to be used with children with autism or children with intellectual disabilities may also be appropriate for a child with SLI. The practitioner chooses a treatment not because the child with communication impairment has a particular diagnosis, but instead the professional matches the intervention to the child's deficits within the language domains of form, content, and use.

Imagine that you are working with a child, Samuel, who is 3 years old and has significant social interaction deficits. He has not been diagnosed with an intellectual disability or autism. However, you know that enhancing social interaction skills is a primary intervention goal and you consider using the Floortime approach (Greenspan & Wieder, 1997; Greenspan & Wieder, 1999). Floortime builds parent-child interactions and facilitates child-initiated communication; it was developed for children on the autism spectrum. You may hesitate to use Floortime because Samuel has a language impairment without a diagnosis of autism. Since Samuel has not been diagnosed with autism, does that mean that Floortime is inappropriate? Absolutely not! As a professional who understands (a) how to evaluate a child's communication disorder within the domains of form, content, and use and (b) how to evaluate a specific intervention program, you may well decide that Floortime is a very appropriate approach to develop Samuel's social communication skills.

In the same vein, you may decide to use an approach described in this chapter with an individual who has a diagnosis other than SLI. Children with SLI talk less than their typical peers, have more difficulty learning vocabulary items, and struggle to learn grammatical morphemes. Other children with different communication disorders also have similar communication challenges. For example, you may decide to use the sentence-combining approach with a high-functioning student on the autism spectrum. The skilled professional understands the specific language skills targeted within each approach and chooses an intervention based on this knowledge.

INTERVENTION APPROACH: ENHANCED MILIEU TEACHING (EMT)

Enhanced milieu teaching (EMT) is a naturalistic approach appropriate for children who (a) are able to imitate sounds and words, (b) have a vocabulary of at least 10 words, and (c) have an MLU between 1.0 and 3.5 words (Hancock & Kaiser, 2006). This MLU level is the language stage when children learn lexical items (i.e., words) and semantic relational combinations (e.g., agent + action [*"Mommy go"*], agent + action + object [*"Daddy throw ball"*]). In the EMT approach, parents are trained to be their child's primary language teacher. EMT also is implemented in preschool classrooms or small-group sessions where the practitioner uses EMT language teaching strategies.

On the continuum of naturalness, EMT is considered a hybrid approach midway between highly child-directed and adult-directed intervention (Yoder, Kaiser, & Alpert, 1991). EMT uses simple questions and requests for child imitation along with adult language modeling techniques; the adult uses the language techniques in response to the child's focus of attention. The EMT hybrid approach differs from (a) highly child-directed modeling-only approaches where the adult models language without placing response demands on the child and (b) adult-controlled interventions where intervention often is skill-based with adult-controlled stimuli presentation (Fey, 1986).

EMT is particularly effective for children with relatively low receptive or expressive language levels (i.e., beginning language learners), while children with higher language ability benefit from either a more didactic (i.e., direct teaching and adult-controlled) approach (Yoder, Kaiser, & Alpert, 1991) or a responsive teaching approach in which adults model and expand language forms and promote topic-continuing talk (Yoder et al., 1995). Three theories explain why EMT is effective for children at the earliest stages of language learning.

First, EMT is appropriate for beginning language learners because it implements language teaching during familiar routines and everyday activities (Delprato, 2001). Beginning language learners learn new language forms most easily in familiar and frequently occurring interactions. A beginning language learner is less likely to be able to generalize language forms learned within decontextualized settings; EMT promotes generalization of newly learned communication strategies.

EMT also is an appropriate intervention for beginning language learners because language-teaching episodes are initiated in response to the child's focus of attention. In a didactic, adult-directed approach, stimulus items are preselected (e.g. the adult decides on the targeted vocabulary). In contrast, EMT language facilitation techniques are linked to the child's interest and motivation. For example, if the child points at an item, the adult begins the mand-model teaching sequence by saying "*What do you want?*" (See Table 5.4 for the definition of *mand-model*). Beginning

Table 5.4 **Enhanced Milieu Teaching (EMT) Definitions and Strategies**

Term	Explanation	Use of technique in EMT to facilitate language for child with language impairment
Modeling (See also Chapter 4)	The language trainer notes the child's focus of attention and provides a language model reflecting the child's interest.	The child wants a block to put into the toy mailbox (the mother has the blocks in her lap). The mother says "*Do you want block?*" and motions to the blocks. If the child imitates the model, the mother provides the block and gives a language expansion, "*I want the red block!*" An incorrect or lack of child response triggers a second language model. After a third incorrect child response, the mother restates "*want the block*" and then gives the block to her child.

(continued)

Table 5.4 **Enhanced Milieu Teaching (EMT) Definitions and Strategies (*Continued*)**

Term	Explanation	Use of technique in EMT to facilitate language for child with language impairment
Mand-model procedure	The language trainer uses a verbal prompt in the form of a question ("*What do you want?*"), choice ("*Do you want ___ or ___?*"), or mand ("*Tell me what you want.*")	The child is focusing on an object or activity (in this example he has a piece of paper but nothing to write with); the language trainer provides a prompt connected to the child's interest. Examples include saying, "*What do you want?*", providing a choice, "*Do you want a crayon or a marker?*", or providing a mand, "*Tell me what you want.*" If the child does not respond, the trainer provides a model: "*Say 'want a crayon.'*" If the child does not repeat the model, the trainer provides a verbal model ("*want a crayon*") and provides the crayon.
Time delay	The language trainer uses a nonverbal prompt and waits before providing desired object or action.	The child and his teacher are tossing a ball back and forth; the teacher says "*throw the ball*" when the child is throwing. After a few throws, when the teacher has the ball, she stops, looks expectantly at the child and waits. If child does not say "*throw (the) ball*" the teacher says, "*Tell me what you want!*" or models "*Say 'throw the ball'*". If the child does not imitate, the teacher provides the model ("*throw the ball*") and throws the ball.
Incidental teaching	The language trainer manipulates the environment so that the child is more likely to talk.	It is snack time and the children are pouring juice. The child is given a cup, but no juice. The adult waits for the child to ask, "*juice*" before pouring juice in the cup. If the child does not respond, the adult provides a model or mand-model training sequence.

Source: From "Enhanced Milieu Teaching," by T. B. Hancock and A. P. Kaiser, 2006. In R. J. McCauley and M. E. Fey (Eds.), *Treatment of Language Disorders in Children* (pp. 203–236). Baltimore, MD: Brookes.

language learners benefit from seeing how communication provides real benefits in everyday interactions. Children with SLI learn a language target most efficiently when they are asked to say the target word to gain access to a favorite toy or activity in contrast to just listening to the language model.

The third and final reason that EMT is appropriate for the beginning language learner is that EMT primarily focuses on vocabulary development and early semantic combinations (e.g., Brown's Stage I). In contrast, other approaches (described below) focus more on grammatical morphological acquisition (e.g., Brown's Stage II and beyond). The more advanced language learner is likely to have mastered the vocabulary and early word combinations emphasized during EMT (Yoder, Kaiser, & Alpert, 1991).

Theoretical Foundations and Teaching Strategies in EMT.   EMT is based on a number of strong theoretical principles. I have emphasized the naturalistic, child-centered focus of EMT. I hope you have reflected back on your knowledge of language theory and connected this approach to the social interaction theories presented in Chapter 1 (Vygotsky, 1962; Bruner, 1975). You may also detect a link to the family systems approach as you consider the role of parents in EMT.

EMT has other theoretical roots, as well. It has a connection to behavior theory in that parents prompt a child's language using an antecedent-behavior-consequence (A-B-C) behavioral sequence (Hart & Rogers-Warren, 1978). The mand-model teaching technique uses this A-B-C progression. For example, a child who is developing typically looks at a cookie jar and says, *"I want cookie."* The child with SLI may fuss or attempt to climb up and open the cookie jar, but may not have the language skill to ask for a cookie. In EMT, the practitioner uses the child's attention on the cookie jar (the antecedent event) to model and prompt a mand: *"Tell me what you want"* (the behavior). Obtaining the cookie is the naturally occurring consequence along with providing an opportunity for a language expansion *"Wow, what a yummy cookie!"* Modeling, with three additional strategies, **mand-model, time-delay,** and **incidental teaching,** are the primary language training methods in EMT. As I described in Chapter 4, modeling includes the adult behaviors of expanding, elaborating, and buildups and breakdowns. In addition to the modeling terminology already familiar to you, in Table 5.4, I provide new definitions for mand-model, time-delay, and incidental teaching.

The practitioner generally needs between 20–30 sessions to train parents to effectively implement EMT tasks. The following steps outline the parent training sequence (Hancock & Kaiser, 2006):

- Parents are trained to choose materials to capture their child's interest and attention. They learn to manage toys so that their child stays engaged and to maximize child communication.
- Parents learn to follow their child's lead, pause to wait for a child's conversational turn, and to maintain balanced adult-child interactions. Interaction balance is documented by computing the following formula: [number of parent verbal turns] − [number of child verbal and nonverbal turns] = X. A balanced interaction results in X = 0.
- Parents practice the EMT training strategies of modeling, mand-model, time-delay, and incidental teaching. By the end of the parent training sessions, parents should be implementing EMT strategies more than 80% of the time.

A decision-tree example of an EMT treatment sequence is shown in Figure 5.3.

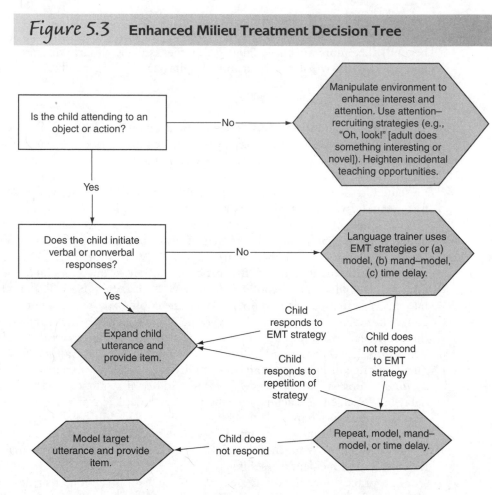

Figure 5.3   Enhanced Milieu Treatment Decision Tree

Source: From "Enhanced Milieu Teaching" by T. B. Hancock and A. P. Kaiser, 2006. In R. J. McCauley and M. E. Fey (Eds.), *Treatment of Language Disorders in Children* (pp. 203–236). Baltimore: Paul H. Brookes.

Data collection is an important part of EMT; data helps the professional modify appropriate intervention treatment goals as the child's communication improves. For example, documentation of parent behaviors might include recording the percentage of parent expansions of child utterances, the average length of parent utterance, and the number of times the parent fails to pause after taking a conversational turn. After analyzing the data, the practitioner sets parent intervention goals. Example EMT parent goals are shown in Figure 5.4; Goals 1 and 2 are potential goals developed to enhance parent language teaching strategies. Goals 3 and 4 in Figure 5.4 reflect child intervention goals. Goals 3 and 4 facilitate specific word combinations, while Goal 5 targets utterance length.

Figure 5.4	**Example Goals for Enhanced Milieu Teaching (EMT)**

Goal 1 Hana's mother will use 3-word utterances during 20-minute shared play interactions with Hana ≥ 80% of her utterances.

Goal 2 Todd's father will pause 5 seconds after an initial model or mand ≥ 80% of his utterances in 4 out 5 consecutive 20-minute play routines.

Goal 3 Abel will produce introducer + X (e.g. *"Hi Mamma," "Hi Pooh-Bear"*) in response to mand (*"What do you say?"*) and visual stimulus (e.g., mother walks in room, playing "peek-a-boo" with stuffed Pooh-Bear) ≥ 90% of opportunities for 8 out of 10 days.

Goal 4 Jackson will spontaneously produce negative + X (e.g., *"No outside," "No ball"*) within appropriate contexts during preschool outdoor play ≥ 70% of opportunities for 8 out of 10 days.

Goal 5 Odell's length of utterance will average 2.5 words when provided an adult model during a 20-minute play intervention for 8 out of 10 days.

Child performance data is also recorded on a regular basis. Table 5.5 demonstrates how child language data could be organized; documentation includes recording the child's utterance length (i.e., the number of 1, 2, 3, and 4+ word utterances) in addition to the child's spontaneous and imitative use of various semantic combinations (e.g., action + object, modifier + noun).

Evidence Supporting the EMT Approach. Experimental investigations of EMT consist of Level II evidence from a number of small-scale studies completed by independent investigators (see Hancock & Kaiser, 2006 for a discussion of research results). Overall, investigators conclude that treatment effects vary depending on child and family characteristics but a majority of children benefit from EMT.

For example, one study considered the effectiveness of novice language trainers in training parents to implement EMT (Kaiser, Hester, Alpert, & Whiteman, 1995). The research team trained parents of three preschool children to implement milieu procedures during five sessions with the support of a novice language trainer (i.e., a student inexperienced with EMT techniques). The children ranged in age from 27 to 37 months. The study was designed to (a) evaluate the effectiveness of novice parent trainers (e.g., Are inexperienced trainers able to effectively teach parents to use milieu techniques?), (b) evaluate parents' abilities to implement milieu procedures, and (c) document child language gain.

Multiple-baseline data documenting frequency of behaviors for trainers, parents, and children showed that:

- With support, novices can become effective parent trainers. In this study the amount of feedback to parents doubled as trainers became more proficient.
- Parents can be trained to use milieu techniques. In this study all three parents reached the criterion of >80% use of targeted milieu techniques.

Table 5.5　**Example of Data Documentation to Establish EMT Intervention Goals**

Measure	Data	
Mean length of utterance	1.83	
Total number of words	145	
Number of different words	62	
Number of one-word utterances	51	
Number of two-word utterances	27	
Number of three-or-more word utterances	22	
Target	Number of utterances produced spontaneously	Number of times prompted
1. Two-word request (e.g., *"Want milk,"* *"Give bubbles"*)	4	2
2. Action + Object (e.g., *"play ball,"* *"blow bubbles"*)	5	1
3. Modifier + noun (e.g., *"red ball,"* *"little bubble"*)	2	1

Source: Based on information from "Enhanced Milieu Teaching" by T. B. Hancock and A. P. Kaiser, 2006. In R. J. McCauley and M. E. Fey (Eds.), *Treatment of Language Disorders in Children* (pp. 203–236). Baltimore: Paul H. Brookes.

- Child performance varied across children. The child with the least language skills did not show clear effects of the intervention. However, the two remaining children showed acquisition of their targets during intervention and generalization to their homes.

This study, although it did not compare EMT with a contrasting intervention, provides reasonably strong evidence for EMT.

INTERVENTION APPROACH: CONVERSATIONAL RECAST TRAINING (CRT)

Practitioners need effective interventions to teach grammatical targets to children with SLI. There is strong evidence that conversational recast training (CRT) is an effective approach facilitating grammatical development in children with SLI (e.g., Fey, Cleave, & Long, 1997; Fey, Cleave, Long, & Hughes, 1993; Nelson, Camarata, Welsh, Butovski, & Camarata, 1996) as well as in children with other developmental disabilities (Scherer & Olswang, 1989; Yoder, Spruytenburg, Edwards, & Davies, 1995). CRT is appropriate for children from age 2 up to early elementary age (Camarata & Nelson, 2005) and is most effective with children above the 2-word level (Yoder, Kaiser, & Alpert, 1991).

A primary technique of CRT is the use of sentence recasts. As I described in Chapter 4, sentence recasts are adult responses to a child's utterance modifying the child's utterance while maintaining the child's meaning. A recast is similar to an expansion; however, CRT varies from traditional language expansion in two ways: (1) sentence recasts vary the sentence modality to heighten the child's awareness of the targeted form and (2) CRT facilitates a higher rate of production as compared to more traditional language expansion techniques.

Consider the following example of an adult using a sentence recast. In this example, the child omits the *be*-auxiliary form (e.g. says *noun + [verb + ing]* instead of *noun + is + [verb + ing]*):

Child: *"Man running."*

Adult: *"Yes, the man is running."*

[Adult points to a picture of a man sitting.]

Adult: *"Is the man running?"*

Child: *"No, man sitting."*

Adult: *"Oh, I see, the man is sitting. The man is not running. The man is sitting!"*

In this example, the adult alternates between statements and interrogative reversals (e.g., *"Is the man running?"*) as well as embedding negative sentence forms (*"The man is not running."*). It is hypothesized that using alternating sentence modality heightens the child's awareness of the targeted grammatical feature and encourages comparison of sentence forms (Fey & Proctor-Williams, 2000). In order to increase the child's exposure to the target forms, Fey and his colleagues (Fey, Cleave, Long, & Hughes, 1993) also embed questions (ADULT: *"What is the man doing?"* CHILD: *"Man sitting."* ADULT: *"Yes, the man is sitting."*), false assertions (ADULT: *"Oh, I think that man is running!"* Child: *"No, is sitting"* ADULT: *"Oh, you are right, the man is sitting!"*), and forced-alternative questions (ADULT: *"Do you think the man is eating or the man is sitting?"*). In several studies, Fey and his colleagues used a cyclic goal-attack strategy selecting multiple grammar goals (e.g., a verb form, *wh* questions, noun modification) for each child. After initially introducing a target during a single session, the practitioner cycled through the goals presenting one or two goals per session. An example of an intervention session in which the practitioner uses sentence recasting is demonstrated in Figure 5.5. An example of sentence recasting intervention goals is demonstrated in Figure 5.6.

A second feature of CRT is that the targeted grammatical feature is produced very frequently during the intervention session—as often as one recast per minute. The example above illustrates how this high target frequency is achieved. It is suggested that the exposure rate should be even more frequent—as much as two recasts per minute—to obtain good results (Proctor-Williams, Fey, & Loeb, 2001).

On the continuum of naturalness, CRT is a hybrid approach. Children are engaged in playlike routines; however, the activities are modified to maintain the child's attention on a specific language target. Activities are selected and the adult output is carefully designed to facilitate specific linguistic targets. An illustration demonstrating a practitioner using CRT is shown in Figure 5.7.

Figure 5.5   Example of Sentence Recasting Intervention Sequence

The adult sets up the zoo. The adult says, *"The animals are hungry and tired. Let's help the zookeeper feed the animals and put them to sleep."*

Dialogue:

Adult: *"Every day, the zookeeper* feeds *the animals. He* feeds *the giraffe. He* feeds *the giraffe every day. What* does *he do?"*

Child: *"He feed giraffe."*

Adult: *"He* feeds *the giraffe, doesn't he? Let's ask the giraffe what he* wants *to eat. What* do *you want to eat? What* do *you want to eat, giraffe? You ask the giraffe what he* wants *to eat."*

Child: *"What you eat?"*

Adult: *"What* do *you eat giraffe? Oh, he* says *he* eats *hay. Does* he eat *bananas? No! The giraffe eats* hay*! The monkey eats* bananas, *doesn't he? Who* do *you think eats these bananas?"*

Child: *"Monkey eats bananas."*

Adult: *"Yes, the monkey* eats *these yellow bananas. Let's help the zookeeper put the giraffe to sleep. Where* does *the giraffe sleep? Does* the giraffe sleep *in a pond?"*

Child: *"No, the frog sleep in pond. The giraffe sleep under tree."*

Adult: *"Oh, I see; the giraffe* sleeps *under this tree and the frog* sleeps *in a pond! You make the zookeeper ask the giraffe* where *he sleeps."*

Child: *"Where you sleep?"*

Adult: *"Where* do *you sleep, giraffe? The giraffe* says *he* sleeps *under the tree."*

Figure 5.6   Example Goals for Conversational Recast Training

- Gavin will spontaneously produce the copula *is* in yes-no questions (*"Is the boy happy?"*) to obtain information in obligatory contexts $\geq 50\%$[1] of the time in a naturalistic[2] 30-minute interaction. Preintervention baseline on (date) was 10%.
- Suzanne will spontaneously produce the possessive (*'s*) to describe ownership (*"This is mommy's purse" "I want the girl's hat"*) $\geq 50\%$ of the time in a naturalistic 30-minute interaction in obligatory contexts. Preintervention baseline on (date) was at 12%[3].

[1] Once a child reaches 50% spontaneous production in a naturalistic setting it is not necessary to emphasize the target as a primary goal. The target can, however, be embedded into other activities and monitored to determine continued mastery (Fey, 1986; Lee, Koenigsknecht, & Mulhern, 1975).

[2] An interaction is considered "naturalistic" even if the adult has to provide stimulus items making it more likely that the target form will be required. Some grammatical forms are low frequency and, without environmental manipulation, the child is not obliged to produce the target. The stimuli should be novel.

[3] Fey (1986) suggests that grammatical forms used between 10–50% in a preintervention baseline should be considered as primary intervention targets.

Figure 5.7 **Conversational Recast Intervention**

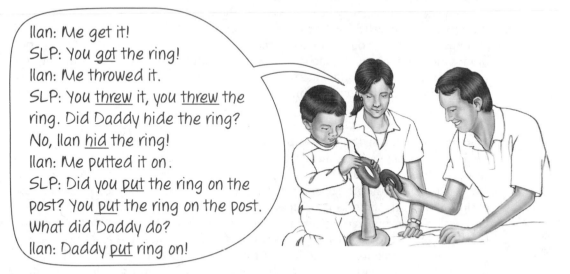

Ilan: Me get it!
SLP: You <u>got</u> the ring!
Ilan: Me throwed it.
SLP: You <u>threw</u> it, you <u>threw</u> the ring. Did Daddy hide the ring? No, Ilan <u>hid</u> the ring!
Ilan: Me putted it on.
SLP: Did you <u>put</u> the ring on the post? You <u>put</u> the ring on the post. What did Daddy do?
Ilan: Daddy <u>put</u> ring on!

Communication Challenge and Intervention Goals: Ilan does not use irregular past tense verbs. The adult uses sentence recasts maintaining Ilan's meaning but incorporating past tense verbs. The adult SLP sometimes alternates sentence modality between declarative and interrogative sentence construction.

An important theory of language learning, the **transactional model** of language learning, underlies CRT. Like the social interaction perspective, the transactional model considers a child's utterances as the antecedent event triggering an adult response (Camarata & Nelson, 2006; Moerk, 1992). The cyclic links between child verbal initiations and adult response is considered a primary feature promoting child language learning.

Implementation of CRT requires that the practitioner target developmentally appropriate grammatical features. During pretreatment assessment, the adult determines the grammatical forms and sentence structures that the child does and does not produce (e.g., Does the child use an auxiliary form in the initiation of a question? ["*Is Daddy outside?*" versus "*Daddy outside?*"]). Since children with SLI frequently have difficulty with verb forms, verb production often is a focus of intervention. However, other grammatical forms including gerunds, passive voice, relative clauses, and *wh* questions also are possible CRT targets (Camarata, Nelson, & Camarata, 1994). Sentence recasts are likely to have their greatest effect after a child already is using a grammatical form at least some of the time (Fey & Loeb, 2002).

CRT is most frequently implemented in individual or small-group sessions. Parents have been trained to use sentence recasts. However, CRT techniques require significant training—up to ten sessions of training—for effective implementation (Fey, Cleave, Long, & Hughes, 1993). Data keeping in CRT consists of regular probes to monitor a child's production of the targeted grammatical form in spontaneous, untrained interactions. In Figure 5.6, preintervention baseline data are incorporated within the intervention goals.

Sentence recasting may be effectively combined with more adult-directed didactic therapy approaches (Fey & Proctor-Williams, 2000). The adult first teaches the grammatical form through modeling and imitation procedures. After a brief period of imitation and modeling practice, the adult introduces sentence recasts during conversational and book-reading interactions. The adult then alternates between modeling/imitation and CRT activities until the child spontaneously produces the target in novel interactions.

Evidence Supporting the CRT Approach.   There is strong empirical evidence that CRT is effective and that children with SLI acquire grammatical forms and are able to generalize production with this procedure. Camarata, Nelson, & Camarata (1994) compared the effectiveness of CRT with an imitative protocol. Twenty-one children with SLI between the ages of 4 and 6 years participated in the study. Grammatical forms were selected as intervention targets if they were (a) consistently in error and (b) developmentally below the child's age level. Two target forms were selected for each child; one form was trained using an imitative procedure and one form with CRT using random assignment. In the imitative procedure, the adult required the child to imitate a sentence with the target form after viewing a picture or object stimuli. CRT consisted of a naturalistic interaction with toys; the child was not required to imitate the sentence recasts and the adult gave no overt reinforcement for the child's productions. You should note that the sentence recasting method described in the Camarata et al. (1994) study differs slightly from the sentence recasting procedure described above where children's responses are directly solicited.

Even without directly requiring child responses, Camarata et al. (1994) reported that CRT prompted the children to produce more generalized spontaneous productions than the imitation protocol. This study, in addition to other studies investigating the use of sentence recasting (e.g., Nelson, Camarata, Welsh, Butkovsky, & Camarata, 1996: Proctor-Williams, Fey, and Loeb, 2001), provides a level of efficacy consistent with Level I evidence. However, a later study (Fey & Loeb, 2002) also evaluated sentence recasting and reported more ambiguous efficacy (i.e., the results were not clear cut). It can be frustrating for students to read about contradictory research results. The process of testing interventions is complex and, until all treatment variables are understood, there will continue to be discrepancies in research results. You will be challenged to continue to interpret varying results produced in intervention studies; this will be a part of your professional training.

INTERVENTION APPROACH: SENTENCE COMBINING

During sentence combining (SC) intervention, the adult gives the student two or more simple sentences and requires the student to combine the simple sentences into a longer, more complex sentence. Typically, the sentences are combined by using relative clauses, conjunctions, or subordinate clauses. Consider the following examples:

Simple Sentence #1: *The boy is running fast.*

Simple Sentence #2: *The boy wears a red hat.*

Simple Sentence #3: *The boy finished the race first.*

Complex sentence #1: *The boy* who is wearing a red hat *is* running fast and finished *the race in first place.*

Complex sentence #2: Because *the boy with the red hat is running fast, he finished the race in first place.*

In the examples above, *who is wearing a red hat,* is a relative clause; *running fast and finished* demonstrates a compound sentence (i.e., two verbs joined with the conjunction *and*), and *because* is a subordinating conjunction. It is interesting to note the two complex sentences vary slightly in meaning; complex sentence #1 emphasizes the description of the boy (*wearing a red hat*) while complex sentence #2 emphasizes the boy's speed (*because he is running fast*).

Students' ability to use complex grammar is improved when they understand how using more sophisticated sentence structure conveys meaning. Sentence manipulation and sentence combining help students see how words can be put into varying patterns. Eisenberg (2006) describes two different forms of sentence combining: **open combining** and **sentence expansion**. During open combining, the student experiments with different ways of combining simple sentences to make a longer, more complex sentence (as shown in the example above). During sentence expansion, the adult provides the student with a kernel sentence and then asks the student to elaborate the sentence. The example below demonstrates this process:

Adult: "*The kernel sentence is* The clown is happy. *Now expand the sentence and tell me why the clown is happy.*"

Student: "*The clown is happy* because *the dog is doing funny tricks.*"

Adult: "*Nice job! Now tell me where the clown is standing; remember to use descriptive vocabulary!*"

Student: "*The clown is happy when he stands under the* giant *tent.*"

Adult: "*Good job. Now make a compound sentence; this time use the word* but."

Student: "*The clown is happy* but *he knows it's almost time to leave the circus.*"

You should note that the examples above demonstrate a sophisticated level of language production. It is unlikely students with language impairment could spontaneously produce sentences at this level. Before asking the student with SLI to complete sentence expansions, generally the practitioner provides a variety of supportive techniques. Example supports include (a) showing pictures to help stimulate possible complex sentences, (b) providing several models before asking the student to produce a sentence, or (c) providing the student with written "scrambled sentences" and asking the student to combine words into varying combinations.

Sentence combining is an appropriate technique for school-age students and has even been used to improve grammar skills in college students (Smith & Hull, 1985). Sentence combining has been documented as an intervention approach for remedial and at-risk students (Weaver, 1996). Generally, brief sessions are better than semester-long drilling on sentence combining (Eisenberg, 2006). The recommended practice is to provide shorter sessions of sentence combining in combination with reminders to use longer sentences during writing practice. Sentence combining (as illustrated above) is an example of an adult-directed intervention technique.

Scott and Nelson (2009) describe the use of sentence combining during the writing process for students with language impairment; the use of SC with student writing samples reflects a more hybrid approach on the continuum of naturalness (Fey, 1986). In this hybrid model of intervention, sentence combining is embedded within the writing process as students are asked to plan, draft, and revise original written stories.

The practitioner initiates a curriculum-based language assessment prior to implementing the SC intervention. To obtain baseline data, the practitioner has the student complete a writing probe. The practitioner then computes the occurrence of complex and compound sentences within the writing sample. The T-unit analysis (see Chapter 2) is a particularly appropriate qualitative approach to document sentence complexity. Periodic writing probes document the student's progress in the SC approach.

Evidence Supporting the Sentence-Combining Approach.   A number of studies document the effectiveness of the SC approach (Andrews et al., 2006). A recent study demonstrates the results of a randomized, control-group design. Saddler and Graham (2005) randomly assigned 44 4th-grade writers to either SC or traditional grammar instruction groups. Practitioners taught the SC group to (a) combine sentences with *and*, *but*, and *because*, (b) embed adverbs or adjectives into sentences (e.g., simple sentences = *They eat food. They eat a lot*; more complex sentence = *They eat a lot of food*) and (c) create complex sentences by creating subordinate clauses. Students practiced the SC skills with their teacher and with a peer.

The control group was called the grammar instruction group. Practitioners taught the control-group students the parts of speech and encouraged students to use descriptive nouns, verbs, adjectives, and adverbs. To assess students' writing development, students (a) provided a first- and second-draft writing sample to a picture prompt, (b) completed a sentence-combining task, and (c) were assessed with a norm-referenced test of writing ability (Test of Written Language-3 [TOWL-3], Hammill & Larson, 1996). Results demonstrated that the students in the SC group were twice as likely to produce complex sentences during the SC task and scored significantly better on the SC subtest of the TOWL-3.

Analysis of the students' writing samples resulted in a more nuanced result. There was no treatment effect for the quality ratings of first drafts; however, the students in the SC group performed better on improving writing when they revised their papers. This result suggests that the SC approach improved the students' metaskills in terms of revising and rewriting. Overall, this level of evidence is consistent with the Level III hierarchy of intervention evidence.

Summary

- Specific language impairment (SLI) is a diagnosis based on exclusionary criteria. A child with SLI has a significant language impairment *without* associated hearing loss, cognitive deficit, neurological, or motor impairments. About 15% of children who are clinically considered to be SLI do not meet all of these exclusionary characteristics. The *Diagnostic and Statistical Manual of Mental Disorders, Fourth Edition–Text Revision* (DSM-IV) (American Psychiatric Association [APA], 2000) lists three major subtypes of SLI: a major delay in receptive language, a major delay in expressive language, or a delay in both receptive and expressive language.

- Before age 4, children who are language delayed are sometimes called late talkers (rather than SLI) because many children who are language delayed as toddlers catch up with their peers in late preschool. It is very important, however, to identify language delay at an early age. The prevalence of SLI is 7%.

- Current research suggests a genetic cause of SLI. Two theories, the extended optional infinitive and the surface theory, describe the inherited deficits underlying SLI.

- A primary focus of intervention is the development of morphosyntax, which is a primary area of difficulty in children with SLI. Young children with SLI have difficulty with verb forms (including auxiliary verbs), possessives, and pronouns, in addition to difficulty learning complex syntax and vocabulary. Pragmatic problems often occur because of problems with interactive communication. Children with SLI more frequently have phonological impairments compared to their peers. Research has documented processing difficulties and the presence of neurological soft signs. Fifty-nine percent of children diagnosed with SLI also are diagnosed with attention-deficit/hyperactivity disorder. Parent-child interactions sometimes require intervention to facilitate language learning for children who have SLI. During the school years, children with SLI often have difficulty with reading and writing development and peer interactions.

- Peer-mediated treatment is a form of intervention that focuses on children's social skills. Three basic paradigms for social skill building are social intervention with peers, peer confederate training, and sociodramatic script training. Interventionists can facilitate children's ability to (a) enter into play with other children, (b) play cooperatively, and (c) interact socially with school-age peers.

- A critical component of the assessment process is language sample analysis (LSA); additionally assessors complete norm-referenced and criterion-referenced assessments on children with SLI. Two criterion-referenced assessments are parent-child interaction observations and curriculum-based language assessments. Both are forms of naturalistic assessment providing multiple opportunities for an individual to perform skills across domains (i.e., social, cognitive, motor, communication).

- Three intervention approaches for children who are SLI include enhanced milieu training (EMT), conversational recast training (CRT), and sentence combining. EMT includes the teaching strategies of mand-model, time-delay, and incidental teaching along with adult modeling. CRT uses a strategy called sentence recasting. Sentence combining is an intervention appropriate for school-aged students who need to improve sentence complexity.

Discussion and In-Class Activities

1. In a small group, role-play a scenario in which you present the results of an assessment to a parent. Imagine that the child is age 4 and is talking in 2- and 3-word combinations; he demonstrates a number of syntax and morphological errors (e.g., *"Me do it!"*). His receptive language is higher than his expressive language, but receptive language is slightly delayed. He has a number of phonological errors, but is about 60% intelligible. He is within normal limits in IQ and has normal hearing. The parent wants to know what is causing his child's impairment. Role-play your answer. Make sure you explain in a way that is meaningful to a parent without background knowledge of language development.

2. Role-play a social group and have one student use poor social communication skills to enter the group interaction. Discuss problems and write 1–2 goals that could be implemented to improve the student's peer interaction.

3. View a videotape of a child with SLI. Use the utterance-level worksheet in Chapter 2 (Table 2.2) to analyze the child's language. Discuss the ways that the child is pragmatically successful or unsuccessful. Discuss the errors demonstrated in morphosyntax. How do these two language domains operate independently in the communication of young children? Write an intervention goal for the child as a result of the language sample analysis.

4. Obtain a case example with a conversational transcript or a videotape of an older student with SLI. Refer back to the information in Chapter 2 on topic control, conversational repair, informativeness, and conjunctive cohesion. Write an intervention goal based on the decision-making process.

5. Obtain a case example with a conversational transcript or a videotape of a young child at Brown's stage I. Use the enhanced milieu decision tree to determine a possible EMT strategy. Write intervention goals based on the decision-making process.

6. Write 2 to 3 additional goals consistent with the conversational recast approaches and the sentence combining approach. Determine a language target appropriate for either younger children, (e.g., present progressive verbs, third person regular verbs, pronoun use, regular past tense) or older students (e.g., subordinate conjunctions, embedded clauses). Also use objects (dolls, trucks, balls, bubbles, bean bags for younger children) or pictures (for older school-age students). Role-play an adult-student interaction representing the two approaches with the items provided.

Chapter 5 Case Study

Zachary is a 10-year-old fifth grader. He is social and well liked by his peers. He is a natural athlete, but doesn't enjoy organized sports. He doesn't easily follow the coaches' verbal instructions and this interferes with his participation. Zachary's interests are rap music and video games. He enjoys talking about his favorite topics but loses interest when the conversation changes to other topics.

Zachary's parents are both attorneys; they work with him daily to help him complete his homework. He was in third grade before he could decode grade-level text. Now, in fifth grade, Zachary is a slow reader and does not easily comprehend what he reads. He works diligently to complete his schoolwork, but his work is generally low average. His writing consists of simple sentences and is produced slowly. Zachary is well behaved in class, but generally doesn't participate in classroom discussions.

Zachary's parents are not sure what, if anything, they should do to help Zachary participate more in class and to improve his reading and writing. Zachary has not been previously assessed for language impairment or learning disabilities.

Questions for Discussion

1. What do you think might be the underlying cause of Zachary's communication style (e.g., avoiding unfamiliar topics)?
2. What classroom-based assessments might you consider to obtain more information about Zachary's abilities?
3. What kinds of information could you provide to Zachary's parents to help them understand their son's abilities?
4. What educational or communication goals could be included in an intervention program for Zachary?

CHAPTER 6

Children with Hearing Loss

—Lori A. Pakulski

Chapter Overview Questions

1. What are the differences between hearing loss (HL) classified as sensorineural, conductive, or mixed?

2. What are APD and AN/AD? How are they different from other types of hearing impairments?

3. What language domains are potentially affected by HL?

4. What paradigm shift has radically changed intervention for children with HL?

5. What factors are of concern at early stages of HL identification?

6. What facilitative counseling strategies are used when working with a family?

7. What are the Cottage Acquisition Scales and the Ling Sound Test?

8. What are "learning to listen" sounds and how are children exposed to these sounds?

This chapter focuses on language learning in the presence of a hearing loss (HL). You will learn about the language challenges associated with hearing loss. Additionally, I will discuss issues surrounding your role as a speech-language pathologist (SLP) or educator as you work with a child with HL, his or her family, audiologists, and educators.

Children with HL are a heterogeneous group, meaning that the cause and severity of the HL varies significantly. The ways that children learn to communicate also will vary. For example, many young children will experience fluctuating and temporary hearing loss caused by infection in the middle ear (known as chronic **otitis media**); other children have permanent hearing loss due to damage in the inner ear. Some families choose to teach their children to listen and talk; other families communicate through sign language. People often assume that if a child has a significant and permanent hearing loss, he or she will need to learn sign language to communicate. However, today most children can learn to listen and talk effectively due to early identification and intervention that includes high-power digital hearing aids and **cochlear implants**. This chapter will help you explore the impact of HL on language. I will present information allowing you to help children and their families maximize their language potential.

Description of the Disorder

PREVALENCE

More than 12,000 children are born each year in the United States with significant permanent hearing loss (3 out of every 1,000; National Institute on Deafness and Communication Disorders [NIDCD, 2007]), making it one of the most common disabilities (Alexander Graham Bell Association [AG Bell], 2005). Hearing loss also occurs after birth. Middle ear infection, or otitis media (OM), is the second-most frequent illness of early childhood after the common cold (Roberts & Hunter, 2002). Otitis media may cause HL in as many as one third of affected children in kindergarten and first grade classrooms on any given day. The prevalence of HL increases with age; it affects approximately 17 in 1,000 children under age 18 (NIDCD, 2007). Because most children learn language by hearing it, a child's early exposure to language is critical in building communication skills. Children with HL are at risk for delays in speech, language, and cognitive development.

TYPES OF HEARING LOSS

Hearing loss is identified by type (**conductive, sensorineural,** or **mixed**) and severity. When the hearing loss occurs in the outer and middle ear, it is called a conductive loss. A conductive loss is typically the result of a medical problem, such as a fluid-filled middle ear (otitis media), or damage, such as a perforated eardrum. Since most conductive disorders are amenable to medical treatment, the hearing loss is typically temporary. Despite the temporary nature of the loss, fluctuating or inconsistent hearing in early childhood may cause problems in the development of auditory brain centers (Gravel et al., 2006; Xu, Kotak, & Sanes, 2007).

Nearly all children will experience at least one episode of otitis media; many will experience repeated episodes. Children who experience repeated (chronic) otitis media may be at risk for other problems. There is emerging data that suggest that recurrent otitis media has a considerable negative impact on the quality of life of children and causes concern to their caregivers. These effects are proportional to the severity of the condition (e.g., Brouwer et al., 2005).

Sensorineural losses are caused by damage to the inner ear structures or auditory nerves. When a child has both a sensorineural hearing impairment and a conductive disorder (e.g., permanent hearing loss due to genetic disorder co-occurring with a middle ear infection), the loss is called *mixed*.

Table 6.1   **Co-Occurring Conditions**

Condition	Percent of children
No additional disorders	48.6%
Visual impairment	3.6
Deaf-blindness	1.4
Developmental delay	3.8
Specific learning disability	8.0
Orthopedic impairment	4.0
Attention deficit disorder	5.1
Speech or language impairment	24.9
Traumatic brain injury	0.3
Cognitive impairments	8.0
Emotional disturbance	1.8
Autism	1.3
Other health impairment	3.6

Source: Regional and National Summary Report of Data from the 2006–2007 Annual Survey of Deaf and Hard of Hearing Children and Youth by Gallaudet Research Institute, 2006, Washington, DC: GRI, Gallaudet University. Used with permission.

Sensorineural hearing loss can be caused by a number of factors, including genetic disorders, birth defects, premature birth, and infections such as meningitis. Typically one third of congenital losses are attributed to genetic disorders, one third to nongenetic disorders, and one third to unknown causation. Disorders that can co-occur with HL are presented in Table 6.1.

VARIATIONS IN HL BY RACE/ETHNICITY

Table 6.2 illustrates the prevalence of HL by race/ethnic background. Varying types of hearing problems impact race or ethnic groups differently. For example, Caucasians are more susceptible to noise-induced hearing loss than African Americans (Jerger, Jerger, Pepe, & Miller, 1986). The Alaska Native and American Indian populations experience more frequent otitis media (Curns et al., 2002).

DEGREE OF HEARING LOSS

Another way to think about HL is to consider the sounds a person can and cannot hear. A person with normal hearing can detect very soft sounds ranging from low frequency sounds to high frequency sounds. Sound **frequency** relates to the perceptual quality we call **pitch**. Most hearing tests measure pitch by exposing the listener to sounds ranging from 250 Hz to 8000 Hz. The sound of a bullfrog is a common

Table 6.2 **Prevalence of Hearing Loss by Race/Ethnicity**

Reported race/ethnicity	Percent of children with hearing loss
Caucasian	47.4
Black/African American	15.1
Hispanic/Latino	28.3
American Indian/Alaska Native	0.7
Asian/Pacific Islander	4.2
Other	1.9
Multiethnic	2.4

Source: Regional and National Summary Report of Data from the 2006–2007 Annual Survey of Deaf and Hard of Hearing Children and Youth by Gallaudet Research Institute, 2006, Washington, DC: GRI, Gallaudet University. Used with permission.

example of a low frequency sound while a bird tweeting is a high frequency sound. In terms of human speech, "oo" is low frequency and "s" is high frequency.

The **degree** or severity of the hearing loss determines which sounds will be inaudible to a person. The degree of hearing loss is determined by measuring the **intensity** level at which a person can detect sounds. Intensity level relates to the perceptual quality of loudness. The degree of loss is determined by identifying an individual's **hearing threshold** and is measured in **decibels** (dB). A person with normal hearing acuity can hear very soft sounds and has hearing thresholds in the range of 0 dB to 15 dB across the frequency range. When a person requires more intensity or loudness to hear a sound, the person is said to have HL. A degree or severity rating (from slight to profound loss) is assigned according to the intensity (in decibels) necessary for a person to detect a particular sound (see Table 6.3). The degree of impairment may vary across the frequency range or between ears. HL can also be characterized in terms of temporary or permanent, fluctuating or progressive, and unilateral (one ear) versus bilateral (both ears). As you can see from the above information, the reasons for, and implications of, a hearing loss are complex. It is important to consider the kinds of questions and concerns parents will bring to you as a professional: in this regard consider the issues posed in Focus 6.1.

AUDITORY PERCEPTUAL PROBLEMS

There is an additional disability type that is related to auditory perceptual problems rather than hearing loss. Auditory perceptual problems are generally caused by **auditory processing disorder** (APD) or **auditory neuropathy/dys-synchrony** (AN/AD). APD or AN/AD are auditory problems, but they cannot be categorized within the domains described above.

Current research suggests that APD is caused by malfunctioning of the auditory pathway to the brain or small defects in the brain's auditory cortex (Jerger, Martin, &

Table 6.3   **Categorizing Degree of Hearing Impairment in Children**

Degree of loss	Decibel level (dB)
Normal	0–15
Slight	16–25
Mild	26–40
Moderate	41–55
Moderately severe	56–70
Severe	71–90
Profound	91+

Source: Based on information from "Uses and Abuses of Hearing Loss Classification,"
by J. G. Clark, 1981, *ASHA, 23,* pp. 493–500.

McColl, 2004). The auditory-neural defects do not result in a true loss of hearing sensitivity—the outer, middle, and inner ear function well. However, the neural or auditory pathway deficits make it difficult for the individual with APD to comprehend spoken language. In other words, the loss is not due to access to sound or audibility—so hearing aids do not help. Instead, the individual may benefit from an assistive device to help highlight the desired signal (speech) so that it can be differentiated from background noise. In other cases, the individual with APD may need to learn speech-decoding strategies. As you can imagine, auditory processing disorders are difficult to identify and may not be diagnosed until the student is school age.

A second auditory processing disorder is auditory neuropathy/dys-synchrony (AN/AD). AN/AD is a different auditory processing deficit; in this case the auditory signal is impeded as it travels from the cochlea to the brain. Like APD, AN/AD is not due to a malfunction in the outer, middle, or inner ear. However, it can be diagnosed early with the appropriate test battery.

The treatment for children with APD and AN/AD can be different—or in some ways similar—to invention programs for children with HL. For example, some children with AN/AD are provided a cochlear implant to bypass malfunctions in the auditory system. However, a cochlear implant is not appropriate for children with APD.

Environmental management is important for children with APD and AN/AD. If listening is challenging, improving the intensity level of the desired sound signal so that it can be differentiated from background noise benefits both APD and AN/AD

FOCUS 6.1 *Clinical Skill Building*

What parent concerns might you hear that might indicate a potential hearing loss? How might the concerns differ for a mild hearing loss, a severe hearing loss, or an auditory processing problem?

listeners. The ratio of the desired sound as compared to background noise level is called the signal-to-noise ratio (SNR). SNR is important for all listeners, but it is particularly important for children with auditory perceptual problems. In most cases, intervention focuses on remediation of the language disorders resulting from the child's auditory processing difficulties.

Causation, Risk Factors, and Communication Impairments

Many factors affect language development in children with HL. The most important factors include age when the hearing impairment occurs (e.g., congenital, or acquired before or after the child learns to speak), age when the hearing loss is identified and treated, the child's auditory and language experience, and the level of parental involvement. I will be presenting more information about these factors within this chapter.

It is important to remember that a child's language development will vary in relation to the severity and type of hearing loss (e.g., mild conductive loss versus a severe sensorineural loss) and other less critical factors. Normal hearing allows auditory access to spoken language from birth and even before birth (i.e., prenatal development). When a permanent hearing loss exists, language acquisition is affected because children cannot access everyday communication interactions. The lack of auditory access also results in a lack of self-monitoring of speech and language productions. For example, children with HL (who are not exposed to amplified sound) begin to make babbling sounds, but their babbling does not continue due to a lack of self-monitoring. The "feedback loop" between sound production and auditory stimulation does not maintain the babbling behavior.

Extensive research has documented the impact of hearing loss on children's language development. Studies have investigated the language proficiency of children with HL who use spoken language and children with HL who use manual communication (e.g., American Sign Language [ASL]). Most recently, research has focused on the benefits of early intervention and early cochlear implantation. Due to technological advances in auditory amplification, the field of deafness and HL has undergone a **paradigm shift**. The term *paradigm shift* refers to a radical change in thinking leading to new approaches.

The paradigm shift that has occurred in the area of deafness and HL can be summarized in this way:

> When family and environmental support are in place and when appropriate and high quality amplification and early intensive intervention is provided, a child with HL who is identified and treated in the first few months of life has the potential of developing language commensurate with normal hearing peers when no other disorders exist (Moeller, 2000, p. E43).

Unfortunately, some children with HL do not access services at early ages or their hearing loss is complicated by other associated conditions (see Table 6.1). In this situation, children with HL are likely to demonstrate language deficits similar to other children with language impairments. The categories of language impairment for

Table 6.4   **Language Problems of Children with Hearing Impairment**

Dimension	Concern
Phonology	Child experiences difficulty with (a) managing breath stream for speech, (b) rotating tongue forward and backward to establish vowel postures, and (c) moving articulators smoothly and continuously from one articulatory posture to the next.
Pragmatics	Has difficulty due to inexperience (e.g., limited conversational partners).
Semantics	May not have sufficient vocabulary variety. May not have complex vocabulary. May not understand subtle differences or figurative language.
Syntax	Child demonstrates unsophisticated grammatical forms and sentence structures. May have a reduced mean length of utterance.

children with HL reflect the domains of language that, by now, are familiar to you. Language domains include morphologic and syntactic deficits as well as semantic, pragmatic, and speech production problems (i.e., articulation and phonological deficits). A summary of specific language problems is provided in Table 6.4. Children with HL who have been identified at older ages or who have associated deficits may experience language problems ranging from mild to severe.

Factors Influencing Outcomes for Children with Hearing Loss

There are a number of factors that strongly affect language outcomes for children with hearing loss. In this section, I discuss three factors: (a) early identification and audiological management, (b) choice of **communication modality**, and (c) family involvement in the remediation process. In 1993, the National Institutes on Health's (NIH) Consensus Development Conference concluded that all infants should be screened for hearing loss, preferably before hospital discharge. More than a decade later, most states have adopted universal newborn hearing screening (UNHS) as part of an early detection of hearing impairment (EDHI) program. EDHI programs provide two critical improvements: (1) children are now identified at birth as opposed to 2 or 3 years of age, and (2) intervention can begin within critical windows of opportunity in the first few months of life. In short, the educational outlook for children born with hearing loss is remarkably better due to universal screening.

EARLY DETECTION

Early detection underlies the paradigm shift that has occurred in the field of deafness and hearing loss. Left untreated, children with HL will have delays in auditory and language development (Moeller, Tomblin, Yoshinaga-Itano, MacDonald-Connor, &

Jerger 2007; Moeller, 2000) and this language gap will widen over time (Geers, 2004; Svirsky, 2000). However, new evidence demonstrates that children who are identified and treated within the first year of life can achieve language levels equivalent to their hearing peers (Dornan, Hickson, Murdoch, & Houston, 2007; Yoshinaga-Itano, Sedey, Coulter, & Mehl, 1998). These are very important data because they demonstrate that hearing impairment in and of itself does not diminish a child's learning and communication ability. However, late identification paired with lack of treatment has profound negative consequences.

NEUROPLASTICITY

The ability to achieve language levels consistent with hearing peers is based on the fact that the auditory system, which supports language development, is "plastic." This phenomenon is known as **neuroplasticity** of the auditory system. Auditory plasticity means that despite damage or disease, the auditory system can develop appropriately with early stimulation. If we remember that we hear with our ears and listen with our brain, it makes sense that if sound does not reach the brain (auditory deprivation) the auditory system development in the brain will be arrested (Gordon & Harrison, 2005).

However, with early stimulation, the brain grows and refines the auditory neural connections needed for spoken language development (Gordon, Papsin, & Harrison, 2003; Sharma, 2007; Sharma, et al., 2004). Importantly, if auditory skills are mastered as close as possible to the normal "biological clock," the neural system experiences **developmental synchrony** (Robbins, Koch, Osberger, & Zimmerman-Philips, 2004). Developmental synchrony is the brain's ability to take advantage of developmental "windows of opportunity" (Flexer, Wray, Sommers, & Schmidt-Robb, 2005; Robbins, Koch, Osberger, & Zimmerman-Philips, 2004). To summarize this important information: A child who receives intervention, particularly auditory stimulation, in the first year of life outperforms children who are identified at later ages (Miyamoto et al., 2007). More importantly, early identified children are likely to have language quotients (language age/chronological age) consistent with their hearing peers by kindergarten (Moeller, 2000; Yoshinaga-Itano et al., 1998). For a more in-depth look at language development in children with HL, you can review the following articles:

- Easterbrooks, S., & Baker, S. (2002). *Language learning in children who are deaf and hard of hearing: Multiple pathways.* Boston: Allyn & Bacon.
- Ling, D. (1989). *Foundations of spoken language for hearing impaired children.* Washington, DC: Alexander Graham Bell Association for the Deaf.
- Paul, P. (2001). *Language and deafness* (3rd ed.). San Diego, CA: Singular/ Thomson Learning.
- Rose, S., McAnally, P., & Quigley, S. (2004). *Language learning practices with deaf children* (3rd ed.). Austin, TX: Pro-Ed.
- Schirmer, B. (2000). *Language and literacy development in children who are deaf* (2nd ed.). Boston: Allyn & Bacon.

CHOOSING A COMMUNICATION MODALITY

You might be aware that there is a controversy between proponents of **Deaf culture** and professionals who believe that children with HL can learn to talk and listen. The situation is complex because 95% of children born with significant hearing loss are raised by parents who can hear (Mitchell & Karchmer, 2004). If parents consider the language used in their home and community, spoken language is the obvious choice for most families. On the other hand, if parents consider the philosophy of the Deaf community—whose members believe that that deafness is not a disorder to be fixed, but a culture to be embraced—parents may consider using sign language as the child's native language and focus on teaching English in its written form as a second language (bilingual). Additional information about the Deaf culture is presented in Focus 6.2.

In order to bridge this difference of opinion, many families choose **total** (simultaneous) **communication,** a mode of communication combining spoken language with sign language. Regardless of the specific communication mode a family chooses for their child, critical components of intervention must be realized, whether child is taught to listen and talk, use sign language and learn English as a second language, or use total communication.

The professional provides information to families to help them make important decisions about their child's communication modality. Each communication modality has positive and negative considerations, and efficacy data must be considered when presenting data to families. As you recall from previous chapters of this book, efficacy data represent research-based documentation of intervention outcomes. Below, I discuss approaches and highlight research data pertaining to two communication

FOCUS 6.2 *Multicultural Issues*

Deaf Culture

For those of us who are hearing, it is sometimes difficult to imagine a culture that celebrates deafness; something we might consider to be a deficit or disability. Culture by definition is a set of learned behaviors of a group of people who have their own language, values, rules of behavior, and traditions. When we consider the definition, it makes sense that a culture may develop when a group of like individuals forms a community around a shared experience: deafness. If they define themselves by their deafness, they may find they have common interests, shared norms of behavior, and similar techniques for facing life challenges. A culture provides social interaction and emotional support.

The cornerstone of Deaf culture is American Sign Language (ASL). Members of the Deaf culture have a sense of pride about their language and its rich culture. Mastery of ASL and skillful storytelling are valued; wisdom, values, and heritage are passed from generation to generation through ASL. When ASL is the primary language for social interactions, written language (English) must be learned as a second language. For this reason, those in the Deaf culture often consider themselves bilingual-bicultural.

modalities: spoken communication (talking and listening) and sign language (total communication approach).

Approaches Focusing on Talking and Listening. Historically, when practitioners implemented talking and listening interventions with HL children, they used either an auditory-verbal or auditory-oral approach. Today, auditory-verbal and auditory-oral approaches have more similarities than differences and lead to similar outcomes (AG Bell, 2009). The AG Bell Academy now recommends using a newer term, **Listening and Spoken Language Specialists (LSLS)** rather than categorizing practitioners with labels like auditory-verbal specialist or auditory-oral specialist. The guiding principles and philosophies guiding listening and spoken language (LSL) terminology are summarized in Table 6.5.

Table 6.5   **Philosophy and Principles for Listening and Spoken Language Specialists (LSLS)**

Philosophy:

a. Listening and Spoken Language Specialists (LSLS) help children who are deaf or hard of hearing develop spoken language and literacy primarily through listening.
b. LSLS professionals focus on education, guidance, advocacy, family support, and the rigorous application of techniques, strategies, and procedures that promote optimal acquisition of spoken language through listening by newborns, infants, toddlers, and children who are deaf or hard of hearing.
c. LSLS professionals guide parents in helping their children develop intelligible spoken language through listening, and coach them in advocating their children's inclusion in the mainstream school. Ultimately, parents gain confidence that their children will have access to the full range of educational, social, and vocational choices in life.

Designations of certification for Listening and Spoken Language Specialists:

a. Certified Auditory-Verbal Therapist (LSLS Cert. AVT; the LSLS Cert. AVT works one-on-one with the child and family in all intervention sessions).
b. Certified Auditory-Verbal Educator (LSLS Cert. AVEd; the LSLS Cert. AVEd involves the family and also works directly with the child in individual or group/classroom settings).

Both types of Listening and Spoken Language Specialists have similar knowledge and skills and work on behalf of the child and family.

Principles:

- Specialists from both designations follow developmental models of audition, speech, language, cognition, and communication.
- Specialists from both designations use evidence-based practices.
- Specialists from both designations strive for excellent outcomes in listening, spoken language, literacy, and independence for children who are deaf or hard of hearing.

Source: Adapted from *AG Bell Academy for Listening and Spoken Language,* Alexander Graham Bell Association, 2009, retrieved March 24, 2009, from www.agbellacademy.org/about-academy.htm. Used with permission.

LSL intervention emerged primarily from parallel work done in the mid-20th century by Doreen Pollack in Colorado and Helen Beebe in Pennsylvania. These pioneers believed that with intensive and appropriate intervention, children could learn to listen and talk. In the early years of the approach, their methods were not consistently supported as some educators considered that LSL approaches "forced" children who were deaf to use their senses in unconventional ways. In reality, their methods were somewhat ahead of their time considering that—at the time—hearing aids were less than adequate and children were typically not identified with an HL until age 2 or 3. The cornerstone of the LSL approach was that children can and must be taught to develop listening function and, with intensive intervention, will be able to develop spoken language.

LSL goals include integration of listening, speech, language, and cognition following the normal developmental sequence. Much like typical children, with LSL approaches, children with HL learn to listen before learning to talk. Early intervention includes development of prespeech and language skills with listening as the foundation, without regard for the child's age. In other words, if Johnny's hearing loss is identified and treated beginning at age 2, his LSLS begins by teaching Johnny to listen to sounds just as if he were a baby. The LSL principle is that Johnny's hearing is like that of an infant. This concept, called **hearing age,** refers to the amount of time that a child has had exposure to sound. In other words, the number of years between the time a person was treated for hearing impairment (e.g., hearing aids fitted and intervention initiated) and his chronological age is called hearing age. Learn more about hearing age in Focus 6.3. In order to engage the child, LSL activities must be interesting and motivating so that the child will attend to and persist in the LSL tasks.

Research Evidence for LSL Approaches.　It is important that your recommendations to parents reflect recent studies that support (or refute) a particular intervention approach. To date, most LSL efficacy studies have been based on retrospective data. Retrospective data reflect information gained by (a) going back and following up on

FOCUS 6.3 *Intervention*

Hearing Age

When comparing children with hearing loss to their typically hearing peers, it is common to compare their developmental skills based on hearing age as opposed to chronological age, much like a premature infant might be compared by gestational age. Hearing age, sometimes called listening age, is used to recognize the important role of audition in the development of language and underscores the expected delay in language until auditory concerns are properly addressed. The closer the chronological age is to the hearing age, the more likely a child's language skills will be on target by the time he or she reaches school age.

clients who have received a particular intervention or (b) evaluating records from prior subjects. A series of retrospective studies on children who received LSL intervention have been completed in recent years. Retrospective studies are considered Level III research (see Chapter 4 for a review of the levels of evidence). Below are some examples:

- Goldberg and Flexer (2001, 1993) surveyed adults who graduated from LSL programs. Results indicated that most respondents were fully mainstreamed and had professions and salaries commensurate with their hearing peers.
- Robertson and Flexer (1993) surveyed parents of LSL graduates and reported that following high school graduation students had average or higher-than-average levels of reading performance as compared to typically hearing peers.
- Children who received LSL during preschool had good academic outcomes. In a group of 19 children, 16 children were participating in regular education classrooms and read at or above grade level (Wray, Flexer, & Vaccaro, 1997).

More recent studies further document positive outcomes for children who receive LSL training; some studies are control-group designs comparing children with HL to hearing peers. For example, Rhoades & Chisolm (2000) reported that 40 children with moderate-to-profound HL in an LSL program experienced 12 months or more of language progress over a year's time; this development favorably compares to typically hearing peers. Similarly, Dornan et al. (2007) reported that a group of 29 children (ages 2 to 6 years old) in an LSL program with a mean hearing loss of 76 decibels had language ability equivalent to hearing peers after a 9-month period of intervention.

Other studies document the language and literacy outcomes of pediatric cochlear implant users. Pediatric cochlear implant users, as a general group, have access to auditory stimuli and children in this group are learning to speak using LSL approaches. Results overwhelmingly support the notion that children who access auditory stimuli through a cochlear implant early in life can develop spoken language and literacy competence commensurate with their hearing peers (Eisenberg, Fink, & Niparko, 2006; Moog, 2002; Nicholas & Geers, 2006; Spencer, Barker, & Tomblin, 2003; Svirsky, Robbins, Kirk, Pisoni, & Miyamoto, 2000). An illustration of a child wearing a cochlear implant is shown in Figure 6.1.

Family and Educational Issues for LSL Communicators. Families consider a number of issues when choosing an LSL approach. The LSL philosophy is founded on the belief that strong auditory skills are critical for language development. In order for children to obtain sufficient auditory experience, parents must (a) maximize auditory input by accessing high-quality and ongoing audiological services, (b) implement all available technology (e.g., hearing aids, cochlear implants), and (c) provide intensive auditory and language experiences in age-appropriate and natural contexts. All of this intervention and management is, of course, guided by professionals.

Once a parent decides to commit to an LSL approach, finding qualified professionals to manage the intensive intervention program is challenging. While the LSLS certification is becoming widely recognized, there are still relatively few certified

---

Figure 6.1   **Child with a Cochlear Implant**

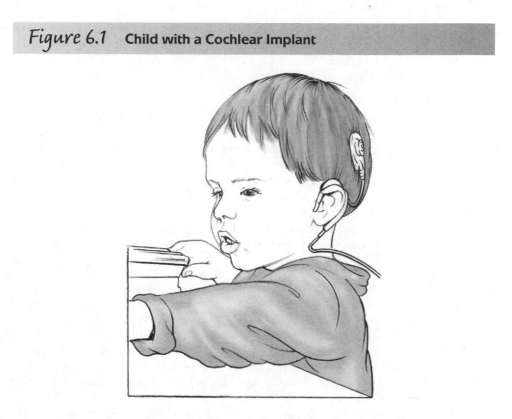

LSL specialists. The new LSLS certification process, begun in 2008, helps more specialists receive the appropriate training. Check out the AG Bell Web site at www.agbellacademy.org/certification.htm, for more information on the certification process for LSL specialists.

Since the overarching goal of LSL is full participation in society for children with HL, inclusion in regular education is expected in LSL approaches. This principle is consistent with the Individuals with Disabilities Education Act (IDEA, 2004). However, achieving complete educational inclusion can be challenging. Common barriers to full inclusion include lack of understanding of the approach on the part of the administrators and educators, the lack of an appropriate auditory learning environment, and the failure to use all available auditory technology. Table 6.6 and Focus 6.4 provide suggestions and highlight issues pertaining to working with teachers.

Approaches Focusing on Visual Learning and Manual Communication.   Sign language has received a great deal of attention as a means of improving the early communication skills of typically developing (normal hearing) infants (e.g., Thompson, Cotnoir-Bichelman, McKerchar, Tate, & Dancho, 2007). This approach has been dubbed in the popular press as "baby signs."

Table 6.6 **Tips for Collaborating with Teachers**

Make sure teachers are well informed. Help teachers understand . . .	• a child's auditory and language-learning needs. • which classroom situations will be challenging. • how to identify auditory and language problems. • how to read an audiogram and understand its implications on classroom performance.
Coordinate inservice training with the audiologist and SLPs so that teachers . . .	• can recognize and troubleshoot amplification device problems. • improve classroom acoustics (e.g., put pads or old tennis balls on table and chair legs).
Provide teachers with instructional tips that improve auditory access to the high language demands in the classroom.	• Outline each day's schedule on the board. • Send home materials for prelearning. • Always face the class when speaking.

In addition to signing with typically developing infants, sign language sometimes is used to enhance expressive language of children with other kinds of communication disorders other than HL (e.g., autism or Down syndrome). However, the use of sign language for children with intellectual disability (ID) or autism spectrum disorder (ASD) must be considered separately from its use related to HL. The underlying cause of language delay in ID or ASD is completely different from the language challenges of children with HL. Consequently, the rationale for choosing sign language as an alternative means of communication for a child with autism or intellectual disability is very different from the rationale for choosing manual communication for children who are HL.

Sign language as a communication approach for children with HL is based on an underlying philosophy: Children who are deaf use sign language because they can see but not hear. Deaf students are primarily visual learners because "they use their eyes as their primary learning channel. They can process some language and environmental information aurally, but this auditory channel is secondary to the visual channel" (Maryland School for the Deaf (MSD Handbook, 2009). If you compare this statement to the findings presented earlier related to the development of

FOCUS 6.4 *Issues for School-Age Children*

Inclusion for Children with Hearing Loss: Working with Teachers

Inclusion is an educational option allowing children with HL to be in the classroom with their typical hearing peers. In this model, support is provided to both students and teachers in order to facilitate optimal access to learning. To improve your clinical decision-making skills, give some examples of how an SLP could work with the teacher if a child with a hearing loss was in a general education classroom.

auditory channels of the brain and the impact on spoken language, it should be evident that there is a clear difference of opinion. The conflicting views in the field of HL challenges parents to make decisions on the best approach for their own child.

There are a number of sign language choices. Children with HL, who are born to deaf parents, are typically immersed in the Deaf culture and learn ASL. As described earlier, ASL is often thought of as a **bilingual-bicultural** approach. According to the Gallaudet (2006) annual survey, approximately 11% of deaf children use sign language as their primary mode of communication.

Total (simultaneous) communication (TC) combines auditory and visual learning and communication strategies; it is the more common manual approach. TC is used more frequently than ASL because, 90% of the time, children with HL are raised by hearing parents who are not part of the Deaf culture. TC may incorporate a variety of different forms of sign language including ASL, **Signing Exact English (SEE)** and **Pidgin**.

TC was developed in the 1960s by David Denton at the Maryland School for the Deaf (MSD) as a middle ground between oralism (i.e., AO) and manualism (i.e., ASL). The term total communication was adopted later as an official name for the school's educational philosophy. Today, however, the school's philosophy is a bilingual approach (ASL and written English). Specifically, the MSD handbook states, "recent research shows that using two languages at the same time compromises both languages, ASL and English" (MSD, 2009, p. 19). As this quote documents, parents receive a great deal of information regarding the "best way" to educate their child with HL. Unfortunately, sometimes the information is conflicting. At present, although most experts do not recommend TC as an educational approach, approximately 33% children using manual communication use TC in the classroom (Gallaudet, 2006).

Family and Educational Issues for Manual Communicators.   Sign language use has specific family implications. Family members, friends, and others who wish to communicate effectively with the child with HL must (a) learn to sign or (b) rely on an interpreter. Initially, parents and other care providers are able to take basic sign courses and learn from videos and books. However, as the child's language becomes more complex, parents and other communication partners must immerse themselves in a sign-language-rich environment to become effective communication partners. Like parents who choose an LSL approach, parents who choose TC should devote considerable time and effort to support their child's manual communication. Unlike LSL approaches, families who choose TC do not ascribe to a set of principles to which they must adhere to maximize success. In fact, in terms of developing language through signing, children using TC may be exposed to varying types or levels of signing and spoken communication (Nusbaum, 2007).

When parents choose TC as a communication modality, they should also consider the greater community and academic system in which their child will be raised. If a child relies primarily on sign language, he should use an interpreter for many routine events (e.g., ordering food at a local restaurant or asking for directions). Initially, the parent may serve as the interpreter, but as the child becomes more independent, the parents should consider ways to increase the child's independence through interpreters.

Academic placement for children who use TC typically depends on local programming. Some school districts have special schools or classes exclusively developed for children with HL who communicate with sign language. In areas where there are fewer students with HL, children often are mainstreamed with an interpreter.

Proponents of sign language often argue that a visual-based communication approach (sign language) is necessary to develop language for most children with HL. According to this line of reasoning, children with HL born to hearing parents are exposed to less linguistically rich environments than their peers for two reasons: (1) the loss of sensory information created by hearing loss and, (2) the lack of a shared native language. Another common thread in this literature is the suggestion that children who are deaf and born to hearing parents generally start learning language later and consequently have less consistent and less useful experiences (e.g., Marschark & Lukomski, 2001).

There is increasing evidence countering this line of thinking. According to the Gallaudet Web site (Nusbaum, 2007), "use of all communication modes, as proposed by a TC approach, does not necessarily guarantee development of either a full spoken language or a full visual sign language." Recent studies have reported that the brain of manual communicators demonstrates structural changes including recruitment of the brain's auditory regions for visual processing (Fine, Finney, Boynton, & Dobkins, 2005; Finney, Fine, & Dobkins, 2001; MacSweeney et al., 2002; Meyer et al., 2007). In contrast, children who begin to use their auditory systems in the first year of life demonstrate neural auditory and language activity consistent with hearing peers (Eisenberg et al., 2006; Geers, Nicholas, & Sedey, 2003; Gordon et al., 2003; Robbins, Koch, Osberger, & Zimmerman-Philips, 2004; Sharma et al., 2004; Werker & Tees, 2005).

FAMILY INVOLVEMENT IN THE REMEDIATION PROCESS

Both IDEA (2004) and the Division of Early Childhood (DEC; Sandall, Giacomini, Smith & Hemmeter, 2006) emphasize the importance of family involvement and parental competence in supporting children's language learning. I will discuss these important factors, which have recently been explored by researchers, only briefly, since they are also covered in the *Connections* section.

When a child is diagnosed with HL, his or her parents must learn to maximize early language experiences (Aram, Most, & Mayafit, 2006; Hart & Risley, 1999; Moeller, 2000; Senechal & LeFevre, 2002; Yoshinaga-Itano et al., 1998). Parents should be taught to use scaffolding, imitation, and closed-ended questions during the first year of life (Yoder, McCathren, Warren, & Watson, 2001). As the child enters the preschool years, parents should use facilitative language techniques reflecting the child's zone of proximal development (Vygotsky, 1978; 1987). See Chapter 4 for descriptions of facilitative language techniques consistent with social-interaction theories of language development. Parents should be trained to use everyday interactions to explicitly teach important language concepts (DesJardin, 2006). Parents also should be supported to engage their child with HL in frequent storybook reading interactions (Aram et al., 2006; Kaderavek & Pakulski, 2007).

Connections

The *Connections* subsections throughout this book are provided to highlight information relevant to a particular domain or disability group. But the information in *Connections* also has broader implications across the speech-language pathology field. In this *Connections* subsection, I present information about (a) the role of a counselor and the process of helping families through emotions triggered by the identification of their child's hearing loss and (b) the important role of family participation in educational decision making and language intervention. While reading this information about children with HL, you should consider the application of this information to children with other disabilities. Almost all parents, even if their child is only mildly impaired, will be affected to some degree by psychological stress after discovering their child has special educational needs. Families with children who are diagnosed with specific language impairment, autism, cognitive disability, and reading/writing deficits also will experience emotional distress and grief. You will play an important role in helping parents cope with their feelings regardless of their child's diagnosis.

I also discuss issues related to family participation in the intervention process. It is important to remember that families play a critical role in the habilitation of all children, whether they have autism, intellectual disability, specific language impairment, or hearing loss. As such, the information presented in this section applies to many different families in your professional career.

COUNSELING PARENTS OF CHILDREN WITH SPECIAL NEEDS

Parents of newly diagnosed children with hearing impairment (or other disabilities) often indicate feeling overwhelmed and inadequate to manage their children's special educational needs (Kurtzer-White & Luterman, 2003). These feelings of inadequacy can trigger feelings of anger. In fact, the cycle of emotions triggered by the identification of a child's disability is similar to the grief process triggered by the death of a loved one. The parent mourns the loss of the hoped-for "perfect" child and cycles through phases of emotions before accepting the fact that his or her child has a disability. Stages of the grief process are briefly described in the next section.

Because understanding a person's psychological state is so important to the habilitation process, SLPs and special educators should develop excellent counseling skills so they can support family member's emotional and psychological concerns (ASHA, 1990). However, in my teaching experience, I have found that beginning clinicians often have difficulty implementing effective counseling skills. One of the difficulties in becoming a good counselor is that counseling behaviors are quite different than typical conversational exchanges. There are several counseling techniques that make counseling different from regular conversation, including (a) tolerating conversational silence, (b) reflecting feeling, and (c) asking open versus closed questions. These techniques are based on humanistic theory (Maslow, 1962; Rogers, 1951) and are useful in that they assume that, given support, individuals will work through emotional crises. The counseling techniques of waiting, listening instead of talking, reflecting feeling, and asking open-ended questions encourage families to talk about their emotions. Family's emotional responses and their coping strategies are directly related to child outcomes (Leigh & Anthony, 1999).

Tolerating Pauses and Listening.   In order to help an individual work through his or her emotions, SLPs and special educators employ a client-centered focus (Shames, 2000). This means that when family members are talking about their feelings, we listen to what they are saying without interjecting our own thoughts and feelings. This sounds easy, but it is harder than you may think. In typical conversations, we are used to a back-and-forth verbal exchange:

> *Speaker A:*   *"I had a terrible day today. I could not find a parking place on campus, I must have driven around for 20 minutes looking for a place to park—and I was late for class."*
>
> *Speaker B:*   *"I know what you mean. Monday mornings on campus are terrible; I can never find anything either!"*
>
> *Speaker A:*   *"He makes me so mad. He always thinks he's right and I'm wrong!"*
>
> *Speaker B:*   *"I've been telling you he's a loser. I think you should dump him!"*

In the first example, Speaker B responds with a shared experience; in the second example, Speaker B gives advice to her friend. Both of these responses are appropriate for a typical conversation, but counseling is different. The counselor stays focused on the speaker's emotional reactions.

The first counseling technique is to learn to wait after an individual begins to talk about his or her emotions. Waiting with relaxed arms and legs (i.e., avoid crossing your arms across your chest) and maintaining a forward-leaning body position (i.e., leaning slightly toward the speaker rather than leaning back in your chair) are nonverbal signals that you are comfortable and open to listening. In the U.S. culture, we typically only wait a few seconds between conversational turns. It will feel very uncomfortable for you to wait after a speaker shares his or her feelings. You will find, however, that if you wait a few more seconds (I recommend slowly counting to 5), the speaker often continues to share feelings and emotions. Sharing negative emotions to a sympathetic listener helps families psychologically adjust to their child's diagnosis.

Reflecting Feeling.   Right about now you might be saying to yourself, "So, I'm just sitting there not talking and waiting for the family member to say something? What if he doesn't say anything else?" When it is apparent to you that the client needs to express emotions, it is helpful to use a technique called **reflecting feeling**. When a professional reflects feelings, he or she responds to the client's emotional expressions rather than to the content of the message. Reflecting emotions is important because family members often hide negative emotional reaction. The use of feeling-related comments is one of the most significant illustrations of empathetic listening and is a powerful means of letting family members know that their feelings are normal and that you are there to support their adjustment to the new situation (Kaderavek, Laux, & Mills, 2004). Here is an example of a reflection of feeling:

> *Family Member:*   *"I thought that something was wrong, but I was afraid to tell anyone about it. I didn't want to accept the fact that he couldn't hear me. But now I feel guilty that I didn't get him tested earlier."*
>
> *Professional:*   (after a long pause) *"It's hard not to feel guilty as a parent, isn't it?"*
>
> *Family Member:*   *"Yes, it's hard not to feel responsible, but I know that I have to let go of the guilt; it doesn't do any good now."*

In the example above, the typical conversational response might be to immediately reassure the family member, *"There's no reason to feel guilty!"* However, by reflecting feelings, you indicate that you understand that families feel a range of emotions including anger, fear, and sadness. Reflecting feelings, rather than providing advice in response to expressed emotions, also indicates your understanding that parents must work through their feelings in their own way.

Open-ended Questions.   Open questions allow family members to respond in a number of different ways while closed questions require a specific response (Cormier & Nurius, 2003; Seligman, 2004). Professionals often use closed questions during an initial interview to obtain specific information. Examples of closed questions include: *"When was your child's hearing loss identified?"* *"How many words does your child use?"* and *"Is your child using amplification all the time?"* Closed questions often are comfortable for beginning students because closed questions are aimed at obtaining factual information rather than emotional responses.

When the professional wants to help families explore the emotions connected with their child's hearing loss, an important technique is to use open-ended questions. Open-ended questions provide more opportunity for the family member to "just talk" and discuss the relevant issues in the way that is most meaningful to him or her. Some examples of open-ended questions include, *"Tell me how the family reacted when you told them about your child's hearing loss."* *"Tell me about your child's experiences at school so far."* and *"What is a typical day like for you at home with your child?"* Open-ended questions provide an opportunity for family members to reveal feelings and communicate that the professional is willing to listen. After posing an open-ended question, the professional waits before responding, tolerates pauses in the conversation, and reflects feelings as appropriate.

THE GRIEF PROCESS

A classic model describing the emotions triggered by death and bereavement is called the stages of grief model (Kubler-Ross, 1969). This model also has been used to describe the emotional reactions of parents after learning that their child has a disability. In a survey of parents, researchers found that parents reported feeling shock (42%), anger (23%), confusion (42%), fear (52%), sadness (16%), frustration (31%), depression (37%), loneliness (16%), and blame (16%) after their child's initial diagnosis of hearing loss (Yoshinaga-Itano & de Uzcategui, 2001). Many of these feelings are associated with the grief model. Keep in mind that parents typically do not pass through emotional stages in a step-by-step fashion. Instead, parents alternate between emotions with a gradual progression toward acceptance, optimism, and hope (Kearney & Griffin, 2001).

The emotions are associated with the grief model include the following:

- *Denial:* Denial is a conscious or unconscious refusal to accept the facts; it is a normal response to a significant negative event
- *Anger:* Sometimes family members are angry with themselves or focus blame on one of the professionals working with their child. Family members may react with anger in ways that appear inappropriate.
- *Depression:* An overwhelming feeling of sadness and loss.
- *Acceptance:* While many individuals pass through periods of grief and loss, in the long term most parents of children with disabilities report that they are "better people" and "feel strengthened" by their experiences, and they describe the joy their child brings to the family (Kearney & Griffin, 2001).

As you perfect your counseling skills and become a sympathetic and supportive listener, you will help families move toward the final stage of acceptance.

FAMILY ROLE IN INTERVENTION

No matter what communication modality a family chooses—teaching the child to listen and talk, sign language, or total communication—parents play a critical role in their child's growth, development, and overall outcomes (Flexer et al., 2005). To develop language, children must be immersed in language—and parents are the child's primary language teachers. Some considerations in working with families:

- Parents are encouraged to develop the skills and knowledge they need to foster their child's communication. The professional avoids taking on the role of the expert who can fix the child's communication. Instead, from the outset, the SLP, audiologist, medical personnel, educator, and family members work together to develop the child's intervention program.
- The professional recognizes that each family has a unique structure. As a professional, you will work with single-parent families, foster families, families with two parents of the same gender, parents who both work full-time, fathers who provide most of the child care, and families headed by grandparents. The professional demonstrates sensitivity and respect for the various values and customs of each child's family (Schirmer, 2000).
- Professionals consider all of the child's daily experiences as potential opportunities for language learning. Encourage everyone possible, including teachers, babysitters, church-school teachers, preschool teachers, coaches, and the child's peers to become involved in communicating with the child with HL.

Assessment and Progress Monitoring

Children with HL experience a great deal of testing during their early years. Audiologists periodically evaluate and monitor the level of hearing loss and evaluate the benefit provided by different amplification systems. The practitioner concentrates on assessing and monitoring the child's speech and evaluating the child's language and literacy development. Practitioners also assess the influence of the child's amplification device on the home and educational environment.

ASSESSMENT TOOLS

There are a number of approaches to assessment for children with HL (see Table 6.7). One frequently used measure is the MacArthur Inventory (Fenton et al., 2007). The MacArthur-Bates Communicative Development Inventory: Words, Gestures, and Sentences includes a questionnaire format and asks parents to identify various words that their child either says or signs. It includes vocabulary relating to home, people, action words, description words, pronouns, prepositions, and question words. The McArthur Inventory also documents the child's use of sentences and grammatical forms. The McArthur scale was not developed specifically for children with HL but is an effective means to document vocabulary growth.

Table 6.7   **Sample Tools for Assessment and Monitoring**

Test	Description
Boehm Test of Basic Concepts—Third Edition (Boehm-3; Boehm, 2000)	Measures the understanding of basic positional concepts of young children and provides information about conceptual development.
Bracken Basic Concept Scale—Third Edition (BBCS-3) (Bracken, 2007)	Evaluates concepts essential to early communication development and school readiness.
Preschool Language Scale—Fourth Edition (PLS-4) (Zimmerman, Steiner, & Pond, 2002)	Measures language and developmental milestones.
Structured Photographic Expressive Language Test—3 (SPELT-3) (Dawson, Stout, & Eyer, 2003)	Provides a means for analysis of specific language structures (e.g., syntax) that may not occur in spontaneous language samples.
Test of Auditory Comprehension of Language (TACL-3) (Carrow-Woolfolk, 1999)	Measures receptive spoken vocabulary, grammar, and syntax.
MacArthur-Bates Communicative Developmental Inventory (CDI-2) (Fenson, L., Marchman, V.A., Thal, D.J., Dale, P.S., Reznick, J.S., & Bates, E. (2006)	Standardized, parent-completed report assists professionals in screening young children's emerging language and communication skills.

Another assessment tool, the Cottage Acquisition Scales for Listening, Language, and Speech (CASLLS; Wilkes & Sunshine Cottage School for Deaf Children, 1999) includes a developmental checklist for assessment and planning for diagnostic therapy. The language section includes steps from preverbal to complex sentences, including pragmatic development. The CASLLS was specifically designed for children with HL and is based on a developmental approach. A developmental approach describes the child's abilities along a continuum of language milestones.

In contrast to the developmental approach used in the CASLLS, other assessment tools take an identification of deficit position typically documented via a norm-based test. This approach typically is used with older children with HL, particularly when the HL has significantly impacted language development. With the deficit approach, the professional compares the language ability of the child with HL to other children with HL and the language development of typical peers. An example of a normative-referenced instrument is the Clinical Evaluation of Language Fundamentals—Preschool (CELF-P; Wiig, Secord, & Semel, 2004). The CELF-P evaluates expressive and receptive language ability focusing on word meanings, word and sentence structure, and recall of spoken language. It is standardized for children with normal hearing abilities from ages 3 years, 0 months to 6 years, 11 months and uses pictures as stimuli for all three areas of language development. In its standardized administration procedure, the CELF-P requires the child to listen to auditory instructions.

Example Assessment Using the CASLLS.   Let's take an example student and think through the process of assessment. Imagine that you are a practitioner who must assess a transfer student midway through the school year. How can you ensure that the child's learning needs are met while simultaneously assessing communication skills?

First and foremost, when working with a child with HL, you (in conjunction with the educational audiologist and other members of the educational team) must insure that auditory learning is accessible. This can be done by completing a **Ling Six Sound Test** (Ling, 1989) at various distances in and across contexts. The Ling Test can be completed by anyone (e.g., parents, SLPs, teachers, audiologists) and is an easy way to determine if a child is hearing sounds in the speech frequency. More information about the Ling test is described in Focus 6.5. The Ling sounds are shown in Figure 6.2.

Next, you must assess the child's communication skills. Diagnostic testing can take weeks to complete, so it is often useful to think of assessment as an ongoing process interspersed with trial intervention. We will start by using the Cottage Scales to complete an observation of a child with HL.

Mary, age 7, was born with a mild, bilateral, sensorineural hearing loss that was not diagnosed until she was a toddler. She is shy but interacts with peers when they initiate the interaction or to meet classroom demands. She uses courtesy language (i.e., *"thank you," "hello"*) without prompting, but does not repair communication breakdowns. Communication repairs are a child's efforts to clarify communication when he or she is not understood as a communicator. For example, a classmate

FOCUS 6.5 *Clinical Skill Building*

Ling Test

When a child presents with an apparent communication deficit, hearing impairment must always be ruled out. Screening is often the first step. A hearing screening can be completed in a physician's office, but is more commonly completed as part of a speech and language evaluation unless the child is under 3 years of age. Before age 3, a child must be screened/assessed by an audiologist. An audiologist also diagnoses and quantifies a child's hearing loss.

Before initiating a diagnostic evaluation (or therapy session), the professional must determine that the child with HL has auditory access. In other words, you must determine if the child's amplification device is working. A simple evaluation tool, developed by Daniel Ling (1989; 2002), is termed the Ling Six Sound Test. The Ling Test evaluates a child's ability to detect and discriminate sounds across the speech spectrum. Figure 6.2 illustrates the relationship between the Ling Six sounds ("m," "ah," "oo," "ee," "sh," and "s") and the speech spectrum. When a child is able to repeat each sound in response to the clinician's request, the adult can be certain that the child has auditory access. In order to ensure that the child is hearing and not seeing the sounds, an acoustic hoop is used to cover the clinician's mouth without interfering with the acoustics of the signal. A simple embroidery hoop with speaker cloth is typically used for this purpose.

A second component of this test is referred to as *circle of hearing* or *listening distance*. Once it is established that the child can hear each sound, the adult determines the distance (usually in feet) at which the child is still able to detect the sound by repeatedly asking the child to discriminate a sound as he or she moves away from the child.

approaches Mary and comments, "*Mary, I'd like to use the pencil sharpener*" to which Mary replies, "*Hi.*" When the first child clearly does not respond to Mary's interaction, Mary does not attempt to continue the conversation or clarify that she did not understand the first child's communication.

Figure 6.2 Approximate Frequency Distribution of Ling Sounds

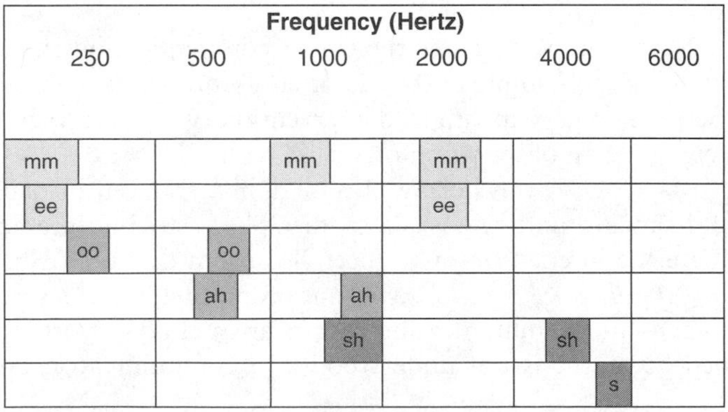

Frequency (Hertz)										
250		500		1000		2000		4000		6000
mm				mm		mm				
ee						ee				
	oo		oo							
		ah		ah						
				sh			sh			
							s			

Mary speaks softly and is moderately intelligible. Her language is approximately a year delayed but is consistent with her hearing age of 5 years, 9 months. Mary has bilateral behind-the-ear hearing aids that should be coupled with an FM system for maximal audition. An FM system is an assistive listening device that delivers the teacher's voice, via a microphone and receiver, directly to Mary's hearing aids. An FM system improves Mary's ability to hear the teacher at a distance and over background noise. However, like many school-age children with mild hearing loss, Mary resists using the assistive listening devices (Reeve, 2005).

As you complete your classroom observations, you observe the following:

- Mary has difficulty with plurals, possessives, and past tense, often omitting the final consonant and using incorrect grammar. For example, when asked, "*How did you get to school today?*" Mary answered, "*I walk.*"
- On her spelling and vocabulary assignments she has trouble with simple words. Mary drew a sled when asked to make a picture of a flag.
- After reading aloud to the class, the teacher asked Mary to answer some basic comprehension questions. When the teacher asked Mary, "*Who did the dog belong to?*" and "*Where did the dog sleep?*" Mary had difficulty describing the central characters in the story and did not understand the story events.

Despite the language difficulties displayed, Mary also demonstrated communication skills consistent with her hearing age. Age-appropriate communication skills included (a) use of subordinate clauses, (b) use of indirect discourse (e.g., "*Mom said I can go.*"), and (c) adverb formation using *ly*. Based on what you know about speech perception, the level of Mary's hearing loss, and her age of identification, do the errors described above seem more or less severe than expected?

To answer this question, we again consider Mary's hearing age of 5 years, 9 months. Mary's hearing age suggests that her speech and language age will be equivalent to a younger child's. Table 6.8 provides Mary's expected language use based on the Cottage Scales. When considering Mary's hearing age of 5:9, however, we see that Mary is making unexpected errors. Plurals, possessives, and past tense are typically mastered between 3 and 4 years of age; vocabulary and her ability to answer questions also should be more developed. Mary is experiencing communication problems that are not consistent with her hearing age.

To understand Mary's difficulties, we must consider again that language development and use is dependent on listening. If someone asks, "*Do you want two or three book?*" (omission of the plural morpheme [*books*]) or states, "*I would like to borrow Emily book,*" [omission of possessive morpheme [*Emily's*]), a typical listener is able to fill in the missing plural or possessive morpheme. In contrast, children with hearing loss are unable to fill in the missing information. Since a child with HL has reduced auditory experience, he or she often is not able to produce or self-monitor important language components.

Vocabulary comprehension also can be challenging for children with HL. In the example of Mary's confusion with *flag* and *sled*, you may have concluded that Mary did not know the words or was inattentive during the task. While these may be causal factors, there are other issues to consider. First, children with mild hearing impairment may mistake one word for another if the sounds (phonemes) in the

Table 6.8   **Select Language Use of 5- to 6-Year-Olds Based on the Cottage Acquisition Scales**

Dimension	Description
Nouns, noun modifiers, and relative clauses	Uses superlative *est*; uses *er* to form nouns (*teach-teacher*); uses gerund (*"Teaching is fun"*); uses relative clauses.
Prepositions and pronouns	Uses reflexive pronoun (*themselves*); uses possessive nominative (*its, ours*); uses *this* and *that* to stand for entire ideas; uses adverbs of time (*within*).
Verbs, adverbs, and infinitives	Uses *ly* to form adverbs; uses specific times (*1 A.M.*); uses indirect discourse; uses infinitive with *wh* word (*"What to do?"*).
Tense, negation, and modals	Uses present perfect, negative + perfect tense, future progressive, present perfect progressive, modal progressive, and negative with *say, ask, tell*.
Coordination, nominals, and adverbials	Produces clauses (e.g., *as soon as, before*); uses *or* to indicate inclusion; uses *neither, do, do too*, and *whether or (not)*; uses subordinate clauses and nominal clauses.
Questions	Asks *wh* questions with *do verb* (*"What does it do?"*).
Discourse	Uses focused chains for narratives; gives threats; issues promises and praise; stays on conversational topic; uses pronoun reference as cohesive device.

Source: Adapted from Cottage Acquisition Scales for Listening, Language, and Speech (CASLLS), by Wilkes & Sunshine Cottage School for Deaf Children, 1999, San Antonio, TX: Sunshine Cottage School for Deaf Children. Used with permission.

word are similar. When we think of similar sounds, we might think of *bat* and *pat*. The sounds /b/ and /p/ are produced similarly, but differ in that /b/ uses vocal fold vibration while /p/ does not.

Other complex acoustic characteristics also make listening difficult for children with HL. For example, the "oo" and "ee" sound have the same first formant (frequency) and differ primarily by their second formant. Because the second formant for "ee" is a high-frequency sound, children with hearing loss often confuse the "ee" and "oo" sounds; they may not be able to distinguish a word with the vowel "ee" from a word with "oo." This vowel confusion may have played a part in Mary's vocabulary error.

As a practitioner, you will learn how to use tools like the CASLLS to guide language assessments of children with HL. With practice and training, you will learn to determine child errors in relation to an individual's overall listening and language-learning environment. The root cause of Mary's language problem likely relates to the inconsistent use of amplification, which causes her to miss important language cues.

Intervention

As a trained professional, you will play a vital role in the education and therapeutic intervention of children with HL. Parents need training and support to guide their child's language and literacy learning. As children enter school, both regular and special education teachers will require your help to meet the special educational and classroom needs of children with HL.

Below I will highlight intervention approaches for children with HL who are learning to listen and talk. Since you may also work with children who use sign language, Table 6.9 provides strategies for maximizing language and literacy development for manual communicators. Intervention considerations for children with auditory processing disorders are addressed in Focus 6.6.

Intervention approaches for children who are hearing impaired often are intertwined with the mode of communication and age of identification. In this section, I discuss the LSL techniques. LSL techniques include "Learning to Listen" sounds, hand cues, acoustic highlighting, sound sandwich, sabotage, and language experience books. The last technique, language experience books, is discussed in a separate section below. LSL techniques are summarized in Table 6.10.

LEARNING TO LISTEN

When initial diagnosis and fitting of amplification devices have been addressed, the interventionist begins periodic family treatment sessions. Parents are coached to build communication through a natural developmental sequence using LSL techniques in meaningful daily experiences.

In the learning to listen (LTL) technique, parents are instructed to play with their child using toys paired with the LTL sounds. LTL sounds are associated with an object (e.g., a transportation vehicle or animal) or a specific action. This type of

Table 6.9 Facilitating Language Development for Children Who Use Sign Language

Technique	Description
Letter calling	Present a word's sign, finger-spell the word, and then draw child's attention to the printed version of the word.
Storybook reading	Expose child to different book genres. Scaffold the reading interaction, activate child's prior knowledge of story themes, support child's story recall, help child identify the main theme, draw conclusions from the story, and provide story details.
Chaining	Explicitly link finger spelling, print, and sign version of the word.
Sign placement	Sign words directly over text when reading to make explicit links between signed and written word.

FOCUS 6.6 *Intervention*

Intervention for Children with Auditory Processing Disorders

In recent years many researchers have shown links between spoken language and auditory development, particularly in the presence of hearing loss (e.g., Sharma, 2007). Much less is understood about the cause-effect relationship between auditory processing disorders and language learning problems. In fact, some research suggests that APD is not the source of language learning problems, but a consequence (Nittrouer, 2002; Uwer, Albrecht, & von Suchodoletz, 2002).

By definition, auditory processing disorder is something that adversely affects a child's ability to decode or interpret auditory information. Since many language-learning and cognitive skills are used in this process (e.g., memory, attention), it is difficult to separate what is truly an auditory function from other language, learning, and cognitive skills (Johnston, 2006). While the specific cause of the APD is not always known, it is known to coexist with many other neurocognitive disorders including autism and specific language impairment. What is clear is that children may have language learning and attention deficits secondary to APD, although it is quite possible that these problems may be more language-based than auditory-related (Nittrouer, 2002; Uwer et al., 2002).

As a future clinician, you may be asking yourself: How do I know which viewpoint to adopt? Future research will likely shed light on these issues. More importantly, you can concern yourself with the functional concerns and outcomes of the children with whom you work. If a child has language-learning problems in the presence of a diagnosis of APD, your most important job will be to determine how these deficits affect communication, language, and learning. Using that information, you will then develop strategies to assist the child in overcoming the deficit. Common strategies related to auditory attention and memory include improving the audibility of the desired signal (e.g., the teacher's voice over the background noise) through preferential seating or amplification devices, minimizing attention demands, and teaching explicit comprehension monitoring (Johnston, 2006).

---

activity is very similar to the auditory experiences parents use with children developing typically. For example, adults often say *"uh-oh"* indicating that they have dropped a toy, or make a motor sound when pushing a toy car. Children are repeatedly exposed to sounds connected to objects or actions in a deliberate and focused intervention program. During parent-child play interactions, parents use acoustic highlighting (i.e., strategies to improve sound audibility such as using a slower rate and increased pitch) and model hand cues (e.g., a technique that signals that the parent is speaking). Below is an example interaction:

> The mother, father, and child with HL sit together on the floor with several toys. The mother makes the sound *"ahhhh"* in a melodic fashion; the father repeats the sound. A toy airplane is introduced and the sound is repeated *"ahhhh"* as the airplane soars through the air. This is repeated. Finally, the mother produces an utterance paired with the LTL sound, *"Mama has the airplane, ahhhh, airplane."*

Table 6.10   **Auditory Verbal Therapy Techniques**

Technique	Description
Learning to listen sounds (LTL)	Sound–object associations used with young children as they learn new sounds and vocabulary. Commonly used LTL sounds are /ahhh/ with *airplane*, "moo" with *cow*, "quack quack" with *duck* and /ssss/ with *snake*.
Acoustic highlighting	Strategies to improve audibility of spoken communication. Examples include slower rate, increased pitch, and providing greater contrast in sets (e.g., *airplane, cookie, dog* versus the stimulus set *dog, hog, frog*).
Hand cue	A technique used to encourage a child to attend to spoken language. The hand is placed near or in front of the mouth to alert new listeners.
Sound sandwich	A way of emphasizing an auditory cue while providing a visual cue when necessary. A word or message is first spoken, and if not understood, then paired with a visual cue (e.g., object, lip reading, sign). The visual cue is followed by a second auditory cue (e.g., say "*apple*," show an apple [or the written word], then say "*apple*" again).
Sabotage	A deliberate mistake is made by the adult to provide a child with the opportunity to recognize and try to repair the mistake.

During similar interactions, parents learn how to encourage and then respond to their child's early communication attempts. During the LTL activities, parents also learn to monitor and adjust the child's listening environment. Too much noise, visual distractions, or other factors affect early language-listening experiences.

As children begin to repeat the LTL sounds and eventually string words together, daily activities (e.g., cooking dinner or driving to school), interactive games, and book reading are used to expose children to important listening and language behaviors. Table 6.11 provides examples of how interweaving language training, listening exposure, and daily activities can be combined to develop foundational language skills. Activities used to teach foundational language concepts are sometimes called extension activities.

LANGUAGE EXPERIENCE BOOKS

The basis for the extension activities presented in Table 6.11 is a widely used tool: the language experience book. Associated with the language experience approach, events and teachable moments in a child's daily experiences are recorded with pictures or illustrations and narrated with varying levels of text (Stauffer, 1970). Parents and the interventionist help the child record experiences and use these books to promote language and literacy.

At the beginning stage of using the language experience book, the book's text usually is based on events in a child's life. For example, a child is shown a picture in

Table 6.11 **Literacy Ideas and Extension Activities Across Different Book Genres**

Genre	Activities
Narrative storybooks	• Choose books that relate to, or can be mimicked in, daily events (e.g., falling asleep in Goodnight Moon [Brown, 2005]). • Role-play subtle nuances of story (e.g., emotions in *Bear Snores On* [Wilson & Chapman, 2001]). • Alter story text to fit child's interests or needs. • If working on specific vocabulary, extend the text into games around the house (e.g., focus on grammar or vocabulary with *Brown Bear, Brown Bear* [Martin & Carle, 2008]).
Manipulative storybooks	• Choose manipulative books that allow child to touch and feel the book (e.g., *In the Ocean* [Wood, 2001]). • Select a few favorite books and make movable features (e.g., add a window with a piece of tape and card stock or cutout characters). • Find corresponding characters from other toys or stuffed animals that can be used to relate elements from play and real life with the story line (e.g., *Little People Cars, Trucks, Planes, and Trains* [Fisher-Price, 2004]). • Rewrite the child's favorite recipes on cards that include pictures of the items and then allow your child to work "hands-on" with items, following the directions.
Role-playing	• Use props to correspond to a book and act out the story (e.g., for beginners, *Blue Hat, Green Hat* [Boyton, 1984]), for older or more sophisticated language users, *Jack and the Beanstalk* [Kellogg, 1997]). • Select books that detail an upcoming event (e.g., *Happy Birthday Maisy!* [Cousins, 2008]). First read the book, then talk about what will happen at the child's party, then practice some aspects such as singing and blowing out candles. • Create or find books that allow you to include the child as a story character (e.g., *Picture Me with Jonah and the Whale* [MacKall, 1997]).
Experience books	• Encourage parents to create experience books and use them at home and in therapy. • Use photos and mementos (e.g., acorns, seashells, a wrapper) to enhance the meaning of an experience book page. Talk about event with child and then decide how to caption it in a way that best represents child's expressions. • Use the experience pages to talk about past and future, abstract concepts, and other language concepts that are difficult for the child to understand.

FOCUS 6.7 *Learning More*

There are dozens of useful Web sites that can provide ideas for therapy with preschoolers. Explore some of these Web sites and create extension activities based on one or more themes.

---

which he is standing in front of the polar bears at the zoo. The adult writes a sentence below the picture: *Andrew went to the zoo for his birthday. The polar bears were eating fish.* Even before the time that the child can read the text, he is encouraged to "read" using emergent reading behaviors (see Chapter 9 for more about emergent reading). Integrating the language experience book into a child's intervention program provides complex language models and provides an opportunity for language expansion (Kaderavek & Pakulski, 2007).

As the child's language develops, the practitioner includes a theme-based language experience approach that combines storybook reading with extension activities. For example, after reading the book, *Head to Toe* (Carle, 2000), the practitioner engages the child in singing, "Hokey Pokey" and "Head, Shoulders, Knees, and Toes." Additional extension activities include discussions on body parts and related concepts. Example activities include (a) baking and decorating gingerbread boy/girl cookies, (b) tracing and coloring the child's body on large paper, (c) examining a skeleton or chicken bones left from dinner, (d) experimenting with muscles and movement, or (e) comparing the child's growth record and changes in height and weight. Focus 6.7 and Focus 6.8 provide more ideas to consider regarding intervention for children with HL.

Throughout a child's education, he or she will require monitoring and intervention. In some cases, as in Mary's example above, audiological management may

---

FOCUS 6.8 *Learning More*

Playgroup for Children with Hearing Loss

A playgroup is an excellent way to implement some of the early literacy and extension activities for preschoolers with HL. A playgroup may incorporate storybook reading, singing and dance/movement, and auditory and language-learning-based games and crafts. When young children are able to listen to stories and say or repeat certain story elements, readers theater can be incorporated. Kerry Moran (2006) provides ideas on adapting readers theater for young children.

solve many of the child's language problems. Other children may require occasional support to develop new skills. For example, as a child's language and thought processes become more complex, he or she may have difficulty with new grammar or perhaps will demonstrate careless speech articulation. Other children, particularly those who did not get early or appropriate intervention, may require ongoing intervention.

Summary

- When the hearing loss occurs in the outer and middle ear, it is called a conductive loss and is typically the result of a medical problem such as a fluid-filled middle ear (otitis media) or damage such as a perforated eardrum.
- Sensorineural losses are those caused by damage to the inner ear structures or auditory nerve, often caused by genetic disorders or birth defects. When a child has both a sensorineural hearing impairment and a conductive disorder (e.g., permanent hearing loss due to genetic disorder co-occurring with a middle ear infection), the loss is called mixed.
- Auditory perceptual problems are generally caused by auditory processing disorder (APD) or auditory neuropathy/dys-synchrony (AN/AD). APD is caused by malfunctioning of the auditory pathway to the brain or small defects in the brain's auditory cortex. AN/AD is an auditory processing deficit that impedes the auditory signal as it travels from the cochlea to the brain. Like APD, AN/AD is not due to a malfunction in the outer, middle, or inner ear.
- Children with hearing loss who did not have early intense auditory training or who have other associated deficits are likely to have language impairments including morphologic and syntactic deficits, in addition to semantic, pragmatic, and speech production problems (i.e., articulation and phonological deficits).
- Due to developing understanding of the potential for auditory development in the brain and advances in amplification, current research demonstrates that when (a) environmental support is in place and (b) appropriate and high-quality amplification and early intensive intervention is provided, a child with HL who is identified and treated in the first few months of life has the potential of developing language commensurate with normal hearing peers when no other disorders exist.
- Factors that families of a child with HL need to consider include (a) early identification and audiological management, (b) choice of communication modality, and (c) family involvement in the remediation process.
- The MacArthur-Bates Communicative Development Inventory: Words, Gestures, and Sentences (Fenson et al., 2007) includes a questionnaire format and asks parents to identify various words that their child either says or signs. It includes vocabulary relating to home and people, action words, description

words, pronouns, prepositions, and question words, and assesses the child's use of sentences and grammatical forms.

- The Cottage Acquisition Scales for Listening, Language, and Speech (CASLLS; Wilkes & Sunshine Cottage School for Deaf Children, 1999) includes a developmental checklist for assessment and planning for diagnostic therapy. The language section includes steps from preverbal to complex sentences, including pragmatic development. The CASLLS was specifically designed for children with HL

- The Ling Six Sound Test (Ling, 1989) is a procedure that can be used by anyone. The phonemes for the Ling Six Sound Test are "m," "ah," "oo," "ee," "sh," and "s." When a child is able to repeat each sound in response to the adult's request, the adult can be certain that the child has auditory access.

- In the Learning to Listen (LTL) technique, parents are instructed to play with their child using toys paired with the LTL sounds. LTL sounds are associated with an object (e.g., a transportation vehicle or animal) or a specific action. In combination with the LTL sounds, parents use acoustic highlighting (i.e., strategies to improve sound audibility such as using a slower rate and increased pitch) and use model hand cues (e.g., a technique that signals that the parent is speaking) during parent–child play interactions.

Discussion and In-Class Activities

1. Before class, obtain a brief case description of a child with a communication impairment. Create a fictional character (mother, father, grandparent, etc.) who is coming to the clinic to discuss his or her child. During class time, in groups of three, take turns being the parent, the trained professional, and the observer. The observer's job is to keep track of open and closed questions, the duration of pause time before the professional responds, the use of appropriate body posture, and the professional's ability to reflect feelings. The professional uses client-centered counseling techniques to encourage the parent to talk. The parent stays "in character," expressing a range of emotions. For case histories and score forms that can be used for this activity, see Kaderavek, Laux, and Mills (2004).

2. In groups of three, discuss and practice LSL techniques. One student should demonstrate use of sabotage at the breakfast table, the second should demonstrate acoustic highlighting for a toddler while playing with play dough, and the third student should design an experience book page for reading *Curious George and the Pizza* (Rey & Rey, 1985) and actually making a pizza with parents.

Chapter 6 Case Study

Katie is a 6 year, 11-month-old female who has just started 2nd grade. She was among the first children in her state to be referred from newborn hearing screening. She was diagnosed with a profound bilateral sensorineural hearing loss and fitted with powerful digital hearing aids within the first few months of life. Katie's parents decided that they would work toward teaching Katie to listen and talk and were proactive in seeking the necessary information and appropriate services to reach this goal. Auditory verbal therapy began when she was 3 months old; manual communication was not introduced. Katie received her first cochlear implant at 20 months of age and a second implant at 5 years. She entered regular preschool at age 3 and has performed at grade level academically. Although her academic performance does meet or exceed grade level, she has difficulty following instructions in the classroom and must work diligently to complete homework and prepare for spelling tests and other assignments.

The SLP administered three norm-referenced tests: the Peabody Picture Vocabulary Test (PPVT; a receptive vocabulary test), the Clinical Evaluation of Language Function-Preschool (CELF-P), and the Phonological Awareness Test (PAT).

Katie received the following standard scores (SS):

Test/Subtest	SS (M = 100)
PPVT	90
CELF-Preschool Total Language Score	85
Receptive CELF-Preschool score	90
Expressive language score	81
PAT	83
Rhyming	68
Syllable blend/segment	64/83
Phoneme isolation	92
Phoneme blend/segment	96/98
Phoneme grapheme	86
Decoding	90

Overall, Katie's normative assessment data indicate that her receptive-expressive language, phonological awareness, and vocabulary knowledge are within normal limits. However, the SLP noted that Katie showed frustration with some of the test instructions, and had difficulty with certain aspects of phonological awareness and maintaining a typically paced conversation.

The SLP consulted with the educational audiologist, who then completed a classroom-based assessment followed by a home visit. The educational audiologist observed that Katie struggles in note taking and following oral directions and that her slower response time often interferes with her ability to take part in classroom discussions. The educational audiologist concluded that Katie has been a high achiever primarily through independent learning, despite the many obstacles she faces in the classroom due to poor classroom acoustics.

The educational audiologist probed Katie's classroom listening skills using criterion-referenced tests (e.g., Listening Inventories for Education (LIFE), Anderson & Smaldino, 1999).

Following the assessment, the SLP and educational audiologist worked with Katie's classroom teacher to develop a plan to improve classroom access to auditory/oral instruction. The developed goals were (1) to provide Katie with preteaching notes that she could use at home with her parents to prepare for new vocabulary and spelling words, (2) to teach Katie to advocate for herself and request that complex directions be restated or broken down when she is not able to synthesize the information quickly, and (3) to improve classroom acoustics by decreasing extraneous noise (e.g., put carpet squares under desks, stop shuffling of papers during important discussions) and encouraging the teacher and classmates to take turns when speaking.

Questions for Discussion

1. Explain why Katie could score reasonably well on standardized tests but find classroom learning so challenging.
2. Examine an audiogram of a child with a cochlear implant and explain how it is different from "normal hearing."
3. Compare language development of children with hearing loss across variables including age of identification, manual versus spoken language use, and parental involvement.

Children with Intellectual Disability

Chapter Overview Questions

1. What is the definition of intellectual disability (ID) and how has the definition changed since the 1960s?
2. What are primary causes and risk factors for ID?
3. What is meant by top-down and bottom-up learning? How is the individual with ID likely to be impacted in his or her bottom-up processing abilities? How does the interventionist modify stimuli and intervention to account for processing differences?
4. Does ID represent a language delay or a language deficit? How are form, content, and use implicated in the various genetic syndromes of ID?
5. Why are criterion-referenced assessments important for individuals with ID? What criterion-referenced assessments should be completed?
6. What are the underlying theory and rationale for two intervention programs for individuals with ID?

T his chapter describes issues, assessments, and interventions appropriate for children with intellectual disabilities. The term **intellectual disability** replaces the less-preferred terms *mental retardation, developmental disability*, and *cognitive impairment* (Executive Act on Intellectual Disabilities, 2003). In this chapter, the term *intellectual disability* (ID) refers to individuals with core deficits encompassing both intellectual and social domains (Schalock & Luckasson, 2005).

Along with changing terminology, there are other significant changes in the field of ID. Current perspectives move beyond identifying and focusing on intellectual deficits of persons with ID. Instead, practitioners evaluate and enhance functional skills, improve personal well-being, identify appropriate support systems within the family and community, and enhance competence through skill development and environmental modification (Schalock, 2004). This chapter will help you learn more about communication interventions that enhance an individual's life quality in profound ways.

Description, Prevalence, Causation, and Major Characteristics

DESCRIPTION OF ID AND THE ECOLOGICAL MODEL

An individual is considered to have ID if the disability

- Originates before age 18.
- Is characterized by significant limitations in intellectual functioning along with limitations in an individual's adaptive behavior as expressed in conceptual, social, and life skills (American Association on Mental Retardation, 2002).

As this definition makes clear, professionals consider an individual's adaptive behavior as well as level of intellectual functioning to determine disability level.

Historically, professionals placed individuals with ID into one of four levels of impairment based solely on IQ levels. The levels consisted of mild (55–69 IQ), moderate (40–54 IQ), severe (25–39 IQ), or profound impairment (IQ below 25 or 20). The use of an IQ-based system was consistent with the general practice of institutional placement for individuals with ID—a practice common prior to 1960. Adaptive behaviors were not viewed as relevant to the diagnostic process since community placement was rarely considered.

However, the current classification system does not use the categories of mild, moderate, severe, and profound IQ levels. This model, visually presented in Figure 7.1, emphasizes the multidimensional aspects of ID (Dimensions I-V), along with highlighting interactions between an individual and his or her support system.

At present, most individuals with ID live and work in community settings; intervention is based on an **ecological model.** The ecological model considers an individual's functioning within the microsystem (i.e., with family and caretakers), the mesosystem (i.e., school, neighborhood, community organizations, work place), and the macrosystem (i.e., the sum of society's cultural views and practices regarding individuals with ID). The levels together influence individual functioning and life quality; this is visually demonstrated in Figure 7.2.

Characteristics of each of the five dimensions within the ecological system include:

- *Dimension I:* **Intellectual ability** is represented by an IQ score of two standard deviations below the mean, an IQ of approximately 70. Professionals typically use this dimension to determine eligibility for services, benefits, or legal services (AAMR, 2002).

Figure 7.1   Theoretical Model of Intellectual Disability

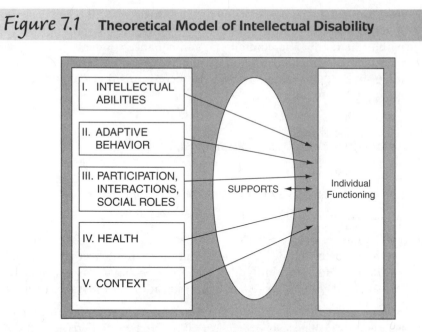

Source: From "American Association on Mental Retardation's Definition, Classification, and System of Supports and Its Relation to International Trends and Issues in the Field of Intellectual Disabilities," by R. L. Schalock and R. Luckasson, 2004, *Journal of Policy and Practice in Intellectual Disabilities, 1*, pp. 136–146. Used with permission.

Figure 7.2   Three-Level Ecological Model of Intellectual Disability

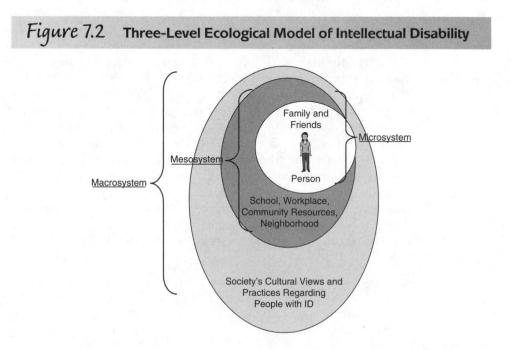

- *Dimension II:* **Adaptive behavior** encompasses an individual's cognitive, communication, and academic skills, social skills, and independent living skills. The professional enhances adaptive behaviors by focusing on the social use of language, use of communication during daily living activities (e.g., making a phone call, buying groceries at the store), and reading and writing skills to facilitate independence, work, and community integration.
- *Dimension III:* Professionals directly observe an individual's participation, interactions, and social roles in everyday activities, because participation in a variety of meaningful activities contributes to life quality. Practitioners concentrate on aspects of communication most likely to improve social interaction.
- *Dimension IV:* Mental and physical health influences functioning in the other four dimensions. There is variation in the degree that health influences an individual's life quality; some individuals have no significant health concerns while others may be significantly affected (e.g., epilepsy, cerebral palsy). An individual's support system influences the impact of health concerns.
- *Dimension V:* Context describes an individual's family, the neighborhood, and community at all three levels of the environment (i.e., microsystem, mesosystem, and macrosystem).
- *Supports:* The ecological model emphasizes the mediating effects of the support system on level of functioning. Support needs vary in intensity in relation to life activities and change across the life span.

As an example of how the systems approach might work, imagine that you are working with an 8-year-old student with ID in a general education class. You communicate with the family and the teacher and discover that the student does not ask or answer questions in class. You collaborate closely with the classroom teacher, obtain lesson plans in advance of the class presentation and, along with the teacher, develop target questions and answers. You and the student practice asking and answering the questions; the teacher provides opportunities for the student to ask and answer target questions in class. This is an example of an ecological approach; you enhanced the student's participation in his community and facilitated communication skills used in everyday life. Think more about how practitioners use the ecological approach by discussing the questions in Focus 7.1.

FOCUS 7.1 *Clinical Skill Building*

Describe how you might use an ecological systems approach to facilitate the communication of (a) an adult who works at his local YMCA who communicates using simple sentences but is very difficult to understand, (b) a teenager who attends classes in general education classrooms at the local high school who would like to participate in an extracurricular activity, and (c) a 3-year-old child with 1-word verbalization enrolled in an inclusive preschool classroom.

PREVALENCE

The prevalence of ID (i.e., the number of persons identified at a given point in time) is 1%–3% of the population; ID occurs more frequently in males than females (World Health Organization, 2001). Children with ID make up 15% of the case-loads of school-based SLPs (Peters-Johnson, 1997); 9% of students ages 6–21 years of age receiving special education in U.S. schools are made up of children with ID (CDC, 2007). According to the 1993 U.S. census, approximately 1.5 million people, ages 6–64, were diagnosed with ID (Harris, 2006). The prevalence rates and the increasing levels of noninstitutionalization imply that most SLPs and educators will work with individuals with ID during their career.

CAUSATION AND RISK

The causes of ID vary in relation to two variables, the timing of the risk factor and the type of risk factor. In terms of timing, risk factors can occur before birth (prenatal), at the time of birth (perinatal), or after birth (postnatal). The types of ID risk factors include biomedical (i.e., physiological in nature), social, behavioral, or educational. Table 7.1 summarizes the various risk factors organized along the dimensions of timing and type.

A child's genetic makeup is a significant prenatal risk factor (Hodapp & Dykens, 2004). Experts have identified more than 750 genetic syndromes resulting in intellectual disabilities (Abbeduto, 2009). Genetic factors are a causative factor in 50% of cases of ID (World Health Organization, 2001). Genetic syndromes can be inherited, but many genetic conditions are caused by genetic mutations. For example, **translocation** occurs when a broken piece of one chromosome attaches to

Table 7.1   **Risk Factors for Intellectual Disability**

Timing	Biomedical	Social	Behavioral	Educational
Prenatal	1. Chromosomal disorders 2. Single-gene disorders 3. Metabolic disorders 4. Maternal illness 5. Parental age	1. Poverty 2. Maternal malnutrition 3. Domestic violence 4. Lack of access to prenatal care	1. Parental drug or alcohol abuse 2. Parental smoking 3. Parental immaturity	1. Parental cognitive disability without support 2. Lack of preparation for parenthood
Perinatal	1. Prematurity 2. Birth injury 3. Neonatal disorders	1. Lack of access to birth care	1. Parental rejection of caregiving role 2. Parental abandonment of child	1. Lack of medical referral for intervention services at discharge

Timing	Biomedical	Social	Behavioral	Educational
Postnatal	1. Traumatic brain injury 2. Malnutrition 3. Meningoencephalitis 4. Seizure disorders 5. Degenerative disorders	1. Impaired caregiver 2. Lack of adequate stimulation 3. Family poverty 4. Chronic illness in family 5. Institutionalization	1. Child abuse and neglect 2. Domestic violence 3. Inadequate safety measures 4. Social deprivation 5. Difficult child behaviors	1. Impaired parenting 2. Delayed diagnosis 3. Inadequate early intervention services 4. Inadequate special-educational services 5. Inadequate family support

Source: From "American Association on Mental Retardation's Definition, Classification, and System of Supports and Its Relation to International Trends and Issues in the Field of Intellectual Disabilities," by R. L. Schalock and R. Luckasson, 2004, *Journal of Policy and Practice in Intellectual Disabilities, 1*, pp. 136–146. Used with permission.

another. In contrast, Down syndrome (DS) sometimes is caused by **gene duplication.** In this instance, chromosome 21 duplicates, resulting in three copies of the chromosome instead of two. Table 7.2 describes the genetic abnormalities contributing to the most common syndromes resulting in ID.

The development of chromosomal maps (**genotypes**) and the influence of genetics on an individual's **behavioral phenotype** (the connection between one's genetic endowment and observable outcome) is a rapidly expanding area of scientific research. Researchers are working to identify and compare language characteristics in relation to ID subtypes (Warren, Brady, & Fey, 2004). The genetic alterations result in a specific pattern of behavioral strengths and weaknesses; awareness of a syndrome's phenotype helps guide the assessment and intervention process. Table 7.2 provides a general description of behavioral characteristics associated with common syndromes. Remember, however, that whether a child has a genetic syndrome or is typically developing, an individual's functioning is due to a complex interaction of genes and environment (Abbeduto, 2009).

In the section above I discussed genetics, a prenatal cause of ID. As demonstrated in Table 7.1, postnatal factors also impact the incidence of ID. A commonly occurring postnatal factor is **traumatic brain injury** (TBI). TBI is defined as an acquired injury to the brain caused by an external physical force, resulting in total or partial functional disability or psychosocial impairment adversely affecting an individual's educational or functional performance.

Unfortunately, the incidence of traumatic brain injury is increasing in infants and preschoolers. Falling, car accidents, and physical abuse are common causes of

Table 7.2   **Syndromes Associated with Genetic Causations of ID**

Syndrome and incidence	Behaviors noted as co-occurring	Genetic characteristics
Down syndrome • 1 in 750 births • 5–6% of all individuals with ID have DS.	1. Better performance on visual-spatial tasks than on verbal or auditory tasks. 2. Adaptive behavior strength relative to IQ. 3. Pleasant and sociable personality. 4. Pragmatic language and lexical skill strength relative to other language abilities.	Three separate chromosomal causes: • Trisomy 21 (child has 47 chromosomes instead of 46; chromosome 21 has 3 copies instead of 2). • An inherited translocation of chromosome pairs.[1] • Uneven division that creates cells varying in chromosome numbers (some having 47 and some having 46).
Williams syndrome 1 in 25,000 births	1. Strengths in language, auditory memory, and facial recognition. 2. Weaknesses in visual-spatial, perceptual, motor, and fine-motor skills. 3. Strength in understanding others' emotions and feelings (i.e., empathizing [see Chapter 8 for more about this term]). 4. Over-friendliness. 5. Pragmatic skills impaired in relation to other language abilities.	A deletion of a small piece of chromosome 7.
Prader-Willi syndrome 1 in 10,000–15,000 births.	1. Food-seeking behavior and obesity. 2. Strength in visual processing. 3. Obsessive-compulsive disorders and poor impulse control are common. 4. Pragmatic difficulties; excessive talking on a narrow range of subjects.	A partial deletion of chromosome 15.
Klinefelter syndrome 1 in 1,000 births	1. Learning disabilities. 2. Delayed expressive speech with phonological, lexical, and morphological skills more impaired relative to other language areas.	Males receive one, two, or three extra X-chromosomes.

Syndrome and incidence	Behaviors noted as co-occurring	Genetic characteristics
Angelman syndrome 1 in 20,000 births	1. Absence or severe reduction in oral language. 2. Bouts of inappropriate laughter. 3. Generally happy disposition at all ages. 4. Hyperactivity and sleep disorders in younger children.	No active copies of a portion of chromosome 15.
Fragile X syndrome 1 in 4,000 males	1. Verbal skills better than visual-spatial skills. 2. Relative strengths in daily living and self-help skills. 3. Can present with inattention, hyperactivity, and autistic-like behaviors. 4. Anxiety disorders common at all ages. 5. Lexical skills are strong relative to other language areas.	Sex-linked inheritance.[2] The disorder is mainly caused by the expansion of the CGG sequence located on the FMR1 gene on the X chromosome. The expansion of this triplet leads to "silencing" of the FMR1 gene[3].

[1] Translocations are structural rearrangements of the chromosomes including breakage and deletions.

[2] Sex-linked disorders: Males have an X and Y chromosome; females have two X chromosomes. Males (XY) are affected by a single recessive gene carried on the X chromosome; females (XX) are affected only if mother is a carrier and father has the disorder. Sex-linked genetic disorders are particularly significant for males.

[3] Penagarikano, Mulle, & Warren (2007).

Source: Information from "Intersyndrome and Intrasyndrome Language Differences," by J. A. Rondal, 2004. In J. A. Rondal, R. M. Hodapp, S. Soresi, E. M. Dykens, & L. Nota (Eds.), *Intellectual Disabilities: Genetics, Behavior, and Inclusion* (pp. 49–113). London: Whurr.

childhood TBI. Approximately 8% of childhood brain injuries are caused by child abuse; the percentage is probably higher as many cases of abuse go unreported (Bryan, 1995). One of the primary forms of abuse is **shaken baby syndrome** (SBS); SBS often is triggered when a caregiver loses control in response to an infant's crying. SBS is a term used to describe the constellation of signs and symptoms resulting from violent shaking or hitting the head of an infant or small child. You can learn more about the signs of potential SBS along with literature for families at www.dontshake.org/

The effects of childhood brain injury are profound since the human brain continues to make primary connections between motor and sensory areas throughout early infancy. Secondary brain development continues through age 5 primarily in the differentiation of verbal and nonverbal functions. Tertiary brain development continues up to age 8; temporal, occipital, and parietal lobes integrate functions resulting in coordinated movement, visual and auditory recognition, and sensory discrimination. The effects of brain injury may include motor, vision, and learning disabilities, communication impairments, and/or intellectual disabilities. Children with TBI sometimes have associated behavior problems including aggression or lethargy (Bryan, 1995).

Although the occurrence of ID cannot always be prevented (as in the case of genetically based risk), professionals continually work to eliminate risk factors such as shaken baby syndrome. Other risk factors that can be prevented include the lack of access to birth care (a social risk factor), poor parenting and poverty (social, behavioral, and educational risk factors), and inadequate early intervention services (social and educational risk factors). You can learn more about the professional's role in prevention of communication disorders and ID in Focus 7.2.

CHARACTERISTICS OF ID AND THE IMPLICATIONS FOR REMEDIATION

Top-Down and Bottom-Up Learning.   Learning occurs via both top-down and bottom-up processes. **Top-down learning** is conceptually driven or guided by higher-level processes (e.g., familiarity with the context and information gained from environmental cues), whereas **bottom-up learning** is guided by perceptual processes interpreted as they are passed up to higher order levels. Bottom-up processing affects top-down processing, and vice versa. The professional considers an individual's bottom-up abilities (e.g., How fast or slow is the individual's visual processing ability? What is the individual's short and long-term memory capacity?) while taking advantage of (and enhancing) top-down learning.

A number of bottom-up skills affect an individual's ability to learn. Bottom-up skills include attention, discrimination, organization, transfer, and memory. The information-processing model (introduced in Chapter 1) is the computerlike model

FOCUS 7.2 *Prevention*

The professional's role in intervention also encompasses the prevention of disabilities. The American Speech-Language-Hearing Association (2004) encourages SLPs to help prevent communication impairments including those caused by intellectual disabilities. A document called *Preferred Practice Patterns for the Profession of Speech-Language Pathology* (available on the Web) lists potential prevention activities:

- identifying and contacting target groups;
- establishing professional relationships with target groups;

- providing consultation and educational strategies to groups:
  - Consultation may be provided to natural support systems, such as the family, or to direct service personnel, organizations, or policy-making groups.
  - Education may provide general information about communication disorders and intervention.
- identifying and/or eliminating risk factors for the onset, development, or maintenance of a communication disorder as well as improving the target groups' ability to cope with communication disorders.

of cognitive processing; this model is helpful in thinking about the bottom-up skills needed for learning and the implications for individuals with ID. As I discussed in Chapter 1, the information-processing model focuses on how an individual processes information from the level of sensory input to final motor output (Drew & Hardman, 2004; Owens, 2002; Sternberg, 2001, 2002). Neurological differences in individuals with ID affect the transfer of information along the neurological "routes" within the system.

Although individuals with ID generally develop underlying information-processing systems along the same developmental path as individuals developing typically, individuals with ID demonstrate variations in the processing system (Drew & Hardman, 2004). A skilled professional understands the underlying skills involved in learning and makes accommodations for the individual's strengths and weaknesses.

The section below lists important underlying skills to be considered when working with a person with ID. Figure 7.3 is a visual representation of these skills and Figure 7.4 provides suggestions for strategies to accommodate individual processing differences.

Bottom-Up Learning Skills. **Attention** is the ability to orient and react to a specific stimulus. Individuals with ID typically have a delayed reaction time in response to stimuli (Baroff, 1999). Accordingly, caregivers should increase wait time, so that individuals with ID have time to respond.

Discrimination is the ability to attend to specific stimuli in a field of similar stimuli. A disturbance of discrimination noted in individuals with ID is **stimulus overselectivity** (selective response to a limited number of stimuli cues). As an example, a student may recognize his name, John, only by attending to the initial letter, *J*. Overselectivity accounts for the fact he selects any name starting with *J* (e.g., Jack or Jill) as his own name (Dube et al., 2003). Stimulus overselectivity also occurs during assessment, as when a student continually responds to an item because of its position (e.g., the upper left corner of a page of pictures) rather than attending to all stimulus features before responding. When overselectivity occurs, the practitioner manipulates the task. For example, if a student only looks at the first letter *J* before selecting his name, the practitioner requires the student to point and say the letters (*J-O-H-N*) before making his selection. If the student consistently points to one picture without looking at all stimuli, the practitioner and student point and look at all four pictures together before the practitioner asks the student to point to a specific picture. Students are also trained to self-monitor a better visual scanning strategy (e.g., *Did I look at all my choices?*) to minimize overselectivity.

Organization refers to the ability to systematize incoming information to speed processing and facilitate retrieval. One organizational strategy, **chunking,** refers to organizing items into familiar manageable units. Individuals with ID have limitations in their ability to organize incoming information (Oross & Woods, 2003). For example, typical learners often use chunking to connect information within similar categories. You may associate words like *sad, morose, pensive*, and *melancholy* as having similar meanings. The individual with ID may learn each new word as a

Figure 7.3 Subskill Processes Needed for Learning

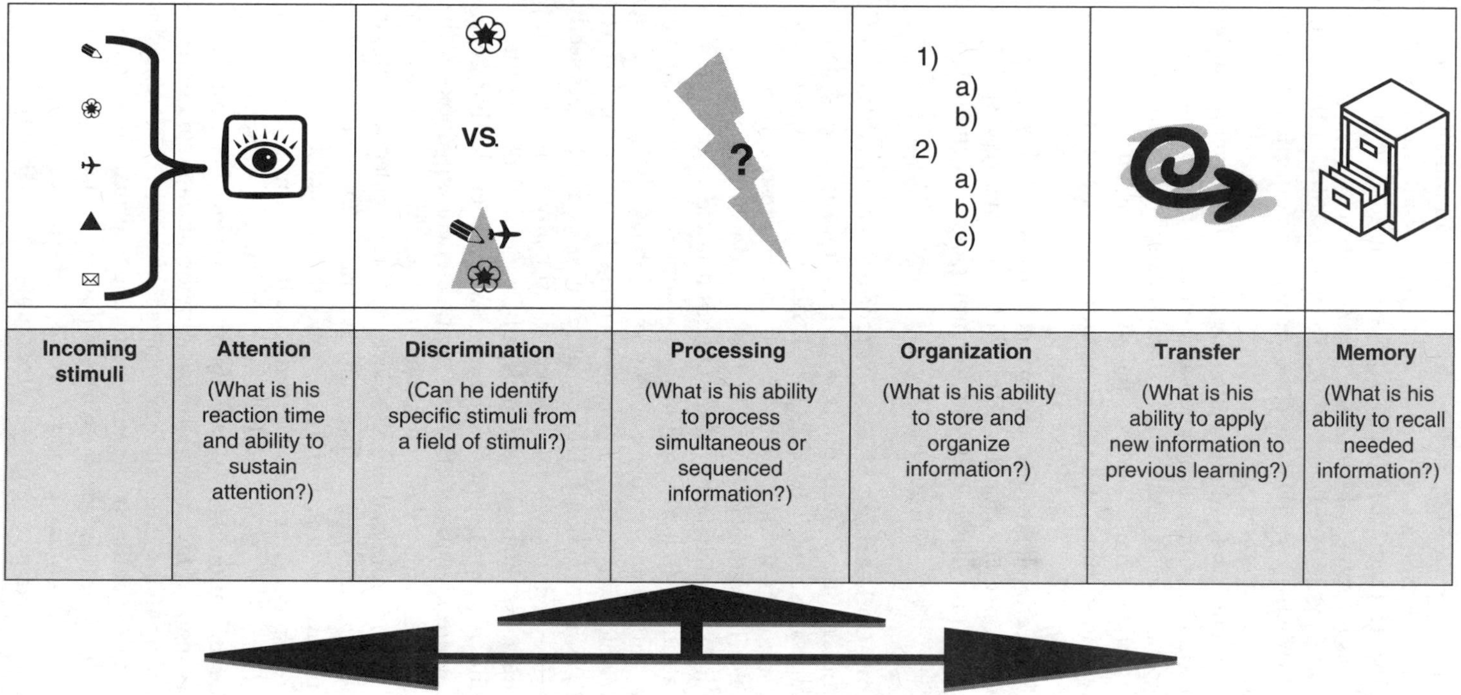

Incoming stimuli	Attention	Discrimination	Processing	Organization	Transfer	Memory
	(What is his reaction time and ability to sustain attention?)	(Can he identify specific stimuli from a field of stimuli?)	(What is his ability to process simultaneous or sequenced information?)	(What is his ability to store and organize information?)	(What is his ability to apply new information to previous learning?)	(What is his ability to recall needed information?)

Subskills interact with each other and alter the individual's ability to process and use incoming information

Figure 7.4	**Strategies for Accommodating Processing Differences**

Facilitate attention and accurate discrimination:

- Manipulate task to encourage the individual to attend to needed information (e.g., point to letters and say them aloud).
- Teach metacognitive techniques to facilitate self-monitoring and attending strategies.
- Give cues alerting the individual that new information is being presented.
- Limit extraneous stimuli to decrease stimuli competition.
- Add new stimuli carefully with attention to stimulus load.

Facilitate simultaneous processing and organization of information:

- Provide additional visual or auditory cues (depending on which sensory avenue is a strength) to assist organization of information.
- Teach individual to organize information into meaningful components (e.g., chunking) and to use association and categorization strategies.
- Teach step-by-step problem-solving strategies.

Facilitate memory:

- Explicitly teach memory strategies and provide increased cues to aid retention (e.g., pictures, symbols, written words, charts).
- Teach rehearsal strategies to aid recall.

Facilitate generalization:

- Highlight similarities between old and new information.
- Teach behaviors in the situation in which they will occur.

completely new semantic concept— without making connections to similar words. The use of metaorganization strategies (like chunking and word association strategies) makes learning and information retrieval faster and more efficient. Some individuals with ID benefit from training in organizational strategies such as mnemonic devices (using letters to remind oneself of the different steps in a process; Beirne-Smith, Ittenbach, & Patton, 2002).

Learning requires both simultaneous and successive processing. **Simultaneous processing** requires coordinating different pieces of information into a linked system. **Successive processing,** on the other hand, requires stimuli to be arranged in a step-by-step or linear sequence. Individuals with ID have difficulty with tasks requiring logic and planning (Baroff, 1999); this difficulty may well stem from difficulty with simultaneous processing. Some individuals with ID benefit from "meta" problem-solving training in which they are taught to (1) break down the problems into simpler elements, (2) generate alternatives, (3) consider the consequences of each alternative, and (4) select a preferred alternative (Tymchuk, Andron, & Rahbar, 1988).

Transfer of information is the ability to apply learned information to novel problems. Transfer includes **near transfer,** learning applied to closely related contexts, and **far transfer,** learning applied to different contexts. Children with ID often have difficulty applying learning to new situations. Simple metacognitive strategies are useful for facilitating skill generalization (Belmont, Butterfield, & Ferretti, 1982; Lee, 1998). A simple metastrategy is the use of self-questioning (*What should I do first? second? last?* and *Did I finish each step?*).

Memory (also called *working memory*) underlies many basic skills such as reading, mathematics, and vocabulary development; it is defined as the current information retained to carry out everyday tasks (Henry & MacLean, 2003). Children with ID use different memory patterns as same age typical peers (Henry & MacLean, 2003) and the memory skills of people with ID lag behind mental age (Numminen et al., 2000). Researchers have studied the memory patterns of individuals with ID and found deficits in nearly every aspect of memory storage and processing (Detterman, Gabriel, & Ruthsatz, 2000).

Rehearsal, or repetition of information, is an effective metaskill to aid memory; however, individuals with ID do not spontaneously rehearse information (Detterman et. al, 2000). Rehearsal strategies include **verbal rehearsal,** in which the individual self-instructs and uses verbal labels to stimulate recall, and **image rehearsal,** in which the individual aids recall by associating task components with pictures (Mercer & Snell, 1977). Chunking (described above) also facilitates memory. For example, the practitioner teaches a student with ID to remember to do three things after arriving at school: (1) *store materials* (hang up coat, put away books, turn in homework), (2) *get ready to work* (sign up for lunch, sit at desk, get out daily schedule), and (3) *start daily work* (begin first daily assignment, don't bother others while they are working). Chunking the information helps information retention; the individual with ID remembers three categories, instead of eight separate items.

Top-Down Learning.   Individuals with ID often are able to demonstrate better communication and functional skills within naturalistic and familiar contexts as compared to their performance on isolated therapeutic tasks (Katims, 2000). This ability to benefit from environmental cues and familiarity reflects the impact of top-down learning. A top-down perspective also encourages professionals to focus on an individual's functional communication. Functional communication emphasizes an individual's use of effective communication strategies during his or her daily activities.

There are many ways that a professional enhances and takes advantage of top-down learning. For example, to improve writing skills, the practitioner targets familiar writing tasks such as writing a shopping list, filling out forms, and taking phone messages. Other strategies facilitating top-down learning include

- Selecting tasks likely to occur in daily life.
- Linking new information to familiar activities and tasks.
- Providing familiar cues to elicit behaviors.
- Using social reinforcement rather than tangible rewards.
- Building on an individual's strengths and interests.

To summarize, professionals recognize that new skills are learned most efficiently when both top-down and bottom-up learning are supported. An individual's ability to perform a specific subskill influences his or her ability to complete a complex skill, while overall task familiarity and meaningful context similarly enhances subskill performance. The skilled professional recognizes that learning is cyclic and requires alternating top-down and bottom-up learning opportunities.

Motivation.   Motivation, sometimes called *mastery motivation*, is the psychological capacity leading people to demonstrate goal-directed behaviors to achieve the positive feelings associated with task competency (Morgan, MacTurk, & Hrncir, 1995). Children with ID demonstrate similar goal-oriented behaviors as children developing typically (Gilmore, Cuskelly, & Hayes, 2003; Hauser-Cram, 1996; Niccols, Atkinson, & Pepler, 2003). However, children with ID sometimes have reduced task mastery motivation in response to difficult tasks. Motivation increases when practitioners modify the tasks to match an individual's ability level (Harris, 2006). High motivation increases children's task persistence and positively correlates with competency in daily activities (Niccols, Atkinson, & Pepler, 2003). Professionals should consider motivational issues when developing intervention for people with ID. Later in this chapter, I present an intervention approach specifically designed to motivate school-age children with ID.

Figure 7.5   **Intervention Activities Should Create Motivating Opportunities for Students to Focus on Improving Their Communication Skills**

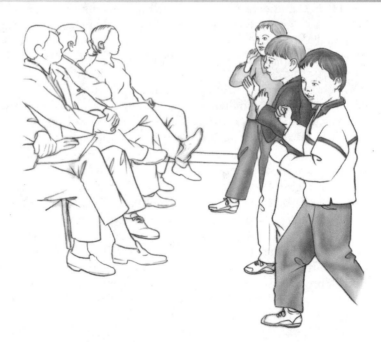

Connections

In this section, I present information linking important concepts discussed previously in this text to their application with ID. I revisit two topics introduced in Chapter 1: (1) a discussion of language delay versus language disorder and (2) the application of Bloom and Lahey's (1978) classification system dividing language into the three domains of form (i.e., syntax, morphology, phonology, prosody), content (i.e., semantics), and use (i.e., pragmatics). Both topics represent important reoccurring concepts discussed in the ID literature. By the end of the *Connections* section, I hope you will be able to explain the two topics and understand the implications for clinical decision making.

LANGUAGE DELAY VERSUS LANGUAGE DISORDER

Is language development delayed or is it fundamentally disordered or deviant in individuals with ID? If one takes the perspective of language delay in ID, the communication behaviors of children with ID mirror the developmental sequence seen in children developing typically—but at a slower rate of acquisition. Ultimately, the individual with ID has the language abilities of a younger person.

Professionals believe that the language delay perspective accurately characterizes individuals with ID during childhood. Before age 10, language output of individuals with ID generally follows the expected developmental sequence except that there is a reduction in the quantity of language. The result is language output with shorter sentences, less grammar sophistication, and reduced vocabulary diversity (Rondal, 2004; Rondal & Comblain, 1996).

However, after age 10, there often are qualitative communication behaviors that suggest a language disorder. A professional defending the language disorder perspective might give an example of an adolescent with ID who asks the same questions repeatedly (*"How old are you?" "What car you drive?"*), in spite of significant efforts to extinguish this behavior. Alternately, the professional might describe a student who whispers continually under her breath, much to the annoyance of family and coworkers. It is unlikely that individuals developing typically would persist in such behaviors.

What would you say during this discussion? I hope that you would introduce several important points. First, you might point out that the population with ID is very heterogeneous. It is impossible to make a single generalization about a population that varies so widely and consists of individuals with very different etiologies (i.e., varying underlying causations).

After making this important point, you might explain (you are sounding quite wise at this point!) that a skilled professional does not see the language delay versus language disorder perspectives as mutually exclusive. You explain that one can use a general developmental framework, particularly with young children, but continually examine the functional use of the communication skills that are the focus of intervention. A broad-based ecological perspective allows the professional to continually consider how an individual's communication differences affect his or her everyday life.

A clinical example demonstrates this decision-making process. You are working with a 10-year-old female child with DS. You have been working on her production of 4- to 5-word sentences; you consider introducing the use of prepositional phrases in conjunction with the basic noun + verb combination (e.g., *"The dog is eating food under the table"*). However, this child's speech intelligibility is reduced when she attempts to produce longer sentences because she has difficulty producing rapidly sequenced motor movements. This is a communication disorder; her oral-motor problems often make her speech unintelligible (i.e., difficult to understand). Rather than introducing longer and more complex sentence structure, you decide to incorporate prepositional phrases within short sentences (e.g., *"The dog is eating. He is under the table."*). You also decide to focus on overall intelligibility as a primary goal of intervention. During this decision-making process, you follow developmental guidelines when choosing your syntax target of prepositional phrases but adapt goals in response to the child's communication disorder.

FORM, CONTENT, AND USE WITHIN SUBTYPES OF ID

How does an individual's nonverbal cognitive ability (i.e., IQ) affect form, content, and use domains? This is a second topic in the ID literature prompted by recent explorations of ID genotypes. Specifically, research demonstrates that within ID subtypes, language domains vary in relation to cognitive ability. In some cases, people with ID have language competencies surpassing expectations given their nonverbal IQ. In other cases, language skills are less than expected. To learn more about nonverbal IQ, see Focus 7.3.

I explore the relationship between cognitive ability and language competencies in the section below in relation to three ID subtypes: DS, fragile X syndrome, and

FOCUS 7.3 *Learning More*

Nonverbal intelligence, sometimes called nonverbal or performance IQ, is a measure documenting a person's ability to carry out motor tasks or analyze and solve problems using visual reasoning. Nonverbal IQ is used to measure general ability for persons with language deficits. Tasks used in nonverbal IQ tests include the following:

- Recognizing and remembering visual sequences
- Understanding the meaning of pictures and recognizing relationships between visual concepts
- Completing visual analogies
- Recognizing causal relationships in pictured situations

It is unfortunate that nonverbal IQ sometimes is used to qualify or deny services to individuals with ID. In many states, SLPs and special educators cannot provide services to a student when his or her language ability and nonverbal IQ are equivalent, a practice called *cognitive referencing* (Casby, 1992; Goldstein, 2006). The assumption is that language skills cannot improve beyond one's language ability. Cognitive referencing oversimplifies the relationship between language and cognition and is a poor indicator of the potential benefit of communication intervention (Greenspan, 2006).

Williams syndrome. Within each syndrome, I compare language abilities to nonverbal IQ and discuss aspects of form, content, and use. Following this discussion, I return to the major topic (How does IQ affect language ability?) and reflect on the clinical implications.

Down Syndrome.   Although overall language acquisition in DS is below expected levels in relation to an individual's nonverbal cognitive ability, there are relative strengths within language domains (Chapman & Hesketh, 2000). Specifically, vocabulary development generally is equivalent to or above nonverbal cognitive levels, while morphosyntax (i.e., sentence length and grammar) skills are more impaired given the individual's nonverbal cognitive ability (Chapman, Schwartz, & Kay-Raining Bird, 1991). Sentences typically lack articles, propositions, pronouns, conjunctions, auxiliary verbs, morphological markings (e.g., verb tense, plural forms), and subordinate clauses (Rondal, 2004). Individuals with DS rarely progress beyond the simple sentence structures exhibited by a typically developing 2-year-old (Fowler, Gelman, & Gleitman, 1994).

From an early age, children with DS evidence communication delay, including slowly developing turn-taking behaviors, delayed babbling, reduced imitation, and delayed use of gestures. Many children with DS do not produce their first words before 2 or 3 years of age (Rondal, 2004).

Children with DS typically have significant phonological deficits (Chapman & Hesketh, 2000). Speech difficulty is due to physiological differences of the articulators and vocal tract, motor programming deficits (Kumin, 2001), and frequent middle ear infections (Rice, Warren, & Betz, 2005). People with DS often have reduced respiratory control resulting in shorter sentences and reduced intelligibility (Miller, 2006).

As mentioned above, individuals with DS have a relative strength in vocabulary development as compared to their more significantly impaired morphosyntactic abilities (Miller, 1996). Figure 7.6 visually demonstrates this relationship. Once word

Figure 7.6   **Language Ability and Nonverbal IQ for Three Subtypes of Intellectual Disability**

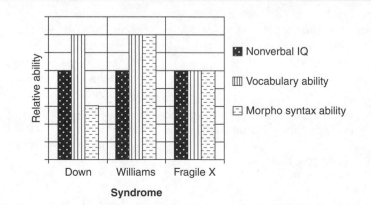

FOCUS 7.4 *Research*

Research demonstrates that individuals with Down syndrome are reading "overachievers." Fowler, Boherty, and Boynton (1995) reported general ability (i.e., a score equivalent to IQ) and reading ability for 33 adults, ages 17–25, with Down syndrome. Participants' reading scores were almost two years *higher* (1.9 years) than general ability level. If typical children were reading a year above overall ability level, they would be classified as overachievers; parents, teachers, and the students themselves, would be amazed and thrilled (Oelwein,

2002)! Researchers interpret this better-than-expected reading ability to be a result of high reading motivation in individuals with Down syndrome (Buckley & Sacks, 1987) and an outcome of reading practice (Oelwein, 2002). These data should encourage you to seek out reading interventions for all individuals with ID and particularly for people with Down syndrome. You will learn about a model of reading for individuals with significant cognitive disabilities in Chapter 9 (the Interactive-to-Independent Model of Literacy Learning).

production begins, children with DS learn new vocabulary, although the rate of acquisition is not equivalent to peers developing typically (Miller, 1999). You many be surprised to know that many children with DS learn to read at functional levels. I highlight some research on reading ability of individuals with DS in Focus 7.4.

Pragmatic abilities are variable. For example, at the 1-word level, children with DS demonstrate an appropriate range of pragmatic function using a variety of speech acts such as requesting, commanding, and question asking (Greenwald & Leonard, 1979). In adolescence, conversational turn taking is appropriate. However, some pragmatic functions are impaired due to difficulty with morphosyntax. For example, children developing typically learn to use an indirect request (e.g., *"Is there any paper available?"*) rather than a direct form (e.g., *"I want paper!"*). An individual with DS is unlikely to use the more complex indirect request.

Fragile X Syndrome. The language ability of children with fragile X is consistent with nonverbal cognitive ability (Abbeduto & Murphy, 2004). This is visually demonstrated in Figure 7.6. Children with fragile X develop receptive skills at one half the rate of children developing typically and expressive ability at one third the rate (Roberts, Mirrett, & Burchinal, 2001). As a result, receptive language is less impaired than expressive language. At the sentence level, individuals with fragile X demonstrate morphosyntax deficiencies and reduced sentence length (Sudhalter, Scarborough, & Cohen, 1991).

Children with fragile X have persistent phonological impairments and difficulties with prosody (e.g., rate, inflection) and voice quality (Abbeduto & Haggerman, 1997; Haggerman, 1999). Some children with fragile X speak with a high-pitched voice (Rondal, 2004).

Content (i.e., semantic or lexical development) is a comparative area of strength with receptive vocabulary being relatively intact. Expressively, however, individuals with fragile X demonstrate word-finding problems (Spinelli, Rocha, Giacheti, & Richieri-Costa, 1995).

The pragmatic skills of individuals with fragile X vary (Abbeduto & Murphy, 2004). Sometimes there are pragmatic deficits in conversational turn taking and topic maintenance (Abbeduto & Hagerman, 1997). Off-topic and stereotypical language production sometimes are present (Belser & Sudhalter, 2001).

Williams Syndrome.   Children with Williams syndrome have better-than-expected verbal abilities given their nonverbal cognitive skills; this pattern is very different from what is seen in most patterns of ID (Landau & Zukowski, 2003; Rice, Warren, & Betz, 2005). Figure 7.6 demonstrates this relationship.

Children with Williams syndrome have delayed verbal skills in early childhood; in fact, early vocabulary development is similar to that seen in children with DS. By adolescence, however, language abilities are equivalent to mental age and some abilities, such as morphosyntax and lexical skills, surpass mental age (Rondal, 2004).

Individuals with Williams syndrome often have a hoarse voice but it generally does not interfere with intelligibility (Rice, Warren, & Betz, 2005). Articulation and prosody are usually good (Rondal, 2004).

Children with Williams syndrome are described as being "overly friendly." Despite this gregarious verbal style, they often have pragmatic weaknesses including inappropriate eye contact, difficulty with topic introduction, poor topic maintenance, and inadequate conversational turn taking. Individuals with Williams syndrome frequently repeat topics and ask excessive questions (Rondal, 2004).

I hope you noted that language impairment varies in relation to nonverbal IQ. For some individuals language is a relative area of strength compared to nonverbal intellectual ability. This is the case with individuals with Williams syndrome. In a second pattern, such as that shown in individuals with fragile X syndrome, language ability is generally equivalent to IQ. In yet a third pattern, seen in individuals with DS, there is a reduced morphosyntactic language ability compared to IQ, but a specific strength in lexical learning.

This information underscores the complexity of the relationship between cognition and language. I hope this discussion has persuaded you to take a multidimensional—rather than one-dimensional—view of language ability. As a practitioner, you will develop the skills to consider independent aspects of form, content, and use in order to appreciate an individual's communication strengths. This perspective will positively impact communication intervention for people with ID.

Assessment

Practitioners typically assess communication skills with a combination of standardized normative tests and criterion-referenced protocols. The role of criterion-referenced assessment is important with people who have ID because particular problems arise in interpreting normative data with this population. In the following sections, I describe the limitations of norm-referenced assessments for individuals with ID, discuss one form of naturalistic assessment called functional assessment, and give an example of an established assessment tool for individuals with ID.

LIMITATIONS OF NORM-REFERENCED ASSESSMENTS FOR INDIVIDUALS WITH ID

Cascella (2006) reviewed 49 language tests published between 1994 and 2004. Students with mild ID were included in the normative sample for only 23 of the tests. When students with ID were included in the normative sample, typically only a few students were tested. For example, the Goldman-Fristoe Test of Articulation, 2nd edition (Goldman & Fristoe, 2000), included only 23 students with ID; the Preschool Language Scale, 4th edition (Zimmerman et al., 2002), included only 1 student with ID. None of the 15 tests met the suggested requirements of at least 100 students in the ID normative sample group (Salvia & Ysseldyke, 1995). Individuals with moderate-severe levels of impairment were not included for any tests.

Only 15 of the tests had separate normative samples for children with mild levels of ID. Separate norms allow comparison of student performance with other children with ID. The majority of the tests evaluated receptive and expressive vocabulary, syntax, and grammar; no recent test evaluated pragmatic ability. The lack of a pragmatic assessment is of particular concern because pragmatic ability often is weak in individuals with ID.

As these data demonstrate, there are obvious limitations with norm-referenced testing for individuals with ID. As a result, skilled professionals always include criterion-referenced protocols during the assessment process. Criterion-referenced protocols should include the following:

- A spontaneous language sample analysis to determine the individual's language skills as compared to typical language development patterns.
- A discourse analysis to identify social communication abilities.
- A classroom-based or workplace assessment to determine needed vocabulary and communication strategies.
- An interview with the individual with ID, family, caregivers, and teachers to identify appropriate communication targets.
- Evaluation of alternative-augmentative communication (AAC) devices, if appropriate (see Chapter 10 for more about AAC).
- Evaluation of reading and writing abilities as appropriate.

FUNCTIONAL ASSESSMENT

During **functional assessment** (sometimes called functional analysis) the professional gathers information about a student's behavior in order to identify the function or purpose of an aversive behavior. This information is used to develop behavioral-change interventions. Functional assessment typically is used with students with ID who have challenging behaviors.

Challenging behaviors are usually classified in one of three areas; they are used (a) to gain attention or obtain a desired item (e.g., tantrums to obtain candy), (b) to avoid or escape an undesired event or demonstrate frustration (e.g., pulls hair when asked to come to the table), or (c) as a sensory stimulus (e.g., rocking, self-biting). The characteristics of the challenging behavior are defined through interviews, rating scales, and direct and systematic observation. After defining the challenging behavior, the practitioner makes a hypothesis regarding the communicative purpose of the aversive behavior and substitutes a more appropriate behavior. I will provide more information on the intervention process in the section on intervention in this chapter.

Functional assessment takes specialized training; often a **transdisciplinary** team completes the assessment process. During a transdisciplinary assessment, families and practitioners from different disciplines work together and make collaborative decisions; members share roles and systematically cross discipline boundaries. Functional assessment draws from behaviorism as well as social/environmental theory. The advantages of functional assessment are that it is an ecological approach (i.e., considers the individual's environment) and that it incorporates all of the stakeholders into the intervention plan. The disadvantages include the level of expertise that is required to provide this type of assessment and the time needed to complete the process.

ACHIEVING COMMUNICATION INDEPENDENCE: A COMPREHENSIVE GUIDE TO ASSESSMENT AND INTERVENTION

Gillete (2003) designed Achieving Communication Independence: A Comprehensive Guide to Assessment and Intervention (ACI) as an assessment tool for AAC users and persons with severe communication disorders. The ACI has several components, including the Communication Opportunities Inventory and the Communication Skill Inventory. The Communication Opportunities Inventory provides a list of 68 opportunities (e.g., eating at a restaurant, following directions, talking on the phone) potentially occurring during daily activities. The assessor uses this list to evaluate the communication opportunities for a particular individual.

The Communication Skill Inventory allows the assessor to rate the individual in 11 communicative skill areas (categorized into four major domains). The four domains allow the assessor to consider if the person with ID can (1) interact (e.g., Can he or she initiate an interaction? Are the interactions socially acceptable?), (2) communicate (e.g., Does he or she use symbolic communication such as words or signs, or nonsymbolic communication such as gestures or sounds?), (3) receive (e.g., Does he or she attend to others' communication?), and (4) express (e.g., Does he or she vary message functions in relation to the communicative context? Is communication intelligible?). Skills within the four domains are rated on a 7-point scale; a score of 1–2 represents no independence in using the skill, 3–5 indicates emerging independence, and 6–7 is scored if the skill is established.

The Communication Skill Inventory measures the individual's independence in interacting, communicating, expressing information, and receiving information (see Figure 7.7). The goal of the Communication Skill Inventory is to collect information about the individual's current communication skills and help identify realistic outcomes for intervention. Each skill is rated based on direct observation, information provided by informants, or information from a client interview. The structure of the entire ASI battery allows the assessor to assess opportunities for communication across domains and a strategy to highlight communication strengths and weakness. The ASI manual suggests ecological intervention goals and provides examples of intervention strategies.

Figure 7.7 Communication Skill Inventory

Name: _____

Directions: Provide a 1–7 score for each skill (see rating scale below)

	N/O	1	2	3	4	5	6	7
Interact								
Participation								
Indication								
Social acceptability								
Emotional control								
Communicate								
Not language-based								
Language-based								
Express								
Vary message functions								
Intelligibility								
Receive								
Attention skills								
Behavioral response skills								
Contextual skills								

Communication Independence Rating Scale:
7 = (Established) Independent
6 = (Established) Independent with certain partners or in certain opportunities
5 = (Emerging) Prompts or interpretations, 2/10 attempts (minimal assistance)
4 = (Emerging) Prompts or interpretations, 4/10 attempts (moderate assistance)
3 = (Emerging) Prompts or interpretations, 6/10 attempts (moderate/maximal assistance)
2 = (Potential skill) Prompts or interpretations, 8/10 attempts (maximal assistance)
1 = (Potential skill) Total prompting and interpreting required (total assistance)
N/O = No opportunity (Do not include N/O items when calculating average.)

Source: From *The Ohio Functional Inventory* by Y. Gillette, 2001, Akron, OH: The University of Akron School of Speech Pathology and Audiology. Used with permission.

Intervention

There are a number of basic principles that guide intervention for individuals with ID:

- Provide intervention from the prelinguistic stage through adulthood. Early and intense intervention is critical to ensure the highest possible functioning (Rondal & Edwards, 1997). Research demonstrates that intervention continues to facilitate communication change into adulthood (Chapman, 2000, 2003; Mattie, 2001).
- Follow a three-pronged approach to intervention programming that considers (1) typical language development patterns, (2) lifespan needs (i.e., What skills and concepts are required at different age levels?) and (3) modifications in response to an individual's communication strengths and weaknesses.
- Approach intervention from an ecological viewpoint by considering the individual's interests and motivation, as well as soliciting input from family, teachers, and employers. Develop intervention approaches that maximize generalization and transfer of communication skills to daily life.

There are a number of good approaches for children with ID consistent with the above-mentioned principles; research-tested approaches include milieu teaching (Yoder & Warren, 2002) and peer-training models (Goldstein & Gallagher, 1992; Goldstein & Kaczmarek, 1992). Both approaches are discussed in other chapters in this book; consider how milieu teaching and peer-training models might be adapted for individuals with ID (see Focus 7.5).

In the following section, I introduce two additional interventions, Functional Communication Training and a newly developed intervention called IT's Fun (Integrated Treatment Is Fun: A Program for Children with DS; Rosin, 2006; Rosin & Miolo, 2005). These two approaches are illustrative of different approaches appropriate for individuals with ID.

INTERVENTION APPROACH: FUNCTIONAL COMMUNICATION APPROACH

The Functional Communication Training (FCT) approach is a behavioral intervention used to replace an individual's maladaptive or problem behaviors (e.g., tantrums, hitting, self-injury) with more socially acceptable communication options. It is built on the concept of functional assessment described above. The underlying assumption

---

FOCUS 7.5 *Intervention*

- Review the milieu teaching and peer training approaches in Chapter 5. What adaptations might be needed for children with ID?
- Make up a case example that describes a student who could benefit from peer training.

What intervention steps would be appropriate? How would you evaluate the impact of the intervention?

is that an individual with ID uses maladaptive behaviors to influence his or her environment, and communicative responses can replace inappropriate behaviors.

The FCT approach was developed in the 1980s. The steps, as originally conceived in the 1980s, include the following:

- Identify the antecedent stimuli (i.e., the time of day, settings, people, activities) triggering maladaptive behavior.
- Determine the purpose of the maladaptive behavior and the reinforcement sustaining inappropriate behaviors via a functional analysis that includes (1) manipulating task demands by altering the discriminative stimuli such as making the task easier or more difficult and (2) changing the reinforcement schedule by presenting and withdrawing the reinforcement while documenting behavior changes.
- Identify a communicative behavior equivalent to the maladaptive behavior (e.g., use of a sign, gesture, pointing response, verbalization) permitting the individual to obtain the desired reinforcement (e.g., attention, task avoidance). The communication response needs to be as easy as, or easier than, the maladaptive behavior.
- Monitor the generalization and use of the communication skill across situations (Bailey, McComas, Benavides, & Lovascz, 2002; Carr, Innis, Blakeley-Smith, & Vasdev, 2004).

The process just described is similar to an experimental design implemented within highly controlled or laboratory-like conditions; this approach represents an outgrowth of Skinner's behavioral theories. Consider the different ways Skinner's theories impact the FCT model (see Focus 7.6).

To clarify the FCT model, imagine that you are a practitioner working with an individual with maladaptive behavior. First, as the trainer, you present two tasks. In the first task, you ask the individual with ID (the trainee) to point to pictures of easy vocabulary items; in the second task, you ask the trainee to point to pictures of difficult vocabulary items. The reinforcement schedule is systematically varied. At times, you provide 100% reinforcement (e.g., praise, shoulder pats) while, in other training sets, you reinforce the trainee after every third response. The occurrence of maladaptive behaviors is noted and interpreted. If, for example, the trainee demonstrates maladaptive behaviors during the more difficult tasks, the maladaptive behavior communicates, *This task is too hard.* On the other hand, if the trainee

FOCUS 7.6 *Learning More*

- Describe how Skinner's principles of behavior modification are demonstrated within the Functional Communication Approach (FCT).

- Describe strengths and weaknesses of Skinnerian-based intervention. How has FCT been modified over the years to account for these weaknesses?

produces more maladaptive behaviors during reduced reinforcement, you interpret the maladaptive behavior to communicate, *I want more attention.* Subsequently, you introduce socially acceptable responses fulfilling the same function, such as coaching the trainee to say, *"This is too hard; help me"* in the first case, or *"Look what I did!"* in the second (Carr & Durand, 1985; Carr, Innis, Blakely-Smith, & Vasdev, 2004).

The use of FCT has changed since its introduction. Originally, FCT was used with nonverbal individuals and the communicative replacement behaviors typically were signed, gestured, or implemented via augmentative communication. At present, individuals with autism, people with varying levels of ID, as well as individuals who are verbal are considered viable FCT candidates (Halle, Ostrosky, & Hemmeter, 2006).

The functional assessment process also has changed. While professionals originally completed FCT within a controlled setting, now it is desirable to consider the person with ID within his or her daily routines. As a result, functional assessment now employs interviews and checklists along with descriptive behavioral observations of everyday interactions. An antecedent-behavior-consequence (ABC; O'Neil et al., 1997) chart (see Table 7.3) is a format helping practitioners capture important environmental components triggering inappropriate behaviors.

Table 7.3   **Example of an Antecedent-Behavior-Consequence (ABC) Analysis: Description of Occurrence of Student's Maladaptive Behaviors**

Questions	Occurred	Did not occur
Who	When working with one teacher and multiple students	When working one-on-one with teacher
What	When asked to do something he did not like to do (e.g., writing). Student draws instead of completing assignment.	
Where	In math, science, and language arts; during class discussions	Art class
When	When asked to read silently in class; when asked to awaken in class	During group reading, during hands-on activities, when he is familiar with content
Why	Uses maladaptive behaviors to avoid completing frustrating or less-preferred work. Behaviors are less likely to occur (a) when student has opportunities for kinesthetic learning, (b) when he gets adult attention, (c) when he is familiar with content.	

Source: From "Positive Behavioral Supports: Creating Supportive Environments at Home, in Schools, and in the Community," by H. Edmonson & A. Turnbull, 2002. In W. I. Cohen, L. Nadel, & M. E. Madnick (Eds.), *Down Syndrome: Visions for the 21st Century* (pp. 357–375), New York: Wiley-Liss (p. 368). Copyright © 2002 by Wiley-Liss. Reproduced with permission of John Wiley & Sons, Inc.

The professional uses the ABC chart to examine the *what, when, why,* and *where* associated with the occurrence of maladaptive behaviors. Typically, once the problem situation is identified, the professional completes a behavioral baseline. For example, the trainer records off-task versus on-task behavior at 10-second intervals during an activity evoking the maladaptive behavior (time sampling), or counts the number of occurrences of a problem behavior within a specific block of time (frequency counts).

Following the baseline data collection, the FCT training begins. Figure 7.8 illustrates an example of a treatment interaction and Figure 7.9 provides examples of intervention goals. The examples demonstrate how the practitioner uses FCT within ecologically valid situations as they occur during classroom, home, or work environments. During intervention, the practitioner remembers to:

- Provide frequent opportunities for the individual to practice the replacement communicative form in context. If needed, the practitioner additionally provides **massed trials,** which are intensive one-on-one training of the targeted behavior (Bambara & Warren, 1993).
- Use behavioral modification techniques including prompting, prompt fading, and reinforcement of successive approximations to teach the replacement communicative behavior (Halle, Osgtrosky, & Hemmeter, 2006).
- Teach tolerance to reinforcement delay so that the trainee does not always require immediate reinforcement. As an example, if a child uses tantrums to obtain a favorite toy, the first step is to teach him to sign, *I want toy!* as an alternative

---

Figure 7.8   **Example of Functional Communication Treatment (FCT) Sequence**

- *Maladapative behaviors:* Mark, a 14-year-old nonverbal boy with ID, engaged in stereotypical arm-flicking behavior and self-injurious fingernail picking. Functional analysis determined that maladaptive behaviors increased under low stimulation conditions and decreased when Mark had access to his radio and other leisure items (e.g., photo album).
- The therapist taught Mark to request access to preferred leisure items by selecting a pictured item from a communication book. For example, if Mark handed the therapist a picture of a radio, he gained access to that item for 2 minutes.
- To demonstrate experimental control, the low stimulation condition was reintroduced, and Mark's problem behaviors resumed at high rates. This reversal procedure was conducted several times demonstrating that the reduction in maladaptive behaviors was a result of treatment.
- Mark was later taught to use his communication book at home and school. Also, he was taught to tolerate delays to reinforcement when an adult was unable to immediately provide an activity.

Source: Information from "Assessment and Treatment of Automatically Reinforced Self-Injurious and Stereotypic Behavior," by D. M. Gadaire, 2000, *Journal of Undergraduate Research, 1.* Retrieved on December 7, 2006 from www.clas.ufl.edu/jur/200002/papers/paper gadaire.html.

response and establish this behavior in everyday situations. As a second step, following the child's request, the practitioner shows a picture of the item and says, *"John, hold on to this picture of the toy, you will get the toy in just _____ seconds."* Initially the delay is very brief, but gradually the delay is increased.

- Monitor the use of the replacement behavior in everyday interactions. If the maladaptive behavior occasionally emerges, the behavior may need to be extinguished by withdrawing reinforcement (e.g., time-out) or giving mild punishment (e.g., frowning or reprimands). Alternately, positive reinforcement of the communicative form may need to be increased.

Evidence Supporting the Functional Communication Approach (FCT).   Published results of FCT interventions appear in peer-reviewed journals demonstrating intervention effectiveness at Level II. Much of this research uses single-subject designs. A single-subject design is an experimental design that focuses on the behavior of an individual subject rather than comparing behaviors of subject groups; an example was completed by Wacker and his colleagues (2005). Wacker's study included 25 children with developmental disabilities between the ages of 1 to 6 years and consisted of 5 phases:

1. Functional analysis.
2. Observation probes to collect baselines of problem behaviors combined into a category called total problem behaviors (i.e., total problem behaviors included destructive behaviors such as aggression and self-injury as well as disruptive behaviors such as crying, task refusal, tantrums, and noncompliance).
3. FCT treatment phase during which parents modeled and reinforced a word, sign, or gesture such as *"help," "done," "play,"* to replace the maladaptive behavior.
4. Evaluation of the occurrence of the replacement behavior in situations other than the training environment
5. Training on a second task (if needed).

Figure 7.9   **Example Goals for Functional Communication Training (FCT)**

- Sasha will produce a signed "take a break" request with a subsequent reduction of off-task behavior. Requesting a break after 15 seconds of completing a demanding task such as stacking blocks will result in a high-quality break (1 minute of interaction with a favorite toy with adult attention); requesting a break without completing the demanding task results in 15 seconds of a low-quality break (no toy, no adult attention).
- Kallie will visually attend and sit through a 1-minute book reading after requesting and being given a favorite toy ("koosh" ball, silly putty) with subsequent elimination of self-stimulating behavior for 7 out of 8 consecutive days.
- Raini will shake her head *no* when given food she does not like for 7 out of 8 consecutive days with subsequent reduction of tantrums. She will request and receive favorite food items using picture cards after finishing a meal without tantrums.

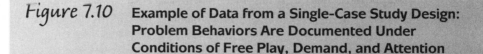

Figure 7.10 **Example of Data from a Single-Case Study Design: Problem Behaviors Are Documented Under Conditions of Free Play, Demand, and Attention**

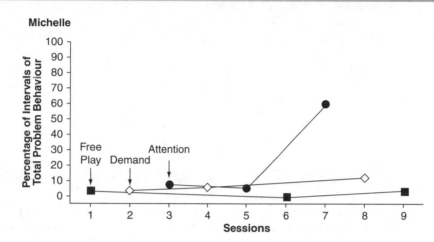

Source: Diagram from "Treatment Effectiveness, Stimulus Generalization, and Acceptability to Parents of Functional Communication Training," by D. Wacker et al., 2005, *Educational Psychology, 25,* pp. 233–256. Copyright 2005 by Taylor & Francis Informa UK Ltd – Journals. Reprinted with permission. Retrieved May 2009 from Academic Search Premier database.

The combined data indicated a decrease in total problem behaviors for 24 of the 25 children. The decrease for one child demonstrated via a single-case study design is visually presented in Figure 7.10.

INTERVENTION APPROACH: IT's FUN PROGRAM

The IT's Fun program (Rosin, 2006; Rosin & Miolo, 2005) is a performance-based intervention designed to emphasize the communicative strengths (i.e., social skills, visual processing, receptive language) of school-age students with DS and faciliate improvement in areas of deficit (i.e., intelligibility, respiratory control, prosody, increased verbal output). During a 3-week "speech camp" intervention format, participants complete theme-based activities including shared book readings, story reenactments, mime and improvisation, vocal and physical warm-ups, singing and dancing, and play rehearsals as well as presenting their skills in a culminating end-of-the-week performance.

Professionals use specific strategies to increase participants' verbal output, vocabulary development, and literacy skills. For example, language facilitators (1) incorporate visual supports (words, pictures, and symbols) to help participants learn song lyrics and lines for the plays, (2) prompt participants to use metacognitive strategies to improve verbal production and organize information (e.g., using pictures, symbols, or a few words as a reminder), and (3) use scripts and routines to increase fluency and verbal output. The participants also are trained to use strategies such as body movement, gesture, and sign to facilitate verbalizations. Some "rules and tools" guiding their performances include: (1) talking slowly, (2) saying all the sounds in words, (3) projecting their voices, and (4) formulating messages before speaking. Participants are given individual daily practice time to speak in front of the group. Dance and movement activities are used to increase and vary vocal quality and enhance the participants' fun and motivation. Figure 7.11 provides an example of a therapeutic interaction and Figure 7.12 an example of communication goals.

Evidence Supporting the IT's Fun Program. The IT's Fun program has a documented Level III efficacy since intervention results are presented via case study examples (Rosin & Miolo, 2005). Experts indicate that the principles underlying the approach are theoretically sound (Miller, 2006).

Figure 7.11 Example of IT's Fun Treatment Sequence

Description of student: Samuel is interested in sports and likes to discuss football. His speech is rapid and often difficult to understand. His communication goal is to increase meta-awareness to improve intelligibility. His talking rules include (1) slow down when talking, (2) stick to one idea at a time, and (3) say all the sounds in the words. He is in front of his peer group during the "In the Spotlight" time and is preparing to discuss Saturday's football game.

Adult: Ok everyone, Samuel is going to tell us about the football game last week! Samuel, what are you going to remember to do when you tell us your story?

Samuel: Talk slow!

Adult: Good! And what else?

Samuel: Say my words.

Adult: Right, you are going to say every sound in all your words. Anything else?

Samuel: (shrugs)

Adult: Look at your talking chart. What is your other talking rule?

Samuel: Say one idea at time.

Adult: That's right! Just tell us one idea before you tell us something new. Watch our faces to make sure we understand.

Samuel proceeds to tell his story with feedback from the adult and his peers. He evaluates his performance by assigning a face to his performance. He keeps his evaluations in his "talking diary."

Faces for Self-Evaluation

Figure 7.12 **Example Goals for IT's Fun Approach**

- Tabitha will tell a story in front of a group using written cues. Story will have a beginning (initiating event), middle (exciting event), and conclusion. Tabitha will achieve a rating of 4–5 on intelligibility (sentences evaluated by interventionist using 5-point scale) for 4 of 5 consecutive days during story telling.

    Rating scale: $5 = \geq 90\%$ of sentences intelligible, $4 = 80\%$ of sentences intelligible, $3 = 70–60\%$ of sentences intelligible, $2 = 50–70\%$ unintelligible, $1 = \geq 80\%$ unintelligible.

- Michael will respond with a complete sentence (noun + verb + noun) on a related topic at least 5 times in a 5-minute group discussion 4 out of 5 consecutive days at a level of 5. Participation will be prompted initially with a nonverbal signal; prompt will be progressively faded.

    Rating scale: $5 = 5$ interactions with no prompting, $4 =$ at least 3 responses with no prompting, $3 =$ produces 4–5 appropriate responses with nonverbal prompt, $2 =$ produces less than 3 responses with nonverbal prompt, $1 =$ produces less than 2 responses with nonverbal prompt or responses are off-topic.

Rosin and Miolo (2005) report pre- and post-intervention data for seven children with DS between the ages of 5 and 12 years. During the IT's Fun program, practitioners developed communication goals for each participant and used a performance rating measure (sometimes called goal attainment scaling) to rate the participants' abilities as follows: $-2 =$ significant deficit, $-1 =$ mild deficit, $0 =$ desired level of functioning, $+1 =$ better than expected ability, $+2 =$ much better than expected performance. Clinical researchers frequently use rating systems to document changes in overall daily functioning in individuals with ID (Jones et al., 2006; Schlosser, 2004).

The seven participants demonstrated improved communication and social skills and showed improved attitudes about talking following the 3-week intervention. Consistent with the Level III levels of evidence rating, the pilot study did not compare the focus intervention to alternative interventions. The authors indicate the intervention approach will continue to be examined with more sophisticated designs (Rosin & Miolo, 2005).

Summary

- The American Association on Mental Retardation (AAMR, 2002) defines intellectual disability (ID) as originating before age 18, characterized by significant limitations in intellectual functioning along with limitations in adaptive behavior as expressed in conceptual, social, and life skills.

- The ecological model of ID considers an individual's functioning in relation to his or her microsystem (i.e., family and caretakers), mesosystem (i.e., school, neighborhood, community), and macrosystem (i.e., society's views and practices regarding individuals with ID). Professionals use this model when developing intervention programs for individuals with ID.
- There are five dimensions considered within the ecological model that include (1) intellectual ability, represented by an IQ two standard deviations below the mean, (2) adaptive behavior, (3) an individual's social interaction in everyday activities, (4) mental and physical health, and (5) an individual's environmental context including all three levels of system support (e.g., micro, meso, macro). The ecological model also emphasizes the mediating effects of the individual's social support system influencing his or her functioning.
- The prevalence of ID is 1%-3% of the population; ID occurs more frequently in males than females. The causes of ID vary in terms of timing and type of risk factors.
- There are varying ID subtypes; each subtype differs with regard to genotype and phenotype. An individual's cognitive processing and language characteristics also vary with respect to genotype. Cognitive processes include attention, discrimination, organization, transfer, and memory. Interventions should accommodate an individual's strengths and weaknesses.
- Prominent debates have centered on several topics, including (1) a discussion of individuals with ID as evidencing language delay vs. disorder and (2) the relationship of nonverbal IQ and language ability. Practitioners consider individual aspects of language form, content, and use with respect to ID genotype.
- Assessment should consider an individual's ecological system. Norm-referenced assessment has limitation for individuals with ID; criterion-referenced assessments are preferred as they describe an individual's functioning. Language sample analysis and functional communication strategy analysis are two important criterion-referenced assessments. Two intervention approaches, Functional Communication Training and the IT's Fun program, offer valuable approaches for working with individuals with ID.

Discussion and In-Class Activities

1. Compare Achieving Communication Independence: A Comprehensive Guide to Assessment and Intervention (ACI; Gillette, 2003) with the observational assessment protocol for children with autism in Chapter 8. How are the assessments similar? How are they different? How is the ACI similar to or different from an assessment protocol for a preschooler with specific language impairment?
2. Look at the data from a single-case study design (Figure 7.10). Examine and describe what might have taken place at different phases of the study and show how they are visually represented in this figure. Complete a literature search and find another communication study using a single-case study design.

Describe the phases of the study (e.g., preintervention, intervention) and show how the phases of the study are visually represented in the data presentation.

3. Make a presentation on shaken baby syndrome (SBS). What are the signs that a family may be under stress and prone to SBS? What happens to the infant brain when it is violently shaken? Call the local Red Cross and obtain literature on their SBS prevention program and present the information in class. What are other possible causes of traumatic brain injury (TBI) in childhood and what can professionals do to help raise community awareness to prevent childhood TBI?

4. Performance rating systems like the one described in this chapter are a viable means to demonstrate behavior change. In a small group, describe a behavior or goal appropriate for an individual with ID and develop a rating system to describe behavior change. Complete a literature search and find other articles on similar rating systems (*Note*: Search for goal attainment scaling, functional communication measures, or performance evaluation). Discuss the pros and cons of performance rating systems.

5. List aspects of the IT's Fun approach that make it an appropriate program for school-age students with ID. In small groups, identify aspects of the program that could be incorporated into other intervention programs. For example, how could aspects of the IT's Fun approach be incorporated into individual therapy sessions for a 12-year-old student with Down syndrome who has difficulty with the /s/ and /l/ phonemes and incorrectly uses pronoun forms (e.g., substitutes *he* for *his* and *she* for *her*)?

Chapter 7 Case Study

Jonah, a 3-year-old male, has Down syndrome. His father is an engineer and his mother is a kindergarten teacher. Jonah has two older sisters, ages 13 and 11. Jonah's hearing has been checked and it is within normal limits. He wears glasses. Otherwise his health is good.

Since birth, Jonah's parents have been reading to him and using simple sign language along with many opportunities for spoken language. A developmental specialist has been visiting Jonah at his home once a month since birth. Jonah will attend an inclusive preschool program in the fall; it is a program with six children who are typically developing and six children with special educational needs.

At present, Jonah has about 20 words; some are spoken, while others are approximations of manual signs. Jonah has difficulty producing words with varying syllables. So, for example, Daddy, is pronounced "*Da-Da*," pudding (a favorite food) is pronounced "*puh*," baby is pronounced "*ba-ba*," and so forth. Jonah likes music and rhythm games (e.g., clapping, pounding a drum, shaking a tambourine). He is more vocal and varies his sound production during rhythm activities.

Jonah has some expressions such as *"What is that?"* and *"Give me that!"* The expressions are always said in the same combination and are primarily prosodic units (i.e., inflection patterns) with poor intelligibility. The individual words (i.e., *what*, *is*, and *that*) are never used in any other combinations or in isolation.

Jonah often points at what he wants and his sisters (who dote on their brother) are eager to figure out what he wants. Jonah's mother has been teaching Jonah to sign *please.* He now uses the sign *please* for almost all his requests throughout the day, rather than labeling the item directly.

You have been asked to work with Jonah. Your plan is to have Jonah, his parents, and his sisters (when they are available) come to your office twice a month and develop a home program.

Questions for Discussion

1. Jonah's parents want to start working on 2- and 3-word combinations because of his use of 3-word phrases such as *"What is that?"* You feel Jonah is at the 1-word stage and would like to see him begin to use some action words, words for appearance/disappearance, modifiers (*big, pretty*). Review the developmental information in Chapter 1 (early word learning stage) and develop an explanation for why Jonah needs to continue to emphasize a variety of word types into his corpus.

2. What environmental factors might be limiting Jonah's word/sign production? With members of your class, develop a mock counseling session in which you make suggestions to the family on how they can help Jonah increase his use of meaningful words and signs. Role-play your intervention session.

3. What do you think might be going on with Jonah's use of phrases? *Hint*: You might want to consider the implication of something called "giant words." **Giant words** are 2- or 3-word combinations that the child hears frequently. When the child says one of these, he or she really is treating the phrase as a polysyllabic single word. At this stage of development the child typically does not use the words separately or in novel combinations with other words. Explain the role of giant words in terms of Jonah's language development.

4. How might you take advantage of Jonah's love of music and rhythm to facilitate his production of two-syllable words with varying sounds (e.g., doggie, bunny, mommy)? With your classmates write an intervention goal to improve Jonah's production of CVCV (consonant-vowel; consonant-vowel) words with varying sound patterns.

Children with Autism Spectrum Disorders

Chapter Overview Questions

1. What overall characteristics are common to all subtypes of autism spectrum disorder (ASD)? What are some characteristics that are specific to the four subtypes discussed in this chapter?

2. What evidence exists to support the genetic link to ASD?

3. How do fundamental skills related to Piagetian theory impact the intervention of children with ASD?

4. What is the difference between communicative functions and communicative means? What differences in communication functions and means might the practitioner expect to see in a child with ASD?

5. What theoretical underpinnings form the basis of the applied behavioral analysis approach and SCERTS intervention approaches? What are examples of intervention goals that reflect the two different interventions?

This chapter describes individuals diagnosed with the disorder of autism. It is designed to help you understand how children with autism are likely to communicate and behave and how practitioners assess and intervene with children in this population. Children on the autism spectrum are one of the most challenging and interesting clinical populations to work with.

One challenging aspect of working with children with autism is their contradictory pattern of ability versus disability. For example, I know of a child with autism who was unable to meaningfully communicate with others but read verbatim from a telephone book. This child demonstrated **hyperlexia,** a precocious reading ability inconsistent with overall ability. He read the words aloud, but did not comprehend what he was reading. An ability discrepancy like hyperlexia is frustrating to families and may prompt seeking novel treatments without proven treatment efficacy. The information in this chapter will help you consider and evaluate assessment and treatment options for children with autism. This set of skills will guide your intervention when you are responsible for helping families make important decisions.

Description of the Disorder

Dr. Leo Kanner, an Australian pediatrician, first described children with autism in 1943. Kanner provided case descriptions of children demonstrating a unique combination of symptoms. One case, Donald T., was noted to "hum and sing many tunes accurately," have an "unusual memory for faces and names," know an "inordinate number of pictures in a set of Compton's encyclopedia," and recite the alphabet "backward as well as forward." However, along with his precocious abilities, Donald T. "almost never cried to go with his mother, did not notice when family or playmates came or went, and was happiest when left alone" (Kanner, 1943, pp. 217-218). Hans Asperger, another Austrian pediatrician, made essentially the same observations at about the same time. He described a form of high-functioning autism, a disorder now known as Asperger syndrome.

The **Diagnostic and Statistical Manual of Mental Disorders, Fourth Edition, Text Revision** (DSM-IV-TR; American Psychiatric Association, 2000) is the published set of standards used for diagnosis of autism spectrum disorders in the United States. The current DSM-IV description describes autism as a qualitative disorder. The term *qualitative* indicates that while one child may demonstrate only a few autistic-like symptoms, another child may demonstrate many significant autistic symptoms. Yet, both children have autism. To account for this disability range, professionals sometimes describe children as being "on the autism spectrum." In this chapter, I use the term **autism spectrum disorder (ASD),** as this is the preferred term.

The DSM-IV lists five types of ASD: autistic disorder (AD), Asperger syndrome (AS), Rett syndrome (RS), childhood disintegrative disorder (CDD), and pervasive developmental disorder—not otherwise specified (PDD-NOS). The clinical symptoms vary somewhat among the five subtypes. However, there are commonalities among all children with ASD. I first discuss ASD commonalities and then discuss unique features found in four of the five ASD subtypes. The fifth subtype, CDD, is a very rare form of autism and is not discussed. Table 8.1 provides the DSM-IV criteria for ASD.

CHARACTERISTIC DEFICITS OF ASD

Communication and Social Differences.   Social interaction and communication impairments are the central deficit of ASD. Parents may describe children with ASD as stiff and unresponsive in infancy, saying they are not "cuddly." As preschoolers, children with ASD may have fewer intentional vocalizations and show limited responsiveness to the interaction and communication attempts of others. Children with ASD sometimes demonstrate **hand leading,** which is using another's body to

Table 8.1   Summary of DSM-IV-TR Criteria for Autistic Disorder

The child must demonstrate a minimum of six items in the domains of (1) social impairment, (2) communication ability, and (3) stereotypical and repetitive behaviors. A child is diagnosed with autism if he or she demonstrates deficits in all three domains before age 3.

Domains	Deficits Within Domains
1. Social impairment	• Impaired nonverbal behaviors (e.g., eye gaze, facial expressions, gestures) • Failure to develop peer relationships • Does not demonstrate happiness or pleasure in response to others • Lack of social or emotional interaction with others
2. Communication ability	• Delayed or absent spoken language • Impaired ability to imitate others or sustain conversation • Use of repetitive or idiosyncratic language forms • Lack of social or imaginative play
3. Stereotypical or repetitive behaviors, interests, and activities	• Preoccupation with stereotypic or abnormal interests • Adherence to compulsive routines or rituals • Repetitive motor mannerisms • Preoccupation with parts of an object (e.g., wheels on a toy car, handle of a basket)

communicate (e.g., moving the mother's hand toward an object), often replacing pointing. Almost all children with ASD have difficulty with peer relationships, a deficit posing a particular challenge in the later elementary school and teenage years. Peers are sometimes incorporated into interventions for students with ASD; learn more about peer intervention in Focus 8.1. Review also the information on peer social communication interventions in Chapter 5.

FOCUS 8.1   *Issues for School-Age Students*

Interventions that incorporate a child's peer group have the potential to positively impact social abilities in school-age children with ASD. Peers developing typically can learn facilitative strategies such as (a) make sure you have your friend's attention, (b) wait for your friend to talk, (c) say something nice (e.g., complement), (d) keep talking, and (e) answer questions. A single-case study design study (see Chapter 7 for an example of single-case study design) demonstrated an improvement in the social skills of five children with ASD after a peer social intervention. Importantly, not only did the children with ASD improve but also the typical peers demonstrated more social acceptance of the children with ASD after the intervention (Thiemann & Goldstein, 2004).

About 75% of children with ASD evidence echolalia (Schuler, 1979). **Echolalia** represents either immediate or delayed imitation. In immediate echolalia, the child imitates the communication partner's utterance; in delayed echolalia, the child produces a previously heard sentence or phrase. Sometimes the child imitates radio or television jingles. Traditionally, experts thought that all echolalia should be eliminated as an aberrant behavior. However, children may use echolalia to communicate. For example, a child may say, "Do the Dew" repetitively (from the Mountain Dew commercial) to indicate his need to change activities. Intervention approaches for echolalia now focus on substituting appropriate verbalizations or gestures (Prizant & Rydell, 1984).

Children with ASD have different communication profiles from other children with language disorders (National Research Council, 2001; Stone, Ousley, Yoder, Hogan, & Hepburn, 1997; Wetherby, Prizant, & Hutchinson, 1998). Specifically, children with ASD use fewer gaze shifts (e.g., lack of alternating gaze between an object and the communication partner), have less positive emotional affect (e.g., less smiling or laughing with communication partner), and demonstrate less-frequent use of conventional gestures and communication strategies during interactions. Many individuals with ASD are nonverbal.

Behavioral Differences.   The sensory impact of taste, smell, and touch are very meaningful for all infants and toddlers. However, with maturity, the senses of sight and sound overshadow olfactory (smell) and tactile (touch) stimulation. A potential explanation for the sensory behaviors exhibited by children with ASD is that the early-developing senses of taste, smell, and touch are neurologically immature or suppressed (Bregman, 2005). Accordingly, children with ASD often are hypersensitive to sensory stimulation and demonstrate discomfort in response to noise, touch, smell, or visual stimulation; this hypersensitivity can make children with ASD anxious in new situations, potentially resulting in an increase in stereotypic behaviors such as rocking or hand flapping. Sometimes these unusual sensitivities may contribute to behavioral symptoms such as resistance to being cuddled or touched.

Children with ASD often have narrow and rigid interests related to physical objects or external stimuli. This interest can become a fixation that limits their ability to interact with others. For example, I worked with a child who was fascinated by clocks. In every interaction the child would seek out, point to, and stare at clocks in the environment. Other children with ASD may focus on visual patterns or motion. For example, some children may like to spin or twist an object while others fixate on light as it refracts through the window. The repetitive physical exploration of toys and objects is another barrier limiting social development and interaction.

Children who have verbal language may talk about an interest without awareness of the need for a back-and-forth conversation between conversational partners. This is an underlying pragmatic language behavior that is characteristic of higher-functioning children with ASD.

Motor and Perceptual Differences.   Many individuals with ASD have delayed motor development and look clumsy or awkward. They may have difficulty performing activities such as throwing a ball, opening a container, or climbing stairs.

Some children with ASD demonstrate a pattern of walking on their toes, a gait descriptively called toe walking. It is likely that some of the motor behavior and body placement difficulty arises because of the individual's limited body awareness with respect to the physical environment (Klin, McPartland, & Volkmar, 2005). The motor deficits also affect the development of self-help skills (e.g., dressing, feeding, toileting).

Learning Differences.   Children with ASD often have significant cognitive and learning differences. For example, memory for meaningful (i.e., symbolic) information is often impaired with the result that individuals with ASD are likely to have significant difficulty remembering where objects are located or recalling daily events (Tsatsanis, 2005). However, tasks that require rote memory, such as simple visual or auditory patterns, may be relatively intact (Sigman, Dissanayake, Arabelle, & Ruskin, 1997). Examples of simple memory tasks include asking a child with ASD to match line drawings or to remember a visual sequence of objects or pictures. Consequently, children with ASD are more likely to recall event sequences when practitioners use visual stimuli as a memory cue.

A deficit in empathizing, a new term for the previously used terms *theory of mind* or *mindblindness,* is considered to occur for many individuals with ASD (Baron-Cohen et al., 2005). **Empathizing** describes the ability to perceive another's motives or thoughts as well as the ability to understand how another person might feel in a particular situation. Children with ASD often have difficulty taking another person's perspective and fail to understand others' emotions. The child with ASD assumes that if he knows something, then everyone knows what he knows. Lack of empathy is demonstrated when a student with high-functioning ASD continues to talk—even when others are bored or disinterested in the conversation.

FIVE DISORDER TYPES WITHIN THE AUTISM SPECTRUM

Autistic Disorder (AD).   In order for children to be diagnosed with autism, they must demonstrate an impairment of social interaction, have a significant communication impairment or marked difficulty initiating and sustaining an interaction with others, and demonstrate unusual stereotypic or repetitive behaviors (American Psychiatric Association, 2000).

Children with AD display differences in social and communication abilities from a very early age. Typical developmental differences include the following:

- Child does not respond when a family member calls his or her name.
- Child does not point at objects spontaneously or in response to adult questions.
- Child uses presymbolic techniques to gain adult attention, such as pulling on a parent's sleeve or hand (i.e., "hand leading") instead of making eye contact and pointing.
- Child does not imitate motor movements such as playing patty-cake or "so big!"
- Child does not engage in pretend or imaginative play (Baranek, Parham, & Bodfish, 2005; Paul, 2005; Rogers, Cook, & Meryl, 2005).

Asperger Syndrome (AS).   Children with AS typically achieve normal language milestones during the preschool years. For example, they talk using single words by age 2, use phrases by age 3, and demonstrate many typical self-help and adaptive behaviors during the preschool years. However, after age 3, children with AS demonstrate specific speech and language impairments and have social difficulty. Communication patterns in children with AS include:

- Differences in prosody and intonation including a too-rapid rate, "jerky" phasing, and too-loud volume.
- Differences in nonverbal communication including limited use of gestures and facial expressions (Klin, McPartland, & Volkmar, 2005).
- Use of unusual phrases and vocabulary.
- One-sided and disorganized conversational style lacking a give-and-take with the listener.

Children with AS also look clumsy, have poor body awareness, and have poor motor skills. They have repetitive and stereotypic patterns of behavior and interests (Bregman, 2005). A common pattern for an individual with AS is an overwhelming interest in a very narrow subject area. Interests sometimes reflect topics fascinating to many children, such as an interest in dinosaurs, video games, or superheroes. However, the individual with AS generally incessantly discusses the topic to the exclusion of other subject areas and lacks awareness of the listener's response to this preoccupation.

An individual with AS often is unable to understand or appreciate others' feelings or perceive social cues. This is evidence of the empathizing deficit described above. The lack of empathy causes significant difficulty for children as they enter the upper elementary and middle school years. The individual with AS has limited ability to make friends and often is socially isolated, bullied, and teased. The situation is compounded since children with AS often have conduct problems such as aggressive and disruptive behaviors, negativity, noncompliance, and anxiety (Klin, McPartland, & Volkmar, 2005; Tonge, Brereton, Gray, Einfeld, 1999).

Focus 8.2 prompts you to consider how a student with Asperger syndrome might be classified using Fey's (1985) assertiveness-responsiveness communication rubric (see discussion in Chapter 4).

FOCUS 8.2 *Clinical Skill Building*

- How would you classify a child with autism using Fey's (1985) assertiveness-respon-siveness communication rubric? Would you change your classification for a child with Asperger syndrome? Why?

- Does a child with autism predominately have a deficit of form, content, or use? Give an example of a communication interaction that demonstrates your answer.

Rett Syndrome (RS).   Rett syndrome occurs in females and presents a much different developmental pattern from what is seen in other ASDs. Children with RS develop normally up to 6 months to 1 year of age. After this period of seemingly typical development, the child begins to regress developmentally within a year or less. During this time, girls with RS deteriorate cognitively to levels of severe-to-profound intellectual disability with a loss of acquired speech and a lack of interest in interacting with others (Van Acker, Loncola, & Van Acker, 2005; Bregman, 2005). Research demonstrates that the brain is 30% smaller than normal in females with RS; however, no obvious malformations, gross abnormalities, or signs of infection are present. Brain neurons are smaller than normal and have reduced branching.

Children with RS has a 95% chance of surviving to age 20–25 years as compared to a 98% survival rate in the general U.S. female population. Between the ages of 25-40, the RS survival rate drops to 69% as compared to 97% in the general female population. The average life expectancy of a female with RS is approximately 47 years.

Along with the cognitive and communication impairments, other patterns of behavior include hand wringing or "washing," hand-to-mouth movements, and irregular breathing. The irregular breathing patterns sometimes result in hyperventilation or breath holding. Figure 8.1 illustrates hand-wringing behavior.

Figure 8.1   **A Child with Rett Syndrome Demonstrating Hand-Wringing Behaviors**

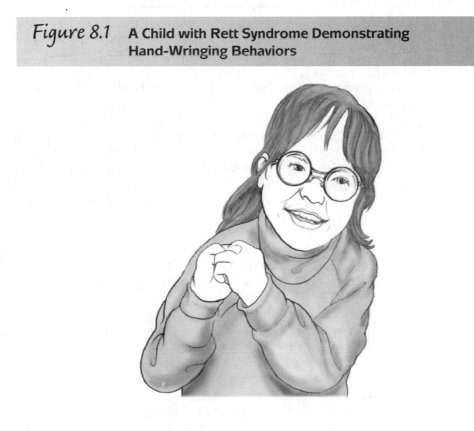

During the elementary years, the rapid decline in ability stabilizes with some improvement in social functioning. However, skeletal and muscular problems may emerge in adolescence, including scoliosis (i.e., a side-to-side curvature of the spine) and muscle spasticity.

Pervasive Developmental Disorder—Not Otherwise Specified (PDD-NOS). Pervasive developmental disorder—not otherwise specified (PDD-NOS) is a diagnostic category for a child who evidences some, but not all, key features of other forms of ASD. Sometimes this label is used to classify a child whose social-communication and cognitive skills are less severely impaired. In other cases, PDD-NOS is used because a child's case history or developmental history is insufficient to classify him or her with child disintegrative disorder or Rett syndrome (Bregman, 2005). PDD-NOS may be an overused diagnostic label in that sometimes it is applied to children who have social phobias, nonverbal learning disability with depression, or a developmental language delay in combination with attention deficit hyperactivity.

Prevalence of Autism and Co-Occurrence of Other Disorders

The Centers for Disease Control and Prevention (CDC, 2007) reported that one out of every 150 children in the United States have an ASD: approximately 560,000 individuals. Children with ASD make up 3% (193,637) of children in special education in U.S. schools. The number of children with ASD receiving school services increased from 22,664 in 1994 to 193,637 in 2005 (CDC, 2007). It is unknown if this upward trend indicates a true increase in autism, if it reflects a change in identification patterns, or if it is a result of more accurate case finding (CDC, 2007; Charman, 2003; Fombonne, 2005; National Research Council, 2001). It may be that physicians now are more likely to diagnose an ASD, whereas previously they may have diagnosed intellectual disability. A recent study in the United Kingdom supports this hypothesis because the incidence of development disabilities has decreased by the same amount as the increase in ASD (Jick & Kaye, 2003). Understanding changes in prevalence statistics for ASD is a central concern of ASD researchers.

More males than females are diagnosed with autism, with an approximate male-to-female ratio of 4:1 (CDC, 2007; Fombonne, 2005). The gender bias strongly points to a genetic basis for autism. I discuss genetic factors in more detail in the section below.

Several associated conditions occur relatively frequently in individuals with autism. The most frequently co-occurring conditions are intellectual disability and seizure disorders. Approximately 30% of individuals with autism have intellectual ability within the average range, 29% have mild-to-moderate levels of intellectual impairment, and 38% have severe-to-profound levels of intellectual impairment (Fombonne, 2005).

Epileptic seizures occur in 20-30% of individuals with ASD (Shea & Mesibov, 2005). A less-frequent medical condition occurring at a higher-than-chance level is tuberous sclerosis, a genetic disease causing benign tumors to grow in the brain and other vital organs.

Causation/Risk Factors

Although experts do not agree on the exact cause of autism, there is a great deal of evidence that autism is a disorder of brain development with a genetic cause (Frith, 2003). I discuss the most compelling and well-documented current theories of autism research in three general categories: (1) neurophysiologic and neurochemical studies, (2) genetic investigations, and (3) environmental factors.

NEUROPHYSIOLOGIC AND NEUROCHEMICAL INVESTIGATIONS

Research suggests that ASD involves the abnormal development of the brain's neural network, and it is thought that the brain is impaired in utero. The neurological patterns seen in ASD are extremely complex; experts from the disciplines of neuropsychology, neuropathology, molecular biology, biochemistry, electrophysiology, neuroimaging, and infrared mapping are using varying research approaches to "untangle" the neurological questions of ASD (Coleman, 2005). Some researchers believe that too many neural connections are formed (i.e., making it difficult for the individual to form a cohesive organization strategy in response to stimuli) while others argue that there is an imbalance between neural inhibition (i.e. blocking attention to unneeded stimuli) and neural excitation.

Neurochemical variations also are observed in individuals with autism including differences in dopamine and serotonin levels. Dopamine facilitates the processing of social cues and affects working memory while serotonin plays an important role in sensory perception, sleep, sexual behavior, motor functioning, learning, and memory (Marazziti et al., 2000; Tsai, 2005). Although pharmacological treatments are unlikely to change the core symptoms of autism, neurobiological research and treatment are critically important and very encouraging (Arnold et al., 2000; Minshew, Sweeney, Bauman, & Webb, 2005; Rutter, 2003). Physicians often prescribe medications as part of a child's overall treatment approach.

GENETIC INVESTIGATIONS

Autism has a strong genetic link. A first-degree relative (e.g., a brother or sister) of an individual with autism is 50 to 100 times more likely to have autism; a second-degree relative (e.g., a cousin) is no more likely to have autism than anyone else in the general population. The increased incidence of ASD in closely related children is evidence of genetic causation. At present, experts believe that two or more genes are involved in the transmission of autism (Autism Genome Consortium, 2007;

Szatmari & Jones, 1998). A deviation in one gene, metC, is seen in one subgroup of ASD; the metC gene also impacts the functioning of the gastrointestinal system; gastrointestinal problems are frequently seen in children with ASD.

ENVIRONMENTAL FACTORS

Despite headlines that "there is living scientific proof that the measles-mumps-rubella vaccine (MMR) causes autism" (Miller, 2004) current epidemiological research has not shown a link between the MMR vaccine and autism (Tsai, 2005). The theory behind the headlines is the MMR inoculation exposes children to mercury, potentially causing impaired intestinal function leading to autism. Careful analysis of the studies linking the MMR vaccine and autism shows that the MMR-autism studies were based on small subject pools and lacked control group comparisons. Before the scientific community vetted and evaluated the evidence, the reports frightened many parents who even decided not to vaccinate their children (Miller, 2004). Many families are understandably concerned about possible environmental causation of ASD. At present, however, experts have not reached a consensus in their interpretation of data linking environmental hazards to ASD.

Many parents consider various alternative treatments for their children with ASD; alternatives include diet restrictions (e.g., gluten [wheat]-free/casein [dairy]-free diet), herbal supplements, and sensory therapies. Professionals should help families evaluate and consider varying treatment options; good resources summarizing effectiveness of alternative treatments are summarized at the Web sites www.autismspeaks.org and www.asatonline.org (Association for Science in Autism Treatment).

Connections

In this section, I examine aspects of ASD in relation to two important concepts introduced in the initial chapters of this book: (1) developmental issues and (2) family involvement.

DEVELOPMENTAL ISSUES

Sensorimotor Skills.   As you recall from the discussion of Piagetian theory, cognitive growth in children developing typically progresses from sensorimotor stages to subsequent development of object permanence, means-end behavior (i.e., demonstration of cause and effect), imitation, and symbolic play. A child's imitation ability facilitates interpersonal relationships and reciprocal (e.g., person-to-person, back-and-forth) interactions (Rogers, 1999).

This developmental sequence from sensorimotor awareness to symbolic play varies in children with ASD. While children with ASD likely develop sensorimotor skills related to objects (i.e., object permanence and means-end), they have difficulty with the sensorimotor skills linked to social interaction and awareness of others (Sigman & Ungerer, 1984). As an example, you may observe a child with ASD demonstrating means-end behavior when he turns the crank on a jack-in-the-box to

FOCUS 8.3 *Learning More*

What does a child's ability to participate in symbolic play tell us about the child's cognitive development? (Clue: Go back to Chapter 1 and re-read "Piaget's Concepts."

make the lid pop open, yet you observe difficulty with a seemingly less-complex task such as imitating a simple motor act like waving "bye-bye." The child also demonstrates little, if any, imaginative or symbolic play. Focus 8.3 prompts you to consider information on Piaget and how it applies to children with ASD.

Professionals accommodate children's learning differences within intervention programs. Imitation skills are taught through techniques such as reciprocal imitation training (RIT; Ingersoll & Schreibman, 2006). Using RIT, the practitioner facilitates imitation by (1) initially imitating the child's actions, gestures, and vocalization while simultaneously describing the behaviors (i.e., describing what the child is doing), (2) initiating bids for child imitation of adult behavior using a duplicate toy (i.e., adult models actions slightly different from the child's and encourages the child to imitate; both the adult and child have the same object), and (3) modeling play with different toys (i.e., generalizing the child's new imitative skills to different objects).

Joint Visual Attention.　Children with ASD have more difficulty in joint visual attention as compared to other children with language delays (Carpenter, Nagell, & Tomasello, 1998). As we discovered in earlier chapters, joint visual attention is the ability of the child to share a common focus of attention and to alternatively lead and follow others' focus. The ability to share others' referential cues precedes the child's ability to name objects and actions. In other words, joint visual attention precedes symbolic understanding and is a skill that typically develops within the first 18 months of life. Joint visual attention skills at older ages facilitate children staying in pretend and social play and using more sophisticated and flexible interactive play routines.

Since children with ASD look, point, and respond less often to adults' communication bids, it is important to target joint visual attention behaviors (Rogers, 1999). To increase joint visual attention, the adult watches the child's gaze and focus of attention, the adult joins the child at eye level, and asks, *"What do you want?"* or *"Look, cookie!"* Waiting and eliciting a verbal or nonverbal response from the child before providing the item facilitates joint visual attention skills.

FAMILY INVOLVEMENT

Family-focused treatment is an important intervention component in a wide range of communication disorders. However, it is particularly important in the treatment of ASD because earlier and more intensive intervention predicts better treatment outcomes (Strock, 2004). Fifty years ago, medical professionals told parents that they "caused" their child's autism. Professionals believed that autism developed in response to cold and rejecting mothers and absent fathers (Bettelheim, 1967). Thankfully, research has clarified the biological causes of autism. Professionals know that rather than causing a child's autism, family support and involvement are key intervention components. Home intervention programs often train parents to:

- Implement behavior modification programs to reduce the child's negative behaviors.
- Involve the child in interactions to enhance the child's social-emotional and communication behaviors, such as facilitating attending skills, child participation during interactions, and the ability to follow commands.
- Facilitate the child's independence, self-monitoring, goal setting, and self-evaluation abilities (Marcus, Kunce, & Schopler, 1997).

As I discussed in Chapter 3, federal laws such as IDEA 2004 mandate that children must be educated in the least restrictive educational environment. Families need to work closely with schools to ensure appropriate educational placement and identify effective interventions. Families often are overwhelmed by the amount of information and terminology involved in the educational process. Parents require support to become effective educational advocates for their child. As the child's speech-language pathologist (SLP) or special educator, you will be an important resource throughout the child's educational process.

As the child matures, the child's family may begin to focus on his or her peer relationships. Even a child with ASD who has normal intellectual ability requires family support and intervention to maximize social inclusion with typical peers. The school years are a challenging and difficult time for adolescents and families (Leblanc, Schroeder, Mayo, 1997; Shea & Mesibov, 2005).

Assessment and Progress Monitoring: Autism

Your first task is to describe and quantify the child's communication and social behaviors. Children with autism often demonstrate a broad range of deficits varying in severity and frequency. The process begins with screening for ASD.

IDENTIFYING CHILDREN WITH POTENTIAL ASD: SCREENING

As you have learned, there are several stages to the assessment process: screening, diagnostic assessment, and progress monitoring. There are a number of screening instruments for ASD. Pediatricians and family physicians generally use a screening tool if a family member voices concern about the child's development or because of observed deficits during the child's regular physical examinations (see Table 8.2 for examples of screening tools). Table 8.2 also provides more information regarding the need for a good screening tool to have both sensitivity and specificity.

A screening tool must be able to identify children requiring a complete assessment battery (i.e., sensitivity); at the same time a screening tool should not overidentify children as having ASD when they do not have the disorder (i.e., specificity). See also Focus 8.4 for clinical skill building related to sensitivity and specificity.

Table 8.2 Examples of Screening Tools for Children with Autism Spectrum Disorders

When evaluating a screening measure the assessor considers the implications of sensitivity and specificity. The assessor must determine how well the screening tool identifies a child with a communication disorder as compared to a more complete test battery (McCauley, 2001). Sensitivity reflects how frequently an individual with the disability is identified by using the screening tool (i.e., Does the tool give a positive result when the individual actually has the disability?). In contrast, specificity makes sure that people who do not have the disorder are not overidentified (i.e., Does the screening tool indicate the person has an impairment when, in actuality, the person does not have a disorder?). In general, screening tests should have a sensitivity $\geq$ .90 (90%) and specificity of $\geq$ .80 (80%) (Plante & Vance, 1995).

Tool	Description
Checklist for Autism in Toddlers (CHAT; Baird et al., 2000; Baron-Cohen, Allen & Gillberg, 1992; Baron-Cohen et al., 1996)	• Parent questionnaire • General population screening administered during regular health examination at 18 months. • Sensitivity ~.75 • Specificity .99
Modified Checklist for Autism in Toddlers (M-CHAT; Robins, Fein, Barton, & Green, 2001)	• Parent questionnaire and observation • Extension of CHAT (e.g., additional items regarding repetitive behaviors) administered at age 24 months. • Sensitivity .96 • Specificity .97
Pervasive Developmental Disorders Screening Test-Stage I (PDDST-Stage I; Siegel, 1996, 1998; Siegel & Hayer, 1999)	• Parent questionnaire • Appropriate for children under the age of 6 years • Questions focus on nonverbal communication, language, temperament, play, and social interaction • Sensitivity .85 • Specificity .71

Source: Adapted from "Screening for Autism in Young Children," by E. E. Coonrod & W. L. Stone, 2005. In F. R. Volkmar, R. Paul, A. Klin, D. Cohen (Eds.), *Handbook of Autism and Pervasive Developmental Disorders. Vol. 2: Assessments, Interventions, and Policy* (3rd ed., pp. 707-729). Hoboken, NJ: Wiley & Sons. Copyright © 2005. Reproduced with permission of John Wiley & Sons, Inc.

FOCUS 8.4 *Clinical Skill Building*

Consider the levels of sensitivity and speci- ficity reported for the screening instruments in Table 8.2. If the tool you are using does not meet this level, how might you adjust your screening process? If sensitivity and specificity are below the optimal level, should you avoid using the screening tool? Discuss this issue in class.

Professionals carefully consider family concerns during the screening and assessment process; 69% to 88% of families with a child with ASD report sensing the problem prior to the child's third birthday (CDC, 2007; see Focus 8.5). Unfortunately, although parents often sense something is wrong at an early age, the median age of identification of ASD is 5.7 years (Shattuck et al., 2009). The large gap between the first signs of ASD and identification underscores the critical need for improved community awareness and professional training. (See Table 8.2 for a list of screening tools.)

Once the child is screened, and if the behaviors are consistent with potential ASD, the physician refers the child for a complete speech-language assessment battery. One of the first goals of assessment is to rule out other diagnoses such as hearing impairment or behavioral issues. In some cases, the SLP may be the first professional suspecting the child is on the autism spectrum. In this case, the SLP completes a speech-language evaluation and then refers the child to the family's physician. The physician, often in conjunction with a team of pediatric specialists, makes the ASD diagnosis.

The assessment protocol includes a variety of evaluative procedures. As in any speech-language evaluation, the assessor obtains a full picture of the child's hearing, oral-motor skills, and speech production (if the child is verbal) including intelligibility, prosody, volume, and fluency (Filipek et al., 1999). Typically, the assessor administers a test resulting in a standardized score in addition to instruments focusing on the core features of autism. Table 8.3 lists examples of evaluation instruments often used to assess children with ASD.

An effective assessment for a child with ASD should include (1) evaluation of the child's ability to demonstrate communication functions both verbally and nonverbally, and (2) observation of the child's abilities during a variety of activities (Crais, 1995; Filipek et al., 1999; Wetherby & Prizant, 1992).

FOCUS 8.5 *Family Issues*

What parent concerns might you hear that might indicate a potential ASD?

Table 8.3 **Examples of Assessment Instruments for Children with Autism Spectrum Disorders**

Tool	Description
Childhood Autism Rating Scale (CARS; Schopler, Reicher, & Renner, 1988)	• 7-point rating scale on 15 items following an observation of adult-child interaction • Some training is required to administrate (a training video tape is available) • Appropriate for assessment of individuals over 2 years old • Has demonstrated internal consistency, its interrater reliability is somewhat variable • CARS is the most widely used rating scale in the United States (Lord & Costello, 2005).
Autism Behavior Checklist (ABC; Krug, Arick, & Almond, 1980)	• A 57-item questionnaire completed by teacher or parent in five domains: sensory, relating, body and object use, language and social interaction, and self-help • Appropriate for children over 3 years old • ABC emphasizes the symptoms of ASD; this provides a different framework as compared to other ASD assessment instruments. It is of limited value because of variable sensitivity (Lord & Corsello, 2005)
Autism Diagnostic Interview-Revised (ADI-R; LeCouteur et al., 1989; Lord, Rutter, & LeCouteur, 1994)	• Semistructured interview to be used during a parent interview; takes from $1\frac{1}{2}$ to 2 hours to administer • Appropriate for children $\geq$ 2 years old • Obtains information in three domains: social interaction, communication and language, and repetitive, stereotypic behaviors • Requires extensive training; examiner must have interviewing experience • Excellent reliability and internal consistency (Lord & Corsello, 2005)

ASSESSMENT OF VERBAL AND NONVERBAL COMMUNICATION FUNCTIONS

The assessor must consider the child's **communicative functions.** Communication functions describe what motivates the child to communicate. Communication functions include requesting, commenting, protesting, turn taking, imitating, and social greeting.

Children developing typically demonstrate communication functions using a variety of communication means. **Communication means** describe how the child communicates. Communication means can reflect either verbal behaviors (e.g., sounds, word approximations, words) or nonverbal behaviors (e.g., gestures, eye contact). As you would suspect, children with ASD typically have a reduced range of communication functions because they are less motivated to interact with others and often demonstrate limited or unusual communication means (e.g., taking a parent's hand rather than making eye contact, using echolalic verbalizations).

Observation of the Child within Play Interactions.   During the assessment protocol, the assessor involves the child in a range of activities and observes the child's ability to participate and imitate during simple turn-taking games. Activities include involving the child in "baby games" like patty-cake, peek-a-boo, and "so big!" The adult also solicits the child's turn taking during back-and-forth motor activities such as rolling a ball, pushing a car, or block building (i.e., the child and the adult take turns building a block tower). In addition to monitoring the child's ability to interact during simple motor-imitation games, the practitioner observes and models simple play routines to determine the child's level of symbolic play. The practitioner knows that a child developing typically begins to participate in simple symbolic play activities, such as rocking and feeding a doll, at around age 2. Throughout the assessment session, the practitioner observes the child's social and affective responses (i.e., his or her facial expression, eye gaze, smiling, laughing) during practioner–child and parent–child interactions. The child's caregiver is included in the assessment because caregivers are an important information source about the child's abilities. Parents indicate if the child's behavior typifies his behavior at home.

The practitioner uses **communication temptations** to entice, surprise, or elicit a child's conversational attempt (Prizant, Wetherby, Rubin, Laurent, & Rydell, 2006; Wetherby & Prizant, 1989). When using a communication temptation, the practitioner "sabotages" the situation, increasing the likelihood of communication (a form of "pragmatic pressure!"). For example, the child and practitioner engage in a play dough activity. During the activity the practitioner uses containers with tight-fitting lids. In order to participate, the child must request adult assistance. Other examples:

To determine if the child can protest	• Give the child an undesired object. • Place the child's hands in something wet or sticky.
To determine if the child can comment	• Have interesting objects or toys in a bag and pull them out one at a time. • Give the child some duplicate objects and then "surprise" him with a different object. • Complete a desired or surprising action (e.g., blowing bubbles, letting the air out of a balloon, playing with a wind-up toy) and watch for the child's response.
To determine if the child can request	• Place a desired toy or object up high or in a jar with a tight lid. • Play a tickle game like "I'm going to get you!" and wait for child to request repetition of the action.

Figure 8.2 provides a simplified version of an assessment protocol suitable for children with ASD. Communication temptations are included in the assessment process.

		Gazes at communication partner	Uses 3-point gaze (partner and objects)	Gestures (Conventional = C, Unconventional = UC)	Vocalizations (Conventional = C, Unconventional = UC)	Speech (E = Echolalic, S = Spontaneous)	Describe
Communication Means (i.e., How does the child communicate?)							
Communication Functions (i.e., What is the child's motivation for communication?)	Comment						
	Request action						
	Request object						
	Social functions (e.g., *Hi, Bye*)						
	Share enjoyment, exclaim, tease						
	Other communication functions						
Response to Communication Temptations	Doing something silly	Describe child response:					
	Bubbles with too-tight lid	Describe child response:					
	Switching toys	Describe child response:					
	Pretending not to understand	Describe child response:					
	Withholding part of toy	Describe child response:					
	Other temptations	Describe child response:					
Receptive Ability							
Responses to Others' Communication	Response to name	Describe child response:					
	Response to yes/no question	Describe child response:					
	Response to *wh* question	Describe child response:					
	Identifies objects?	Describe child response:					

Source: Information from *The SCERTS™ Model: A Comprehensive Educational Approach for Children with Autism Spectrum Disorders. Vol. 1: Assessment*, by B. M. Prizant, A. M. Wetherby, E. Rubin, A. C. Laurent, and P. J. Rydell, 2006, Baltimore, MD: Brookes; and "Assessing Communication in Autism Spectrum Disorders," by R. Paul, 2005. In F. R. Volkmar, R. Paul, A. Klin, and D. Cohen (Eds.), *Handbook of Autism and Pervasive Developmental Disorders. Vol. 2: Assessment, Intervention, and Policy* (3rd ed., pp. 799-816). Hoboken, N J: Wiley & Sons.

During an assessment the assessor observes both expressive and receptive abilities. The receptive portion of the observational protocol allows observation of the child's ability to understand and respond to others' verbal communication.

ONGOING PROGRESS MONITORING

A final component of assessment is the ongoing evaluation of a child's social and communication progress. Progress monitoring documents a child's carryover of targeted skills to the natural environment and generalization of new skills to novel situations. One way to document both the quality and quantity of new behaviors is to use ratings scales. An example of a progress-monitoring tool is shown in Table 8.4. The assessor uses a self-developed tool, like this one, to document the child's use of requests in a novel situation such as snack time. It is important for practitioners to be familiar with developing rating scales; develop your clinical skills by considering the questions in Focus 8.6.

Table 8.4 **Example of a Progress-Monitoring Tool**

Teacher verbal question	*Teacher noverbal cue* (provided at the same time as question)	Child rating
"John, what do you want to drink today?"	Show two drink options.	3 2 1 0
"John, what do you want to eat today?"	Show two food options.	3 2 1 0
"John, after you finish your snack, what would you like to do next?" (Provide stimulus when snack is over.)	Show two pictures of desired activities.	3 2 1 0

Rating scale: 3 = child spontaneously points and verbalizes following teacher question; 2 = child spontaneously points following teacher question; 1 = child points following teacher prompt if child does not respond to initial question (teacher provides prompt ["John, POINT to the one you want"]); 0 = No response following prompt.

FOCUS 8.6 *Clinical Skill Building*

Develop a rating scale to document the child's use of (a) social greetings (a communication function), (b) protesting (a communication function), or (c) pointing (a communication means).

Intervention

There are a number of viable intervention approaches for children with ASD; Table 8.5 lists examples of current approaches. Although the efficacy data demonstrate that early intervention significantly improves overall functioning, current intervention research often does not reflect controlled experimental research. Many controlled ASD research studies are in progress, however, and will be available in the years ahead. Your current

Table 8.5 **Examples of High-Quality Intervention Programs**

Program	Description
Denver model (Rogers & Dilalla, 1991, Rogers & Lewis, 1989)	• Developmental approach with emphasis on interpersonal development • Playschool curriculum • Data of pre- and postintervention studies evidenced better-than-predicted gains (Schafer & Moersch, 1981)
Developmental, Individual Difference, Relationship-based (DIR/Floortime™) approach, (Greenspan & Wieder, 1997; Greenspan & Wieder, 1999)	• Developmental approach, relationship-based • Floortime™ therapy occurs at home or clinic • Data for 200 children with ASD receiving DIR demonstrated that over half the children had good to outstanding outcomes in language, creative and reflective thinking, and social interaction (Greenspan & Wieder, 1999)
Treatment and Education of Autistic and Related Communication-Handicapped Children (TEACCH) model (Schopler & Olley, 1982).	• Developmental and behavioral approach • Focuses on academic, cognitive, and prevocational skills • A 10-hour home-based TEACCH intervention was compared with a discrete-trial classroom-based program; the TEACCH intervention resulted in more improvement on imitation, fine and gross motor skills, and nonverbal concepts (Ozonoff & Cathcart, 1998)
Pivotal response training (Koegel, Koegel, Harrower, & Carter 1999; Koegel, Koegel, Shoshan, & McNerney, 1999)	• Based on ABA methods; structured operant teaching techniques within the child's natural environment, adults follow child's interests and communication attempts • Focuses on communication, academic, social, self-help, and recreational domains • Long term follow-up on ten children using pivotal response model showed good outcomes (Koegel, Koegel, Shoshan, & McNerney, 1999)

(continued)

Table 8.5 **Examples of High-Quality Intervention Programs (*Continued*)**

Program	Description
LEAP (Lifeskills and Education for Students with Autism and Other Pervasive Behavioral Challenges) program (Hoyson, Jamieson, & Strain, 1984)	• A combined approach using applied behavior analysis, discrete trial intervention, incidental learning, errorless teaching, augmentative communication, picture exchange communication systems, sensory diets, and vocational training • Peer-mediated, naturalistic intervention occurring in the home and school environment • Summary of case reports documented positive benefits of LEAP curriculum (Strain & Hoyson, 2000)

goal should include developing the skills needed to critically examine research. Below I present two currently used intervention approaches: Applied Behavioral Analysis (Lovaas, 1987, 1993, 2003) and the SCERTS model (Prizant, Wetherby, Rubin, Laurent, & Rydell, 2006). Understanding two different intervention models, and the theoretical foundation supporting their use, will help you thoughtfully consider new approaches in the future. Learn more about interventions for ASD by considering Focus 8.7.

INTERVENTION APPROACH: APPLIED BEHAVIORAL ANALYSIS (ABA)

To understand the **applied behavioral analysis** approach, keep in mind the behavioral conditioning theories of the 1970s (i.e., links between an initial eliciting stimulus, child behavior, and contingent positive or negative stimuli). ABA developed from the work of Lovaas and his colleagues at the University of California, Los Angeles, and is

---

FOCUS 8.7 *Learning More*

Consider all the interventions listed under the LEAP approach in Table 8.5. To learn more about these terms, complete an Internet search, looking up applied behavior analysis, discrete trial intervention, incidental learning, errorless teaching, augmentative communication, picture exchange communication systems, sensory diets, and vocational training. Discuss your findings in class.

FOCUS 8.8 *Clinical Skill Building*

Ask yourself: What is the theoretical foundation of ABA? What are the behavioral principles likely to be a part of ABA given the theoretical roots? What behaviors and language production are most likely to be facilitated with a highly structured ABA intervention?

sometimes called the Lovaas approach (Lovaas, 1987, 1993, 2003). ABA's operant, learning-based philosophy states that any behavior (even language) can be broken down into separate behaviors, measured in precise terms, and manipulated through principles of reinforcement. Improve your clinical skill and ability to apply theoretical information to clinical practice in Focus 8.8.

Specific instructional techniques or methods emerged from the ABA approach. A primary method is discrete trial therapy (DTT), a method using behavioral techniques to facilitate child behaviors such as (1) receptive identification of objects, pictures, and actions; (2) early play and self-help skills; (3) verbal labeling; (4) early concept development (e.g., recognition and naming of color, shape, size); (5) prepositions; (6) emotion words; and (7) simple carrier phases such as *"I see _____"* and *"I want _____"* (Lovaas, 2003). Behavioral techniques include the use of prompting, cuing, chaining, fading, and differential reinforcement.

Figure 8.3 is an example of a DTT teaching sequence. As Figure 8.3 illustrates, DTT intervention is primarily practitioner-directed and is skill rather than activity based. Typically, parents and trained therapists implement the DTT intervention in the child's home for 20-40 hours per week on an individual basis. Later, after 1 to 3 years of intervention, the intervention takes place with a paraprofessional in an inclusive classroom (Smith, Groen, & Wynn, 2000). Figure 8.4 provides examples of DTT treatment goals.

Figure 8.3 **Example of Discrete Trial Therapy Teaching Sequence**

Steps to Teaching Naming of Actions

- Adult assembles three pictures (e.g., *waving, eating, sleeping*).
- Adult presents one picture and asks, *"What is he (or she) doing?"* Adult immediately prompts the word by saying *"waving."* The adult reinforces the child for each response. The adult continues until the child accurately names all three pictures with high accuracy without prompt.
  - Reinforcement at this stage is often social or includes the use of tokens that the child trades for privileges or prizes.
- Adult intermixes the pictures until the child is 90% accurate in unprompted attempts.
- Adult generalizes labels so that the child describes (a) actions the adult performs, (b) actions the child performs, and (c) actions in books.

Figure 8.4 **Example Goals for Discrete Trial Therapy* (DTT)**

- Without prompting, John will correctly imitate 20 different gross motor behaviors (e.g., waving bye-bye, touching ears) when asked *"do this"* within 2 seconds of request with 90% accuracy.
- John will correctly respond with the response *"happy"* or *"sad"* when the trainer presents a picture of a child either smiling or crying with 90% accuracy when pictures are randomly presented. (Note: child previously demonstrated receptive knowledge of verbs *smiling* and *crying*.)
- John will produce with 90% accuracy without prompting the prepositions *"on top,"* *"under,"* or *"beside"* when asked, *"Where are you?"* while John sits on top of, under, or beside a table or chair.

*All goals in the DTT program require careful sequencing of task presentations; each of the listed goals is introduced as one part in a series of structured intervention steps (Lovaas, 2003).

Evidence Supporting the ABA Approach. Results documenting the effects of ABA-based interventions are published in peer-reviewed journals demonstrating intervention effectiveness at Level II. As you recall from Chapter 4, Level I evidence results from randomized clinical trials while Level II evidence uses control-group design without randomization. In 1987, Lovaas reported data on 38 children who received intervention based on the ABA approach as preschoolers; half of the children received 40 hours of intervention per week while the remaining half received less than 10 hours per week. A comparison group received a different form of intervention at an outside site. The children who received ABA treatment demonstrated more improvement than the control-group children; the children receiving more intervention showed the best results. Subsequently, there is a published follow-up to the children in the study at age 13 (McEachin, Smith, & Lovaas, 1993) In the 1987 study, nine of the children in the intensive intervention group demonstrated an increased IQ score of 20 points and were capable of schoolwork in a general education first grade class. In the 1993 follow-up study, eight of the nine children continued to function within typical education classrooms without special support. Only one of the children in the reduced-intensity intervention demonstrated this result.

This evidence is compelling. However, although most experts do not deny the significance of the ABA approach, there is criticism of the research methodologies used in the ABA efficacy studies (Schopler, Short, & Mesibov, 1989). For example, children receiving high levels of intervention may have been less impaired, and the control-group practitioners may have been less well trained as compared to the ABA practitioners (Gresham & MacMillan, 1997). In spite of the criticisms, ABA approaches continue to be a frequently used intervention for children with autism (National Research Council, 2001).

INTERVENTION APPROACH: SCERTS

The ultimate goal of communication intervention for children with ASD is to help children interact with others in their natural environments. As an alternative to behaviorally based approaches, the **SCERTS approach** is based on social interaction, developmental, and family systems theories. The SCERTS approach emphasizes enhancing children's turn taking, choice making, emotional regulation, and problem-solving abilities (Prizant & Wetherby, 2005). The SCERTS acronym stands for social communication, emotional regulation, and transaction support. The term **transaction support** refers to the interpersonal support provided by the child's adult and peer communication partners, the environmental modifications used to promote social communication and emotional regulation, and enhancement of family support systems (Prizant, Wetherby, Rubin, Laurent, & Rydell, 2006). Transactional goals support learning by reinforcing and motivating the child to use the targeted behavior and integrate new behavior into daily life. Consider how the SCERTS approach is different from the ABA intervention described above by reading Focus 8.9.

The SCERTS approach addresses a child's social communication abilities and social relationships as the primary focus of intervention. Table 8.6 lists the challenges of children with autism at various stages of development. The listed challenges motivate the intervention strategies used in the SCERTS approach.

At the earliest levels, the child needs to establish joint visual attention and improve the frequency of communicative functions such as requesting, commenting/labeling, and negation (Carpenter, Mastergeorge, & Coggins, 1983). At advanced language levels, individuals with ASD need support to improve discourse abilities, repair communication breakdowns, and use language in less familiar social situations. The SCERTS approach uses a facilitative intervention style, as compared to the adult-directive techniques characteristic of ABA methodologies. The SCERTS approach uses the training sequence of:

- Following the child's lead.
- Offering choices and alternatives within the child's daily routines and activities.
- Responding to the child's intent and reinforcing communication attempts.
- Modeling a variety of communication functions at the child's level.
- Elaborating the child's verbal and nonverbal communication attempts (Prizant & Wetherby, 2005).

An example of a SCERTS treatment sequence is shown in Figure 8.5.

In the SCERTS approach, communication partners embed learning sequences within the child's everyday activities. Embedding instruction increases the generalization of the targeted behaviors and encourages the involvement of the child's

FOCUS 8.9 *Intervention*

Refer to the continuum of naturalness in Chapter 4 to refresh your memory regarding clinician- versus child-directed therapy. Describe how the ABA versus SCERTS approach reflects variation in terms of the continuum of naturalness. Can these approaches ever be combined for a particular child?

Table 8.6 **Challenges in Social Communication for Individuals with ASD**

Prelinguistic levels	Emerging and early language levels	Advanced language levels
1. Establishing communication intentionality 2. Problem behavior and communication limitations 3. Establishing nonspeech communication alternatives (e.g., gestures, picture communication, sign language) 4. Establishing joint visual attention and reciprocal action	1. Shift from presymbolic communication to language may be slow 2. Generalization of language to new situations may be slow 3. Language forms are used for limited number of communication functions or purposes 4. Language use strongly influenced by familiarity with context and emotional regulation 5. Considerable difficulty understanding others' communication	1. Difficulty taking the perspective of others (social-cognitive limitation) 2. Discourse difficulty (initiating, maintaining, terminating conversations) 3. Difficulty recognizing need for, and making, communication repairs 4. Difficulty communicating in socially complex and less familiar contexts

Source: Adapted from "Critical Issues in Enhancing Communication Abilities for Persons with Autism Spectrum Disorders," by B. M. Prizant & A. M. Wetherby, 2006. In F. R. Volkmar, R. Paul, A. Klin, & D. Cohen (Eds.), *Handbook of Autism and Pervasive Developmental Disorders: Vol. 2: Assessment, Interventions, and Policy* (3rd ed., pp. 925–945). New York: Wiley and Sons. Copyright © 2005. Reproduced with permission of John Wiley & Sons, Inc.

Figure 8.5 **Example of SCERTS Treatment Sequence**

Communication challenge: Tabitha tends to engage in solitary play and does not typically make eye contact or verbal or nonverbal requests when interacting with others.

- During playtime, the communication partner modifies the toy selection to include toys requiring adult assistance (e.g., wind-up toys, toys with tight lids) or by placing favorite toys in locations requiring Tabitha to initiate a request.
- Communication partner captures Tabitha's interest in toys and then responds to any communicative attempt.
- With Tabitha's more frequent communication attempts, the communication partner delays responding, to encourage vocalization or gestures.

Source: From *The SCERTS™ model: A comprehensive educational approach for children with autism spectrum disorders; Vol. 1: Program planning and intervention,* by B. M. Prizant, A. M. Wetherby, E. Rubin, A. C. Laurent, & P. J. Rydell, 2006, Baltimore, MD: Brookes.

parents, classroom teachers, siblings, and peers. Since intervention aims to improve both the quality and the quantity of interactions, the practitioner uses both frequency counts and behavioral rating systems to document child and communication partner objectives in SCERTS.

For example, if the intervention goal is to increase a student's ability to negotiate more effectively with peers, the professional might document how frequently a classroom peer uses a wipe-off white board to map out negotiations and record compromises during a cooperative science project. In this case, the practitioner has taught the typically developing peer to use this negotiation strategy (Prizant, Wetherby, Rubin, Laurent, & Rydell, 2006). At the same time, the practitioner rates the discourse ability of the student with ASD; conversational initiations and turn taking are recorded with a rating scale (i.e., 3 = all of the time, 2 = some of the time, 1 = none of the time).

Throughout the SCERTS intervention approach there is an effort to increase the child's independent functioning and self-regulation. To accomplish this, intervention often focuses on natural routines with a beginning, middle, and end. For example, during a shared interaction with a puzzle, the puzzle completion signals the end of the interaction, whereas with block play there is not a clear ending point. In this case, the puzzle activity is likely to be easier for a child with ASD as compared to a block activity. The practitioner considers what social routines will challenge—but not overly frustrate—a child with ASD with respect to the event sequence.

There are many different activities with a clear event sequence that can be used to improve social functioning. A very young child in the prelinguistic stage learns the play sequence associated with ring-around-the-rosy. An older child in the emerging language stage learns the interaction routine associated with making a choice during classroom free play. In contrast, a school-age child in the advanced language stage learns the communication skills needed to participate in a group activity in gym class. In all three examples, the practitioner facilitates the child's communication and interaction within reoccurring daily activities.

Communication partners learn to use visual and auditory cues to signal the communication sequences. For example, if the child with autism is practicing asking questions during a shared conversation, the communication partner brings up a topic and then cues an appropriate question with a written sentence (if the child is a reader) or a picture. The adult says, *"I had an exciting weekend!"* and then cues the child with autism to ask, *"What did you do?"* Eventually, the adult promotes additional question types and emphasizes conversational turn-taking strategies; parents and peers also are included in the discourse intervention.

With more linguistically advanced children, practitioners emphasize self-regulation, self-analysis, and self-monitoring of conversational strategies. For example, practitioners videotape shared conversations between children and train the child with ASD to evaluate and modify conversational strategies (Scherer et al., 2001). As you see from the examples above and the goals listed in Figure 8.6, this approach is flexible. The practitioner constantly evaluates the child's current level of functioning and targets skills to improve the child's independence and daily interaction with others. Examples of SCERTS intervention goals are shown in Figure 8.6.

Figure 8.6   **Examples of SCERTS Communication Goals**

- **Child goal:** Child independently will modify communication strategy (use his picture symbols) to obtain desired item when communication partner does not understand vocalized communication attempt in eight out of ten consecutive attempts.
- **Partner goal:** Communication partner will present a series of prompts moving from least directive to more directed (i.e., looking at communication board, pointing to communication board, saying *"Show me what you want"*) to cue child to use picture symbols.
- **Transactional goal:** Communication board is updated to reflect child's current interests and is available throughout the day to promote spontaneous use.

Source: From *The SCERTS™ model: A comprehensive educational approach for children with autism spectrum disorders; Vol. 1: Program planning and intervention,* by B. M. Prizant, A. M. Wetherby, E. Rubin, A. C. Laurent, & P. J. Rydell, 2006, Baltimore, MD: Brookes.

Evidence Supporting the SCERTS Approach.   The SCERTS approach is based on evidence that children learn the most when (1) they are engaged in meaningful activities (Odom, McConnell, & McEvoy, 1992), (2) families are included as a central part of intervention (Dunlap & Fox, 1999), and (3) social interaction and functional communication are central intervention components (National Research Council, 2001).

Prizant, Wetherby, and their colleagues describe children with ASD and the results of SCERTS-based interventions (e.g., Prizant et al., 2005). Published case studies and research supporting the underlying theory of SCERTS intervention places the SCERTS model at a Level III in the scientific studies evidence hierarchy.

Summary

- The *Diagnostic and Statistical Manual of Mental Disorders, Fourth Edition, Text Revision* (DSM-IV-TR; American Psychiatric Association [APA], 2000) describes the diagnostic categories that are considered pervasive developmental disorders.
- Children with autism spectrum disorder demonstrate (a) an impairment of social interaction, (b) significant communication impairment, and (c) unusual stereotypic or repetitive behaviors before the age of 3 years. Children with Asperger syndrome demonstrate normal language milestones at an early age, but evidence pragmatic and prosodic differences after age 3 with narrowly focused and unusual interests. Females with Rett syndrome develop normally up to 6 months to 1 year of age and then rapidly regress in their social and language ability. Pervasive developmental disorder—not otherwise specified classifies children who demonstrate some, but not all, of the symptoms associated with other subtypes on the autism spectrum.
- When all the autism subtypes are considered, 6 out of 1000 children are affected. ASDs affect more males than females at a ratio of 4:1. Intellectual disability and epilepsy are the most frequently occurring associated conditions.

- Autism spectrum disorders are disorders of brain development; current research points to a genetic cause. Pharmaceuticals are increasingly incorporated into the medical intervention treatment programs.
- Deficits in sensorimotor skills, imitation abilities, and the development of joint visual attention are associated with ASD; families play a strong role in the intervention program of children with ASD.
- Intervention approaches vary on the continuum of naturalness; applied behavioral analysis (ABA) and the SCERTS approach demonstrate this variation. ABA draws strongly from behavioral theory and has Level III research data supporting its use. The SCERTS approach is based on development and social interaction theory emphasizing ecological validity.

Discussion and In-Class Activities

1. Your instructor will divide the class into three groups and assign each group a disorder (either Asperger syndrome, Rett syndrome, or pervasive developmental disorder—not otherwise specified). Complete a same different rubric for your assigned disorder comparing it with autistic disorder. In other words, decide how your assigned disorder is the same as or different from autism. Write two intervention goals (refer to Chapter 4 for a review of good goal writing): one for your assigned disorder and one for a child with autism. Explain if your goal targets the language domain of form, content, or use. In what way does the goal target the indicated language domain? How will this goal improve the child's daily life?

2. View videotape clips of children with ASD at www.autismspeaks.org (clips are available in the video glossary of this Web site). Discuss the communications functions and means that you see in the different video clips using the observational tool in this chapter (see Figure 8.2) as a guide. Discuss the decision-making process used to classify the various communication patterns.

3. Develop a series of intervention steps that the professional could use in a behavioral intervention program (like DTT) with the ultimate goal to improve the child's ability to (a) name objects and actions during an adult–child shared book reading, (b) choose a favorite toy during free play, or (c) follow one-step commands.

4. In your small group, take one or more of the communication goals listed below. Develop an intervention to improve the individual's communication functioning in the targeted area via (a) an adult-directed approach and (b) a social interaction intervention (similar to the SCERTS approach). List the pros and cons of each method for improving the specific communication goal.

   - Labeling of objects
   - Requesting toys
   - Answering *wh* questions (e.g., *what, when, where*)

- Labeling actions
- Asking a question
- Following simple one- and two-step directions
- Social greetings
- Maintaining a conversation with a communication partner
- Improving an individual's syntax and semantic skills

5. The SCERTS approach focuses on helping children make real-life changes in their social and communication behaviors. In small groups, discuss how you could document a child's behavioral, social, and communication changes (a) at home during dinner hour, (b) during a family routine such as bath time or bedtime, (c) with peers during free play, (d) in the classroom during an academic activity, (d) during a rule-based game with peers. Consider a variety of methods to document change including rating scales, behavioral sampling, and transcription of child communication. Discuss the pros and cons of each method and brainstorm how documentation could be adapted to make it work for a classroom teacher.

Chapter 8 Case Study

Vijay is a 12-year-old male diagnosed with Asperger syndrome. He attends middle school with his typically developing peers. He is good at math and enjoys his computer class. He spends two periods a day in the resource room where a special educator helps Vijay on his organizational strategies and coaches him in his more difficult subjects (e.g., language arts). You have been working with Vijay on his conversational skills; the focus of intervention has been to work on initiating a conversational topic, staying on topic, and using appropriate discourse strategies to change topics.

Vijay would like to join the chess club. However, he demonstrates inappropriate behaviors (i.e., he "acts out") when he is unfamiliar with the routine or experiencing new situations. He has difficulty with peer interactions when they involve humor, sarcasm, or just kidding around.

Questions for Discussion

1. How can you assist Vijay to conversationally interact and handle chess club?
2. Will your goals more likely reflect an ABA or a SCERTS intervention approach?
3. In small groups, write some intervention goals for Vijay. Describe how you would document progress.
4. Could Vijay's peers be trained to incorporate some facilitating strategies? Describe some possible strategies and a plan for documenting the peers' use of strategies.
5. How could the scheduling or planning for the chess club be modified (or elaborated) to assist Vijay's adaptation to novel situations?

Early Literacy, Reading, and Writing for School-Age Children

Chapter Overview Questions

1. Why does the practitioner working with emergent literacy take a preventative approach? What are the primary emergent literacy targets?

2. What is the embedded-explicit model of emergent literacy intervention? Give examples of embedded and explicit intervention techniques.

3. How does the practitioner assess emergent literacy skills? How does the practitioner assess school-age reading and writing skills?

4. What skills are foundational for school-age readers?

5. What are some intervention strategies for advanced-level phonological awareness skills, narratives, reading comprehension, and writing?

6. What are some target skills within the five levels in the interactive-to-independent model of literacy?

7. What level of evidence exists regarding Gillon's Explicit Phonological Awareness program and Nelson's Writing Lab approach?

This chapter outlines important aspects of written language and literacy development. I discuss early literacy development as well as aspects of later reading and writing development as it pertains to school-age children. I refer to the early stage of reading development as **emergent literacy**. Emergent literacy refers to the skills, knowledge, and attitudes that are precursors to conventional reading and writing (Sulzby, 1985; Whitehurst & Lonigan, 1998). **Conventional reading** refers to the ability of children to decode (i.e., sound out) unfamiliar words and draw meaning from written text. Children with spoken language impairments often have associated difficulties with written language development (Catts, Fey, Tomblin, & Zhang, 2002). The reasons should be obvious to you by now—language development encompasses more than spoken language. A child who is language proficient can, for example, hear and differentiate phonemes, understand complex syntax, infer meaning from vocabulary, and move from less formal conversational-style discourse to more formal academic-sounding language. Skills in each domain—phonological, syntax, vocabulary, and discourse—are needed during reading and writing. Underlying language impairments in language domains have far-reaching effects that negatively impact children's reading and writing abilities throughout their school years (Bishop & Clarkson, 2003).

The Role of the Speech-Language Pathologist in Reading and Writing

The American Speech-Language-Hearing Association (ASHA) strongly advocates that speech-language pathologists (SLPs) indirectly and directly incorporate reading and writing interventions into clinical practice (ASHA, 2001, 2007). Indirect involvement occurs in the early years when SLPs collaborate with classroom teachers and special educators to include literacy-based objectives and activities in prekindergarten programs; it occurs in later school years when SLPs work with general education teachers to provide effective classroom interventions. SLPs are using new approaches to increase their ability to spend more time in classrooms working with teachers (see Focus 9.1). SLPs work directly with students when early literacy, reading, and writing goals are included in language intervention programs.

FOCUS 9.1 School-Based Issues

The American Speech-Language-Hearing Association recommends that SLP school caseloads not exceed 40 students/week; however, the average SLP caseload is 53 students, and some SLPs have school caseloads as large as 110 (ASHA, 2002). Because of large caseload demands, some SLPs question their ability to focus on children with reading and writing deficits.

To overcome the challenge of a large caseload, one approach is to use "workload analysis." Rather than computing workload by counting the number of students served, workload analysis considers face-to-face contact time in addition to time needed for paperwork, classroom visits, collaboration with classroom teachers, and IEP development. This approach gives work credit for SLPs who provide classroom-based support to students with reading and writing deficits. For more information about workload analysis, you can go to the ASHA Web site at: www.asha.org/about/publications/leader-online/archives/2002/q3/020910c.htm

Some SLPs do not feel comfortable including reading and writing goals in their speech and language interventions. Consider the following excerpt sent as a letter to the editor of an SLP journal.

I am an SLP in the schools. I am concerned about stepping into the role of reading specialist/resource teacher when our plate is so full with working within the traditional role of an SLP in oral comprehension, oral expression, articulation, voice, and stuttering. (Jan. 22, 2008; Letters to the Editor, *ASHA Leader*)

The above letter provoked a number of responses from other SLPs. The example below is representative.

We must be cognizant that speech-language pathology is a fluid discipline and continue to keep pace with new perspectives and developments. It was only in the 1970s that we began to consider our role in treating children with language disorders! We need to embrace the range of disabilities that fall under our purview and applaud the fact that our profession allows SLPs to develop specializations across a wide range of communication disorders. (May 6, 2008; Letters to the Editor, *ASHA Leader*)

Needless to say, I agree with the second writer. I understand that it can be difficult to develop new areas of expertise. However, in this case, SLPs are compelled to become knowledgeable in written communication because of current educational policy and research evidence. For example, federal law (IDEA 2004) mandates that SLPs report the academic risk factors for a student receiving school-based SLP services. Further, research evidence overwhelmingly demonstrates the higher-than-expected academic risk factors for students with language impairments (e.g., Catts, Bridges, Little, & Tomblin, 2008).

The professional's role changes when working with younger children as compared to older school-age students. At the earliest ages, the SLP may be the first to detect a child's language impairment. Research demonstrates that the presence of language impairment (LI) in preschool and kindergarten is an important indicator of a potential reading disability. Consequently, prior to school entry, the SLP is likely to be at the forefront in leading an early literacy and language intervention program. I will be talking more about the role of the professional in preventing reading disabilities in the section below.

At later ages (first grade and beyond) the SLP generally works alongside other educational professionals. The education team typically includes the classroom teacher, reading specialist, school psychologist, special education teacher, resource room teacher, and the SLP. The general reading assessment program is typically administered on a schoolwide level and results are monitored by the education team and school administration. The SLP role in assessment and intervention is typically domain specific; for example, targeting the student's narrative ability, spelling abilities, or focusing on written language skills.

This chapter is organized as follows. First, I discuss the role of the SLP and special educator with regard to setting up a prevention program for young children who are at risk for reading disability. In the early literacy section, I describe the primary targets that should be the focus of an early literacy prevention program, including phonological awareness, print concepts, alphabetic awareness, and early writing. I provide information on assessment of early literacy skills. Finally, I outline an intervention model: the embedded-explicit approach. Practitioners use the embedded-explicit approach to implement a literacy prevention program in preschool and kindergarten classrooms.

In the second major subsection, I provide information useful to the SLP and special educator who work with older, school-age children with reading or writing deficits. I describe specific language-focused areas, including narratives, spelling, reading comprehension, and writing. I also describe a literacy model for students with more significant levels of impairment (e.g., children with autism); this approach is called the interactive-to-independent model of literacy. In several subsections in this chapter I describe cultural considerations related to children's literacy development.

In the final major section of this chapter, I present detailed information on two intervention approaches for children with reading impairments. There are dozens (if not hundreds) of intervention approaches for children with reading impairments. I have picked two approaches because (a) both were developed by SLPs, (b) both have peer-reviewed evidence documenting their effectiveness, and (c) the two approaches (one for younger children and one for older school-age children) demonstrate the connections between theoretical knowledge and clinical application.

Emergent Literacy

PREVENTION OF READING DISABILITY IN YOUNG CHILDREN AT RISK FOR READING FAILURE

When practitioners provide literacy interventions to preschoolers, they are participating in a prevention program. A preventative program is like vaccinating a child against a childhood disease. Doctors do not wait until a child has chicken pox to give a vaccination; instead, doctors give the vaccination to prevent chicken pox. Similarly, SLPs and educators participate in emergent literacy preventative interventions to reduce the chance of reading failure in later school years. The goal is to "catch children before they fail" (Torgesen, 1998).

A number of fundamental language skills are required for early literacy development; these skills include a child's phonological awareness, print concepts, alphabetic knowledge, oral language development, and emergent writing. Consequently, much of early language and literacy intervention is focused on these critical domains. Assessment in a prevention program uses the response-to-intervention approach (RTI) introduced in Chapter 3. As you recall, RTI uses scientifically based research to guide intervention. Using a prevention program model, all young children receive evidence-based educational interventions in their preschool classrooms. Next, I describe the primary emergent literacy targets included in a preventative emergent literacy model.

PRIMARY TARGETS OF EMERGENT LITERACY PREVENTION PROGRAMS

Primary Target: Phonological Awareness.   Phonological awareness (PA) is the best predictor of a child's reading ability (Catts, Fey, Tomblin, & Zhang, 2002; Liberman, Shankeiler, & Liberman, 1989). **Phonological awareness (PA)** refers to the ability to reflect on and manipulate phonemic segments of speech (Ehri, 1989; Treiman, 1991). Phonological awareness develops from word and syllable awareness (e.g., rhyming and recognizing and identifying the number of syllables in words) to awareness of individual sounds within words. A child demonstrates awareness at the individual sound level by recognizing that /k/ /æ/ /t/ can be blended together to form the word *cat*. At the beginning stages of PA development the child recognizes larger sound units; he or she learns sentences are made up of words and words are made up of syllables. At more sophisticated levels of PA development, the child demonstrates the ability to sound out and blend individual sounds. The ability to decode at the phoneme level is critically linked to reading development. The term **decoding** is used to describe the ability to read a printed word by relating the letters to corresponding speech sounds (Gillon, 2006). PA instruction should not be confused with **phonics instruction**, which entails teaching students how to use letter-sound relations to read or spell words. You can read more about phonics instruction in Focus 9.2.

Many children begin to develop awareness at the word and syllable levels by the age of 2 years. Specifically, about one in four children at age 2 can complete a rhyming detection task in which they are asked to identify the word that does not rhyme (e.g., *hat, cat, bell;* Lonigan, Burgess, Anthony, & Barker, 1998). Phoneme-level identification (i.e., identification of specific sounds) takes longer. Most children

---

FOCUS 9.2 *Learning More*

What is the difference between phonological awareness (PA) and phonics? *Phonological awareness* describes the broad range of understandings related to the sounds of speech; at beginning levels it includes awareness of words and word parts, at more advanced levels it includes phonemic awareness or understanding of a word's individual sounds. To develop PA, a child learns to pay attention to the sounds within words in an abstract way, learning that sounds (in and of themselves) do not contain meaning.

Phonics is a form of instruction focusing on improving a student's understanding and use of the alphabetic principle. Phonics instruction teaches that there is a predictable relationship between phonemes and graphemes (i.e., letters represent sounds in written language). For example, during phonics instruction a student might be taught that the /aɪ/ sound potentially is represented by different spelling patterns, as in *laid, late,* or *lay*.

Table 9.1   **Developmental Age Levels and Examples of Early Phonological Awareness Skill Areas**

Age at which it is expected to have greater than 75% accuracy	Skills	Examples
Early to late preschool	Word awareness Syllable awareness Rhyming	• *"Can you point to a word on this page?"* • *"Let's clap the syllables in your name."* • *"Can you make a big word from these two words? (cow, boy)"* • *"Let's play a rhyming game. You finish this sentence: The silly old <u>cat</u>, wore a big <u>hat</u>, and sat down on a _____ ."*
Late preschool-early kindergarten	Beginning sound awareness Sound blending Onset-rime	• *"Do these words start with the same sound? (boy, ball) How about these two? (dog, man)"* • *"What word am I saying? /b/ /i/"* • *"Look at these pictures. What word am I saying? b-ubbles"*
Kindergarten	Phoneme identification Sound segmenting	• *"What sound do you hear at the beginning of the word* pig? • *"How many sounds do you hear in the word* boot? *Show me with these blocks."* (Child touches one block at a time as he or she says word phoneme by phoneme.)

Source: From "Embedded-Explicit Emergent Literacy Intervention I: Background and Description of Approach," by L. M. Justice and J. N. Kaderavek, 2004, *Language, Speech, and Hearing Services in Schools,* *35*, pp. 201–211. Reprinted with permission.

do not achieve mastery of phoneme-level awareness until age 5 (Lonigan et al., 1998). Table 9.1 lists the different PA tasks and developmental age guidelines.

You might suspect that children with oral speech and language deficits have more difficulty with PA tasks and later reading development than children with typical language development (Catts, Fey, Tomblin, & Zhang, 2002; Puranik, Petscher, Al Otaiba, Catts, & Lonigan, 2008). You are correct in this assumption. However, you may be surprised to know that some children who do not have obvious oral language deficits sometimes also have difficulty with phonological awareness tasks. "Hidden" PA deficits can significantly impede reading and writing development (Gillon, 2004). Consequently, knowledgeable professionals monitor PA skill development for all children during the early school years; they also support classroom teachers in providing high-quality PA instruction. With SLP assistance, general education teachers learn to provide more explicit and frequent exposure to PA concepts to children whose PA skills are more slowly developing.

Primary Target: Print Concepts and Alphabetic Awareness. The term **print concepts** is used to describe children's understanding of the use and function of print during reading and writing. **Alphabetic awareness** describes children's understanding of letter names. Table 9.2 lists the different skills included within print concepts and alphabetic awareness domains. Like phonological awareness, early awareness of print concepts and alphabetic awareness strongly predict later reading proficiency.

Primary Target: Oral Language Skills. The important skills of phonological awareness, print, and alphabetic concepts are learned within a stimulating oral language environment (Stanovich, 2000). A high-quality oral language environment is fostered when adults frequently engage children in extended conversations. Although this seems obvious, research in preschool classrooms demonstrates that

Table 9.2   **Print Concepts and Alphabetic Awareness Terms, Descriptions, and Teaching Examples**

Term	Description	Teaching example
Environmental print awareness	Children recognize familiar symbols and demonstrate knowledge that print carries meaning.	• Point out signs (e.g., McDonald's sign) and letters in children's daily life. • Ask children to sort items (e.g., put all the similar candy wrappers in one pile).
Concepts of print	Children demonstrate accepted standards of practice for interacting with print.	• Demonstrate left-to-right directionality during reading and writing. • Ask children *"Where do I start reading?"* (front to back directionality of books) • Ask children to *"Show me the big long word on this page!"* Children learn the meaning of *word, letter, sentence, author, title* and recognize that words are set off by the surrounding space. • Involve children and demonstrate the different functions of print (e.g., a newspaper, a letter, a shopping list). • Demonstrate the use of punctuation and ask children to point out different punctuation marks (e.g., *"What do we do when we see a ?"*).

(continued)

Table 9.2   **Print Concepts and Alphabetic Awareness Terms, Descriptions, and Teaching Examples (*Continued*)**

Term	Description	Teaching example
Alphabetic letter knowledge	Children recognize printed letters and understand the letter-sound relationship.	• Play games using letters in children's names; sort and identify letters using blocks, draw and paint letters, play games with magnetic and foam letters. • Help children sort pictures and objects that start with the same letter. • Ask children to find words that have the same first letter as their name. • Sing the alphabet song and have children hold up a letter. • Play "find the hidden letter" or bury plastic letters in the sandbox and have the children find and identify the letters.

Source: From "Embedded-Explicit Emergent Literacy Intervention I: Background and Description of Approach," by L. M. Justice and J. N. Kaderavek, 2004, *Language, Speech, and Hearing Services in Schools, 35*, pp. 201–211. Reprinted with permission.

the majority of teacher talk is "management talk" (Smith & Dickenson, 1994). Management talk includes giving directions and gaining children's attention. Surprisingly, as little as 10% of teacher-child conversation in early childhood classrooms relates to reading and writing (Rosemary & Roskos, 2002).

For many children, opportunities for high-quality oral language discourse are not much better at home. While children in high-income famlilies hear approximately 2100 vocabulary words per hour, children in families who are struggling economically only hear 600 words per hour (Hart & Risley, 1995). Teachers and SLPs promote the importance of an enriched oral language environment during the preschool years, including opportunities to learn sophisticated vocabulary.

Primary Target: Emergent Writing.   Children's writing skills, such as name writing and invented spelling, are one of the strongest predictors of later reading proficiency (Badian, 1998). Early writing puts the child in an active role; children consider how to use a written symbol to communicate meaning. As students' phonics skills develop, they learn to represent sounds with letter combinations. Unfortunately, only 27% of U.S. fourth grade students exhibit proficient writing abilities; 15% have writing abilities at "below basic" levels (U.S. Department of Education, 2002). To improve this poor outcome, practitioners work with early childhood teachers to foster emergent writing (e.g., Kaderavek & Justice, 2004; Torgeson, 1998).

Children's writing development begins with early scribbles and what looks like random marks. These unsophisticated attempts represent children's exploration of writing as a means of communication (Casbergue & Plauché, 2005). In order to compose written language, children draw on their knowledge of the alphabetic principle as well as their language **composition skills.** Composition skills refer to a child's ability to integrate pragmatic, syntax, and semantic language domains to formulate and express thought (Berninger et al., 2006).

Children move from making scribbles and marks to making letter-like shapes. The formation of letter-like shapes is followed by children's beginning attempts to represent the sounds they hear in words. Table 9.3 demonstrates the stages of writing development and describes the important concepts learned at each stage.

Although most children follow a general development in the early stages of writing, children's writing development does not follow a step-by-step path. Children sometimes use less-sophisticated writing (e.g., scribbling) when they attempt a difficult task. In contrast, they may produce a sophisticated writing attempt at other times. For example, a 3-year-old child may painstakingly write her name with accuracy, but in a

Table 9.3 **Writing Development**

Level	Writing	Concepts	Child learns to:
Preschool	Scribble with or without drawing; letterlike forms; random letter strings	• Writing differs from drawing • Print carries meaning • Concept of *letter*	• Pay attention to print • Control a writing implement • "Write" across the page from left-to-right • Produce some letterlike shapes
Late preschool-mid kindergarten	Syllabic writing; writing that the child can "read" (including some conventional letters)	• Chooses own words to make a written text • Concept of word in text • Recognizes own name • Recognizes others' names	• Recognize most letter names • Form and orient many letters • Control letter size • Use letters to make words • Leave spaces between words • Know some letter sounds
Mid kindergarten-mid first grade	Simple texts that can be partially read by others; writing is labored	• Produces messages that others can read • Concept of *sentence* and *story*	• Write name fluently • Organize words into sentences • Use punctuation • Recognize all letter names • Know most letter sounds • Distinguish between upper- and lowercase letters in writing

(continued)

Table 9.3 **Writing Development (*Continued*)**

Level	Writing	Concepts	Child learns to:
Late first grade-second grade	Writing in phrases with greater fluency	• Writes extended and coherent text • Learns vowel patterns in single-syllable words	• Link sentences • Monitor and correct text • Write phrases with fluency • Write simple paragraphs • Apply writing process (brainstorm-compose-proof-revise)

Sources: From *Words Their Way: Word Study for Phonics, Vocabulary, and Spelling Instruction* (4th ed.), by D. R. Bear, M. Invernizzi, S. Templeton, and F. Johnston, 2007, Upper Saddle River, NJ: Pearson; *Teaching Writing: A Workshop Approach,* by A. Fiderer, 1993, New York: Scholastic; "Early Writing and Spelling Development," by J. N. Kaderavek, S. Q. Cabell, and L. M. Justice, in press. In P. M. Rhyner (Ed.), *Emergent Literacy and Early Language Acquisition: Making the Connection.* New York: Guilford; *Literacy Development in the Early Years* (5th ed.) by L. M. Morrow, 2005, Boston: Allyn & Bacon; *Student-Centered Classroom Assessment,* by R. J. Stiggins, 1997, Upper Saddle River, NJ: Prentice Hall.

dramatic play situation, while pretending to write a shopping list, she may scribble and say *"This is my shopping list!"* Both efforts are appropriate and demonstrate important aspects of writing development. The name-writing task represents a child's understanding that writing demands the use of specific letters and that certain letter combinations represent a unique word. On the other hand, a child's scribbled shopping list demonstrates awareness of the function of print in everyday life.

ASSESSMENT OF CHILDREN'S EARLY LITERACY SKILLS

In the section above, I described the early literacy domains most frequently targeted within preschool programs. However, it is important to remember that early literacy development begins in infancy in a child's home (Snow & Ninio, 1986). Consequently, professionals monitor children's early literacy development from an early age and carefully consider the quality and quantity of home literacy experiences. If a child is not demonstrating enjoyment of shared parent-child book reading, the professional works to improve home book-reading practices and monitors the child's literacy growth.

Early literacy assessment tools are typically criterion-referenced rather than norm-referenced assessments (Justice, Invernizzi, & Meier, 2002). This reflects a prevention approach consistent with the response-to-intervention (RTI) model. Consistent with RTI, practitioners do not wait until a child has a literacy delay before implementing a high-quality language-literacy program. Instead, practitioners monitor literacy development for all children and implement intense literacy interventions as needed. As you can see in Figure 9.1, practitioners monitor a broad range of early literacy domains in young children. Along with the literacy features described above, practitioners also consider children's social literacy and literacy orientation.

Figure 9.1 An Early Literacy Observational Checklist

Child's name: _____ Birth date: _____ Chronological age: _____ Observer: _____

Emergent Literacy Accomplishments	Typically Mastered By	Emergent Literacy Component					Child's Accomplishments		Notes/ Comments
		S	O	L	P	PA	Occasionally	Frequently	
(1) Content to stay in lap	Before 12 months								
(2) Asks for books/indicates books are to be repeated	Before 12 months								
(3) Gestures and laughs during book reading	Before 12 months								
(4) Indicates wants favorite book	Before 12 months								
(5) Focuses on picture	Before 12 months								
(6) Makes spontaneous sounds/words/gestures during book reading	Before 12 months								
(7) Independently manipulates, looks at books	Before 18 months								
(8) Enjoys many different stories	Before 18 months								
(9) Handles book properly (pages left-to-right, etc.)	18–36 months								
(10) Names actions of characters (running, etc.)	19–22 months								
(11) Points to pictures when asked	Before 36 months								
(12) Joins in, repeats phrases during book reading	Before 36 months								
(13) Tells stories from books	24–60 months								
(14) Writes attempting to make letters	30–40 months								
(15) Dramatic play (acts out stories)	36–48 months								
(16) Predict plots (what happens next)	36–48 months								
(17) Points to print/knows print is read	36–60 months								
(18) Reads environmental print (cereal boxes, etc.)	36–48 months								
(19) Plays with words (rhymes, etc.)	36 months								
(20) Claps out syllables in words	36–48 months								
(21) Scribbles	36–48 months								
(22) Says scribbles are "writing"	48–60 months								
(23) Recognizes the first sound in words	60–66 months								
(24) Re-tells story (beginning, middle, end)	60–72 months								
(25) Recognizes 12–21 uppercase letters	60 months								
(26) Recognizes 9–17 lowercase letters	60 months								
(27) Writes some real words including first name	60 months								
(28) Names 4–8 letter sounds ("that says /m/")	60 months								
(29) Blends and segments sounds in words	2nd semester kindergarten								
SUMMARY		_/12	_/12	_/11	_/11	_/5			

S = Social literacy; O = Orientation/interest in literacy; L = Language development; P = Print and alphabetic awareness; PA = Phonological awareness

Social literacy considers children's affective (i.e., emotional) response to shared literacy experiences. Parent-child shared book reading is a critically important early learning context. Children who are frequently read to and participate in warm, engaging storybook interactions more frequently become successful readers and writers (Bus & van IJzendoorn, 1997). Further, children's ability to demonstrate joint visual attention and back-and-forth discourse during shared storybook reading supports oral language and literacy development (Snow & Ninio, 1986). Much of what children learn about print and the alphabet is learned through literacy socialization (ASHA, 2001). More information about literacy socialization is provided in Focus 9.3.

Frequent, positive social literacy interactions lead to high literacy orientation. **Literacy orientation** includes aspects of children's temperament, motivation, and attention in response to book reading (Chang & Burns, 2005; Kaderavek & Sulzby, 2000). Most children enjoy shared storybook reading. Some children do not. It is hypothesized that children with language impairments are more likely to have a negative orientation to literacy as compared to children developing typically (Kaderavek & Sulzby, 2000). Literacy orientation impacts the success of literacy interventions because children with high orientation show more improvement in response to treatment in comparison to children with low orientation (Justice, Chow, Capellini, Flanigan, & Colton, 2003). In the observational checklist (Figure 9.1), children's orientation to literacy is documented in items 1-8, 12, 13, 15, and 24.

In addition to informal observational tools, there are other published early literacy assessment tools. A frequently used prekindergarten assessment is the Phonological Awareness and Literacy Screening—Pre-Kindergarten (PALS-PreK: Invernizzi, Sullivan, Meier, & Swank, 2004). The PALS-PreK evaluates a range of early literacy skills including rhyme, beginning sound awareness, name writing, upper- and lowercase letter identification, letter-sound knowledge, and print concepts. The assessor calculates a raw score by summing the points obtained on each subtest and comparing the child's scores with other children the same age. The comparison scores reflect a child's ability in the spring prior to kindergarten enrollment. Total administration time of the PALS-PreK is 20 to 25 minutes.

FOCUS 9.3 *Clinical Skill Building*

Aspects of social literacy can be compared to the description of language *use* in Chapter 1. Discuss how book-reading interactions lend themselves to development of language use.

In the form-content-use model, which language component is involved if a student has lexical deficits contributing to his or her reading problem?

What component is involved if a student has difficulty with structural knowledge?

EARLY LITERACY INTERVENTIONS:
THE EMBEDDED-EXPLICIT APPROACH

The embedded-explicit approach describes a two-faceted intervention model practitioners use to foster children's early literacy development (Justice & Kaderavek, 2004; Kaderavek & Justice, 2004). Through **embedded interventions**, practitioners work to enhance children's oral language, phonological awareness, print and alphabetic concepts, and emergent writing within meaningful activities and classroom interactions. Potential interactions include storybook reading, dramatic play, center-time activities, and even transitional routines (e.g., "signing in" at the beginning of the school day). Teachers learn to take advantage of naturalistic opportunities to target emergent literacy skills.

For example, imagine that you are at the sandbox and children are digging for objects in the sand; prior to the children's arrival you placed objects in the sandbox with the letter *B* in the initial position (e.g., bucket, ball, bat, book, basket, bone). You also buried several plastic letters *B* and *M*. As the children find objects, you say, *"That's a bucket; what sound do you hear at the beginning of* bucket? /b/. *Good, I hear a /b/ sound, too!"* When a child finds a letter *B* or *M* you ask, *"What letter is that?"* Oh, yes, that's a letter B. *It makes the /b/ sound, doesn't it? Is that the sound you heard at the beginning of* bucket?"

As you can see from the example above, during embedded inventions the adult often primes the activity to foster literacy discussions. However, the adult follows the child focus of attention and the context is highly engaging and child-centered. Embedded learning opportunities occur throughout the school day and should be fostered across interactions.

In contrast to embedded approaches, **explicit intervention** emphasizes the importance of structured, sequenced adult-directed instruction. In explicit interventions, the adult selects a particular literacy target and carefully sequences the child's exposure; here the adult takes a more direct route to enhancing literacy. Explicit approaches are less naturalistic because the adult selects the goals and specifies the teaching sequence and materials. In explicit intervention, the adult typically uses modeling, demonstration, prompts for child response, and regular guided practice. Explicit interventions typically occur in individual or small-group sessions for relatively short (e.g., 5-15 minute) periods; sessions are presented intermittently throughout the school day or week.

Children need exposure to both embedded and explicit literacy instruction. Figure 9.2 demonstrates the kinds of embedded and explicit learning that occur in a literacy-rich classroom. As you can see from the activities listed in Figure 9.2, both embedded and explicit early literacy experiences actively engage children as learners; worksheets and drill activities are avoided.

Early Intervention: Phonological Awareness (PA). The sandbox example above demonstrated an embedded PA learning opportunity. Adults also provide embedded PA instruction when they incorporate rhymes and chants into the classroom or read storybooks such as *The Cat in the Hat* and draw attention to rhyming words. Research demonstrates, however, that explicit exposure to PA should also be

Figure 9.2 **Embedded and Explicit Language and Literacy Activities in the Preschool Classroom**

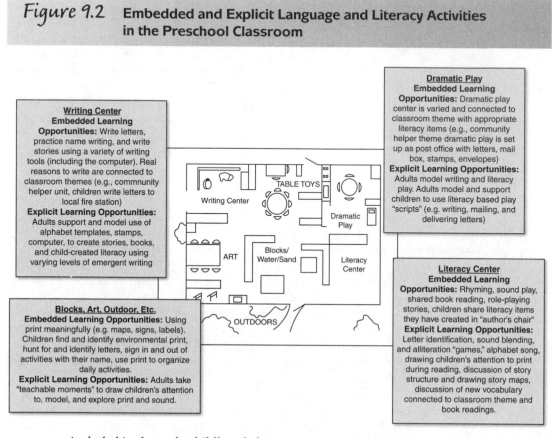

Writing Center
Embedded Learning Opportunities: Write letters, practice name writing, and write stories using a variety of writing tools (including the computer). Real reasons to write are connected to classroom themes (e.g., community helper unit, children write letters to local fire station)
Explicit Learning Opportunities: Adults support and model use of alphabet templates, stamps, computer, to create stories, books, and child-created literacy using varying levels of emergent writing

Dramatic Play
Embedded Learning Opportunities: Dramatic play center is varied and connected to classroom theme with appropriate literacy items (e.g., community helper theme dramatic play is set up as post office with letters, mail box, stamps, envelopes)
Explicit Learning Opportunities: Adults model writing and literacy play. Adults model and support children to use literacy based play "scripts" (e.g. writing, mailing, and delivering letters)

Blocks, Art, Outdoor, Etc.
Embedded Learning Opportunities: Using print meaningfully (e.g. maps, signs, labels). Children find and identify environmental print, hunt for and identify letters, sign in and out of activities with their name, use print to organize daily activities.
Explicit Learning Opportunities: Adults take "teachable moments" to draw children's attention to, model, and explore print and sound.

Literacy Center
Embedded Learning Opportunities: Rhyming, sound play, shared book reading, role-playing stories, children share literacy items they have created in "author's chair"
Explicit Learning Opportunities: Letter identification, sound blending, and alliteration "games," alphabet song, drawing children's attention to print during reading, discussion of story structure and drawing story maps, discussion of new vocabulary connected to classroom theme and book readings.

included in the early childhood classroom; many children will not grasp PA concepts without explicit instruction (Blachman, 2000; Gillon, 2003). I describe several explicit PA learning opportunities below.

One of the easiest PA tasks is syllable recognition. **Syllable recognition** is a child's awareness that a word is made up of syllable subunits. Syllable recognition is considered a word-level task; a child does not need to recognize individual phonemes to recognize syllables. When I engage a child in a syllable recognition task, I ask him or her to clap or tap out word syllables. For example, following a book reading about zoo animals, I may suggest:

"Let's clap out el-e-phant. Now let's clap out ti-ger. Which word has more syllables? Let's clap it again. That's right, el-e-phant has three claps, doesn't it? Elephant has three syllables! Tiger has two claps. Tiger has two syllables!"

Children also should be exposed to phoneme-level tasks such as activities to build initial sound awareness. In the following example, Samantha and I take turns pulling objects out of a "treasure chest."

"Samantha, which of these words starts with the /b/ sound? Snake, boat, sandwich, ball."

I introduce each word individually. I exaggerate and emphasize the initial sound in each word. I go back and let Samantha say the words with me and let her hear the words several times. Note that, at this stage, I only include objects that start with two different sounds (/b/ versus /s/); I avoid choosing objects that start with many different sounds or choosing sounds that are acoustically similar. In this example, to make the task easier, I contrast the stop-plosive sound /b/ with the fricative /s/ sound. I make sure that Samantha stays interested and engaged in the task. Even though it is an explicit intervention, I keep the interaction gamelike rather than a repetitive drill. I provide clues and scaffold the task (i.e., provide as much help as needed) so that Samantha feels successful. I keep the activity brief, approximately 5 minutes.

As Samantha's PA skills improve, I add more sounds, include acoustically similar sound comparisons, and encourage Samantha's independence in completing the PA tasks. Modifying the task also changes the difficulty level. In the example just given, I asked Samantha to identify which word had a target sound (*"Tell me which word starts with /b/"*). This is a beginning-level initial sound awareness task. I can make the task more difficult if I say, *"Tell me the first sound in the word boat,"* or *"Tell me which word does not belong: bus, bun, hat."* During all these activities, I remember that the goal of early PA skill building is exposure to PA concepts, rather than mastery. Children typically demonstrate initial sound awareness by late preschool or early kindergarten (Bradley & Bryant, 1983).

In another example of a different PA skill, I introduce the concept of *onset-rime* to a student by saying, *"Sean, can you tell me what word I am saying? l – amp."* Onset-rime consists of the initial sound (in this case /l/) and the vowel + final consonant combination /æmp/. The ability to recognize onset-rime is connected to rhyming, because a child must have awareness that words "sound the same at the end" in order to rhyme words. After onset-rime skills, children generally learn sound blending and sound segmentation: *"What funny word is the puppet trying to say? /s/ /I/ /t/"* (Answer: *sit).* Sound segmentation is a skill generally demonstrated during kindergarten or first grade.

Practitioners refer to a number of excellent preschool curricula to guide their early literacy interventions. Examples of preschool curricula are listed in Focus 9.4.

FOCUS 9.4 *Clinical Skill Building*

Several early literacy curricula have been evaluated in research programs and have shown clinical efficacy. You can find out more about these curricula by reading about them on the Internet. Make a list of the pros and cons of using an already-developed curriculum in contrast to developing your own goals and activities. Here are two you can investigate:

- *Ladders to Literacy* (Notari-Syverson, O'Connor, & Vadasy, 1998). www.fcrr.org/fcrrreports/PDF/LaddersLiteracyFinal2.pdf
- *Road to the Code: A Program of Early Literacy Activities to Develop Phonological Awareness* (Blachman, Ball, Black, & Tangel, 2000). www.fcrr.org/FCRRreports/PDF/Road Code.pdf

Early Intervention: Print Concepts and Alphabetic Knowledge.   Children are exposed to print concepts and alphabetic knowledge through both embedded and explicit learning opportunities. Adults use an embedded approach when they point out that print can be seen in traffic and store signs. During a discussion of environmental print, a child is likely to learn (a) the meaning of *word, letter, sentence,* (b) readers read the print and not the illustration, (c) readers read from left to right and top to bottom, (d) there are different letters and letters have different names, and (e) letters make sounds and sounds make up words.

Print referencing is an explicit teaching technique that exposes children to print and alphabetic concepts (Justice & Ezell, 2002). For example, during book reading the adult reader includes comments to draw the child's attention to specific print and alphabetic concepts. Below I list several examples of print referencing.

- *"This is the <u>title</u> of the book. Can anyone show me where the <u>author's</u> name is on this front cover? That's right, the <u>author</u> writes the book."* (concepts of print)
- *"Where should I start reading, here or here?"* (adult points to illustration and then text; concepts of print)
- *"What does this sign say in this picture? That's right, it says STOP!"* (awareness of environmental print)
- *"Can anyone find the uppercase* T *on this page?"* (alphabetic awareness)

Early Intervention: Oral Language.   One of the best opportunities for embedded oral language learning is through repeated exposure to shared storybook reading. Children who are frequently read to are more likely to demonstrate literate language. **Literate language** refers to the frequently occurring syntax and morphological features that occur in books and written text (Greenhalgh & Strong, 2001; Westby, 1991). Through repeated readings, children become familiar with the way written language sounds; they internalize word usage, grammatical form, and idiosyncratic features of written language. Consider the following example:

> *"Oh, my!" the small, furry teddy bear exclaimed. "I think I have misplaced my favorite honey jar. Where could I possibly have placed it?" Because the bear could not find his cherished honey pot, he sat down glumly on the closest tree stump.*

In the example above, do you think I was talking to you in a conversational style, or do you think I was reading to you from a book? I imagine you said "reading from a book." What features in the example led you to this decision? There are several clues.

First, I used **dialogic speech**, which is the use of quotation or spoken language by a character in the story. In this example, I used the dialogic marker *exclaimed,* but I also could have used a word like *complained, whined,* or *said.* Dialogic language is rarely used during informal discourse (i.e., conversation) but occurs often within written language (Sulzby, 1985). Children learn to understand dialogic speech when they hear written text.

A second indicator was the use of descriptive vocabulary, such as *small, furry* (teddy bear), *my favorite* (honey pot), *cherished* (honey pot), and *closest* (tree stump). A descriptive adjective before a noun makes a noun phrase (NP). A verb and its modifiers and/or associated auxiliary verbs make a verb phrase (VP). Literate language typically demonstrates more NP and VP elaboration. Children with language impairments have difficulty with descriptive words and they fail to use elaborated NP and VP combinations (Ukrainetz et al., 2005). Written language also uses Tier II vocabulary (see Chapter 4 for a discussion of Tier I, II, and III vocabulary). In the example above, I used the verb *misplaced*, the adjective *cherished*, and the adverb *glumly*. These words are relatively rare and may be unfamiliar to children. When children listen to storybooks they are exposed to Tier II vocabulary.

Literate language also includes more sophisticated verb forms. In the example above, I used past tense verbs. Written text often includes past tense verbs; this contrasts with face-to-face conversations where verb use often reflects present tense. In the example above, I used the past tense verbs *exclaimed, misplaced, could,* and *sat.*

Cognitive verbs, sometimes called mental verbs, are another advanced verb form. **Cognitive verbs** include words like *thought, knew, remembered, decided, imagined, forgot, asked, told, explained, called,* or *yelled.* We use cognitive verbs to describe the actions and thoughts of characters in the text. Oral language uses cognitive verbs less frequently; written text offers more opportunities for exposure to cognitive verbs.

Literate language requires decontextualization and cohesive language devices. **Decontextualized language** allows the listener to understand what is spoken or written without background information or environmental cues. This contrasts with conversational speech. During a conversation, both the speaker and the listener share the same context (i.e., the same environmental stimuli and shared experience) and the listener has the ability to ask questions if there is a need for more information. When one reads a book, it is not possible to ask the author questions; consequently, literate language must be decontextualized.

The use of **cohesive language** devices requires the speaker or writer to use words linking information from one sentence to another. In the example above, after I introduced the main character (the teddy bear), I refer to the bear as *he* in the fourth sentence. This represents a linkage between an introduced referent and the pronoun referring back to the referent. Another cohesive device in the example is the use of the subordinating conjunction *because.* Subordinating conjunctions such as *because, so, then,* and *therefore* make cause-and-effect story connections and highlight the temporal (i.e., time) sequencing of story events (Curenton & Justice, 2004).

Practitioners use embedded opportunities during storybook reading to enhance children's use of literate language features. Practitioners also explicitly increase children's oral language and literate language during story role-plays, storytelling with felt board or puppets, and with child-dictated stories (Justice, Chow, Capellini, Flanigan, & Colton, 2003; Stanovich, 2000).

Early Intervention: Emergent Writing.   Children have embedded opportunities to practice writing during classroom routines and dramatic play. A classroom routine may include children signing out books from the classroom library to take home. Children incorporate writing into dramatic play when literacy objects (e.g., doctor's prescription pad, clipboard, pens, magazines) are included in a play area centering on a specific theme; in this case, the doctor's office. During dramatic play the practitioner uses adult-mediated writing to foster children's emergent writing skills. An example of adult-mediated writing is the adult modeling and demonstrating writing a letter, addressing an envelope, stamping a letter, taking a letter to the post office, and receiving and "reading" a letter. Children's experiences with literacy-rich dramatic play centers (e.g., library, veterinarian's office, grocery store, restaurant) dramatically increase the quality and quantity of children's reading and writing activities (Morrow, 2005; Neuman & Roskos, 1992).

Professionals also use the explicit approach of **story dictation** to foster early writing skills. Story dictation provides children the opportunity to learn that "writing is speech written down." Using the language experience approach (LEA: Stauffer, 1970), the adult writes down a story as the child dictates his or her experiences. The child illustrates the story or supplements the story with photographs. The adult reads the story back to the child and points to each word as it is read aloud.

CULTURAL CONSIDERATIONS IN EMERGENT LITERACY DEVELOPMENT

Young children who must learn English as a second language and children who use African American English face additional challenges learning to read and write. In the past, sometimes teachers, SLPs, and researchers failed to recognize the learning challenges faced by minority students. Other times preconceived notions of "what it takes to be academically successful" are just plain wrong! I will describe two recent studies illustrating both points.

The first example demonstrates the complexity of early language and literacy learning for children who speak Spanish at home and English at school. Cardenas-Hagan, Carlson, and Pollard-Durodola (2007) evaluated the acquisition of early literacy skills for children who are in **dual language programs**.

In dual language programs, the goal is for students to maintain the first language (L1) while learning English as a second language (L2; Cloud, Genessee, & Hamayan, 2000). Teachers use both L1 and L2 at different times of the day; in many programs English is used 50% of the day and Spanish the remaining 50%. Sometimes the ratio of English/Spanish represents a ratio as high as 90%/10%.

Researchers concluded that instructional decisions for L2 learners must include (a) assessment of children's knowledge of letters and letter sounds in both English and Spanish at the beginning of the school year, and (b) careful consideration of instructional time in L1 versus L2. Children with low literacy skills at the beginning of the school may benefit from increased instructional time in Spanish. For other children—children with higher literacy skills in either Spanish or English—the amount of instructional time in L1 versus L2 may not significantly impact literacy development.

The second example demonstrates how preconceived notions of academic readiness are sometimes incorrect. Specifically, I point to findings indicating preschoolers who use many features of African American English (AAE) are *not* necessarily at greater risk for reading failure. This finding contrasts with other reports indicating frequent AAE use in older school-age children is a reading risk factor (Connor & Craig, 2006). What is going on here?

It appears that many young children who enter school with AAE dialect as a primary speaking pattern learn to use General American English (GAE) at school. The movement from primary AAE dialect to GAE is evidence of code switching. As you recall from Chapter 1, code switching refers to an individual's ability to alternate between formal and informal language or between dialectal language patterns and GAE.

Research has revealed some interesting results about code switching in young urban preschool children (Connor & Craig, 2006). At the beginning of formal schooling, urban preschoolers may have minimal exposure to GAE. As a result, at the beginning of the school year, preschoolers may demonstrate high use of AAE features. However, with exposure to GAE, Craig and her colleagues (Connor & Craig, 2006; Craig & Washington, 2004) report that many students learn to code switch with a subsequent decrease in AAE features. The ability to code switch is a sophisticated metalinguistic skill. Children who code switch demonstrate a level of linguistic ability that bodes well for later academic success.

Now, back to the issue I raised earlier. I stated that preschoolers who use many features of African American English (AAE) are not necessarily at greater risk for reading failure. The lack of relationship between high AAE use and early literacy weakness centers on the ability of children to code switch. Young children who are able to code switch and adapt their linguistic patterns once they are exposed to GAE are likely to have good underlying linguistic skills. On the other hand, children who fail to code switch, even though they have exposure to GAE, may have underlying linguistic deficits. In sum, it is not AAE use that limits academic development, but rather underlying language abilities.

School-Age Children with Langauge Impairment

Increasingly, because of the 2001 No Child Left Behind (NCLB) legislation (see Focus 9.5 for more information about NCLB) and our increasing understanding of the connections between oral and written language, practitioners assess and provide intervention for school-age students in reading and writing domains. Research has identified specific skills needed to become a skilled reader (see Figure 9.3); along with the phonological awareness and the ability to match letters and sounds (i.e., phonics), school-age students need to increase reading fluency and develop high-level vocabulary. They also must be able to gain meaning from text; this is called reading comprehension.

FOCUS 9.5 *School-Based Issues*

No Child Left Behind Act of 2001

The No Child Left Behind Act of 2001 (Public Law 107-110), often abbreviated as NCLB, is a U.S. federal law proposed by President George W. Bush. NCLB establishes standards-based education reform based on the belief that setting high standards and establishing measurable goals improves students' educational outcomes. The effectiveness of NCLB has been debated. Specifically, critics argue that NCLB-mandated testing is not appropriate for all students (e.g., students with disabilities, students with limited English proficiency) and/or that teachers "teach to the test" and are less likely to provide best instructional practices to meet students' needs (Forum on Educational Accountability, 2007).

In the section below, I describe information on the literacy domains frequently targeted by practitioners who work with school-age students. I provide an overview of advanced levels of phonological awareness in addition to a discussion on narrative production, spelling, reading comprehension, and writing. At the end of this section on school-age students, I discuss issues related to working with classroom teachers and multi-cultural considerations.

SCHOOL-AGE STUDENTS: PHONOLOGICAL AWARENESS

Many school-age students with language impairments or learning disabilities continue to struggle with PA skills. Consequently, practitioners frequently assess and provide PA intervention for school-age children. Assessment and intervention for older students typically emphasizes sound blending and segmenting.

School-Age Students: Phonological Awareness Assessment.   At young ages the assessor is likely to use informal tests or a screening assessment such as the PALS-PreK to assess PA skills. However, once the student reaches school age, the assessor is more likely to use a norm-referenced assessment (for examples of norm-referenced PA tests see Table 9.4). Whether the assessment is criterion based or norm referenced, PA skills are assessed in the order of developmental sequence and difficulty (see Table 9.1). The practitioner remembers that PA skills can be assessed with a variety of tasks and that some tasks are easier than others. For example, it is easier to identify sounds at the beginning of words (e.g., "*What is the first sound you hear in the word* duck?") as compared to final sound identification. The practitioner also knows that matching tasks (e.g., "*Which words have the same sound at the beginning?* top, man, tin") or a same-different task (e.g., "*Do these words start with the same sound?* pin-fin" are easier for children as compared to a production task ("*Give me a word that rhymes with* cat").

Figure 9.3   **National Reading Panel: Background and Recommendations**

In 1997, Congress asked the director of the National Institute of Child Health and Human Development (NICHD), in consultation with the secretary of education, to convene a national panel to evaluate the research-based knowledge focused on the best methods to help children become skilled readers. The panel evaluated the literature focusing on three areas[1] of reading research

Domain: Phonological Awareness

Definition and rationale for inclusion: Phonemic awareness (PA) involves teaching children to focus on and manipulate phonemes in spoken syllables and words. Correlation studies have identified PA as one of the best school-entry predictors of how well children will learn to read during the first 2 years of instruction.

Findings: Teaching children to manipulate phonemes in words is highly effective under a variety of teaching conditions with a variety of learners across a range of grade and age levels.

Domain: Fluency

Definition and rationale for inclusion: Fluent readers are able to read orally with speed, accuracy, and proper expression. Fluency is one of several critical factors necessary for reading comprehension.

Findings: Guided repeated oral reading procedures have a significant and positive impact on word recognition, fluency, and comprehension. Steps to guided oral reading include (a) adult or peer reads a passage aloud while modeling fluent reading at the student's independent reading level[2], (b) student rereads the text quietly by himself or herself several times, (c) student reads aloud with adult encouragement and feedback, (d) sequence is repeated (typically 3-4 times) until the student can read the passage fluently.

Domain: Reading Comprehension

Definition and rationale for inclusion: Reading comprehension is a student's ability to gain meaning from text and repair misunderstandings when they occur. Deficits in reading comprehension limit children's long-term academic performance.

Findings: Reading comprehension is a complex cognitive process requiring (a) vocabulary development and vocabulary instruction and (b) use of metaskills during reading such as semantic organizers[3], question answering (i.e., readers answer questions posed by the teacher and receive feedback), question generation (i.e., readers ask themselves questions about various aspects of the story), or summarization (readers learn to integrate ideas and generalize from text information).

[1] The panel also looked at the domains of (a) teacher education and (b) computer-based reading instruction but concluded there was not enough research available to draw strong conclusions.

[2] A student's independent reading level is the level at which he can read with 95% word accuracy; it should be "relatively easy" for the student.

[3] Readers make graphic representations (i.e., story maps) to assist comprehension.

Source: From *Report of the National Reading Panel. Teaching Children to Read: An Evidence-Based Assessment of the Scientific Research Literature on Reading and Its Implications for Reading Instruction: Reports of the Subgroups* (NIH Publication No. 00-4754), National Institute of Child Health and Human Development, 2000, Washington, DC: U.S. Government Printing Office.

Table 9.4 Examples of Norm-Referenced Assessments for Older Students for Identification of Reading and Writing Deficits

Language domain	Test	Age range
Narrative development	Test of Narrative Language (TNL). Gillam, R. B., & Pearson, N. A. (2004). Austin: TX: PRO-ED.	5–11:11 years
Phonological awareness	Lindamood Auditory Conceptualization Test–3rd ed. Lindamood, C. H., & Lindamood, P. C. (2004). Austin, TX: PRO-ED.	5–18:11 years
	Test of Phonological Awareness—Second Edition: PLUS (TOPA-2+). Torgesen, J. K., & Bryant, B. R., (2004). Austin, TX: PRO-ED.	K–3rd grade
	Comprehensive Test of Phonological Processing (CTOPP). Wagner, R. K., Torgesen, J. K., Rashotte, C. A. (1999). Austin, TX: PRO-ED.	5:0–24:11 years
Writing	Test of Written Language-3 (TOWL-3). Hammill, D.D., & Larsen, S.C. (1996). Austin, TX: PRO-ED.	7–17:11 years
	Oral and Written Language Scales (OWLS: Written Expression [WE] Scale). Carrow-Woolfolk, E. (1995). Los Angeles, CA: Western Psychological Association.	5–21:11 years
Reading	Woodcock Reading Mastery Tests—Revised/Normative Update (WRMT-R/NU). Woodcock, R. W. (1998). Bloomington, MN: Pearson.	5:0–75+ years
	Test of Reading Comprehension Skills (TORC-4). Brown, V. L., Wiederholt, J. L, & Hammill D. D. (2006). Los Angeles, CA: Western Psychological Service.	7–17:11 years
	Gray Oral Reading Tests–Fourth Edition (GORT-4). Wiederholt, J. L., & Bryant, B. R. (2001). Austin, TX: PRO-ED.	6:0–18:11 years
Spelling	Test of Written Spelling (4th ed.). Larsen, S., & Hammill, D., & Moats, L. (1999). Austin, TX: PRO-ED.	6:0–18:11 years
	Spelling Performance Evaluation for Language and Literacy (2nd ed.) (SPELL-2). Masterson, J. J., Apel, K., & Wasowicz, J. (2002). Evanston, IL: Learning By Design.	Grade 2–Adult
Curriculum-based language assessment	S-MAPS, Rubrics for Curriculum-Based Assessment and Intervention. Wiig, E.H., Lord Larson, V., Olson, J.A. (2004). Eau Claire: WI: Thinking Publications.	K–12th grade

School-Age Students: Phonological Awareness Interventions. When practition-ers work with school-age students; PA skills are targeted with more intensity and activities are less gamelike. It should be clear to older students why they are working on PA. To increase self awareness, practitioners teach metacognitive strategies to use when sounding out words. In the following example, the practitioner works with a student on decoding a word with an initial consonant blend.

"In this word, first you see three consonants grouped together, 'spl'—that's a blend—and we pronounce it like /spl/. The next sound is 'a;' that is a short vowel, /æ/. The next sound, 'sh,' is a digraph; remember a digraph represents two letters together that make one sound. This sound is /ʃ/. Now let's blend the sounds together: /spl/—/æ/—/ʃ/. Splash, the word is splash! You try the next word; look for that 'spl' blend."

Professionals sometimes use Elkonian boxes (see Figure 9.4) to teach students to move tokens and then letter tiles into boxes to represent sounds during phoneme identification, blending, and segmenting tasks. The words are made progressively more difficult to encourage students to listen to subtle sound changes. For example:

"Show me the word /sɪt/. Good. Now, show me the word /sæt/. What sound changed? Right! The middle vowel changed! Now, show me the word /fæt/. What changed? That's right. The first sound changed, didn't it?"

Figure 9.4 **Elkonian Boxes**

SLP: *"Move the colored chips into the boxes. Move one chip for each sound you hear. The word is* sit.*"*

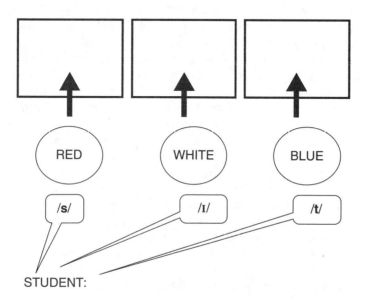

SCHOOL-AGE STUDENTS: NARRATIVES

Children's narratives are an important link between oral and written language development. The **oral narrative** is a monologue describing a real or fictional event organized into linked utterances with specific linguistic features. During a narrative, the speaker describes a "thematic" event; in other words, an event centered around one or more connected actions (Paul, 2007). Children who successfully produce oral narratives have a foundational skill contributing to reading and writing. However, students with language impairments often struggle to produce oral narratives and this impairment negatively impacts literacy development (Catts, Fey, Zhang, & Tomblin, 1999; Gillam & Johnston, 1992; Scott & Windsor, 2000).

Consider this example of an oral narrative from a 6-year-old girl. In this example, the student tells a story in response to a picture showing a spaceship landing in a park with children hiding behind a bush.

> *"A boy and the girl came out of the bushes. And they were in the bushes. And then they saw (an) a spaceship come down. And aliens come out. And then the girl wanted to go out and see them. And, the boy said, 'Don't do it.' And she kept looking. And (um) they came to stay. And the spaceship went up."*

This child demonstrates beginning knowledge of aspects of narrative production, exhibiting both narrative microstructure and macrostructure.

Narrative microstructure features are internal linguistic features occurring within oral narratives. Microfeatures include students' use of increasingly complex syntax along with literate language features (i.e., decontextualized language, cohesive devices, and descriptive vocabulary). As children move from kindergarten to upper elementary school, they increasingly include the required microstructure features needed to produce an effective narrative (Justice et al., 2006).

Narrative macrostructure refers to overall story organization. Stories are not just a random collection of ideas. A story engages the listener by (a) a description of a particular event, (b) the actions that occurred in response to the initial event, and (c) the consequence of the subsequent actions. This linked series of events is called the **story episode** (Stein & Glenn, 1979). A story episode contains three important components. The first component is the **initiating event** (IE) or problem that sets the story in motion. The second component is the **attempt** (A), an action that is undertaken by the story's character to solve the problem. The third component is the **consequence** (C); it is a description of the character's attempt to solve the problem. Children produce a narrative with episodic structure, sometimes called a true narrative, around the age of $4\frac{1}{2}$ to 5 years. Figure 9.5 illustrates a child producing a true narrative. Prior to this point, preschool children often produce a narrative called a two-event narrative. A two-event narrative contains several sentences describing an event (e.g., *"I walked the dog. He pulled me down."*). Alternately, young children may produce a disorganized or leapfrog narrative jumping from one event to another, leaving out major events (McCabe, 1996; McCabe & Peterson, 1991). Table 9.5 demonstrates the typical pattern of narrative development.

Figure 9.5   Three Components of a Narrative Episode

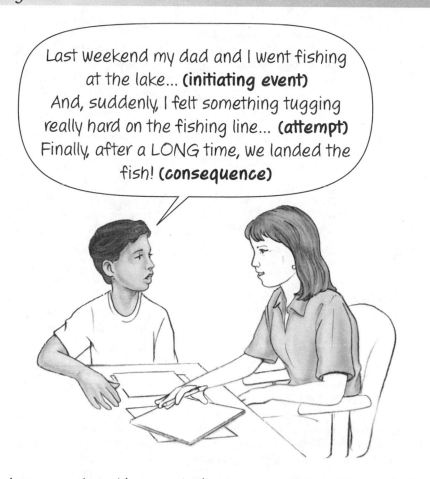

> Last weekend my dad and I went fishing at the lake... **(initiating event)**
> And, suddenly, I felt something tugging really hard on the fishing line... **(attempt)**
> Finally, after a LONG time, we landed the fish! **(consequence)**

A true narrative, with story episodic structure, contains a cause-and-effect relationship between the initiating event, the attempt, and the story consequence. Subordinating conjunctions such as *because, since, then,* and *so* are used to indicate cause and effect. For example, consider the following narrative:

The mother went to the store, but she forgot to bring her purse (IE). After waiting in line for some time, arriving at the cashier's station, she realized that she had no money. In confusion, she dropped her items on the floor and ran out of the store (A). Since she had made such a spectacle of herself, she felt she could never return to her favorite store (C).

In this example, the word *since* highlights the relationship between the attempt (e.g., dropping the items) and the consequence (e.g., her embarrassment at returning to the store). Children with language impairment have difficulty with subordinating conjunctions; this deficit further impairs narrative quality.

Table 9.5 Narrative Development

Age	Terms*	Characteristics
2–3	<u>Additive chains</u>, prenarratives, heap stories, descriptive or action sequences, two-event narratives, leapfrog narratives	• Additive chains: Child describes things he sees or hears in a sequence but does not describe causal relationships. ("*I fall down, Mommy came outside.*") • Heap story: Contains no central theme. • Leapfrog narrative: Disorganized narrative without temporal order; produced by children who are typically developing at young ages and older children with language impairments.
3–5	<u>Temporal stories</u>, sequence stories, primitive narratives, causal chains	• There is some linking of events in a temporal story, but there is typically no resolution and no character motivation.
6–7	<u>True narratives</u>, simple-causal narratives	• Episodic structure emerges (e.g., initiating event, attempt, consequence); the character's motivations are described.
>8	<u>Multi-causal</u>, complex narratives	• The story contains multiple embedded episodes. Narratives typically contain descriptive language.

*Underlined term is most common; other terms also are used to describe narratives.

Sources: From "Assessment and Treatment of Narrative Skills: What's the Story?" (video and manual) by K. Apel and J. J. Masterson, 1998, Rockville, MD: American Speech-Language-Hearing Association; *The Child's Concept of Story: Ages 2 to 17,* by A. Applebee, 1978, Chicago: University of Chicago Press; *Language Disorders from Infancy Through Adolescence: Assessment and Intervention* (3rd ed.) by R. Paul, 2007, St. Louis: Mosby; "An Analysis of Story Comprehension in Elementary School Children," by N. Stein and C. Glenn, 1979. In R. Freedle (Ed.), *New Directions in Discourse Processing* (Vol. 2, pp. 53–120). Norwood, NJ: Ablex.

School-Age Students: Narrative Assessments.   Assessors consider the use of both micro- and macrolevel features during the assessment of children's narrative productions. Professionals sometimes elicit student narratives and complete an analysis much like the language sample analysis discussed in Chapter 2. Sometimes assessors use norm-referenced tests to complete a narrative assessment. An example of a norm-referenced narrative assessment is the Test of Narrative Language (Gillam & Pearson, 2004).

During criterion-referenced assessment, the assessor chooses among a variety of stimuli to elicit student narratives because some narrative tasks are easier than others. For example, in a story-retelling narrative task, the assessor reads or tells a story (with or without illustrations) and asks the student to retell the story. This task is good for younger children or students with limited exposure to narrative language.

A more difficult narrative task is story generation. In this case, the assessor asks the student to make up a story with or without an accompanying illustration. Sometimes the assessor provides examples of narrative story telling prior to soliciting a student's story. The skilled assessor carefully considers the student's age, language abilities, and story-telling experience to appropriately scaffold narrative production.

Once the student produces several narratives, the assessor analyzes both narrative micro- and macrofeatures. As part of microfeature analysis, professionals consider children's use of literate language features including cohesive devices, complex verbs, and descriptive vocabulary. Macrofeature analysis focuses on presence or absence of a story episode; the professional also considers the student's description of story setting and the characters' internal response to the initiating event (i.e., description of a character's feelings). Many children with LI have difficulty telling a sequenced story and their stories often lack detail and cohesiveness (McCabe & Bliss, 2003; Curenton & Lucas, 2007).

School-Age Students: Narrative Interventions.   Narrative intervention focuses on improving students' micro- and macronarrative features. At the beginning stages of narrative intervention, the practitioner selectively targets a single aspect of narrative production. If a student is mastering new macrofeatures (e.g., descriptive vocabulary), the adult asks the student to produce the linguistic features in a familiar narrative task. On the other hand, if story structure is targeted, the practitioner reduces the vocabulary or syntax demands during the story retelling. This dynamic relationship between different aspects of language should remind you of a statement introduced in Chapter 4: *Teach new forms within familiar functions* (Slobin, 1973). Discuss with your classmates how you might apply this idea from Slobin (1973) to develop narrative interventions for school-age students (see Focus 9.6).

Macrostructure is improved when children learn the underlying organization of a story episode. Awareness of macrostructure results in improved reading comprehension and written story organization (Westby, 2005). To facilitate macrostructure, the professional often uses symbols or written words (if the child is a reader) to remind the student to include story setting, a main character, the initiating event, attempt, and consequence. Older children also learn metaskills to self-monitor story organization. Techniques such as using a checklist, story map, or rubric assist metadevelopment. An example of visual cues used to organize story structure is shown in Figure 9.6.

SCHOOL-AGE STUDENTS: SPELLING

Since spelling is a linguistic skill, children with language impairments have more difficulty with spelling tasks as compared to children with typical language (Larkin & Snowling, 2008). Accurate spelling involves skill development in several linguistic and cognitive domains. As demonstrated in Table 9.6, early spelling ability is closely linked to phonological awareness abilities. In later school years, spelling also requires morphological awareness (Rivers, Lombardino, & Thompson, 1996). Both areas are potential areas of weakness for children who are language impaired.

FOCUS 9.6 *Clinical Skill Building*

Balancing Macro- and Microstructure Demands During Narrative Interventions

As children learn a new linguistic task, they may not be able to process additional higher-order tasks at the same time. This idea is exemplified in the "bucket" theory, which suggests there are trade-offs across language domains (Crystal, 1987). For example, there could be trade-offs in syntax production as children produce language containing story structure (e.g., characters, an initiating event). Application of this theory to narrative production suggests a child attempting to produce increasingly complex narrative macrostructure may demonstrate reduced complexity at a microstructural level, and vice versa. As the demands fill the linguistic bucket, the bucket overflows and performance in one or more domains decreases. However, with practice the child learns to produce combinations of linguistic skills. How might the bucket theory affect language intervention for students working on other aspects of language production (other than narratives)? How can a language facilitator modify interventions to account for the bucket theory?

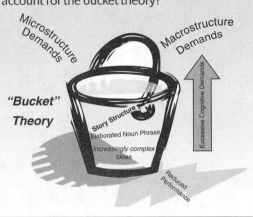

Figure 9.6   Visual Cues to Enhance Narrative Production

SLP: "Describe how this story is organized. You can use shapes and lines to show me. Remember to include the important parts of a story."

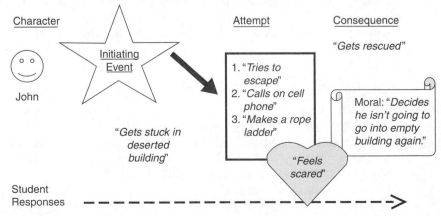

Table 9.6 **Spelling Development**

Age	Spelling	Spelling error examples
Preschool	Emergent/Preliterate Writing bears no letter-sound correspondence; children scribble, make letterlike shapes and some letters.	
Late preschool—mid kindergarten	Semiphonetic Represents salient sounds; represents initial and final sounds in words; typically does not represent vowels.	S (seat) bk (back) Tf (teeth)
Mid kindergarten—mid first grade	Developmental Path Varies Greatly	fale (fail) plat (plate) jriv (drive)
	Phonetic Spelling Represents all or most sounds in words; begins to represent vowels; does not demonstrate all spelling conventions.	
Late first grade—second grade	Within Word Pattern Represents most short vowels correctly, using but confusing long vowel patterns.	back (back) dinisore (dinosaur) chips (chips) driav (drive)
Mid elementary school	Syllable Juncture Stage Children begin to pay attention to patterns such as doubling letters, stressed and unstressed syllable patterns.	funnier (i.e., double the final consonant of a syllable containing a short vowel before adding suffix)
Later elementary school	Derivational Constancy Stage Children understand word roots and use knowledge to spell.	exemption (i.e., derivation from word *exempt)*

Sources: From *Words Their Way: Word Study for Phonics, Vocabulary, and Spelling Instruction* (4th ed.), by D. R. Bear, M. Invernizzi, S. Templeton, and F. Johnston, 2007, Upper Saddle River, NJ: Pearson; "Meeting the Needs of Low Spellers in a Second-Grade Classroom," by J. Brown and D. Morris, 2005, *Reading and Writing Quarterly, 21,* pp. 165–185; "The Development of Spelling Knowledge and Its Role in Reading Acquisition and Reading Disability," by L. Ehri, 1989, *Journal of Reading Disabilities, 22,* pp. 356–365; *Phonological Awareness: From Research to Practice* by G. T. Gillon, 2004, New York: Guilford; *Teaching Spelling* (2nd ed.), by E. H. Henderson, 1990, Boston, MA: Houghton Mifflin; "Learning to Spell: Implications for Assessment and Intervention," by J. J. Masterson and L. A. Crede, 1999, *Language, Speech, and Hearing Services in Schools, 30,* pp. 243–254.

Below, I briefly discuss foundational skills needed to become a proficient speller.

- <u>Phonological awareness</u> is a requirement for spelling as PA knowledge allows the student to segment words into individual phonemes. Phonological awareness proficiency is the best predictor of children's spelling development (Treiman & Bourassa, 2000). When a child spells *night* as *fite*, he or she demonstrates difficulty making a connection between the sounds and the letters representing the sounds.

- A student requires an ability to visually store images of words. <u>Visual storage</u> allows the student to form and maintain visual images for words, morphemes, and syllables. When a child spells the same word differently at different times (e.g., *lite, liet, light*) he demonstrates a weakness in visual storage ability (Masterson & Apel, 2000).

- A student needs <u>orthographic knowledge</u> to be a competent speller. Through development of orthographic knowledge, children learn to recognize that some letter combinations are allowed and other letter combinations are never used. For example, the nonsense word *nuck* is a possible English letter combination, while the nonsense word *ckun* is not a possible letter combination in English because *ck* is never used in the initial position in words (Treiman, 1985).

- <u>Morphological knowledge</u> involves the child's ability to identify base words and their inflected forms (e.g., *confess, confessor, confessional*). Inflectional morphemes are added to words providing additional information about time (e.g., *ed, ing*) or quantity (e.g., plural *s*). Derivational morphemes, either *prefixes* (e.g., *un, re*) or *suffixes* (e.g., *tion, er*) change the word meaning or the word class (e.g., from *learn*, a verb, to *learner*, a noun; Masterson & Apel, 2000).

School-Age Students: Spelling Assessments.   Assessors typically begin a spelling assessment by collecting a sample of a child's spellings (Masterson & Apel, 2000). For example, a simple spelling assessment for young children consists of asking students to write the words *cat, nut, pit, mop,* and *bet*. The practitioner says the word slowly, stretching out the sounds, and then says the word. The student writes down the words; a point is scored for each letter spelled conventionally (i.e., the correct spelling) and a half point is scored for a phonetically acceptable letter (i.e., KAT instead of CAT). There also are a number of norm-referenced spelling assessments. Examples are listed in Table 9.4.

School-Age Students: Spelling Interventions.   The practitioner provides spelling intervention by focusing on the student's deficit areas: PA skills, orthographic knowledge, visual storage, or morphological skills. Deficit in phonological awareness is the most frequent cause of poor spelling; consequently this is a frequently targeted skill for the poor speller. If, on the other hand, a student has weak orthographic knowledge, the practitioner focuses on teaching students to recognize viable and nonviable word combinations (e.g., *qu* is possible at the beginning of a word [*quick, queen, quiet*], but the letter *q* does not appear with any other vowels or in isolation in the word initial position).

To improve visual storage skills, students practice identification of correctly spelled words from a list of foils (i.e., words that are similar to the target word but are spelled incorrectly). Finally, for students with morphological deficits the practitioner focuses on teaching students to recognize and use frequent morphological patterns. Figure 9.7 demonstrates the clinical decision-making process used to identify the appropriate focus for a spelling intervention program.

Figure 9.7 Spelling Intervention Decision Tree

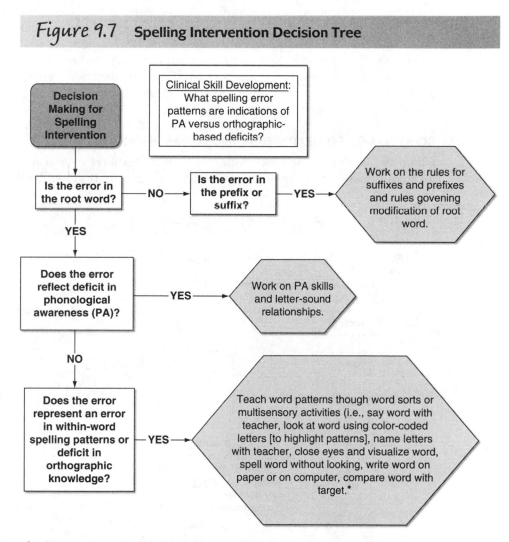

*Multisensory techniques (Beringer et al., 1998) are used to improve visual storage and othographic knowledge.

Source: From "Learning to Spell: Implications for Assessment and Intervention," by J. J. Masterson and L. A. Crede, 1999, *Language, Speech, and Hearing Services in Schools, 30*, pp. 243–254.

The use of word sorts is an effective instructional strategy (Bear, Invernizzi, Templeton & Johnston, 2007). During a word sort activity, the practitioner provides the child with a selection of written word cards demonstrating contrasting spelling patterns. For example, if the practitioner determines that the child does not demonstrate the short-vowel/long-vowel pattern, cards contain short and long vowel words such as *man, main; pan, pain; fin, fine; Tim, time; Sam, same*. Each card contains one word; in the example above, the word sort consists of 10 cards.

To complete the word sort activity, the practitioner asks the child to sort the cards into short vowels and long vowels. A card pair can be placed out on the table to provide an example. In this example, the practitioner places two cards out and says, *"This card is* man—*it has a short vowel; this card is* main—*it contains a long vowel. Now you sort out the rest of these cards into long- and short-vowel piles. I'll help you if you get stuck."* The practitioner supports the child's problem solving, guiding his meta-awareness of the long vowel versus short vowel pattern. Figure 9.8 provides an example of an advanced word sort.

SCHOOL-AGE STUDENTS: READING COMPREHENSION

Comprehension is a complex combination of higher-level mental processes that includes thinking, reasoning, imagining, and interpreting (Kahmi, 2009). Reading

Figure 9.8 **Advanced Spelling Word Sort**

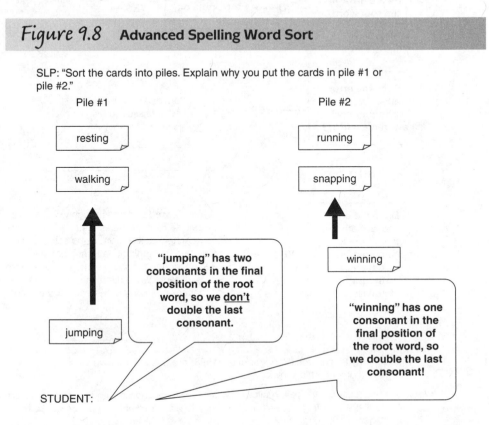

comprehension becomes increasingly important as the reader moves from the early grades into high school. The foundation skills most closely aligned with reading comprehension are vocabulary development, narrative ability, and students' use of metastrategies during the reading process (Catts, 2009; National Institute of Child Health and Human Development, 2000). I have already discussed narrative performance and vocabulary development in this book; in the subsections below I focus on reading comprehension.

School-Age Students: Reading Comprehension Assessments.   To assess reading comprehension, practitioners typically have a student read text and then ask the student to answer questions about the text. McKenna and Stahl (2003) suggest asking questions at three levels of thinking: literal questions, inferential questions, and critical questions.

Literal questions require a student to recall a specific fact explicitly stated in the reading passage. **Inferential questions** are similar to literal questions in that they are fact based; however, the answer to inferential questions must be logically concluded from the text. For example, the practitioner may ask a student, "*What do you think will happen next?*" The student must use facts presented in the passage to make a prediction even though the outcome is not explicitly stated.

Critical questions draw on an individual's value system. To answer a critical question, the student must interpret factual information in keeping with his or her own morals or beliefs. The adult typically uses the word *should* when framing a critical question (e.g., "*Should Mr. Scrooge have given the poor man more money?*").

The SLP and classroom teacher work together to determine if a student meets the reading comprehension state academic standards. As an example of reading comprehension standards from one state, consider the reading comprehension educational standards for Ohio's fifth and sixth graders. I have underlined the changes occurring in the standards from the fifth- to sixth-grade level.

- *Ohio Grade 5 Comprehension Indicators.* The student can:
  - Summarize the information in texts, recognizing that there may be several important ideas rather than just one main idea and identifying details that support each.
  - Make inferences based on implicit information in texts, and provide justifications for those inferences.
  - Answer literal, inferential, and evaluative questions to demonstrate comprehension of grade-appropriate print texts and electronic and visual media.
- *Ohio Grade 6 Comprehension Indicators.* The student can:
  - Summarize the information in texts, recognizing important ideas and supporting details, and <u>noting gaps or contradictions</u>.
  - Answer literal, inferential, evaluative, and <u>synthesizing</u> questions to demonstrate comprehension of grade-appropriate print texts and electronic and visual media.

FOCUS 9.7 *School-Based Issues*

Language Arts State Standards

Every SLP and educator should know how to locate the Language Arts State Standards for his or her own state. Language arts include reading, writing, and oral language at different grade levels.

Here's how I found the state standards for Wisconsin. First I typed, "Language arts state standards Wisconsin" into Google. My search took me to the Wisconsin Department of Public Instruction Web page http://dpi.wi.gov/standards/elaintro.html

On the main Web page, I found links for six contents standards ([A] Reading/Literature, [B] Writing, [C] Oral Language, [D] Language, [E] Media and Technology, and [F] Research and Inquiry); standards were available for Grades 4, 8, and 12. I chose the link to Reading/

Literature for Grade 4 and found the following content standards. Each of the main standards (listed below) included 4-8 subskill competencies (not listed).

By the end of Grade 4, students will:

A.4.1   Use effective reading strategies to achieve their purposes in reading.

A.4.2   Read, interpret, and critically analyze literature.

A.4.3   Read and discuss literary and non-literary texts in order to understand human experience.

A.4.4   Read to acquire information.

Find the content standards for your state. In class, discuss the professional's role in helping students achieve language arts standards.

Professionals should be familiar with the student educational standards for reading comprehension along with other standards for reading and writing skills. Find out more about your state educational standards for reading comprehension (see Focus 9.7).

School-Age Students: Reading Comprehension Metaskills Interventions. Practitioners help students improve reading comprehension strategies by explicitly teaching metaskills (Boardman et al., 2008). When working with students on comprehension metaskills, practitioners help students track comprehension by asking—and answering—literal and inferential questions. Students are taught to (a) make predictions and form questions prior to reading and (b) answer the questions as they read. This question-and-answer technique keeps students actively engaged with the reading task. When students feel confused, they learn to look up difficult words, summarize paragraph by paragraph, and modify predictions as needed.

Practitioners teach students to flexibly combine comprehension strategies. Students learn to activate prior knowledge by briefly listing what they know along with information they predict might be contained within the text. Students begin to use headers and pictures to predict the text's content. Students also look for topic sentences to determine key concepts.

Students learn to use graphic organizers and visual diagrams to organize important concepts. They use graphic organizers before reading to activate prior knowledge and refer to visual organizers to answer questions. After reading short passages, students learn to summarize the main ideas and reread, if necessary, to confirm their summarization. The goal is for students to apply strategies independently and automatically whenever they read (Boardman et al., 2008).

SCHOOL-AGE STUDENTS: WRITING

Writing involves three basic processes: (1) planning what to say and how to say it, (2) translating ideas into the written form, and (3) reviewing writing to edit and improve what one has written. The first step, planning, requires the writer to set goals, generate ideas, and organize ideas into a logical pattern (Graham 2005). Many students with language impairments or learning disabilities do not have the metaskills or executive functions to complete the needed steps for good writing. **Executive functioning** refers to the goal-oriented, purposeful behaviors that allow the individual to take a strategic approach to problem solving. Positive executive functioning includes behaviors such as inhibiting actions, attending selectively to the important information, setting goals, and planning and organizing behaviors (Singer & Bashir, 1999).

A writing assessment can be criterion-based or norm-referenced. Norm-referenced writing assessments are listed in Table 9.4. There are several recommended approaches to criterion-referenced assessment (Espin, Weissenburger, & Benson, 2004). The first method is called primary trait scoring. In primary trait scoring the adult evaluates the student's writing sample for specific traits (e.g., organization, use of topic sentences, grammar, use of cohesive devices) and compares the student's work against a grade-level standard. Typically, the assessor uses a rubric to rate each trait on a 4- or 5-point scale (e.g., 1 = unsatisfactory, 2 = minimal, 3 = satisfactory, 4 = elaborated, 5 = exceptional).

A second writing assessment approach mirrors the oral language sample analysis described in Chapter 2. This analytic approach considers quantitative features of the student's writing such as mean length of utterance, number of different words, and number of complex sentences. Analytic scoring techniques are more sensitive than primary trait scoring, but the disadvantage is that they are more time consuming.

A final recommended approach is consistent with curriculum-based language assessment. In this approach, the assessor obtains a 3- to 5-minute writing sample in response to a curriculum topic. To analyze the writing sample, the assessor considers how well the student reflects curriculum goals in terms of vocabulary, content, sentence structure, spelling, and number of sentences written.

Writing intervention either focuses on specific foundation skills (e.g., spelling, punctuation, syntax) or targets the metaskills and executive function required for the writing process. The goal is to train students to use effective strategies as they complete writing assignments. Practitioners use a number of intervention techniques to enhance students' metaskills and executive functioning abilities:

- Students use story organizers to preplan writing tasks or summarize text. The student learns to organize story ideas or text with circles, boxes, and connecting lines. The use of story organizers facilitates brainstorming, hypothesizing, and prediction, activates prior knowledge, and heightens awareness of the story's underlying structure (Buis, 2004).

- Students learn to improve their self-editing and proofreading skills and learn to use an evaluative rubric. The use of an evaluative rubric or check sheet improves self-evaluation skills and independence (Singer & Bashir, 1999).

I will be discussing more about a specific writing intervention, the writing lab approach (Nelson, Bahr, & Van Meter, 2004; Nelson & Van Meter, 2006), in the final section on evidence-based practices.

WORKING WITH TEACHERS

Literacy intervention for older school-age students focuses on a number of language-based academic skills. The reading and writing targets for older students center primarily on academic areas directly linked to classroom success. As you learned in Chapter 5, curriculum-based language assessment is a key component in this process. Once the student's curriculum-based language assessment is completed, the practitioner develops classroom-based interventions focusing on (a) increasing the student's underlying skills, (b) facilitating the student's meta-awareness of the processes required for successful completion of academic tasks, and (c) modifying academic tasks, instructions, or processes to increase student success.

In the best-case scenario, practitioners provide support facilitating classroom implementation of instructional strategies. I like to think of the school-based practitioner as an academic "coach" for students as well as teachers. When working with teachers, the practitioner balances coaching experiences to (a) develop teachers' content knowledge relating to language-literacy connections, (b) provide opportunities to model instructional strategies within the classroom, and (c) observe teachers implementing target strategies and provide feedback (Walpole & McKenna, 2004). The coaching should be interactive with plenty of time for collaboration and discussion; both the practitioner and classroom teacher continuously reflect on the process. The best collaborative models are developed at a schoolwide level; the coaching is shared among all members of the educational team. The educational team includes the general education teacher, special educator, school psychologist, reading teacher, resource room specialist, SLP, and even school administrators. Expertise is shared and responsibilities are negotiated on a case-by-case basis.

CULTURAL CONSIDERATIONS IN READING AND WRITING DEVELOPMENT FOR SCHOOL-AGE CHILDREN

As students move into later elementary, middle school, and high school grades, educators consider how a student's reading and writing is influenced by his or her culture (Ball, 2006). Experts describe a three-step process—accommodation, incorporation, and adaptation—to provide culturally sensitive education to students from nonmajority cultures (Klingner & Edwards, 2006; Wiley, 1996).

- Accommodation requires practitioners to consider their students' communicative styles and home literacy practices. Practitioners should remember that home literacy, even when there is extreme poverty, is often a rich source of language and print experience (Heath, 1983).

- Incorporation requires reading/writing professionals to study community practices undervalued by schools and incorporate culturally rich literacy learning into the curriculum. It is important to build on communities' "funds of knowledge" (Moll & González, 1994); for example, incorporating family oral storytelling into language arts programs.

- Adaptation requires practitioners help students and families gain access to the language and literacy culture associated with academic success. Culturally and linguistically diverse parents, parents living in poverty, and immigrant parents want to help their children succeed in school, but are sometimes unsure how to work with school practitioners.

Educators sometimes overlook subtle skills affecting literacy learning for school-age children; we may assume children know information we take for granted. For example, even a text's font conveys information. For example, certain font styles may be used in the U.S. in reference to Halloween or a horror movie. Italics are often used to add an air of formality, as in their use on wedding invitations. In contrast, Times Roman font conveys an academic "flavor" to text (Hartley & Harris, 2001) Compare the differences in your interpretation of font styles in Figure 9.9. Skilled readers use cultural knowledge to assist their reading comprehension; if a student lacks cultural knowledge he may be viewed as less intelligent or capable.

Figure 9.9   **Different Fonts Communicate Underlying Meaning**

A font style might be associated with Halloween or horror movies.

Italics may be used to convey a formal tone.

This Roman font is associated with academic text.

Reading and Writing Interventions for Students with Significant Levels of Impairment

Most of this chapter focuses on emergent literacy and reading and writing interventions for students who have mild-moderate communication impairments; the assumption is that mild-moderately impaired individuals can become conventional readers but may require targeted interventions to become proficient.

Professionals also work with individuals with more significant levels of disability. While data suggest that individuals with significant levels of impairment (i.e. individuals with moderate-severe cognitive impairment, individuals with moderate-severe levels of autism) may not become skilled conventional readers, experts suggest that all students should have opportunities to participate in reading and writing activities (Kaderavek & Rabidoux, 2004). When a practitioner is working with an individual with significant learning challenges, literacy goals may look different. For example, an adult with significant cognitive disability may have a literacy goal that includes supported interactive book sharing or functional writing opportunities. However, even if the activities are different, every individual should be able to participate in our society's "literacy culture." Below I describe a model of literacy intervention called the interactive-to-independent (I-to-I) model (Kaderavek & Rabidoux, 2004). The I-to-I model describes an approach to goal writing and intervention for individuals with significant learning challenges.

THE I-TO-I MODEL: OVERVIEW

The I-to-I model is based on Vygotsky's (1978) social interaction theory along with social participation theories (Lave & Wenger, 1991; Rogoff, 2001). Social participation theory suggests literacy is a socially constructed practice that should be accessible to all individuals regardless of ability level. An individual's participation in literacy at any level should be valued and supported. By participating in meaningful interactive literacy experiences, many individuals gradually move toward more independent and conventional reading and writing competency.

A foundation principle of the I-to-I model is the recognition that reading and writing help the individual interact with his or her world. In order to interact with written text, individuals with significant disability are likely to need meaningful, concrete literacy experiences. With the I-to-I model, literacy is viewed as more than teaching individuals with disability to name letters, identify safety signs (e.g., STOP, EXIT, POISON), or repeatedly copy words. As an alternative to completing the rote tasks described above, the I-to-I model proposes that literacy activities, to be meaningful to individuals with significant disability, must center on shared interactions. The I-to-I model consists of five levels of communication partnership facilitating literacy development; each level represents a different level of social and environmental support.

I-TO-I MODEL: LEVEL I

The first level in the I-to-I model focuses on the individual's ability to maintain a joint focus of attention around a shared storybook or other literacy artifact. A literacy artifact can include family pictures, simple line drawings, or other meaningful written or graphic items (e.g., comic books, illustrations, postcard collections). An interaction with a book or literacy artifact provides opportunities for meaningful interaction regardless of an individual's conventional reading ability. As Table 9.7 demonstrates,

Table 9.7 **Interactive-to-Independent (I-to-I) Model of Literacy**

Levels of I-to-I model	Literacy goals associated with each level
Level 1: Attention and responsiveness during literacy interactions	a. Student maintains attention to a literacy artifact and the literacy partner for ___ minutes. b. Student decreases off-task behaviors to no more than 1/minute during a ___ minute storybook interaction. c. Student directs gaze at pictures, turns pages, and interactively manipulates flaps in a lift-the-flap book for ___ minutes. d. Student motorically turn-takes during a shared storybook interaction ___ times during a ___ minute storybook interaction. e. Student uses emergent writing to tell a story or share an experience.
Level II: Balance and turn taking in literacy interactions	a. Student interacts with verbal, gestural, or signed communication within a shared literacy interaction. b. Student initiates communication during a literacy interaction. c. Student demonstrates a range of pragmatic communication skills (describing, requesting, responding, topic initiation and maintenance, etc.) during a literacy interaction.
Level III: Symbolic understanding of written forms	a. Student uses sight words within the school or home setting in functional ways (recognizes own name, follows signs, picks out his own videos, etc.) b. Student matches representational symbols (line drawings) to real objects within a communication exchange. Student uses symbols to communicate needs in functional ways (e.g., pick a lunch menu). c. Student engages in communicative exchange in literacy interactions containing meaningful pictures and written words. d. Student identifies written words with pictures within a communicative literacy exchange (i.e., <u>not</u> rote picture-to-word drill).

(continued)

Table 9.7   **Interactive-to-Independent (I-to-I) Model of Literacy (*Continued*)**

Levels of I-to-I model	Literacy goals associated with each level
Level IV: Conventional literacy supported by social interactions	a. Student uses familiar sight words to create novel sentences within a supported communication exchange. b. Student explains what was read to a naïve listener with support from the communication partner. c. Student dictates words to a communication partner to make a list of daily activities. d. Student writes notes to herself or himself as reminders about daily chores or activities with support. e. Student and communication partner create a scrapbook of favorite written materials (e.g. comic strips, TV guide, sports page) and add to it on a regular basis. f. Student and communication partner interactively read ___ new texts/week. g. Student and communication partner maintain a collaborative written diary illustrated with pictures of the student's activities.
Level V: Conventional literacy at independent level	Conventional literacy activities are introduced with continued emphasis on social and interactive literacy use and function.

Source: From "Interactive to Independent Literacy: A Model for Designing Literacy Goals for Children with Atypical Communication," by J. N. Kaderavek and P. Rabidoux, 2004, *Reading and Writing Quarterly, 20,* pp. 237–260.

at Level I, the literacy goal focuses on keeping the individual with significant levels of disability increasingly engaged with the literacy artifact and encouraging back-and-forth turn-taking behavior by pointing at pictures or turning pages.

I-TO-I MODEL: LEVEL II

In Level II of the I-to-I model, the professional works toward balanced exchange during literacy interactions. Guided by social interaction theory, the literacy partner builds on the individual's actions, vocalizations and/or verbalizations and extends the communication elicited during the shared literacy interaction. Possible intervention goals for Level II are described in Table 9.7. A variety of literacy interactions (i.e., shared writing, looking at different types of written materials) should be included to maintain the individual's interest and engagement.

I-TO-I MODEL: LEVEL III

An individual operating within the I-to-I Model at Level I or II typically does not understand the symbolic nature of written language. Specifically, the individual may not recognize that written words represent meaning. For example, the individual does not recognize that the letters *C-A-T* represent the fuzzy animal that makes a purring sound. A Level III literacy partner begins to recognize some forms of conventional literacy; however, symbolic recognition may vary from that seen in a conventional reader.

For example, students with Down syndrome have achieved reading competency equivalent to that of fifth graders. Reading testing confirmed, however, that students used visual recognition strategies (sight word recognition) as contrasted to a balanced strategic use of PA and visual recognition. Although sight word reading (by itself) is not a route to highly skilled conventional reading, in this case it resulted in functional reading ability. To achieve this level of reading proficiency, educators exposed children to sight words even before the children recognized all the alphabet letters (Layton, 2000).

At Level III, the professional knows the student may recognize increasingly symbolic forms, such as icons, pictures, or sight words. Table 9.7 provides goals to build symbol use at this intermediate level. Typically, at this stage, students require extended practice sessions and daily opportunities to use symbolic forms in real-life interactions.

I-TO-I MODEL: LEVEL IV

At Level IV, children perform conventionally literate tasks when supported by others, but their reading and writing ability will vary according to their strengths and weakness. For example, some children with autism demonstrate hyperlexia. **Hyperlexia** is the precocious ability to recognize written words significantly above an individual's language or cognitive skill level; often children minimally comprehend what they read. In Chapter 8, I mentioned a young preschooler with hyperlexia; the preschooler had minimal ability to communicate with others day to day, but could read aloud from the phonebook for extended periods (Kaderavek & Rabidoux, 2004). A professional worked with the preschooler by facilitating interactive and meaningful communication focusing on illustrations in the phonebook's advertising section.

Students with strengths in sight word reading can be taught to recognize sight words by labeling everyday objects and attaching the written word to specific pictures or icons (Broun & Oelwein, 2007). Through repeated associations between pictures and written words, the sight word repertoire increases. Eventually, the professional encourages the Level IV reader to read beginning-level primer texts or read adult-made books containing familiar sight words. As reading new sight words becomes meaningful and motivating, adults work "backwards" to teach concepts of individual letters and sounds from the known words (Broun & Oelwein, 2007). The range of literacy goals potentially targeted at the Level IV level is shown in Table 9.7.

I-TO-I MODEL: LEVEL V

The Level V reader can read conventionally but requires ongoing and varying levels of support to maintain reading and writing practices. For example, some individuals with cognitive disabilities may demonstrate more reading comprehension when they read aloud to others in contrast to reading silently alone. Writing skills must be continually supported during everyday tasks. Remember that an individual with significant disabilities may vary in his or her literacy ability depending on task familiarity and environmental support. For example, an individual may be able to read a daily schedule once it is familiar, but may need additional support when new items are added to the schedule. Potential goals for a Level V reader and writer are shown in Table 9.7.

Intervention for Students with Reading and Writing Disability: Evidence-Based Practices

There are many different reading and writing programs for students with literacy learning deficits. I present two different programs below. I chose these programs because they were developed by SLPs and have documented efficacy. My goal is to show how a strong intervention has both a clear theoretical foundation and research documenting effectiveness.

EXPLICIT PHONOLOGICAL AWARENESS INTERVENTION

The explicit phonological awareness intervention (EPAI; Gillon, 2000) is based on several theoretical approaches that should be familiar to you. First, the approach is teacher directed and skill based, rather than activity based. Thus, it reflects aspects of behavioral theory. It is a bottom-up approach, breaking down the complex behavior of reading by focusing on an individual component of the reading process.

EPAI, however, also draws from social interaction theory in that the approach engages children in a complex task with the support of a more sophisticated partner. Shared participation in PA activities helps children discover the alphabetic principle.

The EPAI approach targets PA at the phoneme level, rather than the word or syllable level. Gillon (2004) states that awareness at the word and syllable level frequently develops from classroom-based activities. Classroom-based PA activities include rhyming games and clapping syllables. Although children should participate in activities at this level, for many children, implicit learning activities will not be sufficient. Children who are at risk for reading problems usually require more intensive and explicit instruction at the phoneme level to develop needed PA ability.

Gillon (2000) demonstrated the effectiveness of EPAI in a group of 23 children between the ages of 5 and 7 years. All of the children had expressive phonological impairments (i.e., difficulty with producing speech sounds). EPAI was implemented individually 2 hours per week; each child received 20 hours of intervention. Activities included letter-sound knowledge at the phoneme level including phoneme identification, phoneme blending, phoneme segmentation, and tracking sound changes in words.

Two examples of phoneme-level teaching techniques similar to those in the EPAI intervention are demonstrated in Table 9.8. Examples of intervention goals compatible with EPAI are provided in Figure 9.10.

Evidence Supporting the EPAI Approach. Gillon (2000) compared the pre- and postintervention abilities of the 23 children receiving EPAI intervention with two comparison groups. A second cohort of 23 children also received 20 hours of intervention, but their treatment focused on oral speech production and expressive language abilities. A third group of 15 children did not receive treatment due to their inability to access treatment. This last group served as a no-treatment control group.

At the end of the 20-week intervention, the children in the EPAI group demonstrated significantly better ability to decode nonsense words as compared with the children in the other two groups. Importantly, the children in the EPAI group also

Table 9.8 **Example of Phonological Awareness Training Sequences**

Phonological awareness task	Activity	High- and low-support cues*

Recognition of initial sound in words	Show students a "mystery bag." Say, "*We are going to guess whose picture is in the bag. I will give you some clues. The first clue is that the word starts with the /f/ sound. The next clue is that we just read about this animal. Sometimes this animal gets into the chicken coop. Can anyone guess what picture is in the bag?*"
	
	    1st Child: "*Chicken!*"
	    Adult: "*Good thinking, but let's listen to the first sound in that word, /t∫/, /t∫/, /t∫/. We don't hear the /f/ sound in that one, do we?*"
	    2nd Child: "*/f/ /f/ /f/*"
	    Adult: "*Good, you are thinking about that /f/ sound. The word starts with /f/.*"
		• High support: "*Let's listen to this word: cow. Do you hear the /f/ sound? No, you are right, there is not a /f/ sound in cow. It isn't a picture of cow, is it? Listen to this word: fox. Do you hear the /f/ sound? You are right, there is a /f/ sound, and look—here is a picture of a fox in my bag!*"
		• Low support: "*Let me tell you the word slowly and see if you can guess. F-O-X. Does anyone know the word? Good, let's listen for the /f/ sound.*"

Onset-rime	Show children a picture and say, "*Let's play 'I spy.' I will say a word in a funny way and you guess what I am looking at in the picture. I spy: s-un.*"	• High support: "*Do you think I am looking at the sun or the moon? Listen: s-un.*" • Low support: "*The first part of the word is /s/. Does anyone see a picture on this page that starts with /s/?*"

*High support is provided when a child is learning the PA task; low support is provided as a child becomes more proficient in the PA task.

Figure 9.10 Example Goals for Phonological Awareness Intervention

Goal 1 Kirby will blend onset-rime words with picture cues. Kirby will correctly choose a target word from three pictures when given mild support 4/5 times on 3 consecutive days. Mild support includes (a) up to three repetitions of target word and/or (b) saying each of the pictured words with a prolonged initial sound.

Goal 2 Janice will identify the word that does <u>not</u> start with the target sound ("odd man out") 4/5 times on 3 consecutive days given four words. The words will be no longer than three phonemes and the "odd man out" word will be dissimilar in manner and place of articulation. (e.g., man, mouse, car, mom).

Source: From "Phonological Awareness Intervention: A Preventative Framework for Preschool Children with Specific Speech and Language Impairments," by G. T. Gillon, 2006. In R. J. McCauley and M. E. Fey (Eds.), *Treatment of Language Disorders in Children* (pp. 279-308). Baltimore, MD: Brookes.

showed better word recognition, reading accuracy, and reading comprehension. A follow-up assessment 11 months after the intervention indicated that PA, speech production, reading, and spelling development continued for the children in the EPAI group. The children in the other two groups made little or no reading progress (Gillon, 2002). These data demonstrate the effectiveness of PA intervention and underscore the connection between PA and reading ability. The use of a control group, but without randomization, places the level of evidence for EPAI as Level II.

WRITING LAB APPROACH

The writing lab (WL) approach focuses on improving students' writing processes and their oral language communication skills with computer support (Nelson, Bahr, & Van Meter, 2004; Nelson & Van Meter, 2006). The term *writing process* describes the sequence of writing activities used by effective writers: topic selection, planning, organizing, drafting, revising, editing, publishing, and presenting. In the WL approach, SLPs work with general education teachers to facilitate students' meta-ability during the writing process and oral presentations. Students use computer software in many different ways during writing and presentation sequence. Examples of software programs are shown in Table 9.9. Since WL targets a student's oral and written language skills, it is considered a cross-modality or multimodality intervention approach.

Student's writing projects during the writing lab intervention are designed to be authentic; the goal is to have students work on a personally meaningful project that ultimately will be shared with an audience. Throughout the writing sequence, students use small-group interaction, peer and teacher conferencing, rubrics, check sheets/organizers, and computer software to plan, revise, and edit their papers. Each writing cycle is completed when the student presents his or her project orally to the group.

Table 9.9   **Software Examples Used in Writing Lab Approach**

Writing skills	Processes supported	Software programs
Planning and organizing	• Organizing • Outlining • Brainstorming • Illustrating	• Creative Writer 2 [Microsoft] • Ultimate Writing and Creativity Center [Riverdeep/The Learning Company] • Kid Pix Deluxe [Broderbund] • MediaWeaver [Sunburst] • Kidspiration [Inspiration Software]
Drafting	• Word prediction • Word banks • Collaborative writing • Speech recognition	• CollaborEdit [PaperFly Corporation] • Storyspace [Eastgate Systems] • Dragon Dictate [ScanSoft] • ViaVoice [IBM] • Word [Microsoft]
Revising and editing	• Grammar and spelling editing • Thesaurus and rhyming • Spell checkers	• Easybook Deluxe [Sunburst] • Storybook Weaver Deluxe [Riverdeep/ The Learning Company] • The Amazing Writing Machine [Riverdeep/ The Learning Company] • Stationery Studio [Fablevision]
Desktop publishing	• Merge text and graphics • Add drawing and painting tools • Modify text, margins, borders, etc. • Create tables	• Kids Works Deluxe [Knowledge Adventure] • HyperStudio [Knowledge Adventure] • Kids Media Magic [Sunburst] • The Print Shop [Broderbund]

Source: From *The Writing Lab Approach to Language Instruction and Intervention,* by N. W Nelson, C. M Bahr, and A. M. Van Meter, 2004, Baltimore, MD: Brookes.

The WL approach reflects a top-down model. Students attempt to produce a high-quality project that communicates their ideas. Thus, students focus on a meaningful activity. As students revise and edit their papers they focus on language subcomponents such as spelling, syntax, morphology, vocabulary, and story organization. Students are encouraged to use a recursive writing process; they write, share their writing, obtain feedback, and continue to revise and edit until they have a high-quality writing sample. Students practice oral communication skills in their small group and one-on-one feedback sessions and during their final oral presentation. Students self evaluate and receive teacher and SLP feedback on their oral and written communication. The goal is to have students cycle between the "top" (i.e., the written product and oral presentation) and the "bottom" (i.e., language subskills needed for an effective product).

The WL approach draws on two major theoretical approaches. First, social constructivist theory is emphasized in the use of small groups and collaborative partnerships to facilitate students' oral and written communication. Second, the WL approach reflects information processing/connectionism theory. As you recall from Chapter 1, information processing and connectionism theories suggest that language processing is interconnected and requires activation of areas of the brain responsible for specific language components (i.e., phonological, semantic, syntax). The assessment protocols associated with WL are naturalistic assessments, specifically curriculum-based language assessment (see Chapter 5 to review naturalistic/curriculum-based assessments).

The optimal schedule for the WL approach is a 1-hour session scheduled to occur within the general education classroom two or three times per week. Writing projects connect to ongoing classroom instruction potentially including topics related to language arts, social studies, or science. The SLP and teacher present mini lessons lasting no more than 10 or 15 minutes. Mini lessons introduce an aspect of the writing process such as (a) using brainstorming to find a topic, (b) using the computer thesaurus, spell check, or grammar check, or (c) methods of story organization. Students spend the next part of the session writing on their own, peer and teacher conferencing, and revising and editing work in progress.

Students develop author notebooks to organize materials and to maintain organizers to develop metaskills. Some students benefit from keeping word lists of confusing or difficult vocabulary (e.g., coordinating conjunctions, frequently misspelled words). To increase independence, students are encouraged to refer to their notebooks frequently. Completed projects are presented when the student takes the "author chair." Listeners provide feedback and ask questions. A teaching sequence is demonstrated in Figure 9.11. Intervention goals compatible with the WL approach are presented in Figure 9.12.

Evidence Supporting the Writing Lab Approach.   Nelson and her colleagues use a number of different measures to document students' improvement in written language. Some of the measures include (a) a word production fluency measure recording the number of words a student independently writes in a 1-hour written probe, (b) analysis of micro- and macrostructure features of oral and written narratives, (c) documenting the number and type of conjunctions, (d) counting the number of syntactically correct and incorrect sentences, and (e) computing the percentage of words spelled correctly.

In one study, Nelson implemented the WL approach with 53 third-grade students from three different classrooms. The students participated in WL 3 days a week; 2 days in their classroom and 1 day in the school's computer lab. Students were from an inner-city school and included children at risk due to economic disadvantage, special educational status, or nonmajority cultural or racial status.

Assessors completed data probes at three points during the year. Figure 9.13 visually demonstrates the development in narrative story structure (i.e., macrostructure) for four groups of children. All students, regardless of special education status, demonstrated significant growth. Effect size for narrative development and the

Figure 9.11   **Example of Writing Lab Intervention Sequence**

Steps to Teach Student to Self-Evaluate Spelling and Punctuation
Spelling goal: Identification and consistent spelling of prefix words

● The student and adult are conferencing with regard to a student's writing project.

Adult: "What spelling rules have you been working on? Can you go through
your paper and circle any of the words that we might need to take a look at?"
Student: "I have been working on recognizing prefixes."
Adult: "Can you give me some examples of prefixes?"
Student: "Well, I have a list in my notebook. Like auto, and de, and com."
Adult: "Exactly. Why don't you go through your paper and circle any prefix
words and make sure you have spelled them all correctly. I'll come back in a
few minutes and see how you are getting along."

Punctuation goal: Correct use of quotation marks to indicate dialogue

● Two middle-school students (Josh and Sandra) are working together on a script
for a short play to be presented to elementary school students. One of Josh's
writing goals is to correctly use quotation marks to indicate dialogue.

Adult: "What do we call it when two people are talking to each other in a play?"
Josh: "Dialogue."
Sandra: "Like here, where they are talking."
Adult: "Josh, can you explain to Sandra how we use punctuation in dialogue?"
Josh: "We use quotes."
Adult: "Sandy, do you understand how to show dialogue yet?"
Sandra: "No."
Adult: (Supports Josh in his explanation of the use of quotation for dialogue.
Students work together to use correct punctuation in their play with adult
support.)

Figure 9.12   **Example Goals for Writing Lab Intervention**

Goal 1: Oral communication	During author group Sabrina will (a) maintain appropriate eye contact with her group members, (b) provide the peer author with one suggestion to improve his or her work, and (c) provide one positive comment to the author.
Goal 2: Text comprehension	Prior to reading an assignment, Caleb will (a) identify the headings and subheadings in the text and (b) summarize to his group members his ideas of what the article is about. While reading, Caleb will write down key words or sentences to use for his article summary.

Source: From *The Writing Lab Approach to Language Instruction and Intervention,* by N. W Nelson,
C. M Bahr, and A. M. Van Meter, 2004, Baltimore, MD: Brookes.

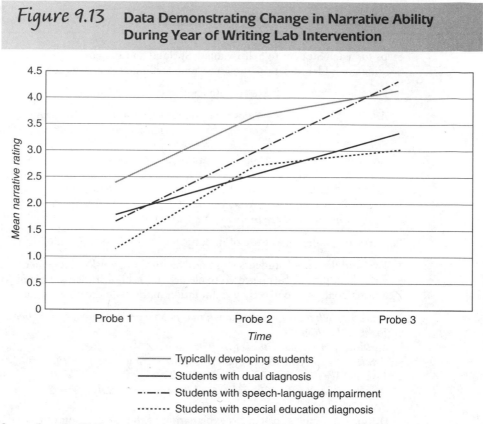

Figure 9.13   **Data Demonstrating Change in Narrative Ability During Year of Writing Lab Intervention**

——— Typically developing students
——— Students with dual diagnosis
–·—·— Students with speech-language impairment
········· Students with special education diagnosis

Source: From *The Writing Lab Approach to Language Instruction and Intervention* (p. 467), by N. W Nelson, C. M Bahr, and A. M. Van Meter, 2004, Baltimore, MD: Paul H. Brookes Publishing Co., Inc.

measure of word production fluency was large (Nelson & Van Meter, 2007). There was growth, but not at the same high level, in the other literacy measures. Since this study did not include a control group, the data reflect Level II evidence.

Summary

- The American Speech-Language-Hearing Association (ASHA) strongly advocates that speech-language pathologists (SLPs) and special educators indirectly and directly incorporate reading and writing interventions into treatment programs. A preventative model of intervention is used with young children in keeping with the response-to-intervention approach.
- The most important emergent literacy targets include phonological awareness, print and alphabetic concepts, oral language skills, and early writing skills.

Phonological awareness develops from word- and syllable-level awareness to awareness of individual phonemes. With awareness at the phoneme level, a child learns to blend and segment words. Print referencing is an explicit teaching technique that facilitates children's development of print and alphabetic concepts. Early writing skills support children's literacy growth.

- The embedded-explicit model of early literacy intervention encourages SLPs to assist teachers in embedding literacy targets within child-directed and engaging classroom activities. SLPs and teachers provide regular explicit, adult-directed literacy activities in individual or small-group sessions to children who need increased learning opportunities.

- Foundational reading skills for school-age students include phonological awareness, reading comprehension, and reading fluency. Research indicates that professionals can improve students' reading comprehension through vocabulary building and by helping students learn comprehension metaskills. Spelling assessment and intervention include analyses of children's phonological awareness, visual storage, orthographic knowledge, and morphological knowledge. Word sorts are an effective intervention approach to improve spelling ability.

- Oral narrative development is an important language skill interrelated to reading and writing development. Children develop both macro- and microstructure narrative features. Macrostructure includes story grammar; a mature narrative demonstrates thematic episode structure and contains an initiating event, an attempt, and a consequence. Microstructure includes literate language features providing decontextualization, cohesion, and descriptive story telling.

- The interactive-to-independent model of literacy intervention targets the individual with significant learning challenges. The model moves from highly interactive, shared literacy experiences (Levels I and II) to increasingly independent reading and writing with varying levels of adult support (Levels III-V).

- Two intervention programs include Gillon's phonological awareness intervention and Nelson's writing lab approach. The PA intervention provides explicit instruction in gamelike activities to enhance PA skills in young children. The writing lab approach uses the writing process to enhance oral and written communication skills of older school-age children.

Discussion and In-Class Activities

1. In small groups, you will be assigned an emergent literacy domain (e.g., phonological awareness, print concepts, alphabetic concepts, oral language, writing) and a classroom theme (e.g., community helpers, seasons, farm and zoo animals, insects, rivers/lakes/streams, plants/flowers, healthy food, our bodies, machines). Develop three different learning opportunities exemplifying your domain. At least one should be an explicit instructional activity and one should

be an embedded instructional activity. Each activity should use vocabulary, pictures, and activities that further the classroom theme. Consider how each activity could be modified for a child who struggles to perform this particular skill, and describe how the activity could be made more challenging for a child with advanced skills.

2. Role-play an adult-student interaction using Elkonian boxes. Start with four boxes and colored blocks or chips. Give instructions for the following:
   - A CVC stimulus word (as in *bed*)
   - A stimulus word in which the client must change the initial or final consonant (e.g., *Ted* or *bet*)
   - A stimulus word in which the vowel is changed (e.g., *Tod*, *beat*).
   - A stimulus word in which a consonant is added to make a consonant blend (e.g., *bleat*).

   Make sure the adult gives appropriate feedback and reinforces the student's demonstration of sound modifications. Try it with different words; have the student leave the chips in place and add or delete chips demonstrating how the sounds in the word change.

   Discuss in class the student skills required to complete this task. How could letters be used in this task instead of chips or blocks? When should letters be introduced? At what age would this type of activity be most useful? How could this activity be used to develop spelling ability?

3. Develop a word-sort activity to teach a spelling rule. You can research spelling rules on the Internet. A good Web site is: www.grammaruntied.com/spelling1.html

4. Record or transcribe a story. Ask a friend or young child, *"Tell me a made-up story; tell me the best story you can."* What narrative features were demonstrated in the oral narrative? What features were omitted? Do you think the story was a good one? Why or why not?

5. Examine elementary textbooks for different grade levels (e.g., science, geography, language arts). Develop strategies that might be used to increase a student's reading comprehension. Role-play with a student taking the role of the professional and another student taking the role of the elementary-age child.

6. Write three additional intervention goals consistent with Gillon's phonological awareness treatment. Then write goals for social communication skill, proofreading, brainstorming, and organizational strategy development for a student using the writing lab approach.

7. View a videotape of preschool children during adult–child book reading. Complete the early literacy observational checklist (Figure 9.1) together in class. What additional activities would you like to see in order to assess additional literacy skills? Develop a list of activities to elicit additional emergent literacy skills. As an outside assignment, you can audiotape or videotape interactions with a preschooler and document the child's ability using the observational form.

Chapter 9 Case Study

Ziquon is a third grader whose oral reading is labored; he often guesses at the word from the first letter. He struggles when he reaches an unfamiliar word. His written work and spelling is poor. Spelling errors noted include PELN (for *plane*), BUP (for *bump*), and SESRT (for *sister*). However, Ziquon knows some sight words and pronounces these immediately and correctly (McKenna & Stahl, 2003).

Questions for Discussion

1. What assessments would you recommend for Ziquon?
2. What reading subskills do you think may be most impaired? Why?
3. Consider Ziquon's spelling errors; what evidence do they provide?
4. Describe an intervention program for Ziquon. What are primary targets for instruction?

Augmentative and Alternative Communication (AAC) and Individuals with Complex Communication Needs

—Julia M. King

Chapter Overview Questions

1. What are complex communication needs?
2. What are the components of an AAC system?
3. What is NOT considered AAC?

4. What assessment components are completed for a potential AAC user?
5. What are some examples of using AAC to address language treatment?

Individuals with language impairments, either receptive or expressive, may have **complex communication needs** (CCNs). Many developmental disabilities such as Down syndrome, autism, and cerebral palsy are associated with communication impairments. People who have a communication impairment affecting daily communication are said to have CCNs. For children, CCNs can occur when there is difficulty with processing, comprehending, or producing language resulting in unmet communication needs. For example, a young child understands his parent when asked what game he wants to play but has difficulty formulating his response because he does not know the name of the game or how to describe it. When semantic, syntactic, morphologic, phonologic or pragmatic impairments impact the success with which a child communicates,

FOCUS 10.1 *Learning More*

Children with Physical Impairments

Children with physical impairments sometimes have CCNs. You will learn more about how to support communication with individuals with physical impairments in other coursework or textbooks on AAC (see Resources at the end of this chapter). Cerebral palsy is a common cause of physical impairments in children.

unmet communication needs prevent successful exchanges. An intervention approach often used to address communication needs is implementation of an **augmentative/ alternative communication (AAC) system**. An AAC system compensates and facilitates, either temporarily or permanently, for the impairment and disability patterns of individuals with severe expressive and/or language comprehension deficits. AAC may be required for individuals demonstrating impairments in gestural, spoken, and/or written modalities.

AAC can benefit children with language impairments as well as those with speech impairments, cognitive impairments, or physical impairments (see Focus 10.1). In this chapter, I focus on aspects of AAC supporting and improving language in children with CCNs.

Background and Description

AAC refers to an area of research in addition to clinical and educational practice (ASHA, 2005b); it addresses temporary or permanent impairments, activity limitations, and participation restrictions of individuals with CCNs. CCNs may stem from language comprehension and production impairments in spoken and written language (ASHA, 2004c). Language impairments may affect the quality and frequency of an individual's communication participation in the activities of daily living (see Focus 10.2 for the WHO model describing activity limitations and participation restrictions).

THE AAC SYSTEM

Recall the different aspects of language form, content, and use presented in Chapter 1. The domains of form, content, and use also are relevant for an AAC system. An AAC system includes rules for combining symbols to create a maximally intelligible and comprehensible (i.e., understandable) message for the broadest audience of communication partners (i.e., form). It also relies on conventions relative to the selection and organization of vocabulary (i.e., content). Finally (and most importantly) AAC systems are directed at maximizing language use in order that the individual communicates effectively and efficiently with as many persons, and in as many circumstances, as possible (ASHA, 2004c).

FOCUS 10.2 *Vocational and Community Issues*

World Health Organization

The World Health Organization (WHO) developed a framework to provide a standard language to describe health-related states (WHO, 2002). This framework is called the International Classification of Functioning, Disability, and Health, or ICF. Although language impairments may not be considered health-related conditions, the impairment could affect the child's ability to use language in various communication activities and participate in life activities. The ICF framework defines activity as the execution of a task or action by an individual, and defines his or her participation as involvement in life situations. The WHO framework focuses on documenting real-life changes in an individual's ability to communicate.

MULTI-MODAL COMMUNICATION

An AAC system is part of a multi-modal view of communication. **Multi-modal** refers to the use of multiple modalities when a person communicates (e.g., gestures, speech, facial expressions, writing, drawing, AAC system). How often do you use gestures or facial expressions to convey a message? Have you used a code when text messaging to represent a message (e.g., B4N for *'Bye for now'*)?

Children often use multiple modes of communication as they develop, even before they produce speech (e.g., crying, cooing, gazing, pointing). The use of pointing with voicing for a young child is very effective. For example, imagine that a child drops a cracker from her high chair, points to the cracker on the floor, and then vocalizes. It is likely that the communication partner will understand this action and vocalization as (a) a request to pick up the cracker or (b) a comment that the cracker is on the floor. We all use multiple modes of communication on a regular basis, sometimes simultaneously and sometimes one mode at a time. AAC systems offer modes of communication for children with impairments supporting their language development and communication needs.

The AAC System Components: What Is AAC?

AAC systems are comprised of four critical components: symbols, aids, strategies, and techniques (ASHA, 2004c, 2005b). **Symbols** can be graphic, auditory, gestural, textured, or tactile representations used to represent language concepts in AAC systems. Figure 10.1 shows examples of different symbols representing the same concept.

AAC SYMBOLS

An individual can use many different symbols to communicate. For example, a young child may use the manual sign for *hello* when he greets a friend on the bus. In other situations, he may point to a drawing representing *hello* to greet someone. The

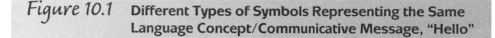

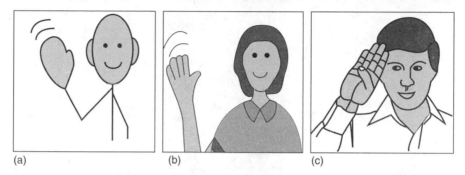

(a)   (b)   (c)

Sources: A. Line drawing, Picture Communication Symbols (© 1981–2009 DynaVox Mayer-Johnson) used with permission. All rights reserved worldwide. B. Line drawing, Picture Communication Symbols (© 1981–2009 DynaVox Mayer-Johnson) used with permission. All rights reserved worldwide. C. Illustration of sign from *Signing Illustrated,* by Mickey Flodin, copyright © 1994 by Mickey Flodin. Used by permission of Perigee Books, an imprint of Penguin Group (USA) Inc.

manual sign and the drawings are both examples of symbols. The first is an example of an **unaided symbol** because the child did not need any prosthetic (or external) support to convey his message. The second example demonstrates the use of an **aided symbol** because the child used a support (i.e., drawing) to convey his message. For a more extensive summary of symbol types, see *Augmentative and Alternative Communication* by Beukelman and Mirenda (2005).

THE AAC AID

The second component of an AAC system is aid. An **AAC aid** refers to a device that can be used to send or receive messages. The aid can be nonelectronic, such as a series of photographs, a collection of objects, or a series of black or color line drawings. Examples of nonelectronic aids are shown in Figure 10.2. Nonelectronic aids are also referred to as low or light technology.

Alternately, an aid can be electronic and refer to simple devices, such as talking photo albums, or complex devices such as speech generating devices (SGDs), as shown in Figure 10.3. Electronic aids are referred to as high technology. Many AAC systems have both low and high technology components. An illustration of a child interacting with his language facilitator with an AAC system is shown in Figure 10.4.

AAC STRATEGIES

The third component of an AAC system is strategy. An **AAC strategy** refers to methods used to communicate effectively and efficiently. AAC strategies support message timing, grammatical formulation, spelling, and communication rate (Beukelman &

Figure 10.2   Examples of Nonelectronic AAC Aids

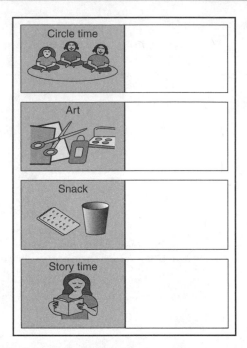

A. Schedule board with line drawings.

Source: Courtesy of Picture Communication Symbols from Mayer-Johnson Boardmaker.

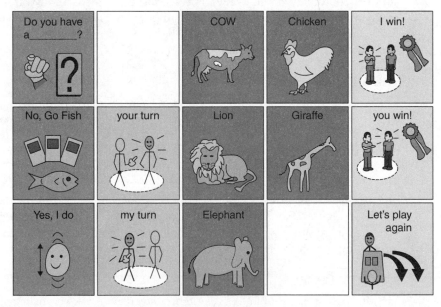

B. Static paper communication display board with line drawings.

Source: The Picture Communication Symbols (© 1981–2009 DynaVox Mayer-Johnson) are used with permission. All rights reserved worldwide.

Figure 10.3 Examples of Electronic AAC Aids

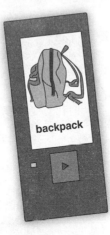

A. Single message low-technology AAC aid.

Source: Courtesy of Attainment Company, Verona, WI; www.attainmentcompany.com

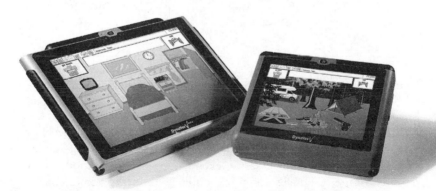

B. Dynamic display high-technology AAC aid.

Source: Courtesy of Dynavox Technologies, Pittsburgh, PA; www.dynavoxtech.com

Mirenda, 2005). Some examples of strategies to enhance communication include prediction and encoding. The prediction strategy is "a dynamic retrieval process in which options offered to the people who rely on AAC change based on the portion of the message that has already been formulated" (Beukelman & Mirenda, 2005, p. 75). An example of prediction is when your computer shows you your most recently accessed files before showing you older or unused files. Young children with language impairments may benefit from letter and word prediction. Letter prediction can support spelling if the child knows the first letter of the word (see Focus 10.3). Word prediction supports syntactical development as the computer program predicts the next word based on syntactic rules.

Figure 10.4   Child Interacting with His AAC Device in His Language Intervention Session

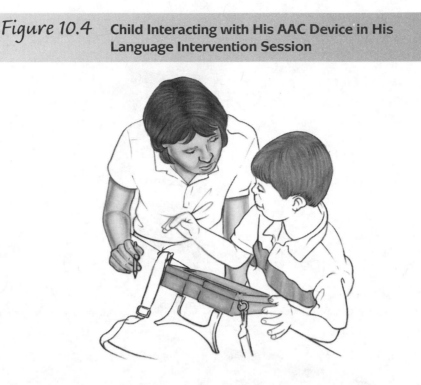

Encoding (i.e., the use of a code) is another effective AAC strategy. Encoding can help an individual quickly express a lengthy message. The most commonly used codes with young children are color coding and symbol coding. With encoding, the user learns to use specific codes for each message. Color coding is used to designate a specific location on a communication display conveying a part of speech (e.g., yellow for nouns). Symbol coding is used for quick communication. For example, if a child wants to tell his friend what he did last weekend, one symbol selection, a photo of his grandparents' home, produces an entire sentence about his experience by encoding the

FOCUS 10.3 *Learning More*

Word Prediction

You may be familiar with word prediction if you program names in your cell phone. The software predicts the name of the person based on the letter you have typed. For example, I start entering the letters *B-a-r* and the predicted name *Barbara* is available for selection. The predicted name saved me 4 keystrokes so I did not have to enter the *b-a-r-a*.

message *"I went to my grandma and grandpa's house this weekend; it was so much fun."* Other encoding systems available in AAC systems, such as number coding and alphanumeric coding, place high demands on the learner to remember the code.

Encoding improves communication efficiency when it is matched with each individual's capabilities (Beukelman & Mirenda, 2005). Research demonstrates that code learning requires a significant investment of intervention time. Also, a child's cognitive ability must be considered when deciding on a coding system (Light et al., 2004). Promising new research in the area of visual scene displays (VSDs) may support encoding for language learning and communication function for young children or for individuals with cognitive impairments (see the Intervention section in this chapter for more on VSDs).

AAC TECHNIQUES

The fourth component of an AAC system is technique. An **AAC technique** refers to how a message is conveyed. Some individuals who have an AAC system use their finger to point to symbols or look directly at their intended object (i.e., eye pointing). This technique is referred to as direct selection because the person directly selects a symbol. This strategy often is the most efficient. However, some individuals who cannot directly select a symbol because of a physical impairment must use another technique called scanning to access their AAC system.

Scanning is most often used for children with physical limitations. Scanning involves a communication partner or an electronic device that displays symbols in a predetermined pattern (Beukelman & Mirenda, 2005). Partner-dependent scanning involves a facilitator scanning through symbol choices until the child indicates his or her choice; the child communicates his or her choice by blinking, pressing a switch, vocalizing, or producing a predetermined physical movement. Electronic aids can also be used to scan choices with lighted displays. Again, the child waits while the device scans through the symbols until the target symbol is illuminated. The child then produces a movement to select the target symbol. Figure 10.5 shows an example of an SGD set up with its scanning system.

AAC SELECTION SET

Many components must be combined to develop an effective communication system. The practitioner creates an AAC system by combining symbols, aids, strategies, and selection set. An **AAC selection set** describes how the components are presented to the communicator using the AAC device (Beukelman & Mirenda, 2005). Many AAC selection sets include a visual display; however, for individuals with visual impairments, auditory and tactile displays can be provided. A selection set can have fixed displays, dynamic displays, hybrid displays, or visual scene displays (Beukelman & Mirenda, 2005).

Fixed displays have symbols and messages that do not change after the person selects the location. Think about ordering at a restaurant. The waiter cannot hear you because of the noise level so you indicate your choice by pointing to the picture

Figure 10.5   Example of Scanning Set-Up on an SGD

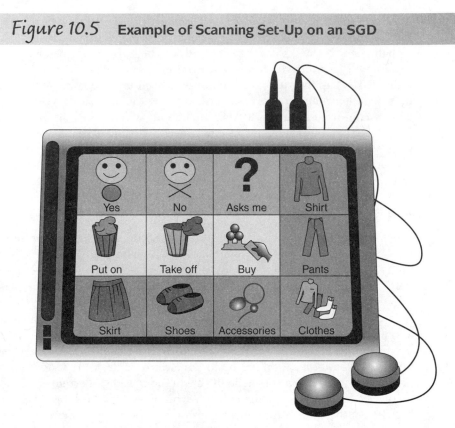

Source: Courtesy of Saltillo Corporation, Millersburg, OH; www.saltillo.com

or words on the menu but nothing changes on the page. You have used a static fixed display to communicate your food choice.

In contrast, **dynamic displays** change after a location is selected. You have likely used dynamic displays on your cell phone, an ATM machine, or possibly your computer. Dynamic displays are "computer screen displays with electronically produced visual symbols [that], when activated, automatically change the selection set on the screen to a new set of programmed symbols" (Beukelman & Mirenda, 2005, p. 85).

There are two additional display types: hybrid and visual scene displays. Hybrid displays are available on a few SGDs. They combine electronic fixed displays with a dynamic feature. The final display type, **visual scene display** (VSD), is "a picture, photograph, or virtual environmental [display] that depicts and represents a situation, place, or experience" (Beukelman & Mirenda, 2005, p. 88). VSD can be used in low technology aids, similar to a fixed display, or in a high technology AAC aid, similar to a dynamic display. I will highlight the use of VSDs in the Intervention section of this chapter.

FOCUS 10.4 *Learning More*

Go to Dr. Dowden's Web site and find a myth and fact about AAC that you had not considered before. How can you help dispel myths about AAC?

WHAT IS NOT AAC?

Now that you understand the definition and components of AAC, I want you to know what AAC is not. Hopefully, as part of this discussion, you also have considered overarching issues about alternative modes of communication. Many professionals (i.e., therapists, teachers, administrators) have misconceptions about AAC. Dr. Pat Dowden at the University of Washington has a Web site dispelling some common myths about AAC by promoting the facts. Check out her Web site at http:// depts.washington.edu/enables/myths/myths_intro.htm. These myths address misconceptions about topics such as intervention strategies that can benefit from AAC and how AAC is more than assistive technology (see Focus 10.4).

AAC is not an intervention approach used to replace speech; instead, it is an approach that augments an individual's available skills and provides alternative communication strategies as needed. AAC is more than the use of "fancy talking computers." AAC enhances input as well as output of language; it can be used in combination with other language intervention approaches.

It is important to remember that *AAC does not hinder language or speech development.* Blackstone (2006) reported, "AAC interventions can have significant benefits on the development of communicative competence and language skills" (p. 3). Blackstone's report and research (see Focus 10.5) reduces anxiety about the implications of AAC interventions. Because "AAC interventions are typically implemented to build communication and language skills through a range of modalities (including signs and aided AAC systems as well as natural speech), rather than to increase speech production alone" (Millar, Light, & Schlosser, 2006, p. 257), concerns about AAC replacing traditional modes of communication are unwarranted. AAC is a tool that facilitates communication.

FOCUS 10.5 *Research*

In 2006, Millar, Light, and Schlosser completed a meta-analysis to determine the effect of AAC on the speech production of individuals with developmental disabilities. The researcher team found 23 studies examining the relationship between speech production and the effects of AAC intervention. The data demonstrated speech increased in a majority of individuals (89%) with AAC intervention and no individuals "showed a decrease in speech production as a result of AAC intervention" (Millar, Light, Schlosser, 2006, p. 254).

Assessment

AAC assessment is a team effort; each team member contributes information about the child's capabilities and needs. Figure 10.6 lists potential AAC team members. Family members are a very important part of the team. Research underscores the importance of family values, lifestyle, and preferences in the AAC assessment and intervention process. An individual's AAC use occurs at home, school, or work place. Accordingly, the family takes on a key role in the intervention process (Granlund, Björchk-Åkesson, Wilder, & Ylvén, 2008).

A comprehensive AAC assessment includes additional components as compared to a standard language assessment (covered in Chapter 2). The additional required components are described in this section. Language capabilities as well as capabilities in the areas of literacy, hearing, vision, oral-motor system, speech, cognition, and physical skills must be documented. Figure 10.7 lists the components of a comprehensive assessment.

The practitioner uses the results from the language and literacy assessment to develop a functional profile of the individual's current language capabilities; this assessment facilitates an appropriate intervention approach (Beukelman & Mirenda, 2005). Adaptations are made if the individual has a physical impairment limiting his participation in the language assessment (see Focus 10.6).

An AAC evaluation must (a) determine an individual's communication needs and participation patterns and (b) identify the best way to represent language in the

Figure 10.6   Potential AAC Team Members

Child
Parents/Family
Speech-language pathologist
Teacher
Occupational therapist
Physical therapist
Rehabilitation engineer
Educational assistant
Nurse/Physician

Figure 10.7   Components of a Comprehensive AAC Assessment

Identification of participation patterns
Identification of communication needs
Capabilities assessment
Symbol assessment
Trials with different AAC system features

FOCUS 10.6 *Clinical Skill Building*

Language tests often require the child to point to pictures. How could you adapt a language test for a child who has a physical challenge and cannot point with his or her finger? How might adapting a language test for a child with physical challenges impact the results, or your interpretation of the results, from a standardized test?

AAC system. AAC assessments are dynamic and ongoing. A skilled assessor begins the assessment by asking a series of questions:

- How does the individual currently communicate?
- Where does the individual communicate?
- With whom does the individual communicate?
- Is the individual successful when he or she communicates?
- If he or she is not successful, what does he or she do?
- How does this individual compare with same-age peers who are developing typically?

To implement a high-quality AAC assessment, the assessor follows the participation model of assessment (Beukelman & Mirenda, 2005). A decision tree demonstrating the participation model is presented in Figure 10.8. The American Speech-Language-Hearing Association endorsed this model in 2004.

The participation model "provides a systematic process for conducting AAC assessments and designing interventions based on the functional participation requirements of peers without disabilities of the same chronological age as the person who may communicate through AAC" (Beukelman & Mirenda, 2005, p. 136). Practitioners use this model to determine both intrinsic and extrinsic factors contributing to an individual's complex communication needs. Using the model, the practitioner assesses an individual's capabilities and constraints (i.e., strengths and challenges) and determines his or her potential as an AAC communicator. The model also illustrates how outside factors can affect complex communication needs.

Why is functional participation important to AAC assessment? In Focus 10.2 I described the ICF framework from the World Health Organization (WHO, 2002). As you recall, the WHO framework considers an individual's everyday functioning in his or her community, school, or job. The WHO framework underscores the importance of an individual's overall communication context.

However, within the confines of a traditional language assessment (using norm-referenced assessments and one-on-one interactions), the assessor may not capture an individual's everyday communication patterns. In contrast, with the AAC participation model, the assessor observes the individual at school, during social activities, and in a variety of interpersonal interactions. Observing everyday communication routines also helps the assessor identify barriers potentially limiting the individual's communication (see Table 10.1).

Figure 10.8 AAC Participation Model

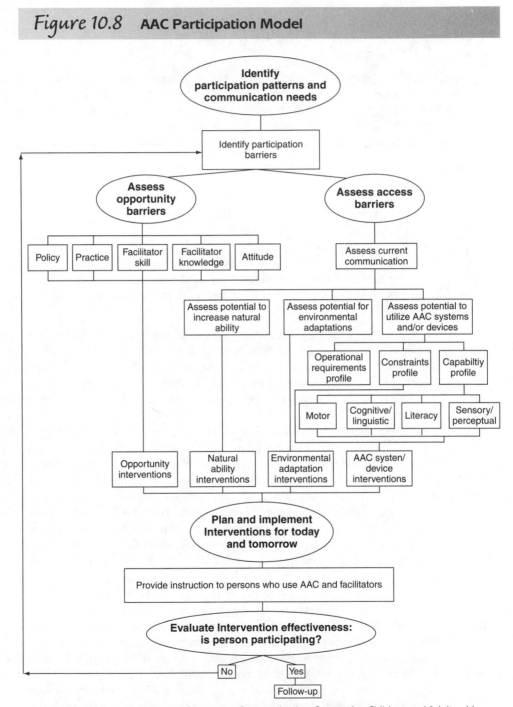

Source: From *Augmentative and Alternative Communication: Supporting Children and Adults with Complex Communication Needs* (3rd ed.), (p. 137), by D. R. Beukelman and P. Mirenda, 2005, Baltimore, MD: Paul H. Brookes Publishing Co. Inc. Reprinted by permission.

Table 10.1 **Barriers to Participation**

Barrier type	Barrier description	Example
Policy barriers	Rules or policies regulating situations and environments	The child does not have access to an AAC system outside of school because of school policy stating systems purchased by the school can not leave school grounds.
Practice barriers	Procedures commonly used in environments	The practitioner was told he or she does not have to provide AAC services because the school district has an Assistive Technology (AT) Consultant
Knowledge barriers	Misinformation or lack of knowledge about AAC	The practitioner does not have knowledge of AAC so he or she does not consider it as a treatment option.
Skill barriers	Professional's clinical skills are not sufficient to appropriately and accurately implement an AAC approach to treatment.	The practitioner has taken an AAC course but has not had practical experience providing AAC services.

Source: From *Augmentative and Alternative Communication: Supporting Children and Adults with Complex Communication Needs* (3rd ed.), by D. R. Beukelman and P. Mirenda, 2005, Baltimore, MD: Brookes.

The ICF framework also guides questioning during an AAC assessment to determine an individual's communication needs. For example, the assessor questions the individual, family, teachers, and/or caregivers to determine:

1. Communication or academic expectations (e.g., silent reading during quiet time in a second-grade classroom).
2. Important communication environments (e.g., Cub Scouts, Special Olympics, school, home).
3. Typical communication partners (e.g., parents, grandparents, siblings, friends, educational assistants, teacher, coach).
4. Activities and routines of daily living (i.e., Does the child participate in kindergarten morning circle time?).
5. Communicative messages regularly required (e.g., messages to support sharing at circle time).

There are two goals underlying the information-gathering protocol listed above; the first goal is to identify the AAC user's participation patterns. A second goal is to compare the potential AAC user's patterns with communication patterns of same-age peers.

To complete the second goal, team members fill out a participation inventory. The participation inventory documents the future AAC user's communication patterns in everyday interactions; team members also describe same-age peers' communication patterns within each interaction. Team members then compare the optimal level of participation to that of the potential AAC user; barriers limiting participation also are identified.

Barriers to communication in each interaction setting are carefully evaluated. In some cases, caregivers unconsciously may be limiting an individual's participation. This is called an opportunity barrier. More examples of opportunity barriers are shown in Table 10.1. At other times, the individual with CCNs may lack access to the interaction; this is an access barrier. The results from the communication assessment may lead to one of the following conclusions:

- The individual's natural communication abilities should be targeted for intervention.
- Environmental changes should be targeted to facilitate communication.
- The individual may benefit from an AAC approach to intervention (Beukelman & Mirenda, 2005).

The conclusions listed above are not mutually exclusive. An individual with language impairment may benefit from an AAC approach in combination with an intervention focusing on improving verbal communication abilities.

SYMBOL ASSESSMENT

A comprehensive AAC assessment also includes a symbol assessment. As you recall from the beginning of the chapter, there are many types of symbols. The goal of a symbol assessment is to "select the types of symbols that will meet the individual's current communication needs and match his or her current abilities, as well as to identify symbol options that might be used in the future" (Beukelman & Mirenda, 2005, p. 191).

AAC symbol assessment considers both unaided and aided symbols. The assessor documents the individual's use of gestures, vocalizations, or manual signs along with the individual's understanding and use of aided symbols. During aided symbol assessment the practitioner typically asks the individual to identify familiar objects. Specifically, the individual is asked to match a target object with (a) other objects, (b) miniature objects, (c) photographs, (d) black line drawings, (e) colored line drawings, and (f) written words. To assess comprehension, the target object or symbol is presented in a series of three (i.e., one target and two foils).

As an example, imagine that you want to determine a student's ability to identify a symbol for *book*. You begin by showing the student a book and asking the student to match the book with a second copy of a book sitting on the table. Next to the second book you have placed two foils (e.g., a cup and a toy car). If the student is able to identify a second copy of the book, you move to the next level of abstraction. Now, you present a miniature hairbrush. You ask the individual to match the miniature hairbrush to one of the items on the table (e.g., real hairbrush, spoon, pencil). If the student is able to match the miniature brush with the real brush, you continue to make the task more abstract. You ask the client to match real objects to photographs, black line drawings, colored line drawings, and written words. Ten items are presented (with foils for each item) to obtain an accurate assessment. With multiple opportunities, you determine which aided symbol type best matches the student's abstraction ability.

As a next step in symbol assessment, you determine the student's ability to use symbols within natural interactions (Beukelman & Mirenda, 2005). To continue with the example above, assume that you determined the student easily recognized language concepts represented by line drawings. You now present opportunities for the student to use the symbols (i.e., drawings) within several communication activities. You prepare a book-reading activity and a music-choice activity because you noted the student enjoyed these activities. You present symbols representing book reading and listening to music and ask the student to choose an activity. With modeling and prompting, you demonstrate how selecting the symbol results in a desired activity.

You point to the book-reading symbol and ask the student *"Would you like to read a book?"* Subsequently, you point to the listening-to-music symbol and ask, *"Would you like to listen to music?"* You train others to offer these opportunities as well. Interactive opportunities extend the assessment process into the student's daily life. This "trial intervention" provides valuable information, allowing you to make recommendations regarding the type of symbols appropriate for the student's AAC system.

AAC assessments can be natural extensions of more traditional communication assessments. Extending symbolic use to represent language for input as well as output eliminates barriers and provides opportunities for children with language impairments to participate in everyday communication activities.

FEATURE MATCH

Another component of a comprehensive AAC assessment includes a match of AAC system features. AAC system features refer to aspects of AAC previously discussed: strategies, display types, selection sets, etc. Specifically, the individual should have opportunities during the assessment to try different types of displays (e.g., static, dynamic) and selection sets. The assessor provides AAC trials with varied features in meaningful, age appropriate contexts. A complete description of a feature-match assessment is beyond the scope of this chapter. However, you can research different options from the resource section at the end of the chapter for more information.

Results from an AAC assessment will include recommendations for an AAC system. The AAC system is part of a multi-modal approach to language intervention to enhance effective communication. See Focus 10.7 for more about assessment protocols for AAC.

FOCUS 10.7 *Learning More*

Social Networks: A Communication Inventory for Individuals with Complex Communication Needs and their Communication Partners (Blackstone & Hunt Berg, 2003) is a commercially available assessment and intervention planning tool that can help you investigate a child's communication needs. The Social Networks tool facilitates and guides the clinician and AAC team to identify (a) the skills and abilities of the child and communication partners, (b) the child's modes of expression, (c) appropriate augmentative and alternative symbols, aids, strategies, and techniques, (d) potential topics of conversation, and (e) levels of support needed to communicate. This information is used to plan ongoing intervention maximizing the child's communicative effectiveness and independence.

Intervention

AAC intervention approaches vary from structured behavioral teaching models to child-centered interactive and social pragmatic models (Beukelman & Mirenda, 2005; Light and Drager 2006). The assessor matches the best intervention strategies for each child based on results from the assessment and AAC system trials. Family members and other communication partners are involved in the AAC intervention. Stakeholders are trained to facilitate the child's language and communication development during everyday interactions (Light & Drager, 2006).

Below I present three AAC intervention approaches; the System for Augmenting Language (SAL), visual scene displays (VSDs), and Picture Exchange Communication System (PECS). For more information on different AAC interventions, you can check out the book, *Pragmatically Speaking: Language, Literacy, and Academic Development for Students with AAC Needs*, edited by Soto and Zangari (2009). You also can (a) read about additional AAC intervention approaches in Focus 10.8 and (b) find additional resources at the end of this chapter.

THE SYSTEM FOR AUGMENTING LANGUAGE (SAL)

The **System for Augmenting Language** or SAL is a total-immersion approach teaching language comprehension and use (Romski & Sevcik, 1996). With the SAL approach, practitioners avoid teaching language in a structured didactic (i.e., structured teacher-student) fashion. Instead, students are encouraged to use the AAC device within realistic spoken communication. The student's communication partners serve as models for AAC use. The five components of SAL are listed in Figure 10.9.

There is evidence supporting the use of SAL. Romski and Sevcik (1996) used the SAL with 13 students who had CCNs secondary to intellectual impairment. The researchers followed the students for two years and reported that all participants

FOCUS 10.8 *Research*

Aided Language Stimulation

SAL is similar to another AAC intervention approach called aided language stimulation (ALS). ALS approach was developed by Carol Goossens' and Sharon Crain and teaches language naturally (see Goossens' & Crain, 1986a, 1986b). During ALS intervention, a communication facilitator points to graphic symbols on a display while simultaneously stating the message (Beukelman & Mirenda, 2005). The symbol display can be on a vest worn by the facilitator, presented on a speech-generating device (SGD), or via a communication board. The facilitator augments language input by (a) pointing to graphic symbols corresponding to the communicative message and (b) supporting the child's independent use of the communication display. This approach takes place during the child's daily routines and activities. ALS has reported efficacy (Binger & Light, 2007; Bruno & Trembath, 2006; Goossens' & Crain, 1986a, b; Harris & Reichle, 2004).

Figure 10.9 **SAL Components and Instructional Strategies**

1. The student is provided with a speech-generating device (SGD) to use within the natural communication environment.
2. Symbols are displayed on the SGD with the English word printed above; the symbols are selected to improve social communication and to meet individual communication needs.
3. The communication partner encourages the child to use symbols by teaching symbol use in loosely structured naturalistic communicative activities (e.g., "Tell me what you want, do you want *water* or *juice?*").
4. Communication partners are trained to use symbols in their communication with the student (i.e., both partners use symbols during interactions).
5. Professional provides ongoing support to the student and his or her communication partners as a resource on using the approach.

Source: From *Breaking the Speech Barrier: Language Development Through Augmented Means,* by M. A. Romski and R. A. Sevcik, 1996, Baltimore, MD: Brookes.

learned to produce referential and **regulatory communication acts** alone or in combination with other modes of communication (e.g., gestures, vocalizations) within different communication environments. Regulatory communication acts are completed when an individual indicates his or her own needs within routines of daily living. The SAL researchers reported that participants learn to communicate with a variety of communication partners, including peers.

In another study, SAL-trained communicators (with five years of AAC experience) were compared with two groups of non-SAL-trained communicators including both "speakers" and "nonspeakers" (Romski, Sevcik, Adamson, & Bakeman, 2005). All three groups consisted of participants with moderate-to-severe intellectual impairment. The results of the study supported the use of the SAL approach. When compared to the nonspeakers, the SAL communicators had higher-quality interactions and a higher level of conversational appropriateness in an interaction with an unfamiliar communication partner.

In comparison with the "speakers," the SAL users were described as being "less fluid." However, the SAL communicators demonstrated an advantage over the speakers in that they used more specific references during their interactions.

The SAL approach also has been used with toddlers with significant developmental delays and complex communication needs (Romski, Sevcik, Cheslock, & Barton, 2006). Initial findings with very young children revealed increased communication using symbols. For example, the subjects in this study learned an average of 62.8 symbols; some toddlers also increased their use of spoken words during the yearlong study.

VISUAL SCENE DISPLAYS (VSDs)

Visual scene displays (VSDs) can be used in an intervention program to support language by organizing vocabulary and communicative messages schematically rather

Figure 10.10 Visual Scene Display on SGD

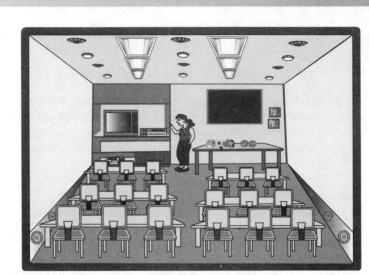

than semantically (Beukelman & Mirenda, 2005). I described VSDs earlier in the chapter when I discussed AAC selection set. VSDs can be used with low-technology or high-technology AAC devices. Visual scenes use photographs or pictures instead of individual line drawings to symbolize language concepts and communicative messages. "Hot spots" within each visual scene are identified areas important for learning and communicating (see Figure 10.10).

Children use the visual scenes to explore, learn, and communicate with parents and other communication partners (Light & Drager, 2006). Beukelman and Mirenda (2005) describe visual scenes as a display that "depicts a set of elements (people, actions, objects) within a coherent, integrated visual image" (p. 88). The arrangement of language concepts and communicative messages in a VSD is very different from the traditional AAC communication board. A traditional AAC display represents language concepts and communicative message with symbols, photos, and words organized into rows and columns. In contrast, as you can see in Figure 10.10, the VSD provides contextual support in comparison to a traditional grid display. In the visual scene, hot spots on the scene are selected so that if a child points to the blocks, the message *I want to play with the blocks* is produced. On a traditional display, the child would express *I want to play with the blocks* by pointing to a block symbol or word. Examples of other VSDs are available at the AAC Web site at the University of Nebraska-Lincoln http://aac.unl.edu/intervention.html.

The advantages of VSD are that the realistic nature of the scenes maximizes meaningfulness and organizes language concepts within categories. Also, VSDs facilitate children's use of speech generation. Young children often find speech generation devices (SGDs) difficult to use (Light & Drager, 2007).

FOCUS 10.9 *Clinical Skill Building*

Remember to consider the child's developmental level and what you would expect other children that age to do when recommending AAC technology as part of an intervention plan. What would a typically developing 3-year-old child be doing? Think of the participation model to keep your expectations and goals realistic and natural.

How do young children developing typically interact with a VSD? Researchers documented that, with only one exposure, three-year-old children initially experience difficulty finding vocabulary items in a visual scene. However, with additional exposure, children locate vocabulary items more quickly with a VSD as compared to finding items in a traditional grid layout. The researchers concluded embedding language concepts in visual scenes is a potentially effective approach for young children (Drager, Light, Carlson, D'Silva, Larsson, Pitkin et al., 2004). Additional ideas to be considered when recommending AAC devices for young children are provided in Focus 10.9. The modes of communication will change as children mature; Focus 10.10 provides questions to further your thinking in this regard.

Light and Drager (2007) introduced an AAC intervention using VSDs to children ages 1-3 years with developmental disabilities. Research demonstrated that the children (a) used the VSDs to participate in social interactions during the initial introduction (with modeling from the adult) and (b) increased the number of independent communication turns during the initial session and in conversations over time. The children in the study eventually learned to use other types of displays, including traditional grid layouts. It was concluded that initial exposure to language concepts and contextual communicative messages via VSDs may serve as a springboard for other forms of communication.

In the sections above, I have stressed the value of SAL and VSD approaches. However, an approach will only be effective if it is introduced and taught using high-quality training techniques. In the example above, I noted how modeling was used to introduce the VSD to young children. Modeling by other communication partners also is important.

FOCUS 10.10 *Clinical Skill Building*

AAC intervention should be multi-modal. What does this mean? What are different modes of communication? What would be appropriate modes of communication for a 2-year-old? How about for a 5-year-old?

Overall Research Results for AAC Interventions.   Light and Drager (2006) described the initial results of a study where very young children (ages 8-40 months) were introduced to appealing, easy-to-use AAC technologies in meaningful social contexts. The children's parents were simultaneously taught to model the use of the AAC device during interactive play, social routines, games, and reading activities. Results were impressive; noted improvements in communication skills occurred with respect to (a) turn-taking behaviors, (b) semantic development, (c) vocabulary acquisition rate, and (d) ability to combine concepts to express complex messages. In addition, the researchers reported the children used their AAC systems to communicate, play, and learn new concepts in addition to developing phonological awareness and literacy skills.

PICTURE EXCHANGE COMMUNICATION SYSTEM (PECS)

The **Picture Exchange Communication System (PECS)** is a popular treatment approach used frequently with children who are on the autism spectrum. In recent years, PECS also has been used with children and adults with other diagnoses (Bondy & Frost, 2009). "The primary goal of PECS is to teach functional communication" (Bondy & Frost, 2009, p. 298). PECS is based on principles of applied behavior analysis (Bondy & Frost, 2009). The protocol has six phases; see Table 10.2 for a summary of each phase of PECS.

Despite its popularity, there is limited research to support the use of PECS as a language intervention approach. Schlosser and Wendt (2007) conducted a systematic

Table 10.2   **Phases of the PECS Protocol**

Phase	Description
I. Teaching the communicative exchange	The child learns how to request by selecting a picture of an item he or she desires and giving it to or exchanging it with a communication partner for the chosen item. The picture is a graphic symbol representing the object.
II. Teaching persistence	The child learns how to exchange pictures with increasing distances to communication partners and/or to the communication pictures.
III. Discrimination training	The child learns how to discriminate between two choices.
IV. Teaching *I want* sentences	The child learns how to use a picture representing *I want* before selecting the desired object.
V. Teaching a response to *What do you want*?	The child learns to respond to the question: *What do you want*?
VI. Teaching use of additional sentence starters	The child learns new sentence starters such as *I see* to develop commenting.

Source: From "The Picture Exchange Communication System," by A. Bondy and L. Frost, 2009. In P. Mirenda and T. Iacono (Eds.), *Autism Spectrum Disorders and AAC* (pp. 279–302). Baltimore, MD: Brookes.

review to determine the effectiveness of PECS instruction on prelinguistic behaviors, speech production, expressive social regulation, and communicative functions of children with ASD. They reviewed 12 studies with a total of 105 participants; their results indicated that PECS only improved the communicative function of requesting in a small number of the studies. As you recall from Chapter 2, requesting is a pragmatic function used to regulate or control the actions of others (Halliday, 1975).

Wendt (2008) conducted another systematic review of research investigating AAC intervention using graphic symbols for children with autism spectrum disorder (ASD). His review of 15 studies found strong evidence that graphic symbols improved children's ability to request; however, no evidence indicated that certain graphic symbols worked better than others. Wendt also concluded the available evidence did not support a specific intervention approach for teaching children to use graphic symbols. Wendt summarized his results by stating that when the interventionist develops graphic symbol intervention for a child with ASD, the interventionist should consider the iconicity of symbols, along with the child's information-processing abilities, learning style, and cognitive abilities.

Summary

- In this chapter, I introduced AAC as an approach for improving children's language and communication treatment. The evidence is clear that children with language concerns and complex communication needs often benefit from an AAC approach. AAC interventions (a) enhance participation in meaningful activities, (b) help meet an individual's communication needs, (c) facilitate language and literacy development, and (d) improve an individual's language skills.
- The benefits of an AAC approach are numerous. Examples include language learning in supported natural activities, increased use of multiple modes of communication, increased participation in communicative interactions, and increased interactions with peers in a variety of different environments.
- When an individual has communication needs that are not being met, these are called complex communication needs (CCNs). CCNs may stem from language comprehension and production impairments in spoken and written language. Language impairments may affect communication opportunities and social participation.
- AAC systems are comprised of four critical components. The components of an AAC system are symbols, aids, strategies, and techniques. Symbols can be graphic, auditory, gestural, and textured or tactile and are used to represent language concepts. An AAC aid refers to a device that can be used to send or receive messages. An AAC strategy refers to methods used to communicate effectively and efficiently. AAC strategies support message timing, grammatical formulation, spelling, and communication rate. Technique refers to how a message is conveyed. Some individuals who have an AAC system use their finger to point to symbols or look directly at the intended object; scanning is another AAC technique. An AAC

system is part of a multi-modal view of communication. Multi-modal refers to the use of multiple modalities when a person communicates.

- AAC is not an intervention approach used to replace speech but rather to augment the skills the child has and to provide alternative strategies and techniques when needed to enhance language development and overall communication skills. It is a common misconception that the use of AAC will hinder speech and language development; recent research demonstrates this is not true.
- Additional assessment components for a potential AAC user include (a) identification of participation patterns, (b) the identification of the individual's communication needs, (c) a capabilities assessment, (d) a symbol assessment, and (e) trials with different AAC system features.
- The System for Augmenting Language (SAL) is a total-immersion approach to teaching language comprehension and use. The SAL approach uses graphic symbols to help students communicate for social purposes. Students who use SAL learn to use referential and social-regulatory symbols in a variety of communication environments. Visual scene displays (VSDs) can be used in an intervention program to support language by organizing vocabulary and communicative messages in a scene display rather than in a grid format. The advantages are that VSDs use scenes representing familiar events and activities; this maximizes meaningfulness and preserves the authenticity of everyday life. There is evidence that the Picture Exchange Communication System (PECS) helps children learn to request by exchanging a picture system for a desired object. There is limited evidence supporting PECS as a language development intervention program.

Discussion and In-Class Activities

1. In the past, AAC was thought of as an approach of last resort. Results from numerous studies provide evidence that using an AAC approach supports language development and provides another mode of communication. Interview a speech-language pathologist. Ask if he or she has used an AAC approach to support language development in addition to supporting expressive communication. How did he or she measure progress? Did he or she have support of the family? Did he or she use any of the AAC interventions introduced in this chapter? What were the outcomes?

2. Check out the Resources section of this chapter. Are these journals or books available at your library?

3. Go to the Web site developed by Drs. Janice Light and David McNaughton at http://aacliteracy.psu.edu/ to learn about the evidence and resources supporting literacy development for children with CCNs.

4. Roleplay a discussion you might have with a classroom teacher. The teacher is concerned that using an AAC device with a child in her classroom may limit the child's efforts at verbal speech.

Resources

Binger, C., & Light, J. (2006). Demographics of preschoolers who require AAC. *Language, Speech, and Hearing Services in Schools, 37*, 200–208.

Blackstone, S. (2006). *Augmentative Communication News*. Monterey, CA: Augmentative Communication, Inc.

Fallon, K., Light, J., & Achenbach, A. (2003). The semantic organization patterns of young children: Implications for augmentative and alternative communication. *Augmentative and Alternative Communication, 19*, 74–85.

Fallon, K., Light, J., & Kramer Paige, T. (2001). Enhancing vocabulary selection for preschoolers who require augmentative and alternative communication (AAC). *American Journal of Speech-Language Pathology, 10*, 81–94.

Goossens', C., & Crain, S. (1987). Overview of nonelectronic eye-gaze communication techniques. *Augmentative and Alternative Communication, 3*, 77–89.

Harris, M., & Reichle, J. (2004). The impact of aided language stimulation on symbol comprehension and production in children with moderate cognitive disabilities. *American Journal of Speech-Language Pathology, 13*, 155–167.

Johnston, S., Reichle, J., & Evans, J. (2004). Supporting augmentative and alternative communication use by beginning communicators with severe disabilities. *American Journal of Speech-Language Pathology, 13*, 20–30.

Light, J. (1997). "Let's go star fishing": Reflections on the contexts of language learning for children who use aided AAC. *Augmentative and Alternative Communication, 13*, 158–171.

Light, J., & Drager, K. (2002). Improving the design of augmentative and alternative technologies for young children. *Assistive Technology, 14*, 17–32.

Light, J., Drager, K., McCarthy, J., Mellott, S., Millar, D., Parrish, C., Parsons, A., Rhoads, S., Ward, M., & Welliver, M. (2004). Performance of typically developing four- and five-year-old children with AAC systems using different language organization techniques. *Augmentative and Alternative Communication, 20*, 63–88.

Light, J., Drager, K., & Nemser, J. (2004). Enhancing the appeal of AAC technologies for young children: Lessons from the toy manufacturers. *Augmentative and Alternative Communication, 20*, 137–149.

Mirenda, P. & Iacono, T. (Eds.) (2009). *Autism spectrum disorders and AAC*. Baltimore, MD: Brookes.

Paul, R. (1997). Facilitating transitions in language development for children using AAC. *Augmentative and Alternative Communication, 13*, 141–148.

Reichle, J., Beukelman, D. R., & Light, J. C. (Eds.) (2002). *Exemplary practices for beginning communicators: Implications for AAC*. Baltimore, MD: Brookes.

Romski, M., & Sevcik, R. A. (2005). Augmentative communication and early intervention: Myths and realities. *Infants & Young Children, 18*, 174–185.

Soto, G., & Zangari, C. (Eds.) (2009). *Practically speaking: Language, literacy, and academic development for students with AAC needs*. Baltimore, MD: Brookes.

Chapter 10 Case Study

Background.   Ben is a 4-year-old boy who lives with his parents and 6-year-old brother. Ben's mother reports a normal pregnancy with no complications and an unremarkable birth at 39 weeks. Ben has a history of multiple ear infections and has been diagnosed with spastic cerebral palsy. Ben is ambulatory with the assistance of a walker. He uses speech to communicate but he has dysarthria which results in imprecise articulation. Ben's parents report they understand his speech about 75% of the time but other communication partners only understand 50% of his speech. Ben's parents are concerned because Ben often gets frustrated when he has difficulty expressing himself or he is not understood. Ben is starting 4-year-old kindergarten soon and the parents are concerned how his communication challenges will impact his academic success and social interactions.

Ben's Assessment.   Ben is referred to you, the school SLP. First you plan your assessment. Refer to the Assessment section of this chapter for the components of a comprehensive AAC assessment. Let's walk through the steps of an AAC assessment together using Ben as an example.

1. Gather case history information. I provided background information in the earlier description. These are questions I ask myself as I prepare for an assessment: When did he get the diagnosis of cerebral palsy? Has he received any services, medical or therapy, for symptoms related to his cerebral palsy? What modes of communication does Ben use (e.g., facial expressions, gestures, signs, speech)? Has he had his hearing tested? How many ear infections has he had? (What do you think when you hear Ben has had multiple ear infections? How can ear infections affect language development?) Does Ben have a motor speech disorder (i.e., dysarthria)? Does Ben have feeding or swallowing difficulty? Who does Ben communicate with? Where does Ben communicate? What does Ben communicate about? Are those topics similar to those of other 4-year-old boys? Other issues are considered in Focus 10.11.
2. Identify participation patterns. How will you do this? Why is it important for you to know about typically developing 4-year-old children? How will you determine if there are any barriers affecting Ben's participation in life situations?

FOCUS 10.11 *Clinical Skill Building*

Can you think of any other questions you would want to ask before you begin the assessment? Why is it important to gather this information before you begin your assessment with Ben?

3. Complete a communication needs assessment. You will need to interview Ben's parents and observe and interact with Ben at his home. Let's say you discover that Ben communicates in the following environments, with the following partners, and about the following topics. What other information might be missing?

Current Partners	Environments	Topics
Parents	Home	Toys
Sibling	Relatives' homes	Food
Grandparents	Parks	Books
Friends	Church	TV
People at church	Stores	Family
People in the community	Restaurants	

4. Complete a capability assessment. For our example, let's assume your capability assessment reveals the following.
   a. Ben passed his hearing screening.
   b. Ben's parents report Ben had his vision checked recently and there are no concerns.
   c. Ben's receptive language skills are at expected levels for his chronological age; his expressive language is delayed with a MLU of 2.2. Examples of Ben's utterances include "*Where doggie?*" "*Doggie running*" and "*Play car*".
   d. Ben recognizes 75% of the letters in the alphabet.
   e. Ben's speech is characterized by imprecise articulation and low volume from a moderate spastic dysarthria.
   f. The occupational therapist (OT) and the physical therapist (PT) report Ben is right-hand dominant but uses both hands for gross- and fine motor tasks. Ben holds and uses large crayons and large pencils with built-up grips. He ambulates with the assistance of a walker. A basket could be mounted on the front of Ben's walker to hold an AAC system.

5. Complete a symbol assessment. You find Ben successfully matches objects to objects, miniature objects, photographs, and both black-and-white and colored line drawings. He is not successful matching the objects to printed words.

6. Remember to include AAC system features trials in your assessment.
   a. Symbols: Interactive play activities are used to teach Ben the meaning of symbols and provide opportunities for him to use the symbols. Given the results of the symbols assessment, colored line drawings with the printed word are used in each activity.
   b. Aids: Different types of aids are used to augment Ben's input (i.e., teach Ben new vocabulary) and facilitate his participation in play activities. A nonelectronic communication board, an SGD with digitized speech (i.e., human-recorded speech), and an SGD with synthesized speech (i.e., computer-generated speech) are all tried with Ben during the assessment. Ben uses all types of aids successfully during the assessment. He independently communicates messages and answers questions using an electronic SGD with speech output.

c. Strategies: Ben is taught and uses symbols to generate sentences using the sequencing of 2-3 symbols, is taught to use symbols to represent entire messages for quick communication (i.e., encoding), and is given opportunities to use VSDs to facilitate understanding of language concepts and expression of ideas.

d. Techniques: Ben is successful with directly selecting symbols and areas on both nonelectronic aids and electronic aids with his right index finger. His accuracy for selection is 100%.

e. Selection set: Ben is successful using static displays during interactive activities to request activities, answer questions, and express his feelings. He also is successful using a dynamic display as he navigates between pages with minimal prompting to talk about his interests, request an activity, and while participating in a card game. Ben also uses VSDs successfully during the assessment session. He demonstrates understanding of language concepts displayed on visual scenes, uses the display to request activities, and initiates a topic regarding a recent family trip (using a family photograph Ben's parents have brought to the assessment).

Writing an Intervention Plan.   You have learned about Ben's current communication. Now it is time to formulate an intervention plan. You know Ben has complex communication needs (CCNs) secondary to his dysarthria and expressive language impairment. Why would Ben benefit from an AAC approach to treatment? An AAC approach would facilitate his expressive language development, meet his current communication needs, and address participation patterns for now and in the future.

Based on the assessment results, a multi-modal communication intervention approach including an AAC system is recommended. Ask yourself: which modes of communication does Ben use; how might an AAC system augment his current modes of communication and add an alternative mode; what AAC features did Ben have success using during the assessment; what AAC features would enhance Ben's communication; and how might an AAC system facilitate participation in life situations for Ben? (see Focus 10.12 for more issues that should be considered). We know Ben successfully uses the following AAC features: color line drawings with the printed word, direct selection, encoding, speech output, and all types of displays. There are several different SGDs with these features available commercially. Your job is to match the features Ben uses successfully with an available SGD and provide a trial period of use for him during your intervention. Remember that AAC assessments are dynamic and ongoing. The best intervention plan will include extensive opportunities for Ben to learn his AAC system and use it in naturalistic situations.

FOCUS 10.12 *Clinical Skill Building*

What do you think when you hear Ben gets frustrated when he experiences difficulty communicating? How is language expression different from speech production? How could difficulty producing speech impact language development?

Multicultural Issues

—Stephanie M. Curenton

Chapter Overview Questions

1. What is the definition of an ethnic group?
2. What are the multicultural challenges for speech-language pathologists (SLPs) and special educators?
3. Describe characteristics potentially occurring in children who are connected to the African American, Latino, Asian American, and Native American cultural groups?
4. Describe the terms *acculturation, individualism, collectivism, bilingualism,* and *bidialectism*
5. How is a child's school achievement impacted by his or her culture and language?
6. How can assessment and intervention practices be modified in response to a child's language and cultural status?

> The important point here is that "My language is me." It is an extension of my being, my essence. It is a reflection and badge of my culture." (Williams, 1997, p. 209).

If you walk through almost any U.S. city or town, you see the diversity of America. U.S. cities, and even some rural hometowns, are the homes for people of many colors, cultures, family practices, ethnic traditions, and languages. Population statistics from Table 11.1 show that this growth in diversity has occurred over the last three decades.

Our country is expected to become even more diverse due to the increase in immigrant families to the United States. In 2005, approximately one out of five American children lived in immigrant families; most of these children are citizens born in the United States (Kids Count, 2007). In the map of the United States

Table 11.1   **Changing Ethnic Demographics in the United States**

Ethnic origin	Percentage of U.S. population				
	1970	1980	1990	2000	2050 (projected)
European (White)	83.7	80	75	70	50
African (Black)	10.6	11.5	12	12*	13
Latino (Hispanic)	4.5	6.4	9	13*	24
Asian	1.0	1.5	3	4*	9
Native American	.4	.6	.7	.9*	1

*In 2000, about 70% of new immigrants to the United States were from Latin America or Asia; a third of all students in U.S. schools are individuals of color.

Source: From Population Reference Bureau (2001). *Migration and Immigration.* Retrieved from www.prb.org/CPIPR/Topics/MigrationImmigration/Trends.aspx?p=1.

presented in Figure 11.1, you can see the vast majority of children born from first-generation immigrants live in California, Nevada, New York, Texas, and New Jersey.

About 25 percent of immigrant children live in **linguistically isolated** households, meaning that no one over the age of 14 living in the household speaks

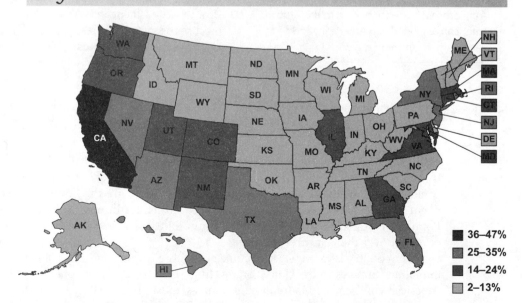

Figure 11.1   **Percentage of Immigrant Children by State**

Legend:
- 36–47%
- 25–35%
- 14–24%
- 2–13%

Source: "The American Community Survey," by Mark Mather, Kerri L. Rivers, and Linda A. Jacobsen, 2005. *Population Bulletin 60, no. 3*, Washington, DC: Population Reference Bureau.

fluent English (Kids Count, 2007). It is important to recognize that not all children living in immigrant families will need the specialized services of language specialists, but some of them, especially those from linguistically isolated households, may need short-term remedial language and literacy interventions to help English language learners. SLPs can partner with teachers to design and deliver these interventions.

Given the diversity of today's environment, practitioners must be knowledgeable and experienced in working with children and families from all cultural, language, and ethnic backgrounds. This chapter provides you with an overview of important concepts and skills you will need to understand and work with ethnically diverse families.

Ethnicity and Culture

An **ethnic group** is a group of individuals who share a common language, heritage, religion, or geography/nationality (Smedley & Smedley, 2005). Commonly, Americans are classified as falling within one of five ethnic groups: European American, Black American, Latino American, Asian American, and Native American. For centuries, these categories were mistakenly believed to represent racial categories related to genetic or biological differences between people. However, today new science using sophisticated techniques to investigate genetic codes and variations reveals there is no scientific basis for believing that people who look different have vastly different genetic codes (Caesar & Williams, 2002; Witzig, 1996). If you take a group of people from different ethnic groups and compare their DNA, scientists report that individuals share over 90% of the same genes (Jorde & Wooding, 2004)!

This new line of genetic research explains that the concept of *race* is a falsehood developed in the 17th and 18th centuries, before scholars accurately understood genetics or evolutionary biology (Witzig, 1996). The truth is that race is a social construct that is based on society's ever-changing historical and political views of its citizens. For example, while searching the historical records for information about my great-great grandmother who was a full-blooded Cherokee Indian, I learned that in the late 1800s Native Americans in South Carolina were classified as Black. This example shows how people might be classified differently depending on when the government is collecting information.

Given this new scientific knowledge, it is best to understand the current classification system of Americans as ethnic groups rather than racial groups. However, defining an ethnic group is more complex than simply considering a person's physical characteristics. The process of defining an ethnic group is difficult because people always fall into multiple ethnic groups. For example, you might be a Catholic (religion) European American (nationality) whose family is from the Appalachian region of the country (geography). In this example, the three ethnic groups you could belong to include Catholic Americans, European Americans, and Appalachian Americans. It is important to understand how ethnic groups are defined because it reminds us that the system of ethnic categorization is multi-layered.

RELATIONSHIP BETWEEN ETHNICITY AND CULTURE

Our current ethnic classification system is useful because it provides a general framework for understanding how cultural traditions are intertwined with ethnicity. **Cultural frameworks** consist of social practices, beliefs, values, and behaviors that members of a group intentionally—and unintentionally—use to communicate and interact (Goffman, 1986). Cultural frameworks are passed down throughout generations. Language is a primary means for transmitting cultural traditions. Through language, we learn our culture's values, expectations, roles, and rules. Language traditions shape our observations, interactions, and interpretations about our environment.

WORKING WITH DIVERSE POPULATIONS

Working with ethnically diverse children and families presents an opportunity for personal growth because it is a chance for each professional to reflect on his or her own culture. Through self-reflection we can expand our attitudes, beliefs, and behaviors by thinking about the strengths and weaknesses of our culture—and learning more about the cultural traditions of others. Being **culturally reflective** means recognizing that you are a product of the beliefs, values, and social-political history of your own ethnic group. Cultural reflection is often difficult to do because it is a common human error to assume that a person acts based on individual beliefs, values, and behaviors. We assume that the way we act is the right or sensible way to do things. We fail to recognize that we are taught our beliefs, values, and behaviors by family and community members. It takes a special effort to examine our actions, values, and beliefs with respect to our cultural heritage. However, it is important for us to go through this cultural reflection because cultural self-reflection ultimately leads to cultural sensitivity.

Cultural sensitivity means being aware and nonjudgmental of the cultural practices of various groups. A culturally sensitive professional understands that his or her way of speaking and interacting is no more right or sensible than the interaction patterns of another cultural group. Cultural sensitivity can be achieved through **cultural dialogue** with people from various ethnic groups. The goal of cultural dialogue is to gather information and knowledge to generate new ideas and insights into people's behavior, values, and life experiences (Gonzalez-Mena, 2008). Cultural dialogue expands our view of the world and reminds us that not everyone does things the way our families, communities, or cultural groups do them, and other ways of doing things are equally as valid and useful. In Focus 11.1, you will find an example of a European American woman's cultural reflection. Take some time to read her reflection, and then use the questions to help guide you through your own cultural reflection.

MULTICULTURAL CHALLENGES

More than half of children in the United States who receive services for speech and language are from ethnic minority groups (U.S. Department of Education, 2002); this trend presents challenges to the field. One challenge is the occurrence of client-practitioner ethnic mismatch; over 90 percent of speech-language pathologists are women of European descent (ASHA, 2006). The match between practitioner and

FOCUS 11.1 *Multicultural Issues*

A European American Woman's Cultural Reflection

As a white, middle-class American with mostly Anglo-Saxon and Celtic heritage, I was surprised to discover that I [even] had a culture. I, like everyone else, moved within a cultural framework every minute of every day. That framework is influenced by and includes many [cultural attributes], some of which I am extremely conscious, but some of which I am barely aware. My life is influenced by my:

- Race
- Gender
- Age
- Abilities and disabilities
- Language
- Social class, including occupational status and income level
- Ethnicity and national origin
- Religion and/or spiritual practice
- Geographic location of where I grew up and where I presently live
- Sexuality, including sexual orientation

My framework influences the way I think, act, feel, and how I interpret the world. So how does my cultural experience as a white, middle-class woman influence my experiences and interactions? It shields me from reality. It gives me a slanted perspective, a narrow view. Besides, it gives me a false impression of importance, letting me believe "my people" are the only ones who count in the world, when in reality, white, middle-class Anglo-Americans like me are a small minority of the world population.

Imagine the harm I can do to both "my people" and to those whose differences I ignore when I carry out my job with this biased attitude. Imagine what my students can do to the children they work with when they define "normality" in the narrow ways they learn from me. What does it do to people who are different from me to have those differences be defined as abnormal? What does it do to the people who are different from me to have those differences ignored?

_____

Source: Based on information from *Diversity in Early Care and Education* (pp. 8–9, 10), by J. Gonzalez-Mena, 2008, Boston: McGraw-Hill.

client is important because although some African American children do not believe the SLP's ethnicity matters (Roseti et al., 2001), there are other children who may mistrust SLPs or teachers who are European American (Terrell, Battle, & Grantham, 1998). So as practitioners, our presence might have a positive or neutral effect on some clients, but a negative effect on others. The field is responding to this challenge of client-practitioner mismatch by recruiting SLPs and teachers from minority ethnic groups.

The second challenge is that all practitioners, regardless of their ethnicity, are unintentionally operating from the European cultural framework because they have been trained to use language philosophies, assessment instruments, procedures, and intervention practices stemming from a European tradition (see Hwa-Froelich & Vigil, 2004). Practitioners must realize that they are operating from European traditions and understand the implications of socioeconomic and regional differences. There is a need for new knowledge that considers the traditions, values, and experiences of multiple cultural groups. The field is making strides in this area by offering courses focusing on the language needs of ethnic minorities; however, programs must make these courses mandatory rather than optional. In addition, the field must make efforts to fund new research investigating the language practices of clients from various ethnic groups.

The third challenge is that, at present, many practitioners are not trained to properly diagnose and treat ethnic minority children from non-English language backgrounds. Forty percent of SLPs report they have only basic knowledge of second language acquisition and its impact on children's academic success (ASHA, 2003). This lack of training results in a disproportionate number of ethnic minority children being represented in special education. While Asian and Latino children are likely to be underrepresented in special education classes, African American and Native American children are overrepresented.

Professionals often are not prepared to treat or intervene with families who live in poverty. Ethnic minorities are more likely to live in poverty than European Americans (Donovan & Cross, 2002). Recent statistics indicate that only 8% of European Americans live in poverty compared to 25% of African Americans, 22% of Latinos, and 25% of Native Americans (Center for American Progress Task Force on Poverty [Center for American Progress], 2007). Figure 11.2 demonstrates that this income disparity has persisted throughout the last two decades. There are also variations in poverty status among Asian Americans. Some nationalities of Asians,

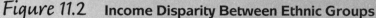

Figure 11.2   **Income Disparity Between Ethnic Groups**

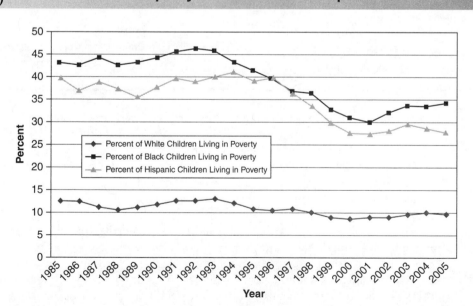

Source: Child Well-Being Index 2007 Report: Key Indicator Figures by Race/Ethnicity. Foundation for Child Development. Retrieved from www.fcd-us.org/resources/resources_show.htm?doc_id=472847. Used with permission.

such as Hmong, Cambodian, and Laotian have rates of poverty similar to the poverty rates reported for African Americans and Native Americans (Ceasar & Williams, 2002).

Families living in poverty are less likely to have access to health care benefits (Center for American Progress, 2007). Often speech and language problems are the result of unaddressed basic health problems. It is important to help families seek needed medical services because ethnic minorities are more likely to develop diseases resulting in communication disorders (Caesar & Williams, 2002).

Description of the Diverse Populations

Below I describe four major American ethnic groups: African, Latino, Asian, and Native American ethnic traditions. I describe these ethnic traditions in terms of "general" language beliefs, values, and socialization traditions. I like to think about it as describing traditions across ethnic groups rather than describing individual children and families.

Remember there is a wide range of diversity within each of the four groups. Although it is true that many children have been socialized into a primary language tradition, some children are exposed to a variety of language traditions. For example, my friend Krista, who is Korean American, has two children who are Korean and Haitian American; their father immigrated to the Unites States from Haiti. Therefore, since birth her children have been spoken to in Korean, English, and Haitian Creole and have been socialized into three language traditions. You can read more about **Creole language** in Focus 11.2.

It is important for professionals to consider a range of factors to sensitively work with families. Two families in your classroom or caseload may be from a similar general language tradition, but have different cultural nuances based on nationality and geography. For example, people from an African-based language tradition include individuals who describe themselves as African American, African, West Indian, and

FOCUS 11.2 *Learning More*

How Does Pidgin Become a Creole Language?

Pidgin develops as "emergency" communication that results from individuals from various language backgrounds being forced together unexpectedly, usually resulting from colonization. In order to communicate, the group develops a **pidgin language**, consisting of rudimentary syntax and vocabulary forms. Initially, pidgin is a very basic system of communication created as the need arises. Subsequently, first generation pidgin speakers teach their children the pidgin language. Due to generation-to-generation teaching, the pidgin becomes a rule-governed system with a set syntax and expanded vocabulary. The pidgin language is then considered a Creole language; all Creole languages have a syntactical structure (Bickerton, 1995).

Afro-Caribbean (e.g., Jamaicans, Haitians, the Bahamians, or others of African descendent who reside in the Caribbean Islands). Many Blacks living in America who are from Africa or the Caribbean are immigrants who face challenges similar to immigrants from other ethnic traditions; challenges include poverty and a lack of health insurance. Table 11.2 shows that many immigrants of African descent come from an African nation. In addition, this figure shows that West Indians make up a small portion of the American population. Most who describe themselves as West Indian are also of African heritage, and their families may have emigrated from counties like Trinidad, Guyana, Barbados, or Belize.

Latinos also come from a variety of nationalities within their larger ethnic group. As Table 11.2 visually demonstrates, Mexicans are the largest group, followed by

Table 11.2 **Racial and Ethnic Categories in the United States, 2000**

Racial or ethnic classification	Approximate U.S. population	Percentage of total population
Hispanic descent	39,305,818	12.5%
Mexican	20,640,711	7.3
Puerto Rican	3,406,178	1.2
Cuban	1,241,685	.4
Other Hispanic	10,017,244	3.6
African descent	34,659,190	12.3
Nigerian	165,481	0.1
Ethiopian	86,918	<
Cape Verdean	77,103	<
Ghanaian	49,944	<
South African	45,569	<
Native American descent	2,475,956	0.9
American Indian	1,815,653	0.6
Eskimo	45,919	<
Other Native American	614,384	0.2
Asian or Pacific Island descent	10,641,833	3.8
Chinese	2,432,585	0.9
Filipino	1,850,314	0.7
Asian Indian	1,678,765	0.6
Vietnamese	1,122,528	0.4
Korean	1,076,872	0.4
Japanese	796,700	0.3
Cambodian	171,937	<
Hmong	169,428	<
Laotian	168,707	<
Other Asian or Pacific Islander	1,173,997	0.4

Racial or ethnic classification	Approximate U.S. population	Percentage of total population
West Indian descent	1,869,504	0.7
Arab descent	1,202,871	0.4
Non-Hispanic European descent	194,552,774	70.9
German	42,885,162	15.2
Irish	30,528,492	10.8
English	24,515,138	8.7
Italian	15,723,555	5.6
Polish	8,977,444	3.2
French	8,309,908	3.0
Scottish	4,890,581	1.7
Dutch	4,542,494	1.6
Norwegian	4,477,726	1.6
Two or more races	6,826,228	2.4

Source: Society: The Basics (10th ed.), by J. J. Macionis, © 2009, p. 308. Reprinted by permission of Pearson Education, Inc., Upper Saddle River, NJ.

Central/South Americans, Puerto Ricans, and Cubans. Mexican Americans primarily live in the Southwest, but Puerto Ricans tend to live in the Northeast, and Cubans tend to live in Florida (Iglesias, 2002). So when working with the Latino population, practitioners must be mindful of the state in which they are working because different nationalities of Latinos will vary in their cultural heritage.

Americans from the Asian tradition may come from Asia or islands in the Pacific Ocean. The largest Asian population in America is from China, followed by Korea, and then Japan (Cheng, 2002). Other nationalities of Asians include those families from Southeast Asian countries like Vietnam, Thailand, Laos, Cambodia, and Burma.

The larger Native American ethnic group consists of numerous tribes, each of which is distinct in terms of tradition. The current population of Native Americans is 2.4 million. Three fourths of Native Americans live out West in rural communities, and about 48% of Native Americans live on, or adjacent to, a Native American reservation (Westby & Vining, 2002). Within the Native American tradition it is important to know whether the family lives within or outside a reservation because resources and community support will vary accordingly.

Issues to Consider When Working with Ethnically Diverse Populations

Working with ethnically diverse families provides an opportunity to understand the complex macrosystem influences on a family. Ethnic minority families operate according to their own cultural traditions while living in a country in which the European ethnic tradition is in power. Before discussing the important issues related to ethnically diverse populations, I want to discuss the terminology I will use to discuss the majority (European) culture in the United States.

The term **dominant culture** has been used to describe the traditions, values, beliefs, and behaviors associated with European American language traditions. However, the term has negative connotations because it signifies this cultural group as having power without acknowledging the pilfering, social injustices, and oppression via colonization and slavery that occurred to gain this power. The term *dominant culture* also places the European American tradition as the gold standard to which all other traditions are compared. As a result, other cultural groups are not examined in their own right as unique and viable cultures. Another issue associated with politics, power, and language is discussed in Focus 11.3.

Another term used to describe the European American tradition is **mainstream culture**. However, this term still regulates other culture groups to the status of

---

FOCUS 11.3 *Learning More*

The Politics of Using African American English in School Systems

The debate surrounding the use of African American English Vernacular (AAEV) as a child's first language in U.S. classrooms has spurred a lot of controversy throughout several decades. This debate has even reached the U.S. Congress.

> *"Too many African-American children have been entering school year-in and year-out speaking different language patterns, something other than Standard English. . . . We should not continue to pretend that this situation does not exist. It does exist. The different language patterns are real . . . The fact of the matter is I think we all want the same thing. We want our students to speak Standard English"* (Maxine Waters, U. S. Congress, 1997, p. 1).

Surprisingly, the debate over AAEV in the classroom is not new. In July of 1979, parents of 11 African American elementary students charged the Ann Arbor public school district with a civil rights violation. Parents claimed that the schools failed to take appropriate actions to teach their children Standard

English, resulting in unequal education (Morgan, 2001). All the plaintiffs' children were African Americans living in public housing. Parents claimed that their children were failing academically because of education inequities; the children spoke "Black dialect" but the school had not taken appropriate action to overcome the barrier. The school district was found to be in violation of the Equal Opportunities Act of 1974 that states that children cannot be denied an equal education due to race, color, sex, or national origin.

Seventeen years later, a school district in California made a very different decision. In 1996, the Oakland school board decided to use AAEV to help children bridge into Standard English; it was felt that initially using AAE in classrooms would facilitate children's learning of Standard English. The Oakland school system adopted the Standard English Proficiency Program (S.E.P.), a cultural-linguistic program that teaches African Americans to recognize differences between home language and school language (i.e., Standard English). The Linguistic Society of America concluded that the Oakland school board decision was a linguistically sound and proper teaching method (Linguistic Society of America, 1997).

However, the media reported that the Oakland school district was teaching AAE instead of Standard English (Williams, 1997). The media reports created heated discussions among politicians and educators.

You should consider your own feelings about this controversy. It could be that the opposition to AAEV is rooted in this country's long history of linguistic chauvinism. It seems perfectly logical that we should use a child's home language system as a foundation for teaching a new language. Many multicultural experts believe that opposition to the idea stems from educators' lack of information about the AAEV language system and unwillingness to adapt teaching styles and assessment measurements to meet students' needs (Newell & Chambers, 1982).

deviant subcultures. So in this chapter, instead of using the terms *dominant* or *mainstream culture,* I refer to the European tradition.

In our discussion of the important issues in working with ethnically diverse families, I will discuss three important issues: (1) acculturation, (2) attitudes of individualism versus collectivism, and (3) the issue of an individual being bilingual versus bidialectal.

ACCULTURATION

The first issue to consider when working with ethnically diverse families is to understand a family's pattern of acculturation. **Acculturation** refers to the extent to which a family feels the need to maintain their own cultural identity while at the same time accepting the values and beliefs of the European American tradition. Table 11.3

Table 11.3   **Patterns of Acculturation**

Does the family value maintaining its own cultural tradition?

		YES	NO
		Integration	*Assimilation*
Does the family value adopting the cultural values, beliefs, and behaviors of the European American (EA) culture?	YES	A family wants to maintain their own culture while adopting the EA culture.	A family wants to adopt the EA and let go of their own culture.
		Separation	*Marginalization*
	NO	A family wants to maintain their own culture and does not want to adopt the EA culture.	A family is not able to maintain their own culture or adopt the EA culture.

Source: From "Consumer Acculturation Process and Cultural Conflict: How Generalizable Is a North American Model for Marketing Globally?" by J. W. Gentry, S. Jun, and P. Tansuhaj, 1995, *Journal of Business Research, 32,* pp. 129–139. Adapted with permission.

shows that the intersection of acculturation and cultural identity results in four acculturation patterns (Berry, 1990).

For some ethnic groups, such as Japanese Americans, Chinese Americans, Cuban Americans, or Mexican Americans, acculturation relates to generational patterns of immigration. **First-generation immigrants,** meaning individuals born in another country and migrating to the United States, typically adopt the pattern of integration because they want to maintain their own cultural traditions while adopting European American traditions. However, when the first-generation immigrants have children, the second generation (i.e., **second-generation immigrants**) often moves toward assimilation. An example of this would be a bilingual adult, who learned to speak Mandarin Chinese as a child, insisting on communicating only in English.

In a different pattern of acculturation, individuals in ethnic groups who did not immigrate to the United States by choice (such as African Americans, Native Hawaiians, or Native Americans) may adopt a separatist pattern. The separatist rejects European American values and clings to cultural traditions to protest the ethnic group's oppression. For example, Native Hawaiians, like the American Indians, are a minority group in their own land: only 6% of inhabitants of the state are full-blooded Native Hawaiians (Cheng, 2002). As a result, some Hawaiians choose to live in areas of the islands that are secluded and deliberately practice old traditions. Families who adopt a separatist pattern are not necessarily against the European American tradition. They are, however, trying to ensure that their ethnic tradition lives on. They believe they can best maintain their culture by being surrounded by members of their own tradition and deliberately carrying out cultural practices.

Like the first-generation immigrants, the majority of families from African American, Native Hawaiian, or Native American traditions want to integrate within the larger American society. This willingness to integrate typically increases from generation to generation due to changes in United States social policies. For instance, as a fifth-generation African American, I realize that I am a product of both African and other American traditions because I have been exposed to the African tradition through my family but I have been exposed to other traditions through school, work, and friendships.

Understanding a family's level of acculturation is important because it not only lets a practitioner know how familiar a family is with the American education and health systems, but it also guides the professional to understand how willing a family might be to accept direct guidance. An understanding of acculturation also provides insight into the family's socialization practices and language preferences.

INDIVIDUALISM VERSUS COLLECTIVISM

Individualist cultures focus on independence within individuals, whereas collectivist cultures focus on interdependence among group members. There are aspects of individualism and collectivism in all cultures, but each culture has a primary orientation. European cultures value individualism, but African, Asian, Latino, and Native American cultures value collectivism.

Individualism versus collectivism has implications for several aspects of family socialization. In an individualist culture, the focus is on the individual and his or her immediate (nuclear) family. In contrast, in a collectivist culture the individual focuses on the well-being of the group and the individual's relation to the family. For example, in most collectivist cultures elders are the leaders of the family (Cheng, 2002). When working with families from a collectivist culture, you might be surprised to find that parents rely on other family members and leaders in the community to help them make decisions about their children's health or education. As a result, you might find yourself in a session in which you are sharing assessment results with parents as well as additional family members whom the parents deem trustworthy and knowledgeable. In instances such as this it is important that you welcome these additional participants to the decision-making process and treat their questions and concerns with respect and consideration because it is quite possible that their opinions will help shape a parent's treatment decisions. The case study at the end of this chapter is an example of this situation. Focus 11.4 illustrates differences in social perceptions between members of a collectivist versus individualist culture.

FOCUS 11.4 *Clinical Skill Building*

Helping Clients Come to Therapy on Time

Many clinicians feel the frustration of working with families who always seem to be late for therapy appointments. As professionals, we learn that time is valuable, so when people are late we sometimes judge them as being inconsiderate and irresponsible. It is possible, however, that a perpetually late family has a different cultural orientation toward time.

Time orientation is one difference between an individualist and a collectivist culture (Hall, 1976; Harris, 1998). In individualist groups, such as the European American culture, there is an emphasis on "clock time" (or monochronic time); a monochronic time orientation means that promptness is a priority and events typically are scheduled and planned. In collectivist cultures, however, there is an emphasis on "event time" (or polychronic time); here event timing revolves around people and interpersonal transactions (Hall, 1976; Harris, 1998). In polychronic time, schedules might change due to family situations and interpersonal needs. For example, clients from collectivist cultures might be late to an appointment because they were obligated to run an errand for a family member or finish dinner as a family. These decisions reflect a cultural tradition that believes that interpersonal interactions and fulfilling group needs outweigh being on time for an appointment. According to a polychronic view of time, events start when the entire group is present, not at a scheduled arbitrary set time.

If practitioners want to ensure that clients come on time, it is best to appeal to them in a way that suggests event time rather than an abstract concept of clock time. Appeal to the

(continued)

family's sense of collectivism and group orientation by explaining how showing up late will mean that another family (who is scheduled following their child's appointment) may miss their therapy session. This explanation supports the polychronic tradition because it focuses on a collectivist versus individualist perspective.

You might also want to consider asking families if they have other important family commitments before or after the appointment. For example, clients may miss therapy sessions because of religious commitments, such as Wednesday night Bible study for Christians or the Muslim day of prayer on Friday evenings (Tellis & Tellis, 2003).

In an individualist society, the goal is to foster children's self-esteem, individuality, and independence; in a collectivist society the goal is to foster interpersonal skills including being polite, well liked, and obedient (Hwa-Froelich & Westby, 2003). Because collectivist cultures emphasize the needs and goals of the group over those of the individual, members of collectivist groups place a high value on personality and social skills because good social skills allow a child to successfully function within a group. This collectivist versus individual cultural focus impacts home-based socialization patterns. In Focus 11.5, you can read about how one family's goals for an intervention differed from the goals set forth from a European tradition.

BILINGUALISM

Approximately 14% of the American population speaks a language other than English (Iglesias, 2002). Spanish is the second most widely spoken language in the United States. Speaking Spanish is one of the major ties that bind the Latino population, and it is spoken by three fourths of Latinos (Iglesias, 2002). Latinos have

FOCUS 11.5 *Family Issues*

Part C of the Individuals with Disabilities Education Act requires that families be involved in the assessment and intervention process of their infants and toddlers. Therefore, practitioners need to recognize family values and beliefs and respect kinship roles. They must understand the traditions of the people. In one example, a young Native American mother brought her son into Indian Health Services for a medical examination. The doctor diagnosed the child with otitis media (OM), and out of what he considered thoughtfulness and consideration, the doctor offered to insert the myringotomies (i.e., "tubes" in the ear) that afternoon in order to save the mother a trip back to the clinic. The nurse recognized the mother's discomfort and in talking with her learned that the mother needed to have a traditional ceremony done for her son before he could have any type of surgery (example adapted from Westby & Vining, 2002).

received a great deal of attention in the past three decades due to the rapid population growth in this group and the community's strong support for bilingualism (Iglesias, 2002). Most members of the Latino language tradition recognize the benefits of being bilingual. Being literate (meaning being able to speak and read fluently) in English provides greater educational and employment opportunities. Being literate in Spanish offers children ethnic pride, cultural tradition, and the ability to communicate with non-English family members, and for recently immigrated families it also allows children to serve critical roles as language liaisons. For example, a bilingual child was able to help her father receive the care he needed while in an emergency room in southern Texas:

> Hace unos meses tuve un accidente en Lakewood. Y en el hospital, ella estaba hablando con las personas. Yo no les entendí nunca nada. Mi hija ha sido para mí muy importante. Para mí, mi hija vale dos personas.

> A few months ago, I had an accident in Lakewood. And in the hospital, she [my daughter] was talking with the people. I didn't understand a thing. My daughter has been very important for me. For me, my daughter is worth two people. (Worthy & Rodriguez-Galindo, 2006, p. 579)

Only a few native languages continue to be spoken by large groups of people. Today the most widely spoken native languages are Cherokee, Navajo, and Teton Sioux/Dakota. By 2020, it is projected that only 20 native languages in total will remain (Westby & Vining, 2002). The Native American Language Act of 1990 recognized the importance of traditional native languages; the act provides funds for language conservation and renewal (Reyhner, 1992). As a result, several tribes have developed education models to teach their native language. Some studies suggest that Native American children achieve best in school when they are taught in their first language through the early school years (Hakuta, 1990).

Using Interpreters. Even though the previous story about the Mexican father in the emergency room provides a poignant example of how family members can bridge language gaps during emergency situations, it is imperative that only trained, professional interpreters be used when working with bilingual clients and families. Family members are not objective interpreters. Sometimes family members might change responses to minimize the client's speech disorder or to present the family more favorably (Kayser, 1995). In contrast, Native American families may fail to report all of their child's strengths and skills because in Native American culture it is inappropriate—and bad luck—to speak highly of an individual (Scollon & Scollon, 1980). In Table 11.4, I describe how Native Americans and European Americans might have different views of communication.

DIALECTS

Dialects are variations of a particular language and are spoken by a large group of people who may share ethnic, regional, or national similarities. A **dialect**, like a language, has distinct syntactic, semantic, and phonetic features, but different dialects

Table 11.4   **Cross-Cultural Difference Between Native Americans and European Americans in Terms of Their Perspective on Communication**

European Americans' views of Native American speakers	Native Americans' views of European American speakers
Viewed as talking too little	Viewed as talking too much
Viewed as being slow to take a conversational turn	Viewed as not giving others a chance to talk during the conversation
Viewed as not wanting to initiate conversation	Viewed as being the first to initiate conversation
Viewed as avoiding direct questions	Viewed as asking too many direct questions
Viewed as only wanting to talk to close acquaintances	Viewed as even wanting to talk to strangers
Viewed as playing down their own abilities	Viewed as bragging about their own abilities
Viewed as acting as if they expect things to be given to them	Viewed as not helping others when they can
Viewed as being reluctant to talk about future planning	Viewed as being eager to talk about future planning

Source: Adapted with permission from a chart in *Interethnic Communication,* by R. Scollon and S. B. Scollon, 1980, Fairbanks, AK: Alaska Native Language Center. The author of this text changed *Athabaskans* to *Native Americans.*

within a particular language are usually comprehensible by people who speak other dialects. In contrast, a language is typically incomprehensible to those who do not speak the language.

The determination of a country's dominant language, or dialect, is based on the status of its users. In the United States, the dominant dialect is referred to as the General American dialect, sometimes called **Standard English.** You can see how the dialects occur geographically within the United States in Figure 11.3.

While two thirds of Americans speak General American English the remaining third speak a regional dialect that is viewed with less prestige (Delaney, 2007). You are likely not surprised to know that the majority of speakers who use lower-prestige dialects tend to be individuals who are poor and/or African Americans.

It is important to understand, however, that everyone in the United States speaks some sort of dialect. The U.S. map presented in Figure 11.3 shows that there are at least 24 regional dialects within the United States. Dialects are often mislabeled as regional **accents;** accents reflect regional differences in phonology (e.g., pronunciation of vowels) and semantics (e.g., use of different words to describe the same object, like *sack* versus *bag*).

Creole is another important term to explain language differences. Creole languages tend to reflect differences in phonology, semantics, and syntax (e.g., verb

Figure 11.3 Patterns of Dialect Use in the United States

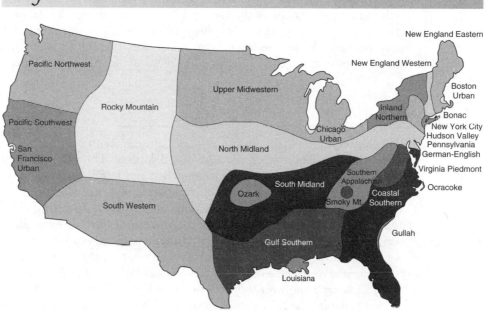

Source: From "American Dialects: Dialect Map of American English" by Robert Delaney, 2000, retrieved November 29, 2007, from www.geocities.com/yvain.geo/dialects.html. Adapted with permission.

tense and usage); a Creole language is adapted from a parent language. Examples of Creole include (a) Hawaiian Pidgin spoken by Native Hawaiians (Cheng, 2002), (b) a Creole that is a mixture of French and a native African language spoken by people from Haiti (see Terrell & Jackson, 2002), and (c) *patois* spoken in Jamaica. African American English Vernacular (AAEV) is a Creole dialect spoken by some individuals who are African American. AAEV is also sometimes called Black English or African American English.

When one dialect is seen as "superior and proper," the result is **linguistic chauvinism.** Linguistic chauvinism often results in speakers of a particular dialect being scorned. It often occurs when a dialect is a result of an ethnic language tradition; it may ultimately result in a student being afraid to express himself or herself verbally because he or she does not want to seem stupid in front of peers. All too often children bear the brunt of linguistic chauvinism and may suffer psychological distress and educational barriers. For instance, imagine a Jamaican American preschooler trying to communicate to his teacher using the patois he was taught at home. Initially, the child may be surprised to understand that his teacher does not understand him, and he may be hurt when he is scolded with, "*That is not the right way to speak.*" Instead of reprimanding the child, a teacher should repeat the child's comment in Standard English. Next, the teacher should briefly explain that it is OK to talk differently at home versus at school.

The teacher's explanation about home language versus school language serves two purposes. First, the explanation facilitates the child's meta-awareness of his speech pattern; it introduces the child to the concept of *code-switching* by explaining that one language or dialect is appropriate at home and another is appropriate at school. Second, the teacher's explanation honors the child's home language and acknowledges that the child has the right to speak with varying dialectal patterns.

Connections

In this section, I discuss the impact of multiculturalism on children's school achievement and identification of communication disorders. The American school system operates from a European cultural framework and has an individualist orientation that values independence and individual achievement (Kalyanpur & Harry, 1999). Teachers of European American descent strongly value fostering children's independence because they believe it leads to self-confidence. For example, a European American Head Start teacher from the Midwest said, "*Taking their coat on and off is my most important thing. I think it's really important for them to be able to be self-sufficient. . . . To have confidence in your abilities and to be able to take care of yourself is a very important thing*" (Hwa-Froelich & Westby, 2003, p. 306).

Unfortunately, the cultural values of the American educational system are out of alignment with the values of some ethnic minority cultures. For example, the Pacific Islander culture values collective work, so individual achievement is not emphasized (Cheng, 2002). In the Pacific Islander school environment, children read, chant, and practice in unison, and most of the education system is based on an oral language tradition.

Asian families typically have a high respect for teachers and they go to great lengths to help their children succeed in school. For example, many Japanese American children are often sent to after-school programs to ensure academic success (Cheng, 2002). Despite the fact that Asian children perform so well in school, surprisingly some Asian cultural themes could be considered contrary to American education environments. A perspective toward learning that may be different from your own is described in Table 11.5.

Communication disorders in the Asian population might often be overlooked because the children are generally quiet during school. Also, teachers may not expect children from an Asian culture to have academic problems; there is a stereotype that Asian children always perform well academically (Cheng, 2002; Lee, 1996). However, we must remember that groups consist of individuals with unique and varying abilities. There are some Asian groups that do not perform as well in school. For example, Pacific Islanders perform at a lower level than their Latino and African American counterparts (Ima & Labovitz, 1990 cited in Cheng, 2002).

Depending on cultural attitudes, parents' reactions may vary when their child has an academic difficulty. For example, when Chinese, Korean, or Japanese children need special education services, parents sometimes believe the academic problems are due to parenting failure (Cheng, 2002).

Table 11.5 **Variations in Attitudes Toward Learning: Families from an Asian Heritage**

Asian cultural themes	Educational implications
Education is formal.	Teachers are formal and expected to lecture.
Teachers are to be highly respected.	Teachers are not to be interrupted. Students are reluctant to ask questions.
Reading of factual information is studying.	Fiction is not considered serious reading.
It is important to have order and be obedient.	Students are to sit quietly and listen attentively.
One learns by observation and by memorization.	Rote memory is considered an effective teaching tool.
Pattern practice and rote learning are studying.	Homework in pattern practice is important and is expected.

Source: From "Asian and Pacific American Cultures," by L. Cheng, 2002. In D. E. Battle (Ed.), *Communication Disorders in Multicultural Populations* (3rd ed.). Boston: Butterworth-Heinemann. Adapted with permission.

Assessment of Ethnic Minority Children

As you learned in prior chapters of this book, there are several stages to the assessment process: screening, diagnostic assessment, and progress monitoring. In the assessment of ethnic minority children there are several additional issues to consider. Your focus for assessing an ethnic minority child is to minimize test bias in the assessment and diagnostic process.

ASSESSING A CHILD IN HIS OR HER NATIVE LANGUAGE

According to the Individuals with Disabilities Act (IDEA, 2004), tests and other evaluation materials must be selected and administered to avoid discrimination in terms of race and/or culture. Tests should be administered in the child's native language, unless it is clearly not feasible to do so.

The rationale behind the IDEA act is that children are penalized on standardized tests when English is not their first language. True language ability is underestimated because the tests are designed to assess children in Standard American English (Cole & Taylor, 1990). Specifically, test items focusing on phonology and syntax should be avoided; syntactical and phonological forms are very likely to be misinterpreted when the speaker does not use Standard English (Ortiz & Kushner, 1997). In some cases, poor test performance results in a child being misclassified as learning disabled because of dialect issues.

In contrast to standardized tests focusing on phonology and syntax, clinicians can use process-oriented measures to assess bilingual and bidialectal children for language impairments. Process-oriented measures are dependent on psycholinguistic processes, such as linguistic mental operations, rather than language knowledge (Campbell, Dollaghan, Needleman, & Janosky, 1997). An example of a process-oriented task is asking a child to repeat numbers (i.e., digit recall). Guideline data is available that allows the assessor to determine if the child's ability to recall a series of numbers is within normal limits or below average. A child who has below-average performance on a process-oriented digit recall task may have an underlying deficit impacting his or her ability to process higher-order language tasks. It should be noted, however, that if a child's digit recall is below average, the practitioner does not focus on improving the child's production of numbers! Instead, the child's performance on the processing task is used as a culture-neutral indicator of more general language abilities. In this case, the practitioner is likely to undertake a process of dynamic assessment to identify functional language targets.

Dynamic assessments are another process-oriented assessment protocol. Dynamic assessment evaluates a child's ability to learn (Gillam & McFadden, 1994). In contrast, typical norm-referenced tests are product-oriented assessments; a product-oriented assessment evaluates a child's output and compares it to normative data. Also, remember that the normative data of most norm-referenced tests typically represents the performance of European American children.

In contrast to using norm-referenced assessment, dynamic assessment has been endorsed as an assessment procedure appropriate for ethnic minority children. In dynamic assessment, the examiner has an opportunity to distinguish disorders from cultural differences due to a child's learning style or exposure (Gutierrez-Clellan, Brown, Conboy, & Robinson-Zanartu, 1998; Lidz & Pena, 1996; Pena, Quinn, & Iglesias, 1992). During dynamic assessment the *test-teach-retest* approach is taken. First, children are tested to get a baseline score. Then the examiner spends time directly teaching the child the skill, known as the **mediated learning** phase; the mediated learning phase is followed by a retest (Ukraninetz, Harpell, Walsh, & Coyle, 2000).

During the mediated learning phase, children are assessed for learning behaviors, such as attention span, planning, self-regulation, motivation, and their response to the intervention. Since some children may not understand the purpose of the test, assessors also use this phase to explain that the goal is to "try" even if it means guessing (Hwa-Froelich & Vigil, 2004). However, the assessor must be careful to explain that the child should make a serious guess, not a playful guess, because in some cultures children are only asked to guess when an adult is playing, joking, or teasing. In this context, children may make farfetched guesses with the intention of maintaining a playful interaction. In contrast, some Asian children may refuse to respond when they are uncertain of the answer (Hwa-Froelich, 2000).

If the child receives positive scores in the mediated learning phase and demonstrates improved scores on the retest, the assessor infers that the low baseline score was likely a result of cultural differences in learning styles. Dynamic assessment has been shown to improve children's performance on intelligence tests (Kaniel, Tzureil, Feuerstein, Ben-Shachar, & Eitan, 1991) and assessors report that dynamic assessment is a valuable approach in achieving more cultural-neutral evaluations.

PRAGMATIC DIFFERENCES

Professionals must also consider differences in children's pragmatic communication styles resulting from a non-European heritage. Important pragmatic aspects to consider are rules about politeness and children's responses in varying social situations. Children from collectivist cultures, as most ethnic minority children are, are socialized to be quiet when communicating with adults (Hwa-Froelich & Vigil, 2004). Consequently, children from collectivist cultures may not be willing to demonstrate their verbal skills with an unfamiliar adult. For example, children from an Asian cultural framework may be unaccustomed to interacting with adults on a one-on-one basis; typically, children in Asian families communicate directly with peers rather than with adults (Cheng, 2002).

Some Native American children may have particular problems with the question-answer format common to standardized testing; they often are unfamiliar with abrupt question-answer sequences and timed responses (Robinson-Zanartu, 1996). African American children also may experience difficulty with direct questions because, in their cultural tradition, adults do not ask children "known" questions. The use of the obvious or known question has been referred as a *test question* (Heath, 1994). The use of test questions (e.g., such as when the adult asks, "*What is that*? during a shared book reading even when the adult and the child know the item's name) is associated with European tradition and may be an unfamiliar or even silly task to a child from a non-European tradition. Figure 11.4 provides more information about the use of the test question.

Eye contact is another pragmatic skill that should be considered. For example, in some African, Latino, and Asian cultural traditions, it is disrespectful for a child to maintain direct eye contact with an adult (Tellis & Tellis, 2003). In this case, a professional unfamiliar with different cultural standards may mistakenly assume a student is disinterested or inattentive.

Intervention

Skilled practitioners carefully consider cultural differences when working with their clients and their clients' families. A lack of cultural sensitivity can make a family feel judged, out of place, and misunderstood. The ability to conduct and design culturally sensitive interventions is important because SLPs and special educators spend most of their time conducting direct interventions with clients and their families (ASHA, 2003b). Two considerations should underlie interventions. I describe both considerations below.

Figure 11.4   Use of the Test Question

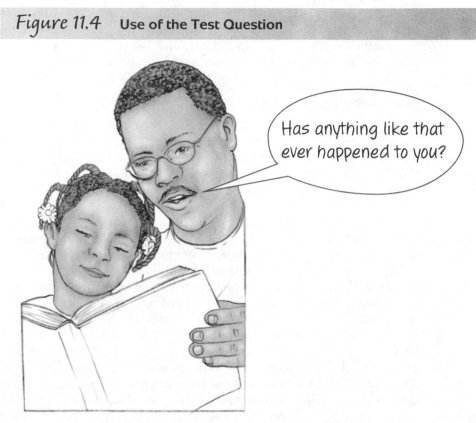

Has anything like that ever happened to you?

African American children may be less familiar with the test question (e.g., "*What is the man doing*?"); instead they may be more familiar with invitations to share a personal experience.

CONSIDERATION #1: CONSIDER THE ROLE OF NUCLEAR AND EXTENDED FAMILY IN FAMILY INTERVENTIONS

The interventionist should consider the family role in the delivery of the child's treatment. Most family interventions involve the parent (or primary caregiver) of a child, and it is assumed that **dyadic** (two person) **interactions** are the primary way the family communicates. However, this assumption may not be true for ethnic minority children who are more commonly socialized into multi-party language interactions consisting of an extended kin network including adults and peers.

Most family interventions assume a parent-child interaction framework; this assumption is rooted in the European cultural tradition of the nuclear household where the mother is primarily responsible for the care giving. However, the nuclear family household is the least frequently occurring family pattern worldwide (Shweder et al., 1998). Instead, an extended kin network is the norm in several cultures, and it is a tradition that has been predominant for many years (Shweder et al., 1998).

In contrast to a nuclear family framework, sibling care is common in African, Native American, Mexican, and Southeast Asian cultures (Shweder et al., 1998; van Kleeck, 1994). Grandmothers also are an important source of language input in an extended family network; throughout the world grandmother care complements maternal care (Shweder et al., 1998). Given these realities among ethnic groups, an intervention program focusing only on parents may not be effective for ethnic minority children. Children in a nonnuclear family may spend a majority of their time communicating with multiple adults, siblings, and other peers (van Kleeck, 1994).

In **multi-party language interactions** children do not typically interact in a face-to-face communication with one primary caregiver. Instead, children are encouraged and reinforced for interacting with multiple people and the primary caregiver's role is to help the child sustain the interaction within the group. Peers play a particularly important role because older siblings "practice" lessons with younger children. This is especially prevalent in families where parents have low literacy levels and do not feel confident in their language abilities (Hwa-Froelich & Vigil, 2004).

CONSIDERATION #2: CONSIDER THE FAMILY VALUES ABOUT CHILD COMMUNICATION NORMS

Often the goal of child language intervention is to increase the amount of child talk. It is assumed that all children live in families that value lots of talk. It is also assumed that children should be encouraged to initiate conversations with adults, and that adults should engage children in prolonged, direct, one-on-one conversations.

In the cultures of the Japanese, groups of Pacific Islanders, Puerto Ricans, and Navajo, adults often encourage verbal restraint and quietness in children. A talkative child is viewed as impolite, self-centered, and undisciplined (see van Kleeck, 1994).

AVOIDING CULTURAL CONFLICTS DURING INTERVENTION

One way to avoid cultural conflicts is by knowing the proper way to address adults in a family. Until told otherwise, the professional should always address family members using Mr., Mrs., or Miss (Hwa-Froelich & Vigil, 2004; Morrow, 1989). Many African Americans consider it rude for a stranger to address them by their first name, so they may be insulted when only a first name is used (Terrell, Battle, & Grantham, 1998; Terrell & Jackson, 2002). Likewise, African American parents may use the practitioner's title and surname when addressing them, and this should be interpreted as a sign of respect and courteous gesture on behalf of the parent. In Asian cultures, often the surname precedes the given same, so practitioners should be sure to understand this nuance and address the family appropriately.

When conflicts arise, as they will, practitioners should make brave and honest attempts to resolve this conflict. For suggestions on how to resolve conflicts see Focus 11.6.

After first meeting with a new family, interview the family to gain insight into their cultural background (Hwa-Froelich and Vigil, 2004). You cannot assume that by knowing where a family lives or what they look like, you will understand the

FOCUS 11.6 *Learning More*

Steps for Negotiating Cultural Conflicts with Families

1. Take it slow. Don't expect to resolve each situation immediately. Building understandings and relationships takes time; some issues won't be resolved, they'll just be managed. You have to learn to cope with differences when there is no common meeting ground or resolution. This sounds hard, but it's possible, if you're willing to accept that resolution is not always the outcome of disagreements.

2. Understand yourself. Become clear about your own values and goals. Know what you believe in. Have a bottom line, but leave space to be flexible.

3. Become sensitive to your discomfort. Tune in to what is bothering you instead of just ignoring it and hoping it will go away. Work to identify what specific behaviors of others make you uncomfortable. Try to discover exactly what creates this discomfort.

4. Learn about other cultures. Books, classes, and workshops help, but watch for stereotypes and biased information. Your best source of information comes from parents. Check out what they believe about their cultures, and see if it fits with other information you receive. Avoid making one person a representative of his or her culture. Listen to individuals, take in the information they give you, but avoid generalizing to whole cultures. Keep an open mind.

5. Find out what the family wants for their children. What are their goals? What are their communication practices? What concerns do they have about their children? Encourage them to talk to you and to ask questions.

6. Be a risk taker. If you are secure enough, you may feel you can afford to make mistakes. Mistakes are part of cross-cultural communication. Ask questions, investigate assumptions, confess your curiosity—but do it all as respectfully as possible. Be humble enough to admit that you need to know more and understand other's point of view.

7. Share power. Empowerment is an important factor [in handling cross-cultural conflicts]. Sharing empowerment means allowing others to experience their own personal power. We all have our personal power, though we can be discouraged or prevented from recognizing or using it. Sharing power enhances everyone.

Source: These guidelines are based on information from *Diversity in Early Care and Education* (pp. 60–61), by J. Gonzalez-Mena, 2008, Boston: McGraw-Hill.

---

family's cultural beliefs. Several questions have been suggested to gain this information (Hwa-Froelich & Vigil, 2004). I list some of them below.

- How would you describe your ethnicity?
- Would you describe your child as spending most of his or her time interacting with just the two of you, interacting with you and other siblings, or interacting with you and other adult friends or family members?
- Would you describe your child as talking too little or needing to talk more?
- When do you and your child do most of your talking—while driving in the car, at the dinner table, at night when getting ready for bed, or at other times of the day?

Questions like these can help you understand a family's ethnic tradition. You can learn whether or not the child is socialized into an extended kin network, the family's view of how much children should talk, and the times and places where families most frequently talk. With this information, your intervention plans are more likely to coincide with a family's language traditions and expectations.

MICRO- AND MACRO-LEVELS OF INTERVENTION

To intervene means to institute a change that is intended to affect an outcome. The change instituted by the intervention may come in the form of an instructional technique, medical procedure, therapy session, social service program, or policy regulation. Typically interventions are designed with the idea that the change will affect the outcome in a positive or healthy manner. However, all interventions have intended (positive) consequences as well as unintended (negative) consequences.

Commonly practitioners intervene at the micro-level of the ecological system, meaning you intervene directly with children or families. However, as practitioners in the field you must also be aware of how macro-level interventions (policy interventions) affect language traditions, service delivery, and assessment within schools and across diverse groups of families. At the macro-level, unintended negative consequences can come into play.

The 2002 No Child Left Behind (NCLB) Act reauthorized and amended the Elementary and Secondary Education (ESE) Act that has been in existence for over four decades. NCLB has become infamous for mandating school testing and offering parents "school choice" in the form of vouchers, but the policy is broader than those two controversial issues. NCLB, in its entirety, addresses policy issues such as family literacy programs, homelessness, migrant children, teacher recruitment, teacher professional development, reading and math curriculum, and standardized testing.

Focus 11.7 provides an outline of the various components of NCLB legislation.

FOCUS 11.7 *Intervention*

Key Components of the No Child Left Behind Legislation

Title I: Improving the Achievement of the Disadvantaged

Part A. Improving Basic Programs Operated by Local Education Agencies

Part B. Student Reading Skills Improvement Grants

Part C. Education of Migratory Children

Part D. Prevention and Intervention Programs for Children and Youth Who Are Neglected, Delinquent, or At Risk

Part E. National Assessment of Title I

Part F. Comprehensive School Reform

Part G. Advanced Placement Programs

Part H. School Dropout Prevention

Part I. General Provisions

Title II: Preparing, Training, and Recruiting High-Quality Teachers and Principals

Part A. Teacher & Principal Training & Recruitment Fund

Part B. Mathematics and Science Partnerships

Part C. Innovation for Teacher Quality

(*continued*)

Title III: Language Instruction for Limited English Proficient and Immigrant Students

    Part A. English Language Acquisition, Language Enhancement, and Academic Achievement Act

    Part B. Improving Language Instruction Educational Programs

    Part C. General Provisions

Title IV: 21st Century Schools

    Part A. Safe and Drug-Free Schools and Communities

    Part B. 21st Century Community Learning Centers

    Part C. Environmental Tobacco Smoke

Title V: Promoting Informed Parental Choice and Innovative Programs

    Part A. Innovative Programs

    Part B. Public Charter Schools

    Part C. Magnet Schools Assistance

    Part D. Fund for the Improvement of Education

Title VI: Flexibility and Accountability

    Part A. Improving Academic Achievement

    Part B. Rural Education Initiative

Title VII: Indian, Native Hawaiian, and Alaska Native Education

    Part A. Indian Education

    Part B. Native Hawaiian Education

    Part C. Alaska Native Education

Title VIII: Impact Aid Program

Title IX: General Provisions

    Part A. Definitions

    Part B. Flexibility in the Use of Administrative and Other Funds

    Part C. Coordination of Programs; Consolidated State and Local Plans and Applications

    Part D. Waivers

    Part E. Uniform Provisions

    Part F. Evaluations

Title X: Repeals, Redesignations, and Amendments to Other Statues

    Part A. Repeals

    Part B. Redesignations

    Part C. Homeless Education

    Part D. Native American Education Improvement

    Part E. Bureau of Indian Affairs Programs

    Part F. Higher Education Act of 1965

Title XI: Teacher Quality Enhancement

    Part A. Teacher Quality Enhancement Grants for States and Partnerships

    Part B. Preparing Tomorrow's Teachers to Use Technology

    Part F. General Education Provisions Act

    Part G. Miscellaneous Other Statutes

    Part J. Certain Multiyear Grants and Contracts

Source: Adapted from Public Law 107–110 115 STAT. 1425, January 8, 2002 (www.ed.gov/policy/elsec/leg/esea02/107–110.pdf).

As you can see, the regulation has specific implications for many cultural language traditions. For example, the regulations and funding guidelines associated with Title I (Improving the Academic Achievement of the Disadvantaged) impacts children living in poverty, most of whom represent ethnic minorities. Title III (Language Instruction for Limited English Proficient and Immigrant Students) has implications for children from cultural traditions speaking a language other than English. Title VII (Indian, Native Hawaiian, and Alaska Native Education) has implications for members of the Native American and Asian cultural language traditions.

Previously I mentioned that NCLB has become notorious for its high-stakes testing and accountability requirements. The testing is considered high-stakes because schools (and districts) can lose government funding if a certain percentage of the school's students are not performing at grade-level proficiency. Under NCLB, 95% of <u>all</u> students must participate in state assessments. This includes ELL students; they also must demonstrate progress toward academic proficiency in math and reading as well as general English language proficiency (Menken, 2006).

In the case of NCLB, the "intervention" is the macro-level policy mandating that all students participate in high-stakes testing. The intended consequence of the intervention is to ensure that educators are providing students with high-quality instruction. However, the unintended consequence is that an individual student may or may not be promoted to the next grade, placed in a college preparatory program, or graduate from high school because of his or her performance on the high-stakes test (Heubert & Hauser, 1999).

If the child is an English language learner, the outcome of the intervention (whether or not the ELL child shows improvement) may not reflect the student's academic gain. A test may be measuring how much English a child knows rather than his or her math or science knowledge (Menken, 2006). The child's ability in various subject areas may not be fairly assessed. In this respect, an unintended consequence is that NCLB (mandating high-stakes testing) could be criticized as being in conflict with IDEA, which mandates that schools modify instruction and assessment to meet children's individual needs.

A third unintended consequence of NCLB is that NCLB regulations may result in loss of federal funding for some school districts. If schools can only assess ELL children with an English achievement test, some schools will have difficulty demonstrating academic progress for the children in their program. A schoolwide, low achievement rating may result in loss of federal dollars for schools or districts serving many ELL children.

Overall, NCLB provides a solid example of how one aspect of a policy intervention results in both positive and negative consequences. As a future SLP or educator, you should consider macro-level interventions because educational policies will impact the schools where you work. It is important to familiarize yourself with the wide-reaching components of educational policy. The most effective professionals speak out against educational policies with negative consequences for children. Knowledgeable professionals want sensitive policies that meet the needs of all families, especially families who may not have the resources to speak for themselves.

Summary

- An **ethnic group** is a group of individuals who share a common language, heritage, religion, or geography/nationality. Americans are classified as falling within one of five ethnic groups: European American, Black American, Latino American, Asian American, and Native American.

- More than half of SLPs' clientele are non-European American ethnic minorities; however, the majority of SLPs are of European-American descent.
- People from an African-based language tradition include those who describe themselves as African American, African, and Afro-Caribbean. Many Blacks living in America face challenges similar to immigrants from other ethnic traditions, such as poverty and lack of health insurance.
- Latinos represent a variety of nationalities within their larger ethnic group, including Mexicans, Central/South Americans, Puerto Ricans, and Cubans.
- Americans from the Asian tradition may come from Asia or islands in the Pacific Ocean. The largest Asian population in American is from China, followed by Korea, and then Japan; other nationalities of Asians include those families from Southeast Asian counties.
- The current population of Native Americans is 2.4 million. The Native American ethnic group consists of numerous tribes, each with distinct traditions.
- Working with ethnically diverse families provides an opportunity to understand the complex influences on a family. Acculturation refers to the extent to which a family feels the need to maintain their own cultural identity while at the same time accepting the values and beliefs of the European American tradition. Individualist cultures focus on independence within individuals, whereas collectivist cultures focus on interdependence among group members. Bilingualism is the ability to read, speak, understand, and write well in two languages. In contrast, bidilectalism refers to an individual who uses two dialects of the same language such as an individual who can use both African American English and General American English.
- The American school system operates from a European cultural framework and has an individualist orientation that values independence and individual achievement; this framework may contrast with the language and practices of children with different cultural experiences.
- Assessors can use process-oriented measures to assess bilingual and bidialectal children for language impairments; one such protocol is called **dynamic assessment**. During intervention planning, assessors should consider if a family interacts in dyadic interactions versus multi-party interactions. The assessor can use cultural interviewing to gain understanding of family communication practices.

Discussion and In-Class Activities

1. Role-play a scenario in which a grandparent, an aunt, and uncle accompany the parents to the child's diagnostic assessment. It is clear that the parents defer to the grandparents and older brother. After the role-play interaction, discuss the session. Brainstorm other alternatives on how the session could have been

handled. Invite an individual from a collectivist culture to class and have him or her view the role-play. Ask for feedback regarding techniques that may have facilitated the interaction.

2. Watch a YouTube clip on African American English (AAE): www.youtube.com/watch?v=Zqohw8nR6qE One of the speakers discusses how and when he decides to code-switch. Does everyone code-switch to some degree? Give examples.

3. Listen to American dialects posted on the Internet at http://dare.wisc.edu/. Have students break into groups and take an area of the country and summarize differences in vocabulary (i.e., word choice), prosody, and phonology. What stereotypes are sometimes associated with the dialect?

4. Break into small groups. Each group will be provided with an age group (preschool, early elementary, middle school, older adolescent) and a cultural heritage. Bring in from a local library books that are multi-culturally sensitive and appropriate for the assigned cultural group. What makes a book appropriate? How could the book be incorporated into language intervention?

5. Labov (1972), one of the founders of sociolinguistics, noted that a person's linguistic behavior changes rapidly as his or her social position changes; he described distinct differences in blue-collar workers, white-collar workers, and professionals. Discuss whether the class agrees or disagrees with Labov's statement. Provide examples.

6. Cohen (1969) postulated functions such as leadership, child care, and rights to money are shared and not assigned via status roles in low-status families. In contrast, decision making and control are based on status roles in high-SES families. In class, discuss your own personal history with regard to family decision making and control. How does status affect adult–child family communication patterns?

Chapter 11 Case Study

The early intervention team for Laurimar, a 3-year-old with a moderate hearing loss, was meeting to discuss her goals for the coming year. Each professional spoke briefly about Laurimar's accomplishments to date, her strengths, and the areas that required continued attention. Laurimar's speech therapist was excited. "I have to admit I was really reluctant at first to meet with Laurimar at her child care center. I thought it would be too distracting, but it's really working out well." Laurimar's father was thrilled, "So you're helping her to talk to the other kids?" The speech therapist looked confused for a moment. "Well, in the long run. But for our weekly sessions, I've arranged to meet in a room down the hall." Laurimar's father rolled his eyes, "That's not the point of having you come to the center. We want her to be able to talk to the other kids, to make friends. You're not helping her do that when you take her out of the room!" Laurimar's mother spoke up as well. "We don't care if she sounds perfect. All that matters is that she's able to play with other kids, that they understand her. What are you going to do about that?"

Questions for Discussion

1. If you were Laurimar's parents, how would you feel during the discussion above?
2. If you were a member of Laurimar's early intervention team, how would you respond to her mother's question?

Source: Information from *Before the ABCs: Promoting School Readiness in Infants & Toddlers*, by R. Partkian, 2003, Washington, DC: Zero to Three Press.

A Tutorial: The Meaning of Standard Scores

1. To begin this example, imagine that I want to find the "worst" softball throwers so that I can provide extra coaching. First, I take the children out of their classroom (by age) and measure how far each child can throw the softball. I find out that 6-year-old girls can throw the softball an average distance of 40 feet (the mean). Some girls are very good throwers; a few girls are very poor throwers (Figure A.1).

2. Then, I have 10-year-old girls throw softballs. They can throw the balls farther; the mean throw for the 10-year-old girls is 60 feet (Figure A.2).

Figure A.1

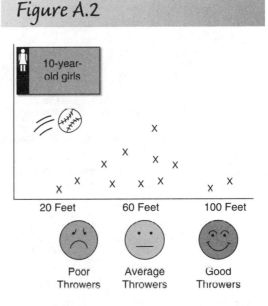

Figure A.2

Now at this point, it is very confusing because I want to identify the girls that need the most help across the age groups. I am going to need to organize the data so that I can easily determine if each girl is a good thrower, an average thrower, or a poor thrower. I decide to give any girl who throws the ball to the mean distance (as compared to other girls her age) a score of 100 (see Figure A.3).

Remember: This *does not indicate* the girl threw the ball 100 feet—instead I am assigning a score of 100 to any girl who throws the softball the mean distance (for 10-year-olds,

Figure A.3

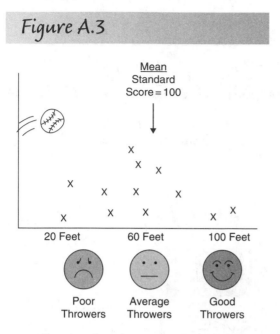

a distance of 60 feet). I then assign scores to all the girls to indicate how close (or far away) each girl threw in relation to the mean.

3. Now, there are several points to consider in Figure A.4. First, of all, I have overlaid a

Figure A.4

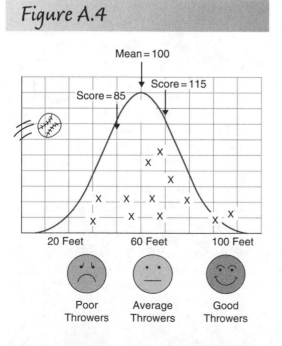

bell-shaped curve over my data points (in "real life" the normative distribution would be statistically computed). If I were to continue to document many throws by many 10-year-olds, I would end up with data that would resemble this curve. The height of the curve at the midpoint (the mean) indicates that more girls threw the ball this distance. As the distance gets longer (moving to the right on my graph), the curve is lower because fewer girls can throw a longer distance; the curve is lower on the left, because only a few girls have significant difficulty throwing the ball. In nature, when individuals are sampled (for any behavior), this is the result. Most of us perform at an average level at most tasks. A few people are somewhat better than average, a few are somewhat worse than average; a very few are much higher than average (i.e., superior performers), and a few individuals will be much lower than average (i.e., individuals with a disability at the targeted task).

Next, in Figure A.4, I have begun to assign scores that represent each girl's throw *relative to the mean for other 10-year-old girls*. A score of 85 is less than average, a score of 115 represents a score that is better than average. These converted scores are called standard scores. So, to reiterate, a standard score (SS) does not indicate the distance the ball is thrown; instead, standard scores are converted scores that allow me to document individual performance relative to same-age peers.

4. In Figure A.5, I have added standard deviations to demonstrate how the measurements are distributed. A standard deviation is the average distance a score falls from the mean score. In a normative sample, approximately 68% of the girls fall ± 1 standard deviation (SD) from the mean. By going to the left approximately 1.5 standard deviations (Figure A.6), I can identify the girls that are performing at the lowest 10th percentile as compared to their same-age peers.

Figure A.5

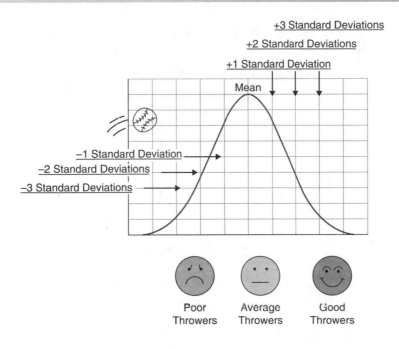

+3 Standard Deviations

+2 Standard Deviations

+1 Standard Deviation

Mean

−1 Standard Deviation

−2 Standard Deviations

−3 Standard Deviations

Poor Throwers　　Average Throwers　　Good Throwers

Figure A.6

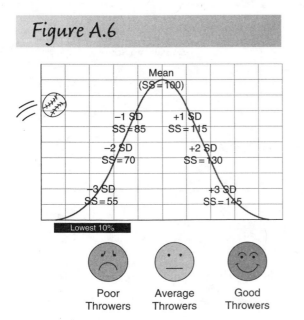

Mean (SS = 100)

−1 SD SS = 85　　+1 SD SS = 115

−2 SD SS = 70　　+2 SD SS = 130

−3 SD SS = 55　　+3 SD SS = 145

Lowest 10%

Poor Throwers　　Average Throwers　　Good Throwers

Many school districts require a student to fall 1.5 standard deviations (SD) below the mean to qualify for special educational services. If the mean of a norm-referenced test is 100, the standard score equivalent for 1.5 SD below the mean would be a standard score 79–80.

As a specific example, consider that a standard score of 98 is a converted score that indicates that the student's performance was very close to average as compared to his peers.

Standard scores also can be converted to percentile rank—an indication of an individual's relative standing in terms of percentage. The percentile rank indicates the percentage of people or scores that fall at or below a specific score on the bell-shaped curve. If an individual achieves a percentile rank of 60%, it means that 40% in the sample had higher scores.

Figure A.7

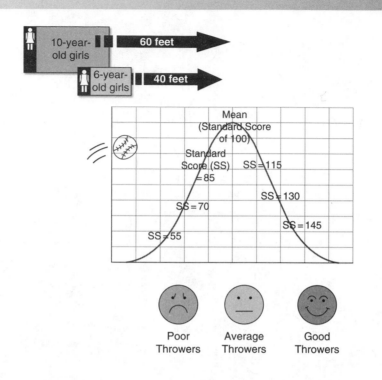

5. I hope it is clear by this point that using standard scores allows me to use the same scoring system for children of different ages. Remember that a score represents where a child performs relative to her peers. So, a score of 100 for a 6-year-old girl indicates that she was able to throw the ball 40 feet (refer back to Figure A.1), whereas a score of 100 for a 10-year-old girl indicates she threw the ball 60 feet (Figure A.7).

In both age groups, if I select the girls that receive a standard score below 80, I will have identified the girls that are the most in need of some additional coaching to improve their skills.

6. In Figure A.8, I demonstrate how this example pertains to children with a language disorder. Using a norm-referenced test, I can identify where a child performs on a tested language skill as compared with children her age. If the standard score

Figure A.8

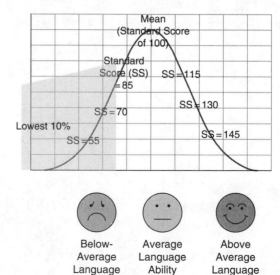

is between 85 and 115 (± 1 standard deviation), I know that the child's language ability is average. If she falls higher than 115, her language ability is higher-than-average. If her standard score is between 80-85, her language ability is somewhat below average. A standard score below 80 indicates that the child is performing at the lowest 10th percentile as compared to other children her age.

It is important to note that not all norm-referenced tests have a mean of 100; some tests, for example, have a mean of 50. Regardless of the conversion that is used, the standard score reflects how close (or far away) the child's performance compares to her same-age peers.

Language Sample Analysis Worksheet

Child's Name:	Chronological Age:	Language Sample Analysis (LSA) Step # 1 (Quantitative Analysis):		
Examiner:	Date of sample:	LSA Step #2 (Qualitative Analysis): Notes:		
List Utterances Below:	(A) Pragmatic Functions (✔ Check one)		(B) Semantic Roles and Relations (Describe)	(C) Bound Morphemes and Brown's Stage Morpheme Typically Appears	# of morp.
	Requests / *Declarations* / *Answer questions* / *Agree/disagree* / *Social speech* / *Imitation* / *Other*		Examples: Agent Action Object Modifier Negation Agent + Action Action + Object Agent + Action Modifier + X Negation + X X + Location	Examples of bound morphemes: Present progressive (*ing*) Prepositions (*in, on*) Plural (*s*) Present tense aux. (*can, will*) Possessive (*'s*) Irregular past tense verb Articles (*a, the*) Copula and auxiliary "*BE*" Regular past tense verbs (*ed*) 3rd person singular verb (*s*)	
			Negation + action + location		
			Agent + action + object		
			Agent + location		

Possible intervention goals include:

Permission is granted by the publisher to reproduce this form for evaluation and record-keeping. From Joan N. Kaderavek, *Language Disorders in Children*. Copyright © 2011 by Pearson Education, Inc. All rights reserved.

Report Writing

SPEECH AND LANGAUGE ASSESSMENT REPORT

	Comments on Report
Client's Name: Thad Smith **Parent's Name:** Ms. Jane Jones **Address:** **Phone Number:** **E-mail:** **Chronological Age:** 5:6 **Date of Birth:** **Date of Evaluation:** **Name of Evaluator:**	• The required demographic information is typically specified by the school, hospital, or clinic. Fill in as required.

I. CASE HISTORY INFORMATION
   AND STATEMENT OF PROBLEM:

Thad is a male 5 years and 6 months old seen for a speech-language evaluation at XXXX clinic. His mother, Ms. Jones, stated that Thad has difficulty understanding others and communicating his ideas. She stated that Thad has problems "putting his words together in a coherent fashion."

Ms. Jones pregnancy was unremarkable. At birth, however, Thad was suspected as having meningitis. He was tube-fed for one week. Final testing for meningitis was negative. At age 2 years, Thad had a high fever virus that caused two consecutive seizures; he was hospitalized for three days. No other medical concerns were noted.

Ms. Jones reported that Thad achieved all physical milestones as expected. She first noted Thad's speech delay when he was 2 years old. Thad began to use single words at age $2\frac{1}{2}$ and two-word combinations at $3\frac{1}{2}$. Presently, Thad uses one- or two-word combinations to communicate. No other members of the family have a history of speech or language delay.

• Be as concise as possible but include all relevant information.

Thad is in a preprimary full-day program for children with special educational needs at XXX school.

EXAMINATION FINDINGS

II. ASSOCIATED AREAS

Thad's hearing was screened and was within normal limits for both ears.

The examiner completed an oral-facial examination to assess Thad's oral mechanism. Structure and function of articulators (lips, tongue, jaw) were normal. Thad was able to rapidly repeat syllables ("*pa-ta-ka*") in imitation of the examiner.

Thad's voice quality was assessed informally and was within normal limits. Fluency and rate of speech were normal. Cognitive abilities were informally assessed in play and with drawing tasks; Thad performed at levels consistent with his chronological age.

Gross and fine motor skills were informally assessed and were within normal limits; Thad was able to hop on one foot, walk a straight line, and hold a pencil in the proper position as he copied a letter T.

- Hearing, oral-motor, voice, fluency, cognitive, and fine/gross motor skills were assessed informally.

III. SPEECH

The examiner administered the Goldman-Fristoe Test of Articulation-Revised to assess Thad's production of consonants in the beginning, middle, and final position in words. Thad substituted /w/ for /r/ in all positions in words and /d/ for /th/ in the beginning of words. Thad achieved a percentile rank of 54% indicating that his ability to produce sounds in words is within normal limits. The noted sound errors are not produced correctly until ages 6 to 7 years for many children developing typically.

- The purposes of the test are described briefly.
- The writer clarifies why the noted speech errors are not considered to be a deficit area.

IV. LANGUAGE

Language use (pragmatics)

Thad's ability to communicate his needs was accomplished both verbally (single words and some word combinations) and nonverbally

- The writer defines pragmatic use and gives examples to clarify terms as appropriate.

(pointing, gesturing, sounds). During play, Thad was able to greet the examiner, label items, request help, comment on actions (he said "*oh-oh*" when the blocks fell down), request information and objects, and deny (said "*no*" when asked if he wanted to play with the doll). He took turns during block play. He stayed in the interaction with the examiner, demonstrated appropriate eye contact, and had appropriate facial expressions and affect (i.e., smiling, laughter). Thad demonstrates appropriate use of early developing pragmatic skills.

Language content (semantics) and following directions

Thad's understanding of word meaning was assessed both formally and informally.

The examiner administered the subtests of the Clinical Evaluation of Language Function-Preschool 2 (CELF-P-2) to evaluate Thad's use and understanding of words and his ability to understand and follow concepts and directions. Subtest scores are as follows:

CELF-P-2 Semantic Subtests	Standard Score (SS) & Percentile	Normal Range Percentile
Concepts & Following Directions (receptive)	4 (SS) 2%	Above 10th percentile
Word Classes Total (receptive & expressive)	4 (SS) 2%	Above 10th percentile
Expressive Vocabulary	3 (SS) 1%	Above 10th percentile

Informal assessment during the play session confirmed the results of the CELF-P-2. Thad was able to follow one-step but not two-step commands. Thad was able to name seven body parts and count to 10 by rote, but had difficulty understanding descriptive words (e.g., "*Show me the*

- The writer included a description of the earliest pragmatic skills (turn taking, eye contact) as well as pragmatic skills typically seen in toddlers and preschoolers (requesting, labeling, etc.)
- Since Thad is at the one-to two-word level, later-occurring discourse skills (e.g., clarifying topic) were not addressed.

- Thad's standard score and percentile are provided. The normal range is given to aid interpretation. On the CELF-P-2 the subtest mean is 10 and one standard deviation is ± 3 (i.e., scores between 7–13 are within 1 standard deviation).
- The results of the informal assessment elaborate and clarify the results of the norm referenced testing. The writer gives examples so that the reader can understand the implication of Thad's difficulties with understanding word meanings.
- Since Thad is a Brown's Stage I (MLU 1-2) his use of word combinations is discussed within this section of language content (i.e., semantics). For an older child who is beginning to use morphology, MLU and the language sample analysis information would be included under language form (i.e., syntax)
- Thad's MLU is used to gauge where he is on Brown's Stages. Comparison information is provided to aid the reader's interpretation
- Number of different words (NDW) is provided.

biggest truck" or "*Show me the old shoe*") or following directions containing prepositions ("*Put the ball under the table*" or "*Show me the book that is on the box.*")

Thad's use of words to communicate and express meaning was noted during the play session. Thad's mean length of utterance (average number of words used to communicate) was 1.9. This mean length of utterance (MLU) places Thad at Brown's Stage I, a level typically achieved by children between 18 and 24 months. Children who are age 5 with typical language development are generally at Brown's Stage V+ and have a MLU of 4+ words.

Thad's vocabulary consisted primarily of concrete nouns (e.g. *truck, block, ball, shoe, tummy, cracker)* with limited verb use. Only the verbs: *want, go, give,* and *night-night* ("*me night-night*") were noted. Modifiers consisted of *my* and *no* (e.g., "*no dolly*," "*my shoe*"). In total, Thad used 45 different words in a 100-utterance language sample. By age 6, children developing typically generally use 117 words in a 100-utterance sample.

Language form (syntax) and morphology

Syntax refers to word order and morphology refers to grammatical forms (plural *s*, past tense *ed*). Thad's spontaneous speech did not contain age-appropriate syntax or morphological complexity. The earliest forms of grammatical complexity produced by children developing typically includes plural *s*, possessive *s* (e.g., "*mommy's shoe*"), the *ing* verb (*walking*), and irregular past tense verbs (*ate, went*). Thad did not use these morphological forms generally produced by children between 2 and 3 years old. Thad used unmarked verbs and nouns (i.e., root word with no morphological endings).

Thad used an early developing pattern for question forms. For example, he used voice inflection ("*Me go?*") rather than the more advanced syntax ("*Can I go?*"). Thad did not use auxiliary verbs (i.e. helping verbs, as in "*Dog is going.*").

- This description of MLU and NDW describes Thad's quantitative data for his language sample analysis.

- This description of Thad's difficulties with morphology and syntax describe the qualitative data from his language sample analysis.
- The morphological structures documented within Brown's Stages are listed for the reader so that the writer can describe Thad's complexity as compared to a child developing typically.

- Interrogative reversals are often very difficult for children with language impairments (LI) as they require a variation of the typical subject-verb-object word order and require the use of the

The following expressive subtests on the CELF-P-2 corroborate the analysis obtained by Thad's spontaneous language sample.

CELF-P-2 Syntax Subtests	Standard Score (SS) & Percentile	Normal Range Percentile
Word Structure (expressive)	4 (SS) 2%	Above 10th percentile
Sentence Structure (expressive)	4 (SS) 2%	Above 10th percentile

Combined scores for the CELF-P-2. Overall, Thad's combined core language score was 71 interpreted as a percentile rank range of 1%–7% (90% confidence interval). His receptive score for the CELF-P-2 was a standard score of 69 and a percentile rank range (90% confidence interval) of 1%–5%. His expressive combined standard score was 67; interpreted as a percentile rank range (90% confidence interval) of 1%–4%.

In summary, Thad's observational assessments, language sample analysis, and results on the CELF-P-2 indicate a severe receptive-expressive language impairment in the areas of semantics (word meaning), syntax (word order), and morphology (grammar forms).

V. CONCLUSIONS AND RECOMMENDATIONS

Thad presents as a child who has cognitive skills that are within normal limits, but with a history of language delay. Formal and informal assessments demonstrate an average level of speech production ability (i.e., ability to produce sounds) but severely impaired receptive and expressive language skills.

Thad is able to use verbal and nonverbal skills to communicate his needs. He does, however, demonstrate significant delays in vocabulary growth. His utterances are reduced in length and complexity.

auxiliary verb *can* (in this example). You will learn more about the syntax problems of children with LI in Chapter 5.

- The summed scores on the CELF-P-2 reinforce the information reported in the rest of the report. If there were discrepancies between subtest scores or if there were inconsistent results between the naturalistic assessments and the norm-referenced findings, the writer clarifies the results.

- The confidence ranges for the percentile score refer to the standard error of measure (SEM). As a student's score is not "absolute," his performance can vary. The testing manual provides a numeric value that is subtracted from and added to the child's standard score to obtain a range of scores at a 90% confidence interval. This means that one can be 90% sure that the child's true score (i.e., the range of possible scores he could obtain if tested repeatedly) would fall between the reported percentile range.

- There should be no surprises in the summary section or in the recommendations. That is to say, the writer cannot make a recommendation for a language domain that has not been justified in the preceeding report. So, for example, in the recommendations it would have been inappropriate to make a recommendation to provide speech intervention since, in the report, the writer indicates that Thad's speech is within normal limits.

Because Thad was able (a) to sustain attention to a task and (b) has positive family support, the prognosis for language improvement is good with regular (2-3 times weekly) intervention and a home language stimulation program.

Recommendations include:

1. Increase production and comprehension of vocabulary, particularly focusing on action words (i.e., verbs), modifiers, and early developing prepositions (*in, on*).

2. Increase word combinations through interactive play and book-reading using modeling, recasting, and elaboration of Thad's productions.

3. Introduce early developing morphemes (*ing, ed*, plural *s*) when Thad begins to produce 2-3 word combinations spontaneously.

4. Continue to monitor Thad's ability to produce sounds in speech and re-evaluate his use of modifiers, auxiliary forms, and pronouns, etc. with periodic language sample analysis

5. Meet with Thad's preschool teacher to coordinate language programming in his preschool program.

- The rationale for any intervention must be substantiated by data results in the body of the report.
- The need for ongoing formative assessment (using language sample analysis) is highlighted. It is likely that once intervention begins, Thad's expressive skills may change rapidly. The professional will monitor his progress and alter the focus of intervention (potentially focusing more on syntax and morphology) as Thad's utterance length improves.

Glossary

AAC aid A device used to send or receive messages. The aid can be nonelectronic (such as a series of photographs, a collection of objects, or a series of black-and-white or colored line drawings) or electronic.

AAC selection set How the visual symbols are presented; a selection set can include fixed displays, dynamic displays, hybrid displays, or visual scene displays.

AAC strategy Methods used to communicate effectively and efficiently; used to support message timing, grammatical formulation, spelling, and communication rate (Beukelman & Mirenda, 2005). Some examples of strategies to enhance communication include prediction and encoding.

AAC technique How a message is conveyed. Some individuals point or look at their symbol, other individuals use techniques such as scanning.

Accent Speech and language patterns that reflect regional differences in phonology and semantics.

Accommodation Piagetian concept of cognition demonstrated when prior schemata are adjusted to incorporate new information.

Acculturation The extent a family maintains their own cultural identity while at the same time accepting the values and beliefs of the European American tradition.

Achieving Communication Independence A comprehensive assessment for individuals with moderate–severe ID.

Adaptive behaviors Conceptual, social, and life skills.

Adult-directed intervention An intervention in which the adult leads the interaction by (a) choosing the stimulus items, (b) regulating how the child will respond, (c) prompting particular responses through pointing, modeling, or the use of questions, and (d) providing direct feedback on the child's performance.

Aided symbol A symbol that requires a support (i.e., drawing) to convey the message.

Alphabetic awareness An individual's understanding of letter names and the connection between letters and sounds.

Applied behavioral analysis (also called *discrete trial, Lovaas therapy*) A set of principles guiding behavior-based intervention for individuals on the autism spectrum.

Asperger syndrome (also called Asperger disorder) One of the five subtypes within the autism spectrum. Children with Asperger syndrome have verbal language but exhibit difficultly with social interaction and pragmatic skills.

Assertiveness-responsiveness scheme Profiles an individual according to levels of social participation; an assertive communicator initiates conversational turns, a responsive communicator responds to others' communication attempts.

Assimilation Piagetian concept of cognition demonstrated when a child takes in new information and incorporates it into his or her existing schemata.

Attempt A component of a narrative story episode; it is the action that is undertaken by the story's character to solve the problem.

Attention The ability to orient and react to a specific stimulus.

Attention-deficit/hyperactivity disorder (ADHD) Disorder in which a student exhibits behaviors of impulsivity, high activity, and distractibility.

Auditory neuropathy/dys-synchrony (AN/AD) A disorder of the auditory nerve fibers at the connection point with the cochlea (synapse) or higher which causes variable hearing thresholds and reduced word recognition.

Auditory processing disorder (APD) Impaired ability to make use of spoken language and other auditory signals, despite normal hearing thresholds.

Augmentative and alternative communication systems Systems that compensate and facilitate, temporarily or permanently, for the impairment and disability patterns of individuals with severe expressive and/or language comprehension deficits. AAC may be required for individuals demonstrating impairments in gestural, spoken, and/or written modalities.

Autism spectrum disorder The preferred term used to describe the range of disorders in social and communication functioning within the diagnostic category of Pervasive Developmental Disorders.

Autism, autistic disorder (AD) One of the subtypes within the autism spectrum. Children with AD have difficulty with social interaction, display problems with verbal and nonverbal communication, and exhibit repetitive behaviors or narrow, obsessive interests.

Autistic savant An individual within the autism spectrum with a unique talent. The unique ability is likely to be in mathematics (e.g., "lightning calculation"), memory, geography facts, or artistic/musical ability.

Backward design An approach to decision making that advocates considering the desired results for a particular student before setting an intervention goal; after describing the ultimate goal, the SLP identifies interventions needed to equip students to achieve the ultimate goal.

Baseline The data obtained prior to intervention; documentation of the occurrence of the target behavior before intervention.

Behavioral chaining Reinforcement of a number of linked substeps with the goal of training a complex behavioral sequence.

Behavioral phenotype The connection between one's genetic endowment and observable outcome.

Behaviorism A theory that learning occurs when an environmental stimulus triggers a response or behavior.

Bilingual-bicultural Persons who align themselves with the Deaf culture and communicate via sign language, learning written English as a second language.

Bilingualism The ability to read, speak, understand, and write in two languages.

Blinding A process whereby the individual who assesses subjects in a research study is not the same individual who directs the study or provides treatment.

Bottom-up learning Learning guided by perceptual processes interpreted as they are passed up to higher-order levels; specific subskills needed to accomplish an overall task.

Buildup/breakdown A language modeling technique in which the adult deconstructs a sentence into its separate components (e.g., noun phrase, verb phrase, prepositional phrase, adverb and adjective clauses) and then builds the sentence back to its original form.

Case grammar A semantic theory proposed by Fillmore; children's semantic use of words precedes syntax and is guided by universal concepts.

Case history A review of the written documentation of a child or student to obtain background information on developmental, medical, and educational history.

Child-directed intervention An intervention in which the adult follows the child's lead, responds contingently to the child's responses, and waits for the child to respond before initiating another conversational sequence.

Chronic otitis media Repeated or ongoing inflammation of the middle ear caused by infection.

Chunking Organizing items into familiar manageable units.

Cochlear implant Device implanted in the cochlea of an individual with significant hearing loss enabling access to auditory signals.

Code switching An individual's ability to alternate between formal and informal language; it also refers to an individual's ability to vary between dialectal language patterns and General American English.

Cognitive perceptual processing skills Attention, discrimination, organization, transfer, and memory.

Cognitive theory Based on the writings of Jean Piaget; a proposed sequence of progressively more sophisticated cognitive abilities from sensorimotor stage to advanced cognitive ability in the formal operations stage.

Cognitive verbs Used to describe the actions and thoughts of characters in the text; includes words like *thought, knew, remembered, decided, imagined, forgot, asked, told, explained, called,* or *yelled.*

Cohesive language Language features that require the speaker or writer to use words linking information from one sentence to another. Includes linkage between an introduced referent and a pronoun referring back to the referent and subordinating conjunctions such as *because, so, then,* or *therefore.*

Collectivist culture Focuses on interdependence among group members.

Communication forms (also called *communication means*) The way in which the child communicates, including gestures, nonlinguistic sounds, spoken or signed word or pictured symbols, or combinations of words or signs.

Communication functions (also called *communication intentions* and *communication acts*) The goal of a communication attempt, such as requesting, commenting, refusing, protesting, sharing emotion, initiating a topic, or continuing a topic.

Communication intent Demonstrated when an individual exhibits (a) gestures, vocalization, and/or eye contact to direct the attention or actions of a communication partner, (b) joint visual attention, (c) waiting after a communication attempt (i.e., expecting the partner to respond), or (d) persisting in a communication attempt that is not understood.

Communication means see *Communication forms.*

Communication modality The method in which one exchanges information or ideas. May include spoken language and/or sign language.

Communication temptations Orchestrated situations in which the situation is "sabotaged," heightening the child's need to communicate (e.g., favorite toys are placed out of reach, desired items are placed in containers requiring adult assistance).

Communication Transfer of symbolic and non-symbolic information (i.e., facial expressions, body language, gestures) between interaction partners.

Complex communication needs (CCNs) Occur when children have difficulty with processing, comprehending, or producing language, resulting in unmet communication needs.

Composition skills An individual's ability to integrate pragmatic, syntax, and semantic language domains to formulate and express thought.

Conductive hearing loss A hearing loss that results from diseases or obstructions in the outer or middle ear.

Consequence A component of the story episode underlying narrative structure; the result of the character's attempt to solve the problem.

Construct validity The underlying theory on which an assessment instrument is based.

Content validity The degree to which test items represent a defined domain.

Contingency The semantic and pragmatic links between the language facilitator's communication and the child's output.

Continuous reinforcement Every correct response is followed by an event increasing the probability the response will be repeated.

Continuum of naturalness A continuum of behaviors describing treatment intervention ranging from a strong adult (clinician)-directed approach (typically in a one-to-one adult–child interaction) to an approach that is child directed and takes place within the child's everyday interactions.

Conventional reading An individual's ability to decode unfamiliar words and draw meaning from written text.

Conversational discourse The unstructured or unplanned spoken interactions that occur between two individuals.

Conversational recast treatment (CRT) An intervention in which the targeted grammatical feature is produced very frequently during the intervention session; adult uses sentence recasts.

Conversational repair strategies Verbal behaviors exhibited by a speaker or listener during a communication breakdown.

Coordinating attention Following an infant's focus of attention and matching a child's communication to his or her eye gaze.

Creole language Reflects differences in phonology, semantics, and syntax (e.g., verb tense and usage) drawn from a parent language.

Criterion-referenced assessments Assessment that is used to evaluate an individual's ability relative to a predetermined level of performance, often used to measure progress in intervention.

Criterion-related validity The degree to which test results on one test align with another test measuring the same construct.

Critical question A question that demands that an individual draw on his or her value system for an answer.

Cultural dialogue Gathering information and knowledge to generate new ideas and insights into people's behavior, values, and life experiences.

Cultural frameworks Social practices, beliefs, values, and behaviors that members of a group use to communicate and interact.

Cultural sensitivity Being aware and nonjudgmental of the cultural practices of various groups.

Culturally reflective Recognizing that everyone is a product of the beliefs, values, and social-political history of his or her own ethnic group.

Curriculum-referenced language assessment An assessment process that considers the academic content and social interaction demands of the curriculum, the skills the student brings to the curriculum, the knowledge and skill needed to succeed academically, and identification of instructional modifications to enhance the student academic success.

Cyclic goal attack strategy A strategy in which several goals are targeted, each for a specified time period independent of accuracy with a repeating sequence.

Data collection Clinical procedures that (a) allow the SLP to track a student's progress from one session to another, (b) document the effectiveness of an intervention approach, and (c) maximize the effectiveness of the intervention.

Deaf culture Customs and beliefs shared by individuals with prelingual hearing loss.

Decibel (dB) Unit of measurement related to hearing threshold.

Decision tree A graphic illustration of the alternatives in the decision-making process.

Decoding The ability to translate a word from print to speech, usually by employing knowledge of sound-symbol correspondences. It is also the act of deciphering a new word by sounding it out.

Decontextualized language Language features that allow the listener to understand what is spoken or written without background information or environmental cues.

Deep structure Chomsky's principle describing the underlying meaning of the sentence the speaker wants to produce.

Degree of hearing loss The severity of the hearing loss (e.g., mild, moderate, severe, profound).

Descriptive-developmental approach An approach that describes an individual's language use by focusing on his/her level of language development and functioning within natural contexts.

Developmental synchrony Cumulative practice of auditory and language brain centers to perfect a developing skill such as listening.

Diagnostic and Statistical Manual of Mental Disorders, Fourth Edition, Text Revision (DSM-IV-TR) The handbook, published by the American Psychiatric Association, used most often in diagnosing mental disorders in the United States.

Dialect Has distinct syntactic, semantic, and phonetic features, but dialects within a language are usually comprehensible by those who speak other dialects.

Dialogic speech A linguistic form found in text; quoted or spoken language by a character in the story.

Differentiated instruction An approach to teaching that includes planning and executing various educational approaches to meet individual learning needs of students.

Direct service model classroom-based approach The practitioner (a) collaborates with the teacher using a team-teaching method or (b) takes turns with the teacher providing specific lessons to the entire class.

Directive language Adult-directed language that occurs when a parent requests a child to say or do something or asks many questions.

Disability The reduced ability of an individual to meet the needs of daily living; determined by the severity of the impairment, the person's lifestyle, or the extent to which the individual can compensate.

Discourse The connected and contingent flow of language between two or more individuals.

Discrepancy criterion model The discrepancy model requires that a child have a significant difference between IQ (i.e., overall cognitive ability) and school achievement.

Discrete trial (see *Applied behavioral analysis*)

Discrimination The ability to attend to specific stimuli in a field of similar stimuli.

Disequilibrium A Piagetian term that describes a cognitive process in which the child recognizes that two schemata are contradictory. Reorganization to higher levels of thinking is motivated by this disequilibrium.

Distributed practice An intervention approach that provides children with opportunities to practice a skill frequently throughout the day; associated with classroom-based intervention approach.

Dominant culture The traditions, values, beliefs, and behaviors associated with European American culture (also called *Mainstream culture*).

Drill play An intervention activity that is somewhat more natural than drill, but still highly structured; in drill play, an element of a play routine is used to increase motivation.

Drill An adult-directed intervention approach eliciting a high number of child responses; typically produced in response to adult questions and followed by adult reinforcing statements and feedback.

Dual language programs An academic program in which the goal is for students to maintain the first language (L1) while learning English as a second language (L2).

Dyadic interaction A two-person communication.

Dynamic assessment A process-oriented measure that evaluates a child's ability to learn via a test-teach-retest approach.

Dynamic displays Refers to an augmentative communication device in which the symbol position changes after a location is selected (e.g., a prediction device allows the more frequently chosen symbols to occur at the top of the possible items to be selected).

Dysarthria A motor speech disorder in which the muscles of the mouth, face, and respiratory system may become weak, move slowly, or not move at all after a stroke or other brain injury; the type and severity of dysarthria depend on the area of the nervous system affected.

Echolalia The repetition or echoing of verbal utterances made by another person.

Ecological approach Theory that acknowledges variation in individual, family, community, and cultural modes for dealing with challenges; considers the impact of an individual's communication impairment in relation to functioning and relationships within the family and community.

Effectiveness A term that is used to describe experimental research; it refers to the extent to which a specific intervention results in positive outcome when it is used in routine practice.

Effect-size estimates Metrics designed to characterize results in more functional and meaningful ways; effect-size data indicate the magnitude of an effect in addition to estimates of probability.

Efficacy A term that is used to describe experimental research; efficacy documents the extent to which a specific intervention, procedure, or service produces a beneficial result under ideal conditions.

Efficiency Documents the resources that are required to produce a beneficial result within the domain of evidence-based practice.

Embedded intervention A contextualized, child-centered activity that takes place during ongoing classroom routines.

Embedded learning opportunity Intervention that takes place as part of children's self-initiated, naturalistic, and contextualized interactions as they occur in the classroom.

Emergent literacy The skills, knowledge, and attitudes that are precursors to conventional reading and writing.

Empathizing Also referred to as *theory of mind* or *mindblindness*. Empathizing describes the ability to perceive another's motives or thoughts as well as the ability to understand how another person might feel in a particular situation. Empathizing deficits are characteristic of autism spectrum disorders.

Engagement Refers to a child's duration and complexity of play and quality of interaction with others.

Enhanced milieu teaching (EMT) A naturalistic approach appropriate for children who are able to imitate sounds and words, have a vocabulary of at least 10 words, and have an MLU between 1.0 and 3.5 words.

Epidemiology, Epidemiological The scientific study of factors affecting the health and illness of populations; epidemiologic studies are descriptive or analytic with the goal of identifying causal factors.

Equilibrium A balance between assimilating new information into old schemata and developing new schemata through accommodation.

Ethnic group A group of individuals who share a common language, heritage, religion, or geography/nationality.

Etiology The cause of a disorder or disease.

Exclusionary criteria Other possible causes of language impairment must be eliminated as possible reasons for a child's language delay to meet criteria for specific language impairment.

Executive functioning Goal-oriented, purposeful behaviors that allow the individual to take a strategic approach to problem solving.

Expansion A modeling technique in which the adult repeats the child's preceding verbalization along with adding one or more morphemes or words to make the sentence an acceptable adult sentence.

Explicit intervention Structured, sequenced, adult-directed instruction; the adult selects a particular language/literacy target and carefully sequences the child's exposure.

Expository narrative An informational narrative genre; the individual describes a sequential event within a domain of academic content (e.g., science experiment or historical incident).

Expressive language An individual's ability to express himself or herself and communicate meaning with language.

Expressive vocabulary The words a child produces.

Extended optional infinitive theory Theory that young children with language impairment persist in using unmarked verbs (e.g., *walk* versus *walking, walks,* or *walked*) well beyond the point when children with normal language discontinue this pattern

Extension A language modeling technique in which the adult repeats the child's preceding verbalization and adds additional information related to the ongoing event.

Extinction Lack of reinforcement with the goal of elimination of an unwanted behavior.

Fading A technique in which an adult's prompting is reduced and the behavior is gradually shaped to occur naturally within a social context.

Far transfer Learning applied to different contexts.

Fidelity The degree to which the intervention in a research study is carried out as described.

Figurative speech Words or expressions that are used nonliterally, such as metaphors, idioms, and proverbs.

First-generation immigrants Individuals born in another country and migrating to the United States.

Fixed displays Symbols and messages that do not change after the person selects the location on an AAC device.

Focused stimulation A modeling procedure in which a child is exposed to multiple examples of a linguistic target within a meaningful communication context.

Frequency The number of vibrations or the number of repetitions of a complete wave form in cycles per second; an acoustic measure that correlates to the perceptual quality we call *pitch.*

Functional assessment (also *functional analysis*) An assessment in which the professional gathers information about a student's behavior in order to identify the function or purpose of an aversive behavior and uses the information to develop behavioral-change interventions.

Functional communication training (FCT) A behavioral intervention replacing maladaptive behaviors with more socially acceptable communication options.

Gene duplication A portion of a whole chromosome or a whole chromosome is repeated, resulting in a genetic syndrome.

Generalization probe The interventionist evaluates the use of the target behavior as it occurs in a natural context or as it is independently produced by the student.

Generalization Refers to the ability of an individual to take a learned skill and apply it in a novel situation.

Genotype An individual's genetic endowment.

Giant words 2- or 3-word combinations that the child hears frequently; a phrase treated as a polysyllabic single word. The words are not used separately or in novel combinations with other words.

Goal attack strategy The way in which multiple goals are approached or scheduled within an intervention session.

Goal attainment scale (GAS) An individualized, criterion-referenced approach; it documents a student's baseline performance and numerically records behavioral changes from a -2 to +2 level.

Goal attainment scaling (also called *functional communication measure; performance rating system*) A rating system documenting changes in overall daily functioning.

Goal An intervention goal is made up of three components: the *do* statement, the *condition* statement, and the *criterion* statement.

Graph A visual representation of the occurrence of a behavior over time.

Hand leading Using another's body to communicate (e.g., moving the mother's hand toward an object), often replacing pointing.

Handicap The social disadvantage that an individual experiences because of an impairment and resulting disability.

Hearing age The number of years between the time a person was treated for hearing impairment (e.g., hearing aids fitted and intervention initiated) and his or her chronological age.

Hearing threshold Lowest level at which a sound signal is audible.

Horizontal goal attack strategy A strategy in which several goals are repeatedly targeted within every session.

Hybrid intervention An intervention approach in which the clinician focuses on a small subset of language behaviors and focuses a great deal of attention on identified targets within the intervention session; a midpoint intervention approach on the continuum of naturalness.

Hyperlexia The precocious ability to recognize written words significantly above an individual's language or cognitive skill level; often children with hyperlexia minimally comprehend what they read.

Image rehearsal A learning strategy in which the individual aids recall by associating task components with pictures.

Imitation One communication partner copies another's actions or sounds.

Impairment Any loss or abnormality of psychological, physiological, or anatomical structure or function.

Incidental teaching A strategy in which the language facilitator manipulates the environment to increase the likelihood the child will communicate.

Inclusion Children with disabilities are educated in the same context as nondisabled peers.

Indirect service model classroom-based approach The SLP or special educator serves as a consultant to the classroom teacher so that instructional methods can be adjusted to meet a child's special needs.

Individualist culture Focuses on independence within individuals.

Individualized education program (IEP) A plan outlining special education and related services specifically designed to meet the unique educational needs of a student with a disability.

Individuals with Disabilities Education Act (IDEA) The Individuals with Disabilities Education Act is the law that guarantees all children with disabilities access to a free and appropriate public education.

Infant-directed talk (also called *motherese*) The characteristics of child-directed communication enhancing infants' ability to learn language.

Inferential question A question form that demands that the individual make a logical conclusion from the text in order to answer the question.

Information-processing theory (also called *connectionism*) A model of cognition and language that compares the human brain to a computer and considers that cognitive ability is achieved by linked neuronal components.

Initiating event A component of the story episode underlying narrative structure; the initiating event is the problem that sets the story in motion.

Intellectual ability Mental capability that involves an individual's ability to reason, plan, solve problems, think abstractly, comprehend complex ideas, learn quickly, and learn from experience; a capacity often represented by an IQ score. Also defined as the ability to apply knowledge in order to perform better in an environment.

Intellectual disability (ID) A disorder originating before age 18 and characterized by significant limitations in intellectual functioning along with limitations in adaptive behavior.

Intensity Measured in decibels or other scales; psychological correlate is loudness.

Intermediate-level intervention goal A goal highlighting grammatical categories, operations, or processes.

Intermittent reinforcement Only some correct responses are followed by the reinforcing event; sometimes called *partial reinforcement*.

IT's Fun program A performance-based intervention for school-age students with ID.

Joint visual attention Following the direction of a communication partner's gaze or pointing or showing an object with the intention of drawing the communication partner's attention to the object or event.

Language content Semantics.

Language delay Language development mirroring typical development but at a delayed rate of acquisition.

Language difference A variation of a symbol system used by a group of individuals that reflects and is determined by shared regional, social, or cultural/ethnic factors.

Language disorder Impaired comprehension and/or use of spoken, written, and/or other symbol systems.

Language form Phonology, morphology, and syntax.

Language function or language use Pragmatics

Language sample analysis (LSA) An evaluation of an individual's spontaneous or self-generated speech; has both quantitative and qualitative components.

Language A complex and dynamic system of conventional symbols used for thought and language expression can be expressed orally, through writing, pictured symbols, or manually.

Late talker A young child under the age of 4 with a language delay.

Least restrictive environment (LRE) A learning plan that provides the most possible time in the regular classroom setting.

Level I evidence Evidence resulting from randomized experimental research; this is considered the best or "gold standard" research design in the levels of evidence for scientific studies.

Level II evidence Evidence reflecting high quality, but nonrandomized, experiments in the levels of evidence for scientific studies.

Level III evidence Evidence reflecting well-designed nonexperimental studies and case studies in the levels of evidence for scientific studies.

Level IV evidence Evidence representing experts' opinions in the levels of evidence for scientific studies.

Ling sound test A method of determining hearing aid, cochlear implant, or other device function based on a person's responses to six sounds that span the human speech frequencies. Named after Daniel Ling, who described the approach. Sounds include /oo/, /ah/, /ee/, /sh/, /s/, and /m/.

Linguistic chauvinism When one dialect is seen as "superior and proper."

Linguistically isolated households Homes in which no one over the age of 14 living in the household speaks fluent English.

Listening and spoken language specialists (LSLS) Specialists who help children who are deaf or hard of hearing develop spoken language and literacy primarily through listening.

Literacy orientation Aspects of children's temperament, motivation, and attention in response to book reading or other literacy interactions.

Literacy socialization A learning opportunity that includes activities such as shared book reading and shared writing activities.

Literal question A question form that requires a student to recall a specific fact explicitly stated in the reading passage.

Literate language Frequently occurring syntax and morphological features that occur in written text or formal spoken language.

Loudness The perceptual correlate of *volume*; relates to the decibel level of the acoustic signal.

Macrosystem Part of the ecological model summarizing society's cultural views and practices regarding individuals with ID.

Mainstream culture see *Dominant culture*.

Mainstreaming When students with disabilities spend a portion of their school day in the general education program and a portion in a separate special education program (this is not a preferred term).

Maladaptive behaviors Socially inappropriate or self-injurious behaviors such as tantrums, hitting, or head banging.

Mand-model A strategy in which the language facilitator uses a verbal prompt in the form of a question *("What do you want?")*, choice *("Do you want ___ or ___?")*, or mand *("Tell me what you want.")*.

Massed practice A term that indicates that students are provided intervention in less-frequent and longer sessions.

Massed trials An intervention approach in which the individual participates in intensive one-on-one training to increase accuracy and recall of a targeted behavior.

Mean A statistical average of all the scores in a sample.

Means-end Piagetian principle in which the child demonstrates intentionality; it occurs when the child identifies a problem and makes a plan to solve the problem.

Mediated learning phase The middle phase of dynamic assessment (i.e., test, teach, retest) during which the assessor teaches the child a skill; the child is monitored for attention span, planning, self-regulation, motivation, and response to the intervention.

Mediation The adult's manipulation of the task to increase the learner's success and self-efficacy.

Memory (also called *working memory*) Current information retained to carry out everyday tasks.

Mesosystem Part of the ecological model that includes school, neighborhood, community organizations, and work place.

Meta-analysis A specialized form of systematic review in which the results from several studies are summarized using a statistical technique resulting in a single weighted estimate of their findings.

Meta-awareness The ability to be self reflective; demonstration of the learning process.

Metacognition Conscious awareness of the thinking process.

Metalinguistics An individual's ability to focus on and talk about language.

Microcephaly Abnormally small head.

Microsystem Part of the ecological model that includes family and caregivers.

Mixed hearing loss A hearing loss that refers to a combination of conductive and sensorineural loss and means that a problem occurs in both the outer or middle and the inner ear.

Modeling A technique in which the adult talks and the child listens; provides an opportunity for the child to induce linguistic structures because the communication partner provides multiple examples of the language target. The language facilitator notes a child's focus of attention and provides a language model reflecting the child's interest.

Morphology The language domain that governs the structure of words and the construction of word forms.

Morphosyntax The combined features of morphology and syntax.

Motivation (also called *mastery motivation*) Goal-directed behaviors undertaken to achieve positive feelings associated with task competency.

Motor apraxia The inability of a person to perform voluntary and skillful movements of one or more body parts, although there is no evidence of underlying muscular paralysis.

Multi-modal The use of multiple modalities when a person communicates (e.g., gestures, speech, facial expressions, writing, drawing, AAC system).

Multi-party language interaction Interactions that take place with multiple people at the same time.

Narrative macrostructure The overall organization of a narrative; the story structure.

Narrative microstructure Internal linguistic features occurring within narratives; includes the syntax, vocabulary, and literate language used within narratives.

Nativist theory Connected to the writings of Noam Chomsky; proposes that children have an innate ability to learn language.

Naturalistic assessment An assessment in which the observer provides multiple opportunities for an individual to perform skills across domains (i.e., social, cognitive, motor, communication).

Near transfer Learning applied to closely related contexts.

Negative reinforcement An unpleasant stimulus that is removed when the targeted behavior is performed.

Neural maturation An accumulating body of science explaining the relationship between language and brain development in young children.

Neurological soft signs Behaviors consistent with a neurological impairment; however, the brain scan of an individual with neurological soft signs does not show hard evidence of neurological damage.

Neuroplasticity The brain's capacity (e.g., the neural auditory system) to be molded or reshaped.

Nonverbal IQ (also called *performance IQ*) A measure of one's ability to carry out motor tasks or analyze and solve problems using visual reasoning.

Nonword repetition tasks Repetition of nonsense words; used as a nonlinguistic processing task to diagnose language impairment.

Norm-reference assessments (also called *normative referenced assessment*) Assessment where ability is compared to a larger standardization group, usually resulting in a standard score, often used to determine eligibility for services.

Object constancy A Piagetian principle that describes how the child learns that he or she is viewing the same object regardless of distance, light, or different viewing angle.

Object permanence A Piagetian principle that describes the child's realization that an object exists even when it cannot be seen.

Objective data Data that are based on observable phenomena (e.g., ratings scales, behavioral/classroom observations, test scores).

Onset-rime An onset is the initial consonant sound of a syllable (the onset of *bag* is *b*-; of *swim* is *sw*-). Rime is the part of a syllable containing the vowel and all that follows it (the rime of *bag* is -*ag*; of *swim* is -*im*).

Open combining A sentence-combining approach in which the student combines simple sentences to make a longer, more complex sentence.

Oral narrative A monologue describing a real or fictional event organized into linked utterances with specific linguistic features.

Organization The ability to systematize incoming information to speed processing and facilitate retrieval.

Otitis media Inflammation of the middle ear caused by infection.

Paradigm shift Refers to a radical change in thinking leading to new approaches.

Parallel talk A modeling technique in which the adult uses language to describe what the child is thinking, feeling, and doing.

Parent-child communication routines Play routines that involve action patterns facilitating child participation.

Peer confederate training Students with typical language are trained to use strategies to encourage communication from students with communication disorders.

Pervasive Developmental Disorder (PDD) According to the Diagnostic and Statistical Manual of Mental Disorders, the fifth of the five autism spectrum disorder types.

Phenotype The observable characteristics or physical manifestation of one's genotype.

Phonics instruction Letter-sound relationships needed to read or spell words.

Phonological assessment An evaluation of the rules that govern the sound combinations in speech production; considers sound error patterns.

Phonological awareness deficits Problems detecting, segmenting, and blending sounds.

Phonological awareness The ability to reflect on and manipulate phonemic segments of speech; highly correlated with early reading skill.

Phonology The sound system of a language and the rules that govern the sound combinations.

Phrase structure grammar Chomskian description of the basic syntax structure of a sentence regardless of the language being spoken.

Piaget, Piagetian theory Developmental theory based on the work of Jean Piaget (1896–1980), who developed principles of cognitive processes.

Picture exchange communication system A six-phase intervention program designed to teach functional communication.

Pidgin language A communication pattern formed as a result of individuals with different languages needing to communicate; consists of rudimentary syntax and vocabulary forms.

Pitch The perceptual correlate of acoustic frequency (e.g., the individual perceives a tone as high pitch versus low pitch).

Play-based assessment A form of naturalistic assessment that considers the child's ability to use objects in functional ways, play symbolically, and communicate within a familiar context.

Positive reinforcement A stimulus that increases the frequency of a particular behavior using pleasant rewards.

Practice The repetition of a task to gain proficiency.

Pragmatics Context-related features of language; principles governing language use.

Predictive validity How well a test score will predict a student's performance on a future criterion-referenced task.

Primary prevention   The elimination of the onset and development of a communication disorder by altering susceptibility or environment for susceptible persons.

Print concepts   An individual's understanding of the uses of print and print functions needed during reading and writing.

Print referencing   An explicit teaching technique that exposes children to print and alphabetic concepts; often used during shared book reading interactions.

Process-oriented measures   Measures that are dependent on psycholinguistic processes such as linguistic mental operations rather than language knowledge.

Progress monitoring   Data that represent the student's communication progress during intervention and guide decisions and programmatic changes.

Prompts   Instructions or cues ensuring a child responds correctly (e.g., tactile, written, gestural cues).

Pullout model   A service delivery model where the SLP works with an individual or small groups of children in an area outside of the students' classroom.

Punishment   A negative response making it less likely that the unwanted behavior will occur.

Qualitative data   Data describing the attributes or properties that an object possesses. Although qualitative data can be organized into categories and assigned a number, the numbers do not have value by themselves, but rather represent descriptive attributes.

Quantitative data   Numeric data expressing quantity, amount, or range of a targeted behavior.

Race   A social construct based on historical and political views.

Randomized research design   After individuals consent to participate in a study they are randomly assigned to be in the treatment group or the control group.

Reading decoding   The various skills an individual uses to decipher and understand printed words (e.g., sounding out and spelling words during reading and writing).

Receptive language   An individual's ability to understand and process language.

Receptive vocabulary   The words the child understands, both in spoken and written form.

Reflecting feeling   A strategy used in counseling when a professional responds to the client's emotional expressions rather than to the content of the message.

Regulatory communication acts   Pragmatic communication acts that indicate an individual's needs within routines of daily living.

Rehearsal strategies   Learning strategies the individual uses to self-instruct to stimulate recall; includes verbalization of sequential steps and image rehearsal.

Reinforcement   Behaviors that follow the target behavior that increase the probability a behavior will reoccur.

Reliability   The degree to which a test is free from errors of measurement across forms, raters, time, and within an instrument.

Research bias   When an examiner unconsciously inflates a student's abilities because of knowledge that the student participated in a prior intervention.

Resource allocation   A term from the information-processing model suggesting the way in which energy is distributed in a cognitive system is affected by the number of parallel stages operating at one time.

Response to intervention (RTI)   Response to intervention is a model whereby students who are identified as at-risk have their progress monitored and receive increasingly intense, multi-tiered, research-based interventions.

Rett syndrome   One of the ASD disorders affecting females exclusively; characterized by normal early development followed by loss of purposeful use of the hands, distinctive hand movements, slowed brain and head growth, gait abnormalities, seizures, and intellectual disability.

Root word   A fundamental or unmarked part of a word (e.g., *walked*, *walks*, and *walking* all contain the root word *walk*).

Routine   A term that is used is describe times of day and/or familiar activities such as eating, bathing, bedtime, hanging out, going to the store, traveling in the car.

Rubric   A data system for qualitative behavior documentation; a set of criteria and standards used to assess an individual's performance on a specific task.

Scaffolding The graduated assistance provided to novice learners in order to help them achieve higher levels of conceptual and communicative competence; adult support allows a child to engage in a challenging activity.

Scanning Used for children with physical limitations. Scanning involves a communication partner or an electronic device displaying symbols in a predetermined pattern.

SCERTS approach An educational approach for children with autism based on social interaction, developmental, and family systems theories.

Schema Piagetian concept that describes a concept, mental category, or cognitive structure.

Scripts Predictable patterns of interaction facilitating the participation of language learners.

Secondary prevention The early detection and treatment of communication disorders. Early detection and treatment may lead to the elimination of the disorder or the retardation of the disorder's progress, preventing further complications.

Second-generation immigrants The children of first-generation immigrants.

Self talk A modeling technique in which the adult describes what he or she is thinking, feeling, or seeing.

Semantic transparency Words or phrases in which meaning is easily observed or intuited.

Semantics The language domain that governs the meanings of words and sentences.

Sensitivity In relation to an assessment tool, sensitivity refers to how frequently an individual with the disability is identified by using the tool (i.e., Does the tool give a positive result when the individual actually has the disability?).

Sensorineural hearing loss A hearing loss that results from damage to the sensory hair cells of the inner ear or the nerves that supply them.

Sentence expansion A sentence-combining approach in which the adult provides the student with a kernel sentence and then asks the student to elaborate the sentence.

Sentence-combining (SC) intervention An intervention in which the adult gives the student two or more simple sentences and requires the student to combine the simple sentences into a longer, more complex sentence.

Shaken baby syndrome (SBS) A term used to describe the constellation of signs and symptoms resulting from violent shaking or hitting the head of an infant or small child.

Shaping A behavioral concept that describes the production of closer approximations to the behavioral target prior to reinforcement; the language trainer facilitates easy, small steps gradually approximating the goal behavior.

Significance tests Statistical analyses reflecting the probability that the reported outcome being due to chance or random fluctuation is adequately small.

Signing Exact English (SEE, sometimes *Signed Exact English* or *Signed English*) A system of manual communication that strives to be an exact representation of English vocabulary and grammar.

Simultaneous processing The coordination of different pieces of cognitive information into a linked system.

Single-subject research designs Stimuli are presented individually and behavioral responses for stimuli are examined and compared.

Social communication problem Limitations in an individual's social, cognitive, and language skills necessary for contextually appropriate, meaningful, and effective interpersonal communication.

Social interaction theory A theory that proposes that communication interactions play a central role in children's acquisition of language.

Social intervention Focuses on teaching specific social skill strategies and facilitating the student's use of peer communication.

Social literacy An individual's affective (i.e., emotional) response to shared literacy experiences.

Social script A repeated social interaction likely to occur in daily life.

Sociocultural theory A language acquisition theory based on the writings of Vygotsky proposing that initially a child learns to solve problems with a more capable partner but eventually the child internalizes the process and functions independently.

Sociodramatic script training Engaging children in opportunities to role-play social scripts.

Specific language impairment (SLI) A language deficit but without accompanying factors such as hearing loss, low intelligence scores, or neurological damage.

Specificity The extent that an individual without a disorder is correctly identified as such, using a screening or assessment tool.

Speech/articulation assessment An evaluation of the child's motor ability to produce phonemes; considers sound production in isolation, syllables, words, sentences, and running speech.

Speech The articulation of speech sounds and the rate and quality of an individual's voice.

Speech-motor assessment An evaluation of (a) facial symmetry, (b) structure and function of the lips, tongue, jaw, and velopharnx (i.e., the soft palate), and (c) the resonance, phonatory, and respiratory systems used for speech.

Standard deviation A statistical calculation that describes the spread of scores around the mean.

Standardized scores Transformed scores measured in standard deviation units.

Stimulus overselectivity Selective response to a limited number of stimuli cues.

Story dictation A teaching technique in which the adult writes down text to a child's dictation. Often child illustrates the story. The adult reads the story back while pointing to the text.

Story episode The basic narrative structure that includes an initiating event, attempt, and consequence.

Subjective data Data that represent an individual's opinion.

Successive processing Arrangement of incoming cognitive information in a step-by-step or linear sequence.

Surface structure A Chomskian term that describes the actual sentence the speaker produces (i.e. the words that are heard).

Surface theory Theory proposing that morphemes' short duration and unstressed pronunciation contribute to learning difficulties for children with SLI.

Syllable recognition An individual's awareness that a word is made up of syllable subunits.

Symbolic play A Piagetian concept that describes the representational actions of a child when he or she uses one object to represent another.

Symbols Graphic, auditory, gestural, and textured or tactile representations used to represent language concepts in AAC systems.

Syntax The language domain governing the order and combination of words to form sentences, and the relationships among the elements within a sentence.

System for augmenting language (SAL) An AAC intervention consisting of (1) a speech-generating device, (2) visual-graphic symbols chosen to help the individual communicate, (3) encouragement of symbols as a means to communicate in everyday life, (4) modeling symbol use by communication, and (5) provision of feedback to family members.

Telegraphic speech Language that typically includes only content words, such as nouns, verbs, and a few adjectives/adverbs, with few or no function words (e.g., auxiliary verbs, articles, conjunctions, and prepositions).

Tertiary prevention The reduction of a disability by attempting to restore effective functioning.

Test question The use of the obvious or known question.

Time delay A strategy in which the language facilitator uses a nonverbal prompt and waits before providing the desired object or action.

Top-down learning Learning that is conceptually driven or guided by higher-level processes (e.g., familiarity with the context and information gained from environmental cues).

Total communication (also *simultaneous communication*) A mode of communication combining spoken language with sign language.

Total number of different words (TNW) A frequently used measure of lexical diversity; computed by counting the number of different root words in a 100-utterance language sample.

Transactional model Considers a child's utterances as the antecedent event triggering an adult response

Transdisciplinary An approach to assessment in which families and practitioners from different disciplines work together and make collaborative decisions; members share roles and systematically cross discipline boundaries.

Transfer of information Ability to apply learned information to solve novel problems.

Transformational grammar A Chomskian term describing the grammar rules specific to each language.

Translocation A genetic deficit that occurs when a broken piece of one chromosome attaches to another resulting in a genetic syndrome.

Traumatic brain injury (TBI) An acquired injury to the brain caused by an external physical force, resulting in total or partial functional disability or psychosocial impairment adversely affecting an individual's educational or functional performance.

Treatment efficacy Refers to a change under highly controlled conditions; differs from treatment effectiveness, which is the extent that the intervention results in favorable outcomes in everyday conditions.

Unaided symbol Symbol that does not require any prosthetic or external support to convey message.

Validity Degree to which a test procedure accurately measures what it was designed to measure.

Verbal rehearsal A learning strategy in which the individual self-instructs and uses verbal labels to stimulate memory and recall of information.

Vertical goal attack strategy A strategy in which one goal at a time is targeted until some predetermined level of accuracy is achieved.

Visual scene displays (VSDs) Depiction of a set of elements (people, actions, objects) within a coherent, integrated visual image.

Writing process The sequence of writing activities used by effective writers, including topic selection, planning, organizing, drafting, revising, editing, publishing, and presenting.

Zone of proximal development (ZPD) A Vykotskian term that describes the competence that a child demonstrates with minimal assistance. The ZPD is the area between the zone of competence (what a child can do independently) and the zone of incompetence (what a child is unable to do, even with assistance).

References

Abbeduto, L. (2009). Forward: Language, literacy, and genetic syndromes. *Topics in Language Disorders, 29,* 109–110.

Abbeduto, L., & Hagerman, R. (1997). Language and communication in fragile X syndrome. *Mental Retardation and Developmental Disabilities Research Reviews, 3,* 313–322.

Abbeduto, L., & Murphy, M. M. (2004). Language, social cognition, maladaptive behavior, and communication in Down syndrome and fragile X syndrome. In M. L. Rice & S. F. Warren (Eds.), *Developmental language disorders: From phenotypes to etiologies.* Mahwah, NJ: Erlbaum.

Adams, C. (2002). Practitioner review: The assessment of language pragmatics. *Journal of Child Psychology and Psychiatry, 43,* 973–987.

Adams, C. (2005). Language and social competence: An integrated approach to intervention. *Seminars in Speech & Language, 26,* 181–188.

Adamson, L. B., Romski, M. A., Deffebach, K., & Sevcik, R. A. (1992). Symbol vocabulary and the focus of conversations: Augmenting language development for youth with mental retardation. *The Journal of Speech and Hearing Research, 35,* 1333–1343.

Albertini, J. (1980). The acquisition of five grammatical morphemes: Deviance or delay? *Proceedings of the Symposium on Research in Child Language Disorders, 1,* 94–111. Madison: University of Wisconsin, Madison.

Alexander Graham Bell Association (2005). *Facts about hearing loss.* Retrieved May 14, 2007 from www.agbell.org/DesktopDefault.aspx?p=Facts_About_Hearing_Loss.

Alexander Graham Bell Association (2009). *AG Bell Academy for listening and spoken language.* Retrieved March 24, 2009 from www.agbellacademy.org/about-academy.htm.

Alt, M., & Plante, E. (2006). Factors that influence lexical and semantic fast mapping of young children with specific language impairment. *Journal of Speech, Language, and Hearing Research, 49,* 941–954.

ALTEC, University of Kansas (2009). RubiStar: *Creating rubrics for project-based learning.* Accessed June 17, 2009 at http://rubistar.4teachers.org/index.php.

American Academy of Pediatrics, Committee on children with Disabilities (2001). Technical report: The pediatrician's role in the diagnosis and management of autistic spectrum disorder in children. *Pediatrics, 107.* Retrieved August 8, 2006, from www.pediatrics.org/cgi/content/full/107/5/e85.

American Association on Mental Retardation (AAMR) (2002). *Mental retardation: Definition, classification, and systems of supports* (10th ed.). Washington, DC: Author.

American Occupational Therapy Association (1997). Statement: Sensory integration evaluation and intervention in school-based occupational therapy. *The American Journal of Occupational Therapy, 51,* 861–863.

American Psychiatric Association (2000). *Diagnostic and statistical manual of mental disorders–Text Revision* (4th ed.). Washington, DC: Author.

American Psychological Association (1999). *Standards for educational and psychological testing.* Washington, DC: Author.

American Speech-Language-Hearing Association (ASHA) (1990). Scope of practice: Speech-language pathology and audiology. *ASHA, 30*(8), 23–25.

American Speech-Language-Hearing Association (ASHA) (1991). *Prevention of communication disorders tutorial* [Relevant paper]. Available from www.asha.org/policy.

American Speech-Language-Hearing Association (ASHA) (1993). *Definitions of communication disorders and variations [Relevant paper].* Available from www.asha.org/policy.

American Speech-Language-Hearing Association (ASHA) (2000). *Guidelines for the roles and responsibilities of the school-based speech-language pathologist* [Guidelines]. Available from www.asha.org/policy.

American Speech-Language-Hearing Association (ASHA) (2001). *Roles and responsibilities of speech-language pathologists with respect to reading and writing in children and adolescents* [Guidelines]. Rockville, MD: Author.

American Speech-Language-Hearing Association (ASHA) (2002). *A workload analysis approach for establishing speech-language caseload standards in the schools: Technical report.* Available from www.asha.org/policy.

American Speech-Language-Hearing Association (ASHA) (2003a). *American English dialects [Technical report].*

Retrieved December 26, 2007 from www.asha.org/policy.

American Speech-Language-Hearing Association (ASHA) (2003b). *2003 Omnibus survey caseload report: SLP.* Rockville, MD: Author.

American Speech-Language-Hearing Association (ASHA) (2004a). *Preferred practice patterns for the profession of speech-language pathology.* Retrieved December 5, 2006, from www.asha.org/members/deskref-journals/deskref/default.

American Speech-Language-Hearing Association (ASHA) (2004b). Admission/discharge criteria in speech-language pathology. *ASHA supplement, 24,* 65–70.

American Speech-Language-Hearing Association (ASHA) (2004c). *Roles and responsibilities of speech-language pathologists with respect to augmentative and alternative communication: Technical report.* Available from www.asha.org/policy.

American Speech-Language-Hearing Association (ASHA) (2005a). *Evidence-based practice in communication disorders [Position statement].* Available from www.asha.org/policy.

American Speech-Language-Hearing Association (ASHA) (2005b). *Roles and responsibilities of speech-language pathologists with respect to augmentative and alternative communication: Position statement.* Available from www.asha.org/policy.

American Speech-Language-Hearing Association (ASHA) (2006a). *Responsiveness-to-intervention technical assistance packet.* Available at www.asha.org.

American Speech-Language-Hearing Association. (2006b). *2006 Schools survey report: Current issues.* Rockville, MD: Author.

American Speech-Language-Hearing Association (ASHA) (2007a). *Scope of practice in speech-language pathology.* Available from www.asha.org/policy.

American Speech-Language-Hearing Association (ASHA) (2007b). *Augmentative communication: A glossary.* Accessed March 10, 2008 from www.asha.org/public/speech/disorders/accPrimer.htm.

Anderson, K., & Smaldino, J. (1999). Listening inventories for education: A classroom measurement tool. *The Hearing Journal, 52,* 74–76.

Andrews, R., Torgerson, C., Beverton, S., Freeman, A., Locke, T., Law, G., et al. (2006). The effect of grammar teaching on writing development. *British Educational Research Journal, 32,* 39–55.

Apel, K., & Masterson, J. J. (1998). *Assessment and treatment of narrative skills: What's the story?* (video and manual). Rockville, MD: American Speech-Language-Hearing Association.

Apel, K., Masterson, J. J., & Niessen, N. L. (2004). Spelling assessment frameworks. In C. A. Stone, E. R., Silliman, & B. J. Ehren (Eds.), *Handbook of language and literacy: Development and disorders* (pp. 644–660). New York: Guilford Press.

Applebee, A. (1978). *The child's concept of story: Ages 2 to 17.* Chicago, IL: University of Chicago Press.

Aram, D., Most, T., & Mayafit, H. (2006). Contributions of mother-child storybook telling and joint writing to literacy development of kindergarteners with hearing loss. *Language, Speech, and Hearing Services in Schools, 37,* 209–223.

Arnold, L. E., Aman, M. G., Martin, A., Collier-Crespin, A., Vitiello, B., Tierney, E., et al. (2000). *Journal of Autism and Developmental Disorders, 30,* 99–111.

Athanasiou, M. S. (2007). Play-based approaches to preschool assessment. In B. Braken & R. Nagle (Eds.), *Psychoeducational assessment of preschool children* (4th ed.) (pp. 219–238). Mahwah, NJ: Earlbaum.

Autism Genome Project (AGP) Consortium (2007). Mapping autism risk loci using genetic linkage and chromosomal rearrangements. *Nature Genetics, 39,* 319–328.

Ayers, A. J. (1979). *Sensory integration and the child.* Los Angeles; Western Psychological Services.

Badian, N. A. (1998). A validation of the role of preschool phonological and orthographic skills in the prediction of reading. *Journal of Learning Disabilities, 31,* 472–481.

Bailey, J., McComas, J. J., Benavides, C., & Lovascz, C. (2002). Functional assessment in a residential setting: Identifying an effective communicative replacement response for aggressive behavior. *Journal of Developmental and Physical Disabilities, 14,* 353–369.

Baird, G., Charman, T., Baron-Cohen, S., Cox, A., Swettenham, J., Wheelwright, S., et al. (2000). A screening instrument for autism at 18 months of age: A 6-year follow-up study. *Journal of the American Academy of Child and Adolescent Psychiatry, 39,* 694–702.

Baldwin, D., & Meyer, M. (2007). How inherently social is language? In E. Hoff & M. Shatz (Eds.), *Blackwell handbook of language development* (pp. 87–106). Malden, MA: Blackwell.

Ball, A. F. (2006). Teaching writing in culturally diverse classrooms. In C. A. MacArthur, S. Graham, & J. Fitzgerald (Eds.), *Handbook of writing research* (pp. 293–310). New York: Guilford.

Bambara, L. M., & Warren, S. F. (1993). Massed trial revisited: Appropriate applications in functional skills training. In R. A. Gable & S. F. Warren (Eds.), *Advances in mental retardation and developmental disabilities* (pp. 165–190). Philadelphia: Jessica Kingsley Publishers.

Baranek, G. T., Parham, L. D., & Bodfish, J. W. (2005). Sensory and motor features in autism: Assessment and intervention. In F. R. Volkmar, R. Paul, A. Klin,

& D. Cohen (Eds.), *Handbook of autism and pervasive developmental disorders: Vol. 2. Assessment, intervention, and policy* (3rd ed., pp. 831–862). Hoboken, NJ: Wiley & Sons.

Baroff, G. S. (1999). *Mental retardation: Nature, cause, and management* (3rd ed.). Philadelphia, PA: Taylor-Francis.

Baron-Cohen, S., Allen, J., & Gillberg, C. (1992). Can autism be detected at 18 months? The needle, the haystack, and the CHAT. *British Journal of Psychiatry, 161,* 839–843.

Baron-Cohen, S., Cox, A., Baird, G., Sweettenham, J. Nightingale, N., Morgan, K., et al. (1996). Psychological markers in the detection of autism in infancy in a large population. *British Journal of Psychiatry, 168,* 158–163.

Baron-Cohen, S., Wheelwright, S., Lawson, J., Griffin, R., Ashwin, C., Billington, J., et al. (2005). Empathizing and systemizing in autism spectrum conditions. In F. R. Volkmar, R. Paul, A. Klin, D. Cohen (Eds.), *Handbook of autism and pervasive developmental disorders: Vol. 1. Diagnosis, development, neurobiology, and behavior* (3rd ed., pp. 628–639). Hoboken, NJ: Wiley & Sons.

Baroody, A. J., Lai, J., & Mix, K. S. (2006). The development of young children's early number and operation sense and its implications for early childhood education. In B. Spodek & O. N. Saracho (Eds.), *Handbook of research on the education of young children* (2nd ed., pp. 187–222). Mahwah, NJ: Erlbaum.

Bates, E., Dale, P. S., & Thal, D. (1995). Individual differences and their implications for theories of language development. In P. Fletcher & B. MacWhinney (Eds.), *The handbook of child language* (pp. 96–151). Oxford: Blackwell.

Battle, D. E. (2002). *Communication disorders in multicultural populations* (3rd ed.). Boston: Butterworth-Heinemann.

Baum, W. M. (2005). *Understanding behaviorism: Behavior, culture, and evolution.* Maiden: Blackwell.

Bear, D. R., Invernizzi, M., Templeton, S., & Johnston, F. (2007). *Words their way: Word study for phonics, vocabulary, and spelling instruction* (4th ed.). Upper Saddle River, NJ: Pearson.

Beck, I. L., & McKeown, M. G. (1985). Teaching vocabulary: Making the instruction fit the goal. *Educational Perspectives, 23,* 11–15.

Beck, I. L., & McKeown, M. G. (2007). Increasing young low-income children's oral vocabulary repertoires through rich and focused instruction. *The Elementary School Journal, 10,* 251–271.

Beck, I. L., McKeown, M. G., & Kucan, L. (2002). *Bringing words to life: Robust vocabulary instruction.* New York: Guilford Press.

Beirne-Smith, M., Ittenbach, R. F., & Patton, J. R. (2002). *Mental retardation* (6th ed.). Upper Saddle River, NJ: Merrill/Prentice Hall.

Beitchman, J. H., Hood, J., Rochon, J., & Peterson, J. (1989). Empirical classification of speech and language impairment in children: II. Behavioral characteristics. *Journal of the American Academy of Child and Adolescent Psychiatry, 28,* 118–123.

Beitchman, J. H., Hood, J., Rochon, J., Peterson, M., Mantini, T., & Majumdar, S. (1989). Empirical classification of speech and language impairment in children: I. Identification of speech-language categories. *Journal of the American Academy of Child and Adolescent Psychiatry, 28,* 112–117.

Beitchman, J. H., Nair, R., Clegg, M., Ferguson, B., & Patel, P. (1986). Prevalence of psychiatric disorders in children with speech and language disorders. *Journal of the American Academy of Child Psychiatry, 25,* 538–535.

Bellugi, U., Bihrle, A., Neville, H., Doherty, S., & Jernigan, T. L. (1992). Language, cognition, and brain organization in a neurodevelopment disorder. In M. Gunnar & C. Nelson (Eds.), *Developmental behavioral neuroscience: The Minnesota Symposia on Child Psychology* (pp. 201–232). Hillsdale, NJ: Erlbaum.

Belmont, J. M., Butterfield, E. C., & Ferretti, R. P. (1982). To secure transfer of training instruct self-management skills. In D. K. Detterman & R. J. Sternberg (Eds.), *How and how much can intelligence be increased?* (pp. 147–154). Norwood, NJ: Ablex.

Belser, R., & Sudhalter, V. (2001). Conversation characteristics of children with fragile X syndrome: Repetitive speech. *American Journal on Mental Retardation, 106,* 28–38.

Benigno, J. P., & Ellis, S. (2004). Two is greater than three: Effects of older siblings on parent support of preschoolers' counting in middle-class families. *Early Childhood Research Quarterly, 19,* 4–20.

Berard, G. (1993). *Hearing equals behavior.* New Canaan, CT: Keats.

Berk, L. E. (1997). *Child development* (4th ed.) Boston, MA: Allyn & Bacon.

Berninger, V. W., Abbott, R. D., Jones, J., Wolf, B. J., Gould, L., Anderson-Youngstrom, M., et al. (2006). Early development of language by hand: Composing, reading, listening, and speaking connections; three letter-writing modes; and fast mapping in spelling. *Developmental Neuropsychology, 29,* 61–92.

Berry, J. W. (1990). Psychology of acculturation. In J. J. Berman (Ed.), *Cross-cultural perspectives: Proceedings of the Nebraska symposium on motivation* (pp. 201–234).

Bertrand, J., Mars, A., Boyle, C., Bove, F., Yeargin-Allsopp, M., & Decoufle, P. (2001). Prevalence of autism in a United States population: The Brick Township, New Jersey, investigation. *Pediatrics, 108*, 1155–1161.

Bettelheim, B. (1967). *The empty fortress: Infantile autism and the birth of the self.* New York: Free Press.

Beukelman, D. R., & Mirenda, P. (2005). *Augmentative and alternative communication: Supporting children and adults with complex communication needs* (3rd ed.). Baltimore, MD: Brookes.

Bickerton, D. (1990). *Language and species.* Chicago, IL: University of Chicago Press.

Bickerton, D. (1995). Creoles and the bankruptcy of current acquisition theory. In H. Wekker (Ed.), *Creole languages and language acquisition* (pp. 33–44). Berlin: Walter de Gruyter & Co.

Binger, C., & Light, J. (2007). The effect of aided AAC modeling on the expression of multi-symbol messages by preschoolers who use AAC. *Augmentative and Alternative Communication, 23*, 30–43.

Bishop, D. V. M., & Snowling, M. J. (2004). Developmental dyslexia and specific language impairment: Same or different? *Psychological Bulletin, 130*, 858–886.

Bishop, D. V. M., Adams, C. V., & Rosen, S. (2006). Resistance of grammatical impairment to computerized comprehension training in children with specific and nonspecific language impairments. *International Journal of Language and Communication Disorders, 41*, 19–40.

Bishop, D. V. M., Price, T. S., Dale, P. S., & Plomin, R. (2003). Outcomes of early language delay: II. Etiology of transient and persistent language difficulties. *Journal of Speech, Language, and Hearing Research, 46*, 561–575.

Bishop, D., & Clarkson, B. (2003). Written language as a window into residual language deficits: A study of children with persistent and residual speech and language impairments. *Cortex, 39*, 215 –237.

Blachman, B. A. (2000). Phonological awareness. In M. K. Kamil, P. B. Mosenthal, P. D. Pearson, & R. Barr, (Eds.), *Handbook of reading research: Vol. III* (pp. 483–502). Mahwah, NJ: Erlbaum.

Blachman, B. A., Ball, E. W., Black, R., & Tangel, D. M. (2000). *Road to the code: A phonological awareness program for young children.* Baltimore, MD: Brookes.

Blackstone, S. (2006, June). Young children: False beliefs, widely held. *Augmentative Communication News, 18*(2), 1–4.

Blackstone, S., & Hunt Berg, M. (2003). *Social networks: Communication inventory for individuals with complex communication needs and their communication partners.* Monterey, CA: Augmentative Communication, Inc.

Blake, I. K. (1995). Language development and socialization in young African-American children. In P. M. Greenfield & R. R. Cocking (Eds.), *Cross-cultural roots of minority child development* (pp. 167–195). Hillsdale, NJ: Erlbaum.

Bloom, L., & Lahey, M. (1978). *Language development and language disorders.* New York: Wiley.

Bloom, P. (2001). Précis of "How children learn the meanings of words." *Behavioral and Brain Sciences, 24*, 1095–1103.

Boardman, A. G., Roberts, G., Vaughn, S., Wexler, J., Murray, C. S., & Kosanovich, M. (2008). *Effective instruction for adolescent struggling readers: A practice brief.* Portsmouth, NH: RMC Research Corporation, Center on Instruction.

Bodrova, E., & Leong, D. J. (2007). *Tools of the mind: The Vygotskian approach to early childhood education.* Upper Saddle River, NJ: Pearson.

Boehm, A. E. (2000). *Boehm Test of Basic Concepts – 3rd Edition (BTSC-3).* San Antonio, TX: The Psychological Corporation.

Bondy, A., & Frost, L. (2009). The picture exchange communication system. In P. Mirenda & T. Iacono (Eds.), *Autism spectrum disorders and AAC* (pp. 279–302). Baltimore, MD: Brookes.

Botting, N., Simkin, Z., & Conti-Ramsden, G. (2006). Associated reading skills in children with a history of specific language impairment (SLI). *Reading and Writing, 19*, 77–98.

Botwinik-Rotem, I., & Friedmann, M. (2009). Linguistic bases of child language disorders. In R. G. Schwartz (Ed.), *Handbook of child language disorders* (pp. 143–173). New York: Psychology Press.

Bowen, M. (1978). *Family therapy in clinical practice.* Northvale, NJ: Jason Aronson.

Bowers, L., Huisingh, R., & LoGiudice, C. (2008). *The Social Language Development Test—Elementary.* East Moline, IL: Lingua Systems.

Boyton, S. (1984). *Blue hat, green hat.* New York: Little Simon.

Bowers, L., Huisingh, R., LoGiudice, C., & Orman, J. (2004). *The WORD Test-2-Elementary.* East Moline, IL: Lingua Systems.

Bracken, B. (2007). *Bracken Basic Concept Scale Third Edition (BBCS-3).* San Antonio, TX: Harcourt Assessment.

Brackenbury, T., & Pye, C. (2005). Semantic deficits in children with language impairments: Issues for clinical assessment. *Language, Speech, and Hearing Services in Schools, 36*, 5–16.

Bradley, L., & Bryant, P. E. (1983). Categorizing sounds and learning to read—a causal connection. *Nature, 301*, 419–421.

Bregman, J.D. (2005). Definitions and characteristics of the spectrum. In D. Zager (Ed.), *Autism spectrum disorders: Identification, education, and treatment* (3rd ed., pp. 5–46). Mahwah, NJ: Erlbaum.

Brinton, B., & Fujiki, M. (1995). Conversational intervention with children with language impairment. In M. Fey, J. Windsor, & S. Warren (Eds.), *Language intervention: Preschool through the primary school years.* (pp. 183–212). Baltimore: Brookes.

Brinton, B., & Fujiki, M. (2005). Improving peer interaction and learning in cooperative learning groups. In T. A. Ukrainetz (Ed.), *Contextualized language intervention: Scaffolding K–12 literacy achievement* (pp. 289–318). Eau Claire, WI: Thinking Publications.

Brinton, B., Fujiki, M., & McKee, L. (1998). Negotiation skills of children with specific language impairment. *Journal of Speech, Language, Hearing Research, 41,* 927–940.

Brinton, B., Robinson, L. A., & Fujiki, M. (2004). Description of a program for social language intervention: If you can have a conversation, you can have a relationship. *Language, Speech, and Hearing Services in Schools, 35,* 283–290.

Bronfenbrenner, U. (1979). *The ecology of human development: Experiments by nature and design.* Cambridge, MA: Harvard University Press.

Broun, L., & Oelwein, P. (2007). *Literacy skill development for students with special educational needs: A strength-based approach.* Port Chester, NY: National Public Resources.

Brouwer, C. N., Rovers, M. M., Maille, A. R., Veenhoven, R. H., Grobbee, D. E., Sanders, E. A., & Schilder, A. G., (2005). The impact of recurrent acute otitis media on the quality of life of children and their caregivers. *Clinical Otolaryngology, 30,* 258–265.

Brown, J. D., & Hudson, T. (2002). *Criterion-referenced language testing.* New York: Cambridge University Press.

Brown, J., & Morris, D. (2005). Meeting the needs of low spellers in a second-grade classroom. *Reading and Writing Quarterly, 21,* 165–185.

Brown, L., Sherbenou, R., & Johnsen, S. (1997). *Test of Nonverbal Intelligence-3.* Austin, TX: PRO-ED.

Brown, M. W. (2005). *Goodnight moon* [Hardcover edition]. New York: HarperCollins.

Brown, R. (1973). *A first language: The early stages.* Cambridge, MA: Harvard University Press.

Brown, V. L., Wiederholt, J. L, & Hammill D. D. (2006). *Test of reading comprehension skills* (TORC-4). Los Angeles, CA: Western Psychological Association.

Browne, M. N., & Keeley, S. (2007). *Asking the right questions: A guide to critical thinking* (8th ed.). Upper Saddle River, NJ: Prentice Hall.

Bruner, J. (1975). The ontogenesis of speech acts. *Journal of Child Language, 2,* 1–19.

Bruner, J. S. (1981). The social context of language acquisition. *Language and Communication, 1,* 155–178.

Bruner, J. S. (1982). The organization of action and the nature of adult-child transaction. In G. D'ydewalle, J. Nuttin, W. Lens, & J. W. Atkinson (Eds). *Cognition in human motivation and learning* (pp. 1–44). Mahwah, NJ: Erlbaum.

Bruno, J., & Trembath, D. (2006). Use of aided language stimulation to improve syntactic performance during a weeklong intervention program. *Augmentative and Alternative Communication, 22*(4), 300–313.

Bryan, M. R. (1995). The preschool child sustains a traumatic brain injury: Developmental and learning issues. *NeuroRehabilitation, 5,* 323–330.

Buckley, S. J., & Sacks, B. I. (1987). *The adolescent with Down syndrome: Life for the teenager and the family.* Portsmouth: Portsmouth Polytechnic.

Buis, K. (2004). *Making words stick: Strategies that build vocabulary and reading comprehension in the elementary grades.* Portland, ME: Stenhouse.

Bus, A. G., & van IJzendoorn M. H. (1997). Affective dimension of mother-infant picturebook reading. *Journal of School Psychology, 35,* 47–60.

Caesar, L. G., & Williams, D. R. (2002). Socioculture and the delivery of health care: Who gets what and why. *The ASHA Leader, April,* 6–8.

Calandrella, A. M., & Wilcox, M. J. (2000). Predicting language outcomes for young prelinguistic children with developmental delay *Journal of Speech, Language, and Hearing Research, 43,* 1061–1071.

Camarata, S. M., & Nelson, K. E. (2005). Conversational recast intervention with preschool and older children. In R. J. McCauley & M. E. Fey (Eds.), *Treatment of language disorders* (pp. 237–264). Baltimore, MD: Brookes.

Camarata, S. M., Nelson, K. E., & Camarata, M. N. (1994). Comparison of conversational-recasting and imitative procedures for training grammatical structures in children with specific language impairment. *Journal of Speech and Hearing Research, 37,* 1414–1423.

Campbell, T., Dollaghan, C., Needleman, H., & Janosky, J. (1997). Reducing bias in language assessment: Processing-dependent measures. *Journal of Speech, Language, and Hearing Research, 40,* 519–525.

Cantwell D., & Baker, L. (1987). *Developmental speech and language disorders.* New York: Guilford Press.

Cardenas-Hagan, E., Carlson, C. D., & Pollard-Durodola, S. D. (2007). The cross-linguistic transfer of early literacy skills: The role of initial L1 and L2 skills and language of instruction. *Language, Speech, and Hearing Services in Schools, 38,* 249–259.

Carle, E. (2000). *Head to toe.* New York: Scholastic.

Carpenter, A., & Strong, J. (1988). Pragmatic development in normal children: Assessment of a testing protocol.

National Student Speech-Language-Hearing Association Journal, 12, 40–49.

Carpenter, M., Nagell, K., & Tomasello, M. (1998). Social cognition, joint attention, and communicative competence from 9 to 15 months of age. In R. K. Clifton & M. W. McCall (Eds.), *Monographs of the Society for Research in Child Development, 63*(4, Serial No. 255).

Carpenter, R., Mastergeorge, A., & Coggins, T. (1983). The acquisition of communicative intentions in infants 8 to 15 months of age. *Language and Speech, 26,* 101–116.

Carr, E. G., & Durand, V. M. (1985). Reducing behavior problems through functional communication training. *Journal of Applied Behavior Analysis, 18,* 111–126.

Carr, E. G., Innis, J., Blakeley-Smith, A., & Vasdev, S. (2004). Challenging behavior: Research design and measurement issues. In E. Emerson, C. Hatton, T. Thompson, & T. R. Parmenter (Eds.), *The international handbook of applied research in intellectual disabilities* (pp. 423–441). West Sussex, UK: Wiley.

Carr, E., & Wixon, K. K. (1986). Guidelines for evaluating vocabulary instruction. *Journal of Reading, 29,* 588–595.

Carrow-Woolfolk, E. (1995). *Oral and written language scales (OWLS: Written expression [WE] scale).* Los Angeles, CA: Western Psychological Association.

Carrow-Woolfolk, E. (1999). *Test of Auditory Comprehension of Language (TACL-3).* Bloomington, MN: Pearson.

Casbergue, R. M., & Plauché, M. B. (2005). Emergent writing: Classroom practices that support young writers' development. In R. Indrisano & J. R. Paratore (Eds.), *Learning to write, writing to learn: Theory and research in practice* (pp. 8–25). Newark, DE: International Reading Association.

Casby, M. (1992). The cognitive hypothesis and its influence on speech-language services in schools. *Language, Speech, and Hearing Services in Schools, 23,* 198–202.

Cascella, P. W. (2006). Standardized speech-language tests and students with intellectual disability: A review of normative data. *Journal of Intellectual & Developmental Disability, 31,* 120–124.

Caselli, M. C., Casadio, P., & Bates, E. (2001). Lexical development in English and Italian. In M. Tomasello & E. Bates (Eds.), *Language development: The essential readings* (pp. 76–110). Malden, MA: Blackwell.

Catts, H. (1991). Early identification of dyslexia: Evidence from a follow-up study of speech-language impaired children. *Annals of Dyslexia, 41,* 163–177.

Catts, H. W. (2009). The narrow view of reading promotes a broad view of comprehension. *Language, Speech, and Hearing Services in Schools, 40,* 178–183.

Catts, H. W., Bridges, M., Little, T., & Tomblin, J.B. (2008). Reading achievement growth in children with language impairments. *Journal of Speech-Language-Hearing Research, 51,* 1569–1579.

Catts, H. W., Fey, M. E., Tomblin, J. B., & Zhang, Z. (2002). A longitudinal investigation of reading outcomes in children with language impairments. *Journal of Speech, Language, and Hearing Research, 45,* 1142–1157.

Catts, H. W., Fey, M. E., Zhang, X., & Tomblin, J. B. (1999). Language basis of reading and reading disabilities: Evidence from a longitudinal investigation. *Scientific Studies of Reading, 3,* 331–361.

Catts, H., & Kahmi, A. (2005). *The connections between language and reading disabilities.* Mahwah, NJ: Erlbaum.

Center for American Progress Task Force on Poverty (2007). *From poverty to prosperity: A national strategy to cut poverty in half.* Washington, DC: Author.

Centers for Disease Control and Prevention (2004). *Hearing loss.* Retrieved on May 14, 2007 from www.cdc.gov/NCBDDD/EHDI/FAQ/questionsgeneralHL.htm#prev.

Centers for Disease Control and Prevention (CDC, 2007). *Prevalence of autism spectrum disorders, autism and developmental disabilities monitoring network, 14 sites, United States, 2000,* MMWR SS 2007, 56 (SS-1) (1). Retrieved February 9, 2007, from www.cdc.gov/ncbddd/autism/documents/AutismCommunityReport.pdf.

Cepeda, N. J., Pashler, H., Vul, E., Wixted, J., & Rohrer, D. (2006). Distributed practice in verbal recall tasks: A review and quantitative synthesis. *Psychological Bulletin, 132,* 354–380.

Chang, F., & Burns, B. M. (2005). Attention in preschoolers: Associations with effortful control and motivation. *Child Development, 76,* 247–263.

Chapman, R. S. (2000). Children's language learning: An interactionist perspective. *Journal of Child Psychology and Psychiatry, 41,* 33–54.

Chapman, R. S. (2003). Language and communication in individuals with Down syndrome. In L. Abbeduto (Ed.), *International review of research in mental retardation: Language and communication* (pp. 1–34). New York: Academic.

Chapman, R. S., & Hesketh, L. (2000). Behavioral phenotype of individuals with Down syndrome. *Mental Retardation and Developmental Disabilities Research Reviews, 6,* 84–95.

Chapman, R. S., Schwartz, S. E., & Kay-Raining Bird, E. (1991). Language skills of children and adolescents with Down syndrome: I. Comprehension. *Journal of Speech and Hearing Research, 34,* 1106–1120.

Charman, T. (2003). Epidemiology and early identification of autism: Research challenges and opportunities. In G. Bock & J. Goode (Eds.), *Novartis Foundation Symposium on Autism: Neural basis and treatment possibilities* (pp. 10–25). Chichester, UK: Wiley.

Cheng, L. (2002). Asian and Pacific American Cultures. In D. E. Battle (Ed.), *Communication disorders in multicultural populations* (3rd ed., pp. 71–112). Boston: Butterworth- Heinemann.

Cheour M., Imada T., Taulu S., Ahonen A., Salonen J., & Kuhl, P. (2004). Magnetoencephalography (MEG) is feasible for infant assessment of auditory discrimination. *Experimental Neurology, 190,* 44–51.

Chiang, B., & Rylance, B. (2000). *Wisconsin speech-language pathologists' caseloads: Reality and repercussions.* Oshkosh: University of Wisconsin-Oshkosh.

Chomsky, N. (1965). *Aspects of the theory of syntax.* Cambridge: MIT Press.

Chomsky, N. (1990a). Language and mind. In D. Mellor (Ed.), *Ways of communicating* (pp. 56–80). The Darwin College Lectures. Melbourne: Cambridge University Press.

Chomsky, N. (1990b). On the nature, use, and acquisition of language. In M. Putz (Ed.), *Thirty years of linguistic evolution: Studies in honor of Rene Dirven on the occasion of his sixtieth birthday* (pp. 3–29.) Amsterdam and Philadelphia: John Benjamin Publishing.

Chow, B. W., & McBride-Chang, C. (2003). Promoting language and literacy development through parent-child reading in Hong Kong preschoolers. *Early Education and Development, 14,* 233–248.

Chow, D., & Skuy, M. (1999). Simultaneous and successive cognitive processing in children with nonverbal learning disabilities. *School Psychology International, 20,* 219–231.

Cirrin, F. M., & Gillam, R. B. (2008). Language intervention practices for school-age children with spoken language disorders: A systematic review. *Language, Speech, and Hearing Services in Schools, 39,* 110–137.

Cirrin, F., & Penner, S. (1995). Classroom-based and consultative service delivery models for language intervention. In M. Fey, J. Windsor, & S. Warren (Eds.), *Language intervention: Preschool through elementary years* (pp. 333–362). Baltimore: Brookes.

Clahsen, H. (1999). Linguistic perspectives on specific language impairment. In W. C. Ritchie & T. K. Bhatia (Eds.), *Handbook of child language acquisition* (pp. 675–704). San Diego, CA: Academic Press.

Clancy, B. & Finlay, B. (2001). Neural correlates of early language learning. In M. Tomasello & E. Bates (Eds.), *Language development: The essential readings* (pp. 307–330). Malden, MA: Blackwell.

Cleary, L., & Peacock, T. (1998). *Collected wisdom.* Boston. Allyn & Bacon.

Cleave, P., & Rice, M. L. (1995). *Acquisition of BE: A detailed analysis.* Poster presented at the Convention of the American Speech-Language-Hearing Association, Orlando, FL.

Cloud, N., Genesee, F., & Hamayan, E. (2000). *Dual language instruction: A handbook for enriched education.* Boston: Heinle & Heinle.

Cochran, P. S., & Masterson, J. J. (1995). Not using a computer in language assessment/intervention: In defense of the reluctant clinician. *Language, Speech, and Hearing Services in Schools, 26,* 213–222.

Cohen, J. (1988). *Statistical power analysis for the behavioral sciences* (2nd ed.). Hillsdale, NJ: Erlbaum.

Cohen, R. (1969). Conceptual style, culture conflict and non-verbal tests of intelligence. *American Anthropologist 71,* 840–861.

Cole, K., Coggins, T., & Vanderstoep, C. (1999). The influence of language/cognitive profile on discourse intervention outcome. *Language, Speech, and Hearing Services in Schools, 30,* 61–67.

Cole, P. A., & Taylor, O. L. (1990). Performance of working class African-American children on three tests of articulation. *Language, Speech, and Hearing Services in Schools, 21,* 171–176.

Coleman, M. (2005). *The neurology of autism.* New York: Oxford University Press.

Connell, P. (1987). An effect of modeling and imitation teaching procedures on children with and without specific language impairment. *Journal of Speech and Hearing Research, 30,* 105–113.

Connor, C. M., & Craig, H. K. (2006). African American preschoolers' language, emergent literacy skills, and use of African American English: A complex relation. *Journal of Speech, Language, Hearing Research, 49,* 771–792.

Conti-Ramsden, G. & Jones, M. (1997). Verb use in specific language impairment. *Journal of Speech and Hearing Research 40,* 1298–313.

Coonrod, E. E., & Stone, W. L. (2005). Screening for autism in young children. In F. R. Volkmar, R. Paul, A. Klin, D. Cohen (Eds.), *Handbook of autism and pervasive developmental disorders: Vol. 2. Assessments, interventions, and policy* (3rd ed., pp. 707–729). Hoboken, NJ: Wiley.

Corkum, V., & Moore, C. (1995). Development of joint visual attention in infants. In C. Moore & P. J. Dunham (Eds.), *Joint attention: Its origins and role in development* (pp. 61–84). Hillsdale, NJ: Erlbaum.

Cormier, S., & Nurius, P. S. (2003). *Interviewing and change strategies for helpers: Fundamental skills and cognitive behavioral interventions* (5th ed.). Pacific Grove, CA: Brooks/Cole.

Cousins, L. (2008). *Happy birthday Maisy!* Cambridge, MA: Candlewick.

Crago, M. (1990). Development of communicative competence in Inuit children: Implications for speech-language pathology. *Journal of Childhood Communication Disorders, 13*, 73–83.

Craig, H. (1993). Social skills of children with specific language impairment. *Language, Speech, and Hearing Services in Schools, 24*, 206–215.

Craig, H. K., & Washington, J. A. (1994). The complex syntax skills of poor, urban, African-American preschoolers at school entry. *Language, Speech, and Hearing Services in Schools, 25*, 181–190.

Craig, H. K., & Washington, J. A. (2004). Grade-related changes in the production of African American English. *Journal of Speech, Language, and Hearing Research, 47*, 450–463.

Craig, H., & Washington, J. (1993). The access behaviors of children with specific language inmpairment. *Journal of Speech and Hearing Research, 36*, 322–337.

Craig, H. K., & Washington, J. A. (2000). An assessment battery for identifying language impairments in African American children. *Journal of Speech, Language, and Hearing Research, 43*, 366–379.

Crain-Thoreson, C., Dahlin, M. P., & Powell, T. A. (2001). Parent-child interaction in three conversational contexts: Variations in style and strategy. *New Directions for Child and Adolescent Development, 92*, 23–38

Crais, E. R. (1995). Expanding the repertoire of tools and techniques for assessing the communication skills of infants and toddlers. *American Journal of Speech-Language Disorders, 4*, 47–59.

Cross, T. (1978). Mothers' speech and its association with the rate of syntactic acquisition in young children. In N. Watson & C. Snow (Eds.), *The development of communication* (pp. 199–216). New York: Wiley.

Crystal, D. (1987). Towards a "bucket" theory of language disability: Taking account of interaction between linguistic levels. *Clinical Linguistics and Phonetics, 1*, 7–22.

Crystal, D., Fletcher, P., & Garman, M. (1989). *The grammatical analysis of language disability: A procedure for assessment and remediation* (2nd ed.). London: Whurr Publishers.

Culatta, B., & Horn, D. (1982). A program for achieving generalization of grammatical rules to spontaneous discourse. *Journal of Speech and Hearing Disorders, 47*, 174–180.

Curenton, S. M., & Justice, L. M. (2004). African American and Caucasian preschoolers' use of decontexualized discourse: Literate language features in oral narratives. *Language, Speech, and Hearing Services in Schools, 35*, 240–253.

Curenton, S. M., & Lucas, T. D. (2007). Assessing narrative development. In K. L. Pence (Ed.), *Assessment in emergent literacy* (pp. 377–432). San Diego, CA: Plural.

Curns, A. T., Holman, R. C., Shay, D. K., Cheek, J. E., Kaufman, S. F., Singleton, R. J., et al. (2002). Outpatient and hospital visits associated with otitis media among American Indian and Alaska Native children younger than 5 years. *Pediatrics, 109*, 41.

Dawson, J., Stout, C. E., & Eyer, J. A. (2003). *Structured Photographic Expressive Language Test-3 (SPELT-3)*. DeKalb, IL: Janelle.

Delaney, R. (2007, March 27). American dialects: Dialect map of American English. Retrieved on November 29, 2007, from www.geocities.com/yvain.geo/dialects.html.

Delpit, L. (1995). *Other people's children*. New York: The New Press.

Delprato, D. (2001). Comparison of discrete-trial and normalized behavioral language intervention for young children with autism. *Journal of Autism and Developmental Disorders, 31*, 315–325.

Denes, P. B., & Pinson, E. N. (2001). *The speech chain: The physics and biology of spoken language*. New York: Macmillan.

Deno, S. L. (1992). The nature and development of curriculum-based measurement. *Preventing School Failure, 36*, 5–10.

DesJardin, J. (2006). Family empowerment: Supporting language development in young children who are deaf or hard of hearing. *The Volta Review, 106*, 275–298.

Determan, D., Gabriel, L., & Ruthsatz, J. (2000). Intelligence and mental retardation. In R. J. Sternberg, *Handbook of intelligence* (pp. 141–158). New York: Cambridge University Press.

Dinnebeil, L., Pretti-Frontczak, K., & McInerney, W. (2009). A consultative itinerant approach to service delivery: Considerations for the early childhood community. *Language, Speech, and Hearing Services in Schools, 40*, 435–445.

Dollagen, C. A. (2007). *The handbook of evidence-based practice in communication disorders*. Baltimore, MD: Brookes.

Dollaghan, C. A., & Miller, J. (1986). Observational methods in the study of communicative competence. In R. Schiefelbusch (Ed.), *Language competence: Assessment and intervention* (pp. 99–129). San Diego: College-Hill.

Dollaghan, C. A., Campbell, T. F., Paradise, J. L., Feldman, H. M., Janosky, J. E., Pitcairn, D. N., et al. (1999). Maternal education and measures of speech and language. *Journal of Speech, Language, and Hearing Research, 42,* 1432–1443.

Donovan, S., & Cross, C. T. (Eds.). (2002). *Minority students in special and gifted education.* Washington, DC: National Academy Press.

Dore, J. (1974). A pragmatic description of early language development. *Journal of Psycholinguistic Research, 3,* 343–350.

Dore, J. (1975). Holophrases, speech acts and language universals. *Journal of Child Language, 3,* 13–28.

Dornan, D., Hickson, L., Murdoch, B., & Houston, T. (2007). Outcomes of an auditory-verbal program for children with hearing loss: A comparative study with a matched group of children with normal hearing. *Volta Review, 107,* 37–54.

Drager, K. D. R., Light, J. C., Carlson, R., D'Silva, K., Larsson, B., Pitkin, L., et al. (2004). Learning of dynamic display AAC technologies by typically developing 3-year-olds: Effect of different layouts and menu approaches. *Journal of Speech, Language, and Hearing Research, 47,* 1133–1148.

Drew, C. J., & Hardman, M. L. (2004). *Mental retardation: A life-span approach to people with intellectual disabilities* (8th ed). Upper Saddle River, NJ: Pearson.

Dube, W. V., Lombard, K. M., Farren, K. M., Flusser, D. S., Balsamo, L. M., Fowler, T. R., et al. (2003). Stimulus overselectivity and observing behavior in individuals with mental retardation. In S. Soraci Jr. & K. Murata-Soraci (Eds.), *Visual information processing* (pp. 107–123). Westport, CT: Praeger.

Dunlap, G., & Fox, L. (1999). A demonstration of behavioral support for young children with autism. *Journal of Positive Behavior Interventions, 1,* 77–87.

Dunn, L. M., & Dunn, D. M. (2006) *Peabody Picture Vocabulary Test-4 (PPVT-4).* Bloomington, MN: Pearson.

Dunn, M., Flax, J., Sliwinski, M., & Aram, D. (2001). The use of spontaneous language measures as criteria for identifying children with specific language impairment: An attempt to reconcile clinical and research incongruence. *Journal of Speech, Language, and Hearing Research, 39,* 643–654.

Durand, V., & Merges, E. (2001). Functional communication training: A contemporary behavior analytic intervention for problem behaviors. *Focus on Autism and Other Developmental Disabilities, 16,* 110–121.

Easterbrooks, S., & Baker, S. (2002). *Language learning in children who are deaf and hard of hearing: Multiple pathways.* Boston: Allyn & Bacon.

Edmonson, H., & Turnbull, A. (2002). Positive behavioral supports: Creating supportive environments at home, in schools, and in the community. In W. I. Cohen, L. Nadel, & M. E. Madnick (Eds.), *Down syndrome: Visions for the 21st century* (pp. 357–375). New York: Wiley-Liss.

Edmunds, K. M., & Bauserman, K. L. (2006). What teachers can learn about reading motivation through conversations with children. *The Reading Teacher, 59,* 414–424.

Edwards, D., & Mercer, N. (1987). *Common knowledge: The development of understanding in the classroom.* London: Methuen.

Ehren, B. J. (2007, May 8). SLPs in secondary schools: Going beyond survival to "thrival." *The ASHA Leader,* 22–23.

Ehren, B. J., Montgomery, J., Rudebusch, J., & Whitmire, K. (2006). *Responsiveness to intervention: New roles for speech-language pathologists.* American Speech-Language-Hearing Association. Retrieved June 3, 2008 from www.asha.org/members/slp/schools/profconsult/NewRolesSLP.htm.

Ehri, L. (1989). The development of spelling knowledge and its role in reading acquisition and reading disability. *Journal of Reading Disabilities, 22,* 356–365.

Eisenberg, L. S., Fink, N. E., & Niparko, J. K. (2006). Childhood development after cochlear implantation: Multicenter study examines language development, *The ASHA Leader, 11,* 5, 28–29.

Eisenberg, S. L. (2006). Grammar: How can I say that better? In T. A. Ukrainetz (Ed.), *Contextualized language intervention: Scaffolding preK-12 literacy achievement* (pp. 145–194). Greenville, SC: Thinking Publications.

Eisenberg, S. L., Fersko, T. M., & Lundgren, C. (2001). The use of MLU for identifying language impairment in preschool children: A review. *American Journal of Speech-Language Pathology, 10,* 323–342.

Elman, J. L. (2001). Connectionism and language acquisition. In M. Tomasello & E. Bates (Eds.), *Language development: The essential readings* (pp. 295–306). Malden, MA: Blackwell.

Espin, C. A., Weissenburger, J. W., & Benson, B. J. (2004). Assessing the writing performance of students in special education. *Exceptionality, 12,* 55–66.

Executive Order No. 12994, Executive Act on Intellectual Disabilities, (2003).

Feeney, Cynthia (2008). SLPs as reading specialists? [Electronic Version] *The ASHA Leader Online,* January 22, 2008. Retrieved March 27, 2009, at www.asha.org/about/publications/leader-online/LettersArchive/2008Letters/ltr080122a.htm.

Fenson, L., Dale, P. S., Reznick, J. S., Thal, D., Bates, E., Hartung, J. P., Pethick, S., & Reilly, J. S., (2007). *MacArthur Communicative Development Inventories* (2nd ed.). Baltimore, MD: Brookes.

Fernald, A., Pinto, J. P., Swingley, D., Weinberg, A., & McRoberts, G. W. (2001). In M. Tomasello & E. Bates (Eds.), *Language development: The essential readings* (pp. 49–56). Malden, MA: Blackwell.

Fernald, D. (2008). *Psychology: Six perspectives.* Los Angeles: Sage.

Fey, M. E. (1986). *Language intervention with young children.* Boston: Allyn & Bacon.

Fey, M. E. (2006). Commentary on "Making evidence-based decisions about child language intervention in schools" by Gillam and Gillam. *Language, Speech, and Hearing Services in Schools, 37,* 316–319.

Fey, M. E., & Loeb, D. F. (2002). An evaluation of the facilitative effects of inverted yes-no questions on the acquisition of auxiliary verbs. *Journal of Speech, Language, and Hearing Research, 45,* 160–174.

Fey, M. E., & Proctor-Williams, K. (2000). Recasting, elicited imitation and modeling in grammar intervention for children with specific language impairments. In D. V. M. Bishop & L. B. Leonard (Eds.), *Speech and language impairments in children: Causes, characteristics, intervention, and outcome* (pp. 177–194). East Sussex, UK: Psychology Press.

Fey, M. E., Cleave, P. L., & Long, S. H. (1997). Two models of grammar facilitation in children with language impairments: Phase 2. *Journal of Speech, Language, and Hearing Research, 40,* 5–19.

Fey, M. E., Cleave, P. L., Long, S. H., & Hughes, D. L. (1993). Two approaches to the facilitation of grammar in children with language impairment: An experimental evaluation. *Journal of Speech and Hearing Research, 36,* 141–157.

Fey, M. E., Long, S. H., & Finestack, L. H. (1993). Ten principles of grammar facilitation for children with specific language impairments. *American Journal of Speech-Language Pathology, 12,* 3–15.

Fiderer, A. (1993). *Teaching writing: A workshop approach.* New York: Scholastic.

Filipek, P. A., Accardo, P. J., Baranek, G. T., Cook Jr., E. H., Dawson, G., Gordon, B., et al. (1999). The screening and diagnosis of autism spectrum disorders. *Journal of Autism and Developmental Disorders, 29,* 439–484.

Fillmore, C. J. (1968). The case for case. In E. Bach & R. T. Harms (Ed.), *Universals in linguistic theory* (pp. 1–88). New York: Holt, Rinehart & Winston.

Fine, I., Finney, E. M., Boynton, G. M., & Dobkins, K. R. (2005). Comparing the effects of auditory deprivation and sign language within the auditory and visual cortex. *Journal of Cognitive Neuroscience, 17,* 1621–1637.

Finney, E. M., Fine, I., & Dobkins, K. R. (2001). Visual stimuli activate auditory cortex in deaf. *Natural Neuroscience, 12,* 1171–1173.

Fisher-Price (2004). *Little people cars, trucks, planes, and trains.* Bath, England: Reader's Digest Children's Books.

Fletcher, P., & Peters, J. (1984). Characterizing language impairment in children: An exploratory study. *Language Testing, 1,* 33–49.

Flexer, C., Wray, D., Sommers, R., & Schmidt-Robb, B. (2005). Early intervention for children with cochlear implants: A paradigm shift in expectations. *Hearsay, 17,* 15–27.

Flodin, M. (1994). *Signing illustrated.* New York: Penguin Putnam.

Fombonne, E. (1998). Epidemiological surveys of autism. In F. R. Volkmar (Ed.), *Autism and pervasive developmental disorders,* pp. 32–63. Cambridge, UK: Cambridge University.

Fombonne, E. (2005). Epidemiological studies of pervasive developmental disorders. In F. R. Volkmar, R. Paul, A. Klin, & D. Cohen (Eds.), *Handbook of autism and pervasive developmental disorders. Vol. 1: Diagnosis, development, neurobiology, and behavior* (3rd ed., pp. 628–639). Hoboken, NJ: Wiley & Sons.

Forum on Educational Accountability (2007). *Assessment and accountability for improving schools and learning: Principles and recommendations for federal law and state and local systems (Executive Summary).* Retrieved April 6, 2007 from www.edaccountability.org/AssessmentExecSumm061207.pdf.

Fowler, A. E., Boherty, B. J., & Boynton, L. (1995). The basis of reading skills in young adults with Down syndrome. In L. Nadel & D. Rosenthal (Eds.), *Down syndrome: Living and learning in the community* (pp. 121–131). New York: Wiley-Liss.

Fowler, A. E., Gelman, R., & Gleitman, L. (1994). The course of language learning in children with Down syndrome. In H. Tager-Flusberg (Ed.), *Constraints on language acquisition: Studies of atypical children* (pp. 91–140). Hillsdale, NJ: Erlbaum.

Fox, A. V., Dodd, B., & Howard, D. (2002). Risk factors for speech disorders in children. *International Journal of Language & Communication Disorders, 37,* 117–131.

Friederici, A.D. (2007). Neuroplasticity of sign language: Implications from structural and functional brain imaging. *Restorative Neurology and Neuroscience, 25,* 335–351.

Frith, C. (2003). What do imaging studies tell us about the neural basis of autism? In G. Bock & J. Goode (Eds.) *Novartis Foundation Symposium on Autism: Neural basis and treatment possibilities* (pp. 149–176). Chichester, UK: Wiley.

Fromkin, V., Krashen, S., Curtiss, S., Rigler, D., & Rigler, M. (1974). The development of language in Genie: A case of language acquisition beyond the 'critical period'. *Brain and Language, 1,* 81–107.

Fujiki, M., & Brinton, B. (2009). Pragmatics and social communication in child language disorders. In R. G. Schwartz (Ed.), *Handbook of child language disorders* (pp. 406–423). New York: Psychology Press.

Gadaire, D. M. (2000). Assessment and treatment of automatically reinforced self-injurious and stereotypic behavior. *Journal of Undergraduate Research, 1.* Retrieved on December 7, 2006 from www.clas.ufl.edu/jur/200002/papers/paper_gadaire.html.

Gallaudet Research Institute (2006). *Regional and national summary report of data from the 2006–2007 annual survey of Deaf and hard of hearing children and youth.* Washington, DC: GRI, Gallaudet University.

Ganea, P. A., Bloom-Pickard, M., & DeLoache, J. S. (2008). Transfer between picture books and the real world by very young children. *Journal of Cognition and Development, 9,* 46–66.

Gardner, M., & Brownell, R. (2000). *Expressive One-Word Picture Vocabulary Test-2000 Edition.* Novato, CA: Academic Therapy.

Gauger, L. M., (2008, May 6). *More on SLPs and literacy [Letters to the editor]. The ASHA Leader, 13*(6), 2.

Gavin, W. J., Klee, T., & Membrino, I. (1993). Differentiating specific language impairment from normal language development using grammatical analysis. *Clinical Linguistics and Phonetics, 7,* 191–206.

Geers, A. E. (2004). Speech, language, and reading skills after early cochlear implantation. *Archives of Otolaryngology, Head and Neck Surgery, 130,* 634–638.

Geers, A. E., Nicholas, J. G., & Sedey, A. L. (2003). Language skills of children with early cochlear implantation. *Ear and Hearing, 24,* 46S-58S.

Gentner, D. (2006). Why verbs are hard to learn. In K. Hirsh-Pasek & R. Golinkoff (Eds.), *Action meets word: How children learn verbs* (pp. 544–564). New York: Oxford University Press.

Gentry, J. W., Jun, S., & Tansuhaj, P. (1995). Consumer acculturation process and cultural conflict: How generalizable is a North American Model for marketing globally? *Journal of Business Research, 32,* 129–139.

Gillam, R. B., & Pearson, N. A. (2004) *Test of Narrative Language.* Austin, TX: PRO-ED.

Gillam, R. B., & Johnston, J. (1992). Spoken and written relationships in language/learning impaired and normally achieving school-age children. *Journal of Speech and Hearing Research, 35,* 1303–1315.

Gillam, R. B., Loeb, D. F., Hoffman, L. M., Bohman, T., Champlin, C. A., Thibodeau, L., et al. (2008). The efficacy of Fast ForWord language intervention in school-age children with language impairment: A randomized controlled trial. *Journal of Speech, Language, and Hearing Research, 51,* 97–119.

Gillam, R., McFadden, T. U., & van Kleeck, A. (1995). Improving narrative abilities: Whole language and language skills approaches. In M. E. Fey, J. Windsor, & S. F. Warren (Eds.), *Language intervention: Preschool through the elementary years* (pp. 145–182). Baltimore: Brookes.

Gillam, R. B., & Johnston, J. R. (1985). Development of print awareness in language-disordered preschoolers. *Journal of Speech and Hearing Research, 28,* 521–526.

Gillam, R. B., & Johnston, J. R. (1992). Spoken and written language relationships in language/learning-impaired and normally achieving school-age children. *Journal of Speech and Hearing Research, 35,* 1303–1315.

Gillam, S. L., & Gillam, R. B. (2008). Teaching graduate students to make evidence-based decisions: Application of a seven-step process within an authentic learning context. *Topics in Language Disorders, 28,* 212–228.

Gillberg, C., & Wing, I. (1999). Autism: Not an extremely rare disorder. *Acta Psychiatrica Scandinavica, 99,* 399–406.

Gillette, Y. (2001). *The Ohio Functional Inventory.* Akron, OH: The University of Akron, School of Speech Pathology and Audiology.

Gillette, Y. (2003). *Achieving communication independence: A comprehensive guide to assessment and intervention.* Eau Claire, WI: Thinking Publications.

Gillam, R., & McFadden, T. U. (1994). Redefining assessment as a holistic discovery process. *Journal of Childhood Communication Disorders, 16,* 36–40.

Gillon, G. T. (2000). The efficacy of phonological awareness intervention for children with spoken language impairment. *Language, Speech, and Hearing Services in Schools, 31,* 126–141.

Gillon, G. T. (2002). Follow-up study investigating benefits of phonological intervention for children with spoken language impairment. *International Journal of Language and Communication Disorders, 37,* 381–400.

Gillon, G. T. (2004). *Phonological awareness: From research to practice.* New York: Guilford Press.

Gillon, G. T. (2006). Phonological awareness intervention: A preventative framework for preschool children with specific speech and language impairments. In R. J. McCauley & M. E. Fey (Eds.), *Treatment of language disorders in children* (pp. 279–308). Baltimore, MD: Brookes.

Gilmore, L., Cuskelly, M., & Hayes, A. (2003). A comparative study of mastery motivation in young children with Down's syndrome: Similar outcomes, different processes? *Journal of Intellectual Disability Research, 47,* 181–190.

Goffman, E. (1986). *An essay on the organization of experience frame analysis.* Boston: Northeastern University Press.

Goldberg D., & Flexer, C. (1993). Outcome survey of auditory-verbal graduates: study of clinical efficacy. *Journal of the American Academy of Audiology, 12,* 189–200.

Goldberg D., & Flexer, C. (2001). Auditory-verbal graduates: Outcome survey of clinical efficacy. *Journal of the American Academy of Audiology, 12,* 406–414.

Goldman, R. (2000). *Goldman-Fristoe Test of Articulation-2.* Circle Pines, MN: American Guidance Service.

Goldman, R., & Fristoe, M. (2000). *Goldman-Fristoe Test of Articulation,* 2nd ed. Upper Saddle River, NJ: Pearson.

Goldstein, H. & Cisar, C. (1992). Promoting interaction during sociodramatic play: Teaching scripts to typical preschoolers and classmates with disabilities. *Journal of Applied Behavior Analysis, 25,* 265–280.

Goldstein, H. (1984). Effects of modeling and corrected practice on generative language learning of preschool children. *Journal of Speech and Hearing Disorders, 49,* 389–398.

Goldstein, H. (2006). Language intervention considerations for children with mental retardation and developmental disabilities. *Perspectives on Language Learning and Education: American Speech-Language-Hearing Association, Special Interest Division 1, 13,* 21–26.

Goldstein, H., Schneider, N., & Thiemann, K. (2007). Peer-mediated social communication intervention: When clinical expertise informs treatment development and evaluation. *Topics in Language Disorders, 27,* 182–199.

Goldstein, H., & Gallagher, T. M. (1992). Strategies for promoting the social-communication competence of young children with specific language impairment. In S. L. Odom, S. R. McConnell, & M. A. McEvoy (Eds.), *Social competence of young children with disabilities: Issues and strategies for intervention* (pp. 189–213). Baltimore: Brookes.

Goldstein, H., & Kaczmarek, L. (1992). Promoting communicative interaction among children in integrated intervention settings. In S. Warren & J. Reichle (Eds.), *Causes and effects in communication and language intervention* (pp. 81–111). Baltimore: Brookes.

Gonzalez-Mena, J. (2008). *Diversity in early care and education.* Boston: McGraw-Hill.

Goossens', C., & Crain, S. (1986a). *Augmentative communication assessment resource.* Wauconda, IL: Don Johnston.

Goossens', C., & Crain, S. (1986b). *Augmentative communication intervention resource.* Wauconda, IL: Don Johnston.

Gopnick, M. (1990). Feature blindness: A case study. *Language Acquisition, 1,* 139–164.

Gordon, K. A., Papsin, B. C., & Harrison, R. V. (2003) Activity-dependent developmental plasticity of the auditory brainstem in children who use cochlear implants. *Ear and Hearing, 24,* 485–500.

Gordon, K. A., & Harrison, R. V. (2005). Changes in human central auditory development caused by deafness in early childhood. *Hearsay, 17,* 28–35.

Graham, S. (2005). Strategy instruction and the teaching of writing: A meta-analysis. In C. A. MacArthur, S. Graham, and J. Fitzgerald (Eds.), *Handbook of writing research* (pp. 187–207). New York: Guilford Press.

Granlund, M., Björchk-Åkesson, E., Wilder, J., & Ylvén, R. (2008). AAC interventions for children in a family environment: Implementing evidence in practice. *Augmentative and Alternative Communication, 24,* 207–219.

Gravel, J. S., Roberts, J. E., Roush, J., Grose, J., Besing, J., Burchinal, M., Neebe, E., Wallace, I. F., & Zeisel, S. (2006). Early otitis media with effusion, hearing loss, and auditory processes at school age. *Ear and Hearing, 27,* 353–368.

Gray, S. (2004). Word learning by preschoolers with specific language impairment: Predictors and poor learners. *Journal of Speech, Language, and Hearing Research, 47,* 1117–1132.

Gray, S. (2005). Word learning by preschoolers with specific language impairment: Effect of phonological or semantic cues. *Journal of Speech, Language, and Hearing Research, 48,* 1452–1467.

Green, L. (2009). The nature of writing difficulties in students with language/learning disabilities. *Perspectives on Language Learning and Education, 16,* 4–8.

Greenhalgh, K. S., & Strong, C. J. (2001). Literate language features in spoken narratives of children with typical language and children with language impairments. *Language, Speech, and Hearing Services in Schools, 32,* 114–125.

Greenspan, S. (2006). Functional concepts in mental retardation: Finding the natural essence of an artificial category. *Exceptionality, 14,* 205–224.

Greenspan, S. I., & Wieder, S. (1997). Developmental patterns and outcomes in infants and children with disorders in relating and communicating: A chart review of 200 cases of children with autistic spectrum diagnoses. *Journal of Developmental and Learning Disorders, 1,* 87–141.

Greenspan, S. I., & Wieder, S. (1999). A functional developmental approach to autism spectrum disorders.

Journal of the Association for Persons with Severe Handicaps, 24, 147–161.

Greenwald, C., & Leonard, L. (1979). Communicative and sensorimotor development of Down's syndrome children. *American Journal of Mental Deficiency, 84,* 296–303.

Gresham, F. M., & MacMillan, D. L. (1997). Autistic recovery? An analysis and critique of the empirical evidence on the Early Intervention Project. *Behavior Disorders, 22,*185–201.

Gutierrez-Clellan, V. F., Brown, S., Conboy, B., & Robinson-Zanartu, C. (1998). Modifiability: A dynamic approach to assessing immediate language change. *Journal of Children's Communication Development, 19,* 31–42.

Haager, D., Klingner, J., & Vaughn, S. (2007). *Evidence-based reading practices for response to intervention.* Baltimore, MD: Brookes.

Hadley, P. A., & Schuele, C. M. (1998). Facilitating peer interaction: Socially relevant objectives for preschool language intervention. *American Journal of Speech-Language Pathology, 7,* 25–36.

Hadley, P., & Rice, M. (1996). Emergent uses of BE and DO: Evidence from children with specific language impairment. *Language Acquisition, 5,* 209–243.

Haggerman, R. J. (1999). Fragile X syndrome. In R. J. Hagerman (Ed.), *Neurodevelopment disorders* (pp. 61–132). Oxford: Oxford University Press.

Hagopian, L. P., Fisher, W. W., Sullivan, M. T., Acquisto, J., & LeBlanc, L. A. (1998). Effectiveness of functional communication training with and without extinction and punishment. *Journal of Applied Behavior Analysis, 26,* 23–36.

Hahne, A., Eckstein, K., & Friederici, A. D. (2004). Brain signatures of syntactic and semantic processes during children's language development. *Journal of Cognitive Neuroscience, 16,* 1302–1318.

Hakuta, K. (1990). *Bilingualism and bilingual education: A research perspective. Focus No. 1.* Washington, DC: National Clearinghouse for Bilingual Education.

Hall, E. T. (1976). *Beyond culture.* New York: Doubleday.

Halle, J. W., Ostrosky, M. M., & Hemmeter, M. L. (2006). Functional communication training: A strategy for ameliorating challenging behavior. In R. J. McCauley & M. E. Fey (Eds.), *Treatment of language disorders in children* (pp. 509–545). Baltimore, MD: Brookes.

Halliday, M. A. K. (1975). *Learning how to mean: Explorations in the development of language.* London: Edward Arnold Publishers Ltd.

Hammill, D. D., & Newcomer, P. L. (2008). *Test of Language Development Intermediate-3.* Bloomington, MN: Pearson.

Hammill, D., & Larsen, S. (1996). *Test of Written Language—3.* Austin, TX: PRO-ED.

Hancock, T. B., & Kaiser, A. P. (2005). Enhanced milieu teaching. In R. J. McCauley & M. E. Fey (Eds.), *Treatment of Language Disorders in Children* (pp. 203–236). Baltimore, MD: Brookes.

Haring, T. G., & Breen, C. G. (1992). A peer-mediated social network intervention to enhance the social integration of persons with moderate and severe disabilities. *Journal of Applied Behavioral Analysis, 25,* 319–333.

Harm, M. W., & Seidenberg, M. S. (1999). Phonology, reading acquisition, and dyslexia: Insights from connectionist models. *Psychological Review, 106,* 491–528.

Harris, G. A. (1998). American Indian cultures: A lesson in diversity. In D. E. Battle (Ed.), *Communication disorders in multicultural populations* (pp. 117–156). Boston: Butterworth-Heinemann.

Harris, J. C. (2006). *Intellectual disability: Understanding its development, causes, classification, evaluation, and treatment.* New York: Oxford University Press.

Harris, M. D., & Reichle, J. (2004). The impact of aided language stimulation on symbol comprehension and production in children with moderate cognitive disabilities. *American Journal of Speech-Language Pathology, 13,* 155–167.

Hart, B. M., & Rogers-Warren, A. K. (1978). Milieu teaching approaches. In R. L. Schiefelbusch (Ed.), *Bases of language intervention* (Vol. 2, pp. 193–235). Baltimore: University Park Press.

Hart, B., & Risley, T. (1999). Observing children and families talking. In B. Hart & T. Risley (Eds.), *The social world of children learning to talk* (pp. 7–29). Baltimore, MD: Brookes.

Hart, B., & Risley, T. R. (1995). *Meaningful differences in the everyday experiences of young American children.* Baltimore, MD: Brookes.

Hartley, J., & Harris, J. L. (2001). Reading the typography of text. In J. L. Harris & A. G. Kamhi (Eds.), *Literacy in African American Communities* (pp. 109–126). Mawhah, NJ: Erlbaum.

Hauser-Cram, P. (1996). Mastery motivation in toddlers with developmental disabilities. *Child Development, 67,* 236–248.

Haynes, W. O., & Pindzola, R. H. (2008). *Diagnosis and evaluation in speech pathology* (7th ed.). Boston, MA: Allyn & Bacon.

Heath, S. B. (1983). *Ways with words: Language, life, and work in communities and classrooms.* New York: Cambridge University Press.

Hegde, M. N., & Maul, C. A. (2006). *Language disorders in children: An evidence-based approach to assessment and treatment.* Boston: Allyn & Bacon.

Henderson, E. H. (1990). *Teaching spelling* (2nd ed.). Boston: Houghton Mifflin.

Henry, L. A., & MacLean, M. (2003). Relationships between working memory, expressive vocabulary and arithmetical reasoning in children with and without intellectual disabilities. *Educational and Child Psychology, 20,* 51–64.

Heubert, J., & Hauser, R. (Eds.) (1999). *High stakes testing for tracking, promotion, and graduation.* Washington, DC: National Academy Press.

Hodapp, R. M., & Dykens, E. M. (2004). Genetic and behavioral aspects: Application to maladaptive behavior and cognition. In J. A. Rondal, R. M. Hodapp, S. Soresi, E. M. Dykens, & L. Nota (Eds.), *Intellectual disabilities: Genetics, behavior, and inclusion* (pp. 13–49). London: Whurr.

Hodson, B. W. (2004). *Hodson Assessment of Phonological Patterns (3rd ed.).* Austin, TX: PRO-ED.

Hoff, E. (2006). How social contexts support and shape language development. *Developmental Review, 26,* 55–88.

Horner, R. H., & Budd, C. M. (1985). Teaching manual sign language to a nonverbal student: Generalization of sign use and collateral reduction of maladaptive behavior. *Education and Training of the Mentally Retarded, 20,* 39–47.

Howlin, P., Mawhood, L., & Rutter, M. (2000). Autism and developmental receptive language disorder-—A follow-up comparison in early adult life. II: Social, behavioral, and psychiatric outcomes. *Journal of Child Psychology and Psychiatry, 41,* 561–578.

Hoyson, M., Jamieson, B., & Strain, P. S. (1984). Individualized group instruction of normally developing and autistic-like children: A description and evaluation of the LEAP curriculum model. *Journal of the Division for Early Childhood, 8,* 157–172.

Hresko, W. P., Herron, S. R., & Peak, P. K. (1996). *Test of Early Written Language-Second Edition.* Austin, TX: PRO-ED.

Huang, R., Hopkins, J., & Nippold, M. A. (1997). Satisfaction with standardized language testing: A survey of speech-language pathologists. *Language, Speech, and Hearing Services in Schools, 28,* 12–29.

Huguenin, N. H. (2000). Reducing overselective attention to compound visual cues with extended training in adolescents with severe mental retardation. *Research in Developmental Disabilities, 21,* 93–113.

Huisingh, R., Bowers, L., LoGiudice, C., & Orman, J. (2005). *The WORD Test-Adolescent.* East Moline, IL: Linguisystems.

Hulit, L. M., & Howard, M. R. (2006). *Born to talk: An introduction to speech and language development.* Boston: Pearson.

Hunt, K. W. (1965). *Grammatical structures written at three grade levels.* Urbana, IL: National Council of Teachers of English.

Hwa-Froelich, D. A. (2000). *Frameworks of education: Perspectives of Asian parents and Head Start staff.* Unpublished doctoral dissertation, Wichita State University, Witchita, KS.

Hwa-Froelich, D., & Vigil, D. C. (2004). Three aspects of cultural influence on communication: A literature review. *Communications Disorders Quarterly, 25,* 107–118.

Hwa-Froelich, D. A., & Westby, C. E. (2003). Frameworks of education: Perspectives of Southeast Asian parents and Head Start staff. *Language, Speech, and Hearing Services in Schools, 34,* 299–319.

IDEA (2004). *Reauthorization of the Individuals with Disabilities Education Act: Guidance with Respect to State and Federal Regulations Implementing the Individuals with Disabilities Education Act of 2004.* Retrieved November 17, 2007 from www.ed.gov/policy/speced/guid/idea/idea2004.html.

Idol, L. (2006). Toward inclusion of special education students in general education: A program evaluation of eight schools. *Remedial and Special Education, 27,* 77–94.

Iglesias, A. (2002). Latino culture. In D. E. Battle (Ed.), *Communication disorders in multicultural populations* (3rd ed., pp. 179–204). Boston: Butterworth-Heinemann.

Imada, T., Zhang, Y., Cheour, M., Taulu, S., Ahonen, A., & Kuhl, P. (2006). Infant speech perception activates Broca's area: A developmental magnetoencephalography study. *NeuroReport, 17,* 957–962.

Individuals with Disabilities Education Act (IDEA) Amendments of 1997, Pub. L. No. 105–17, 20 U.S.C., 1400 et seq.

Ingersoll, B., & Schreibman, L. (2006). Teaching reciprocal imitation skills to young children using a naturalistic behavioral approach: Effects on language pretend play and joint attention. *Journal of Autism and Developmental Disorders, 36,* 487–505.

Ingram, D. (1972a). The acquisition of questions and its relation to cognitive development in normal and linguistically deviant children: A pilot study. *Papers and Reports on Child Language Development, 4,* 13–18.

Ingram, D. (1972b). The acquisition of the English verbal auxiliary and copula in normal and linguistically deviant children. *Papers and Reports on Child Language Development, 4,* 79–91.

Invernizzi, M., Sullivan, A., Meier, J., & Swank, L. (2004). *Phonological Awareness Literacy Screening—Pre-Kindergarten.* Charlottesville: University of Virginia.

Jerger, J., Jerger, S., Pepe, P., & Miller, R. (1986). Race difference in susceptibility to noise-induced hearing loss. *American Journal of Otology, 7,* 425–49.

Jerger, J., Martin, J., & McColl, R. (2004). Interaural cross correlation of event-related potentials and diffusion tensor imaging in the evaluation of auditory processing disorder: A case study. *Journal of the American Academy of Audiology, 15,* 79–87.

Jick, H., & Kaye, J. A. (2003). Epidemiology and possible causes of autism. *Pharmacotherapy, 23,* 1524–1530.

Joanisse, M. E. (2009). Model-based approaches to language disorders. In R. G. Schwartz (Ed.), *Handbook of child language disorders* (pp. 257–278). New York: Psychology Press.

Johnston, J. (2006). *Thinking about child language: Research to practice.* Eau Claire: Thinking Publications.

Jones, M. C., Walley, R. M., Leech, A., Paterson, M., Common, S., & Metcalf, C. (2006). Using goal attainment scaling to evaluate a needs-led exercise program for people with severe and profound intellectual disabilities. *Journal of Intellectual Disabilities, 10,* 317–335.

Jorde, L. B., & Wooding, S. P. (2004). Genetic variation, classification and 'race'. *Nature Genetics Supplement, 36,* S28–233.

Joyce, B., & Showers, B. (1996) The evolution of peer coaching. *Educational Leadership, 53,* 12–16.

Justice, L. M. (2002). *The syntax handbook: Everything you learned about syntax . . . but forgot.* Eau Claire, WI: Thinking Publications.

Justice, L. M. (2006). Evidence-based practice, response to intervention, and the prevention of reading difficulties. *Language, Speech, and Hearing Services in Schools, 37,* 284–297.

Justice, L. M., & Ezell, H. K. (2002). Use of storybook reading to increase print awareness in at-risk children. *American Journal of Speech-Language Pathology, 11,* 17–29.

Justice, L. M., & Fey, M. E. (2004, Sept. 21). Evidence-based practice in schools: Integrating craft and theory with science and data. *The ASHA Leader,* pp. 4–5, 30–32.

Justice, L. M., & Kaderavek, J. N. (2004). Embedded-explicit emergent literacy intervention I: Background and description of approach. *Language, Speech, and Hearing Services in Schools, 35,* 201–211.

Justice, L. M., Bowles, R., Eisenberg, S. L., Kaderavek, J. N., Ukrainetz, T. A., & Gillam, R. B. (2006). The index of narrative micro-structure (INMIS): A clinical tool for analyzing school-aged children's narrative performance. *American Journal of Speech-Language Pathology, 15,* 177–191.

Justice, L. M., Chow, S. M., Capellini, C., Flanigan, K., & Colton, S. (2003). Emergent literacy intervention for vulnerable preschoolers: Relative effects of two approaches. *American Journal of Speech-Language Pathology, 12,* 1–14.

Justice, L. M., Invernizzi, M. A., & Meier, J. D. (2002). Designing and implementing an early literacy screening protocol: Suggestions for the speech-language pathologist. *Language, Speech, and Hearing Services in Schools, 33,* 84–101.

Kaderavek, J. N., & Rabidoux, P. (2004). Interactive to independent literacy: A model for designing literacy goals for children with atypical communication. *Reading and Writing Quarterly, 20,* 237–260.

Kaderavek, J. N., & Justice, L. M. (2002). Shared storybook reading as an intervention context: Practices and potential pitfalls. *American Journal of Speech-Language Pathology, 11,* 101–110.

Kaderavek, J. N., & Justice, L. M. (2004). Embedded-explicit emergent literacy intervention II: Goal selection and implementation in the early childhood classroom. *Language, Speech, and Hearing Services in Schools, 35,* 212–228.

Kaderavek, J. N., & Pakulski, L. M. (2007). Facilitating literacy development in young children with hearing loss. *Seminars in Speech and Language, 28,* 69–78.

Kaderavek, J. N., & Sulzby, E. (1998). Parent-child joint book reading: An observational protocol for young children. *American Journal of Speech-Language Pathology, 7,* 33–47.

Kaderavek, J. N., & Sulzby, E. (2000). Issues in emergent literacy for children with specific language impairments: Language production during storybook reading, toy play and oral narratives. In L. R. Watson, T. L. Layton, & E. R. Crais (Eds.), *Handbook of early language impairment in children: Assessment and treatment* (pp. 199–244). New York: Delmar.

Kaderavek, J. N., Cabell, S. Q., Justice, L. M. (2009). Early writing and spelling development. In P. M. Rhyner (Ed.), *Emergent literacy and early language acquisition: Making the connection* (pp. 104–152). New York: Guilford Press.

Kaderavek, J. N., Laux, J. M., & Mills, N. H. (2004). A counseling training module for students in speech-language pathology training programs. *Contemporary Issues in Communication Science & Disorders. 31,* 153–163.

Kahmi, A. G. (2009). The case for the narrow view of reading. *Language, Speech, and Hearing Services in Schools, 40,* 174–177.

Kahmi, A. G., & Catts, H. W. (2002). The language basis of reading: Implications for classification and treatment of children with reading disabilities. In K. G. Butler & E. R. Silliman (Eds.), *Speaking, reading, and writing in children with language learning disabilities: New Paradigms in research and practice* (pp. 45–72). Mahwah, NJ: Erlbaum.

Kail, R., & Leonard, L. B. (1986). *Word-finding abilities in children with specific language impairment. Monographs of the American Speech-Langauge-Hearing Association,* No. 25. Rockville, MD: American Speech-Language-Hearing Association.

Kaiser, A. P., & Hancock, T. B. (2003). Teaching parents new skills to support their young children's development. *Infants & Young Children, 16,* 9–21.

Kaiser, A. P., & Hester, P. P. (1994). Generalized effects of enhanced milieu teaching. *Journal of Speech and Hearing Research, 37,* 1320–1340.

Kaiser, A. P., & Trent, J. A. (2007). Communication intervention for young children with disabilities: Naturalistic approaches to promoting development. In S. Odom, R. Horner, M. Snell, & J. Blacher (Eds.), *Handbook of developmental disabilities* (pp. 224–246). New York: Guilford Press.

Kaiser, A. P., Hester, P. P., Alpert, C. L., & Whiteman, B. C. (1995). Preparing parent trainers: An experimental analysis of effects on trainers, parents, and children. *Topics in Early Childhood Special Education, 14,* 385–414.

Kalyanpur, M., & Harry, B. (1999). *Culture in special education.* Baltimore: Brookes.

Kamhi, A. G. (1988). A reconceptualization of generalization and generalization problems. *Language, Speech, and Hearing Services in Schools, 19,* 304–313

Kamhi, A. G. (2003, April 15). The role of the SLP in improving reading fluency. *The ASHA Leader, 8*(7), 6–8.

Kamhi, A. G. (2009). Prologue: The case for the narrow view of reading. *Language, Speech, and Hearing Services in Schools, 40,* 174–177.

Kaniel, S., Tzuriel, D., Feuerstein, R., Ben-Shachar, N., & Eitan, T. (1991). Dynamic assessment: Learning and transfer abilities of Ethiopian immigrants to Israel. In R. Feuerstein, P. Klein, & A. Tannenbaum (Eds.), *Mediated learning experience* (pp.179–209). London: Freund.

Kanner, L. (1943). Autistic disturbances of affective contact. *Nervous Child, 2,* 217–250.

Katims, D. (2000). *The quest for literacy: Curriculum and instructional procedures for teaching reading and writing to students with mental retardation and developmental disabilities.* Reston, VA: The Council for Exceptional Children.

Kayser, H. (1995). Interpreters. In H. Kayser (Ed.), *Bilingual speech-language pathology* (pp. 207–222). San Diego, CA: Singular.

Kearney, P. M., & Griffin, T. (2001). Between joy and sorrow: Being a parent or a child with developmental disability. *Issues and innovations in nursing practice, 34,* 582–592.

Kellogg, S. *Jack and the beanstalk* [Paperback]. New York: Harper Collins.

Kerry Moran, K. J. (2006). Nurturing emergent readers through readers theater. *Early Childhood Education Journal, 33,* 317–323.

Khan, L., & James, S. (1983). Grammatical morpheme development in three language disordered children. *Journal of Childhood Communication Disorders, 6,* 85–100.

Kids Count (2007, March). *One out of five U.S. children is living in an immigrant family.* (Data Snapshot No. 4). Baltimore, MD: Annie Casey Foundation.

Klin, A., McPartland, J., & Volkmar, F. R. (2005). Asperger syndrome: In F. R. Volkmar, R. Paul, A. Klin, & D. Cohen (Eds.), *Handbook of autism and pervasive developmental disorders: Vol. 1. Diagnosis, development, neurobiology, and behavior* (3rd ed., pp. 88–125). Hoboken, NJ: Wiley.

Klingner, J. K., & Edwards, P. A. (2006). Cultural considerations with Response to Intervention models. *Reading Research Quarterly, 41,* 108–17.

Koegel, L. K., Koegel, R. L., Harrower, J. K., & Cater, C. M. (1999). Pivotal response intervention I: Overview of approach. *Journal of the Association for Persons with Severe Handicaps, 24,* 174–185.

Koegel, L. K., Koegel, R. L., Shoshan, Y., & McNerney, E. (1999). Pivotal response intervention II: Preliminary long-term outcome data. *Journal of the Association for Persons with Severe Handicaps, 24,* 186–198.

Kovarsky, D., & Duchan, J. F. (1997). The interactional dimensions of language therapy. *Language, Speech, and Hearing Services in Schools, 28,* 297–307.

Krug, D. A., Arick, J. R., & Almond, P. J. (1980). *Autism screening instrument for educational planning.* Portland, OR: ASIEP Educational.

Kubler-Ross, E. (1969). *On death and dying.* New York: MacMillan.

Kuhl, P. K. (2004). Early language acquisition: cracking the speech code. *Nature Reviews Neuroscience, 11,* 831–844.

Kuhl, P. K., & Rivera-Gaxiola, M. (2008). Neural substrates of language acquisition. *Annual Review of Neuroscience, 31,* 511–534.

Kumin, L. (2001). Speech intelligibility in individuals with Down syndrome: A framework for targeting specific factors for assessment and treatment. *Down Syndrome Quarterly, 6,* 1–8.

Kurtzer-White, E., & Luterman, D. (2003). Families and children with hearing loss: Grief and coping. *Mental Retardation and Developmental Disabilities Research Reviews, 9,* 232–235.

Labov, W. (1972). *Sociolinguistic patterns.* Oxford: Blackwell

Lahey, M. (1988). *Language disorders and language development*. New York: Macmillan.

Landau, B., & Zukowski, A. (2003) Objects, motions, and paths: Spatial language of children with Williams Syndrome. *Developmental Neuropsychology, 23*, 105–138.

Landry, S. H., Smith, K. E., & Swank, P. R. (2006). Responsive parenting: Establishing early foundations for social, communication, and independent problem-solving skills. *Developmental Psychology, 42*, 627–642.

Larkin, R. F., & Snowling, M. J. (2008). Comparing phonological skills and spelling abilities in children with reading and language impairments. *International Journal of Language and Communication Disorders, 43*, 111–124.

Larsen, S., Hammill, D., & Moats, L. (1999). *Test of written spelling* (4th ed.). Austin, TX: PRO-ED.

Lave, J., & Wenger, E. (1991). *Situated learning: Legitimate peripheral participation*. Cambridge: Cambridge University Press.

Law, J., Campbell, C., Roulstone, S., Adams, C., & Boyle, J. (2008). Mapping practice onto theory: The speech and language practitioner's construction of receptive language impairment. *International Journal of Language & Communication Disorders, 43*, 245–263.

Layton, T. (2000). Young children with Down syndrome. In T. Layton, E. Crais, & L. Watson (Eds.), *Handbook of early language impairment in children: Nature* (pp. 193–232). Albany, NY: Delmar Publishers.

Leadholm, B., & Miller, J. (1992). *Language sample analysis: The Wisconsin guide*. Madison, WI: Wisconsin Department of Public Instruction.

LeBlanc, J. M., Schroeder, S. R., & Mayo, L. (1997). Life-span approach in the education and treatment of persons with autism. In D. Cohen & F. R. Volkmar (Eds.), *Handbook of autism and pervasive developmental disorder* (2nd ed., pp. 934–944). New York: Wiley.

LeCouteur, A., Rutter, M., Lord, C., Rios, P., Robertson, S., Holdgrafer, M., et al., (1989). Autism Diagnostic Interview: A standardized investigator-based instrument. *Journal of Autism and Developmental Disorders, 19*, 363–387.

Lee, A. Y. (1998). Transfer as a measure of intellectual functioning. In S. Soraci & W. J. McIlvane (Eds.), *Perspectives on fundamental processes in intellectual functioning: A survey of research approaches, Vol. 1* (pp. 351–366). Stamford, CT: Ablex.

Lee, L., Koenigsknecht, R., & Mulhern, S. (1975). *Interactive language development teaching*. Evanston, IL: Northwestern University Press.

Lee, L. (1996). Developmental sentence types: A method for comparing normal and deviant syntactic development. *Journal of Speech and Hearing Disorders, 31*, 311–330.

Lee, S. J. (1996). *Unraveling the "model minority" stereotype listening to Asian American youth*. New York: Teacher's College Press.

Leigh, I., & Anthony, S. (1999). Parent bonding in clinically depressed deaf and hard-of-hearing adults. *Journal of Deaf Studies and Deaf Education, 4*, 28–36.

Leonard, L. B., McGregor, K., & Allen, G. (1992). Grammatical morphology and speech perception in children with specific language impairment. *Journal of Speech and Hearing Research, 35*, 1076–1085.

Leonard, L. (1981). Facilitating linguistic skills in children with specific language impairments. *Applied Psycholinguistics, 2*, 89–118.

Leonard, L. B. (1991). Specific language impairment as a clinical category. *Language, Speech, and Hearing Services in Schools, 22*, 66–68.

Leonard, L. B. (1998). *Children with specific language impairment*. Cambridge, MA: MIT Press.

Leonard, L. B., Bortolini, U., Caselli, M. C., McGregor, K., & Sabbadini, L., (1992). Morphological deficits in children with specific language impairment: The status of features in the underlying grammar. *Language Acquisition, 2*, 151–179.

Leonard, L. B., Eyer, J., Bedore, L., & Grela, B. (1997). Three accounts of the grammatical morpheme difficulties of English speaking children with specific language impairment. *Journal of Speech and Hearing Research, 40*, 741–753.

Lepola, J., Salonen, P., & Vauras, M. (2000). The development of motivation orientations as a function of divergent reading careers from preschool to second grade. *Learning and Instruction, 10*, 153–177.

Liberman, I. Y., Shankweiler, D., & Liberman, A. M. (1989). *The alphabetic principle and learning to read*. Reprinted from Phonology and reading disability: Solving the reading puzzle, *International Academy for Research in Learning Disabilities Monograph Series*. Retrieved March 17, 2006, from www.pattan.k12.pa.us/files/Newsletters/EBP-Sum01.pdf.

Lidz, C. S., & Pena, E. D. (2009). Responsiveness to intervention: New opportunities and challenges for the speech-language pathologist. *Seminars in Speech & Language 3*, 121–133.

Lidz, C., & Pena, E. (1996). Dynamic assessment: The model, its relevance as a nonbiased approach, and its application to Latino American preschool children. *Language, Speech, and Hearing Services in Schools, 27*, 367–372.

Light, J., & Drager, K. (2006). Beginning communicators: Improving AAC outcomes. *Augmentative Communication News, 18* (1), 8–10.

Light, J., & Drager, K. (2007). AAC technologies for young children with complex communication needs: State of the science and future research directions. *Augmentative and Alternative Communication, 23,* 204–216.

Light, J., Drager, K., McCarthy, J., Mellott, S., Millar, D., Parrish, C., et al. (2004). Performance of typically developing four- and five-year-old children with AAC systems using different language organization techniques. *Augmentative and Alternative Communication, 20,* 63–88.

Lindamood, P. C., & Lindamood, P. (2004). *Lindamood Auditory Conceptualization Test (LAC-3) – Third Edition.* Austin, TX: PRO-ED.

Ling, D. (1989). *Foundations of spoken language for hearing-impaired children.* Washington, DC: Alexander Graham Bell Association for the Deaf.

Ling, D. (2002). *Speech and the hearing-impaired child: Theory and practice* (2nd ed.). Washington, DC: Alexander Graham Bell Association for the Deaf.

Linguistic Society of America (1997). Linguistic Society of America resolution on the Oakland "Ebonics" issue, January, 3, 1997. Retrieved www.lsadc.org/info/lsa-res-ebonics.cfm.

Loban, W. (1976). *Language development: Kindergarten through grade twelve.* Urbana, IL: National Council of Teachers.

Loeb, D. F., & Leonard, L. B. (1988). Specific language impairment and parameter theory. *Clinical Linguistics & Phonetics, 2,* 317–327.

Loeb, D. F., Kinsler, K., & Bookbinder, L. (2000, November). *Current language sampling practices in preschools.* Poster presented at the Annual Convention of the American Speech-Language-Hearing Association, Washington, DC.

Lombardino, L. J., Lieberman, R. J., & Brown, J. J. C. (2005). *Assessment of literacy and language.* San Antonio, TX: Harcourt.

Lonigan, C. J., Burgess, S. R., Anthony, J. S., & Barker, T. A. (1998). Development of phonological sensitivity in 2- to 5-year-old children. *Journal of Educational Psychology, 90,* 294–311.

Lord C., & Corsello, C. (2005). Diagnostic instruments in autistic spectrum disorders. In F. R. Volmar, A. Klin, & D. Cohen (Eds.), *Handbook of autism and pervasive developmental disorders* (Vol. 2, 3rd ed., pp 730–771). New York: Wiley.

Lord, C., & Corsello, C. (2005). Diagnostic instruments in autistic spectrum disorders. In F. R. Volkmar, R. Paul, A. Klin, D. Cohen (Eds.), *Handbook of autism and pervasive developmental disorders. Vol. 2: Assessments, interventions, and policy* (3rd ed., pp. 730–771). Hoboken, NJ: Wiley.

Lord, C., Rutter, M. L., & Le Couteur, A. (1994). Autism Diagnostic Interview-Revised: A revised version of a diagnostic interview for caregivers of individuals with possible pervasive developmental disorders. *Journal of Autism and Developmental Disorders, 24,* 659–685.

Losardo, A., & Notari-Syverson, A. (2001). *Alternative approaches to assessing young children.* Baltimore, MD: Brookes.

Lovaas, O. I. (1977). *The autistic child: Language development through behavior modification.* New York: Irvington.

Lovaas, O. I. (1987). Behavioral treatment and normal educational and intellectual functioning in young autistic children. *Journal of Consulting and Clinical Psychology, 55,* 3–9.

Lovaas, O. I. (1993). The development of treatment-research project for developmentally disabled and autistic children. *Journal of Applied Behavior Analysis, 26,* 617–630.

Lovaas, O. I. (2003). *Teaching individuals with developmental delays: Basic intervention techniques.* Austin, TX: PRO-ED.

Lovelace, S., & Stewart, S. R. (2009). Effects of robust vocabulary instruction and multicultural text on the development of word knowledge among African American children. *American Journal of Speech-Language Pathology 18,* 168–179.

MacDonald J. D. (2004). *Communicating partners: 30 years of building responsive relationships with late talking children including autism, Asperger's Syndrome (ASD), Down Syndrome, and typical development.* London: Jessica Kingsley Publishers.

Macionis, J. J. (2008). *Society: The basics* (10th ed.). Upper Saddle River, NJ: Prentice Hall.

MacKall, D. D., (1997). *Picture me with Jonah and the whale.* Akron, OH: Playhouse Publishing.

MacSweeney, M., Woll, B., Campbell, R., McGuire, P. K., David, A. S., Williams, S. C., et al. (2002). Neural systems underlying British Sign Language and audio-visual English processing in native users. *Brain, 125,* 1583–1593.

Marazziti, D., Muratori, F., Cesari, A., Masala, I., Baroni, S., Giannaccini, G., et al. (2000). Increased density of the platelet serotonin transporter in autism. *Pharmacopsychiatry, 33,* 165–168.

Marcus, G. F., & Fisher, S. E. (2003). FOXP2 in focus: What can genes tell us about speech and language? *Trends in Cognitive Sciences, 7,* 257–262.

Marcus, L. M., Kunce, L. J., & Schopler, E. (1997). Working with families. In C. J. Cohen & F. R. Volkmar (Eds.),

Handbook of autism and pervasive developmental disorders (2nd ed., pp. 631–649). New York: Wiley.

Margolis, H., & McCabe, P. P. (2006). Improving self-efficacy and motivation: What to do, what to say. *Intervention in School and Clinic, 41,* 218–227.

Marschark, M., & Lukomski, J. (2001). Understanding language and learning in deaf children. In M. D. Clark, M. Marschark, & M. A. Karchmer (Eds.), *Context, cognition, and deafness* (pp. 71–87). Washington DC: Gallaudet University Press.

Martin, B., & Carle, E. (2008). *Brown bear, brown bear, what do you see?* [40th anniversary edition]. New York: Henry Holt.

Maryland School for the Deaf (MSD) *Handbook for Parents and Students* (2009). Retrieved from www. msd.edu/forms/cc_handbook.pdf.

Mashburn, A. J., Justice, L. M., Downer, J. T., & Pianta, R. C. (2009). Peer effects on children's language achievement during pre-kindergarten. *Child Development, 80,* 686–702.

Maslow, A. H. (1962). *Towards a psychology of being.* Trenton, NJ: van Nordstrand.

Masterson, J. J., & Apel, K. (2000). Spelling assessment: Charting a path to optimal intervention. *Topics in Language Disorders, 20,* 50–65.

Masterson, J. J., & Crede, L. A. (1999). Learning to spell: Implications for assessment and intervention. *Language, Speech, and Hearing Services in Schools, 30,* 243–254.

Masterson, J. J., Apel, K., & Wasowicz, J. (2002). *Spelling performance evaluation for language & literacy* (2nd ed.) (SPELL-2). Evanston, IL: Learning By Design.

Mather, M., Rivers, K. L., & Jacobsen, L. A. (2005). The American community survey. *Population Bulletin 60,* 3. Washington, DC: Population Reference Bureau.

Mattie, H. D. (2001). Generalization effects of cognitive strategies conversation training for adults with moderate to severe disabilities. *Education and Training in Mental Retardation and Developmental Disabilities, 36,* 178–187.

McCabe, A. (1996). Evaluating narrative discourse skills. In K. Cole, P. Dale, & D. Thal (Eds.), *Assessment of communication and language* (pp. 121–142). Baltimore, MD: Brookes.

McCabe, A., & Bliss, L. S. (2003). *Patterns of narrative discourse: A multicultural, life-span approach.* Boston: Allyn & Bacon.

McCabe, A., & Peterson, C. (Eds.) (1991). *Developing narrative structure.* Hillsdale, NJ: Erlbaum.

McCaleb, P., & Prizant, B. (1985). Encoding of new versus old information by autistic children. *Journal of Speech and Hearing Disorders, 50,* 230–240.

McCauley, R. J. (2001). *Assessment of language disorders in children.* Mahwah, NJ: Erlbaum.

McEachin, J. J., Smith, T., & Lovaas, O. I. (1993). Long-term outcome for children with autism who received early intensive behavioral treatment. *American Journal of Mental Retardation, 97,* 359–72.

McFadden, T. U., & Gillam, R. B. (1996). An examination of the quality of narratives produced by children with language disorders. *Language, Speech, and Hearing Services in Schools, 27,* 48–56.

McGinty, A. S., & Justice, L. M. (2006). Classroom-based versus pullout speech-language intervention: A review of the experimental evidence. *EBP Briefs, 1,* 1–25.

McGregor, K. (2009). Semantics in child language disorders. In R. G. Schwartz (Ed.), *Handbook of child language disorders* (pp. 365–387). New York: Psychology Press.

McKenna, M. C., & Stahl, S. A. (2003). *Assessment for reading instruction.* New York: Guilford Press.

McTigue, E. M., Beckman, A. R., & Kaderavek, J. N. (2007). Assessing literacy motivation and orientation. In K. Pence (Ed.), *Assessment in emergent literacy* (pp. 481–518). San Diego, CA: Plural.

McWilliam R. A., & de Kruif, R. E. L. (1998). *Engagement Quality Measurement System III: E-Qual III.* Accessed June 10, 2008 at www. vanderbiltchildrens.com/.

McWilliam, R. A., & Casey, A. M. (2007) *Engagement of every child in the preschool classroom.* Baltimore, MD: Brookes.

McWilliam, R. A., & Clingenpeel, B. (2003, August). *Functional intervention planning: The routines-based interview.* National Individualizing Preschool Inclusion Project, Vanderbilt Medical Center. Accessed June 15, 2008 at www.collaboratingpartners.com/docs/R_Mcwilliam/RBI%20 Flyer%20April%202005.pdf.

McWilliam, R. A., Scarborough, A. S., & Kim, H. (2003). Adult interactions and child engagement. *Early Education & Development, 14,* 7–28.

Menken, K. (2006). Teaching to the test: How No Child Left Behind impacts language policy, curriculum, and instruction for English Language Learners. *Bilingual Research Journal, 30(2),* 521–546.

Mercer, C. D., & Snell, M. E. (1977). *Learning theory research in mental retardation: Implications for teaching.* Upper Saddle River, NJ: Merrill/Prentice Hall.

Merrell, A., & Plante, E. (1997). Norm-referenced test interpretation in the diagnostic process. *Language, Speech, and Hearing Services in Schools, 28,* 50–58.

Meyer, J. (1997). Models of service delivery. In P. O'Connell (Ed.), *Speech, language, and hearing programs in schools: A guide for students and practitioners* (pp. 241–288). Gaithersburg, MD: Aspen Publishers.

Meyer, M., Toepel, U., Keller, J., Nussbaumer, D., Zysset, S., & Friederici, A. D. (2007). Neuroplasticity of sign language: Implications from structural and functional brain imaging. *Restorative Neurology and Neuroscience, 25,* 335–351.

Millar, D. C., Light, J., & Schlosser, R. W. (2006). The impact of augmentative and alternative communication intervention on the speech production of individuals with developmental disabilities: A research review. *Journal of Speech, Language, and Hearing Research, 49,* 248–264.

Miller, C. G. (2004). *MMR kids—Living scientific proof that MMR causes autism.* Accessed on August 18, 2008 from http://whale.to/a/mmr_kids.html.

Miller, J. (1996). The search for the phenotype of disordered language performance. In M. L. Rice (Ed.), *Toward a genetics of language* (pp. 297–314). Mahwah, NJ: Erlbaum.

Miller, J. (1999). Profiles of language development in children with Down syndrome. In J. Miller, M. Leddy, & L. Leavitt (Eds.), *Improving the communication of people with Down syndrome* (pp. 11–39). Baltimore, MD: Brookes.

Miller, J. (2006). Language and communication development in children with Down syndrome. *Perspectives on Language Learning and Education: American Speech-Language Hearing Association, Special Interest Division 1, 13,* 17–20.

Miller, J. F. (1991). Quantifying productive language disorders. In J. F. Miller (Ed.), *Research on child language disorders: A decade of progress* (pp. 211–220). Austin, TX: PRO-ED.

Miller, J. F., & Yoder, D. E. (1972). A syntax teaching program. In J. E. McLean, D. E. Yoder, & R. L. Schiefelbusch (Eds.), *Language intervention with the retarded* (pp. 191–211). Baltimore: University Park Press.

Mills, D. L., Plunkett K., Prat C., & Schafer G. (2005). Watching the infant brain learn words: Effects of vocabulary size and experience. *Cognitive Development, 20,.*19–31.

Minshew, N. J., Sweeney, J. A., Bauman, M. L., & Webb, S. J. (2005). Neurological aspects of autism. In F. R. Volkmar, R. Paul, A. Klin, & D. Cohen (Eds.), *Handbook of autism and pervasive developmental disorders: Vol. 1. Diagnosis, development, neurobiology, and behavior* (3rd ed., pp. 473–514). Hoboken, NJ: Wiley.

Mintz, T. H., & Gleitman, L. R. (2002). Adjectives really do modify nouns: The incremental and restricted nature of early adjective acquisition. *Cognition, 84,* 267–293.

Mitchell, R., & Karchmer, M. (2004). Chasing the mythical ten percent: Parental hearing status of deaf and hard of hearing students in the United States. *Sign Language Studies, 4,* 138–163.

Miyamoto, R. T., Hay-McCutcheon, M. J., Kirk, K. I., Houston, D. M., & Bergeson-Dana, T. R. (2007, August). *Speech and language skills of profoundly deaf children implanted under 12 months of age: Preliminary results.* Oral presentation at the Collegium Oto-Rhino-Laryngologicum Amicitiae Sacrum, Seoul, Korea.

Moats, L. (2000). *Speech to print.* Baltimore, MD: Brookes.

Moeller, M. P. (2000). Early intervention and language development in children who are deaf and hard of hearing. *Pediatrics, 106*(3), E43.

Moeller, P., Tomblin, B., Yoshinaga-Itano, C., MacDonald-Connor, C., & Jerger, S. (2007). Current state of knowledge: Language and literacy of children with hearing impairment. *Ear and Hearing, 28,* 740–753.

Moerk, E. (1992). *A first language taught and learned.* Baltimore, MD: Brookes.

Moerk, E. L. (2004). The guided acquisition of first language skills. Westport, CT: Greenwood Publishing Group.

Moll, L. C., & González, N. (1994). Critical issues: Lessons from research with language minority children. Journal of Reading Behavior (*JRB*): A Journal of Literacy, 26, 439–456.

Moog, J. S. (2002). Changing expectations for children with cochlear implants. *The Annals of Otology, Rhinology, and Laryngology, 111,* 138–142.

Morehead D., & Ingram, D. (1973). The development of base syntax in normal and linguistically deviant children. In D. Morehead and A. Morehead (Eds.), *Normal and Deficient Children* (pp. 209–238). Baltimore: University Park Press.

Morgan, G. A., MacTurk, R. H., & Hrncir, E. J. (1995). Mastery motivation: Overview, definitions, and conceptual issues. In R. H. MacTurk & G. A. Morgan (Eds.), *Mastery motivation: Origins, conceptualizations, and applications* (pp. 1–18). Norwood, NJ: Ablex.

Morgan, M. H. (2001). The African-American speech community: Reality and sociolinguists. In A. Duranti (Ed.), *Linguistic anthropology: A reader* (pp. 74- 94). Maiden, MA: Blackwell Publishers Inc.

Morrow, L. M. (2005). *Literacy development in the early years* (5th ed.). Boston: Allyn & Bacon.

Morrow, R. D. (1989). What's in a name? In particular, a Southeast Asian name? *Young Children, 44,* 20–23.

Nagy, W. W. (1988). *Teaching vocabulary to improve reading comprehension.* Urbana: IL: National Council of Teachers of English; and Newark, DE: International Reading Association.

Nail-Chiwetalu, B. J., & Ratner, N. B. (2006). Information literacy for speech-language pathologists: A key to evidence-based practice. *Language, Speech, and Hearing Services in Schools, 37*, 157–167.

National Institute of Child Health and Human Development (2000). *Report of the National Reading Panel. Teaching children to read: An evidence-based assessment of the scientific research literature on reading and its implications for reading instruction: Reports of the subgroups* (NIH Publication No. 00–4754). Washington, DC: U.S. Government Printing Office.

National Institute on Deafness and Communication Disorders (NIDCD) (2007). Statistics about hearing, balance, ear infections, and deafness. Retrieved May 14, 2007 from www.nidcd.nih.gov/health/statistics/hearing.asp.

National Reading Panel. (2000). *Report of the National Reading Panel: Teaching children to read*. Washington, DC: National Academy Press.

National Research Council (2001). *Educating children with autism*. Committee on Educational Interventions for Children with Autism. Division of Behavioral and Social Sciences and Education. Washington, DC: National Academy Press.

National Scientific Council on the Developing Child. (2007) *The Science of Early Childhood Development*. Retrieved December 18, 2007 at www.developingchild.net.

Nelson, K. E., Camarata, S. M., Welsh, J., Butkovsky, L., & Camarata, M. (1996). Effects of imitative and conversational recasting treatment on the acquisition of grammar in children with specific language impairment and younger language-normal children. *Journal of Speech and Hearing Research, 39*, 850–859.

Nelson, N. W. (1998). *Child language disorders in context: Infancy through adolescence* (2nd ed.). Boston: Allyn & Bacon.

Nelson, N. W., & Van Meter, A. M. (2006). Finding the words: Vocabulary development for young authors. In T. A. Ukrainetz (Ed.), *Contextualized language intervention: Scaffolding PreK-12 literacy achievement* (pp. 95–143). Greenville, SC: Thinking Publications.

Nelson, N. W., & Van Meter, A. M. (2006). The writing lab approach for building language, literacy, and communication abilities. In R. J. McCauley & M. E. Fey (Eds.), *Treatment of language disorders in children* (pp. 383–422). Baltimore, MD: Brookes.

Nelson, N. W., Bahr, C. M., & Van Meter, A. M. (2004). *The writing lab approach to language instruction and intervention*. Baltimore, MD: Brookes.

Neuman, S. B., & Roskos, K. (1992). Literacy objects as cultural tools: Effects on children's literacy behaviors in play. *Reading Research Quarterly, 27*, 202–225.

Niccols, A., Atkinson, L., & Pepler, D. (2003). Mastery motivation in young children with Down's syndrome: Relations with cognitive and adaptive competence. *Journal of Intellectual Disability Research, 47*, 121–133.

Nicholas, J. G., & Geers, A. E. (2006). Effects of early auditory experience on the spoken language of deaf children at 3 years of age. *Ear and Hearing, 27*, 286–298.

Nittrouer, S. (2002). What clinicians need to understand about speech perception and language processing. *Language, Speech, and Hearing Services in the Schools, 33*, 237–252.

Notari-Syverson, A., O'Connor, R., & Vadasy, P. F. (1998). *Ladders to literacy: A preschool activity book*. Baltimore: Brookes.

Nsamenang, A. B., & Lamb, M. E. (1994). Socialization of Nso children in the Bamenda grass fields of northwest Cameroon. In P. M. Greenfield & R. R. Cocking (Eds.), *Cross-cultural roots of minority child development* (pp. 133–146). Hillsdale, NJ: Erlbaum.

Numminen, H., Service, E., Ahonen, T., Korhonen, T., Tolvanen, A., Patja, K., et al. (2000). Working memory structure and intellectual disability. *Journal of Intellectual Disability Research, 44*, 579–590.

Nusbaum, D., (2007). Communication choices with Deaf and hard of hearing children. Laurent Clerc National Deaf Education Center. Retrieved November 10, 2007, from http://clerccenter.gallaudet.edu/KidsWorld DeafNet/e-docs/EI/appendix.html.

O'Neil, R. F., Horner, R. H., Albin, R. W., Sprague, J. R., Storey, K., & Newton, J. S. (1997). *Functional assessment and program development for problem behavior*. Pacific Groves: Brookes/Cole.

Oberecker, R., Friedrich, M., & Friederici, A. D. (2005). Neural correlates of syntactic processing in two-year-olds. *Journal of Cognitive Neuroscience, 17*, 1667–1678.

Ochs, E., & Schieffelin, B. (2001). Language acquisition and socialization: Three developmental stories and their implications. In A. Duranti (Ed.), *Linguistic anthropology: A reader* (pp. 263–301). Oxford, UK: Blackwell.

Odom, S., McConnell, S., & McEvoy, M. (1992). *Social competence of young children with disabilities: Nature, development, and intervention*. Baltimore: Brookes.

Oelwein, P. L. (2002). Liberation from traditional reading and math teaching methods and measurements. In W. I. Cohen, L. Nadel, & M. E. Madnick (Eds.), *Down syndrome* (pp. 421–436). New York: Wiley Liss.

Oetting, J., & Rice, M. (1993). Plural acquisition in children with specific language impairment. *Journal of Speech and Hearing Research, 40*, 62–74.

Oetting, J. B., & Hadley, P. (2009). Morphosyntax in child language disorders. In R. G. Schwartz (Ed.), *Handbook of child language disorders* (pp. 341–364). New York: Psychological Press.

Olswang, L., & Bain, B. (1991). Intervention issues for toddlers with specific language impairments. *Topics in Language Disorders, 11,* 69–86.

Oross, S., & Woods, C. B. (2003). Exploring visual perception abilities in individuals with intellectual disabilities: Assessment and implications. In S. Soraci Jr. & D Murata-Soraci (Eds.), *Visual information processing* (pp. 35–79). Westport, CT: Praeger.

Ortiz, A. A., & Kushner, M. I. (1997). Bilingualism and the possible impact on academic performance. In L. Silver (Ed.), *Child and adolescent psychiatric clinics of North America: Academic difficulties* (pp. 657–679). Philadelphia: W. B. Saunders Company.

Owens, R. E. (2010). *Language disorders: A functional approach to assessment and intervention* (5th ed.). Boston: Allyn & Bacon.

Owens, R. E. Jr. (2002). Mental retardation: Difference and delay. In D. K. Bernstein & E. Tiegerman-Farber (Eds.), *Language and communication disorders in children* (5th ed., pp. 436–509). Boston: Allyn & Bacon.

Ozonoff, S., & Cathcart, K. (1998). Effectiveness of a home program intervention for young children with autism. *Journal of Autism and Developmental Disorders, 28,* 25–32.

Parker, S., Zuckerman, B. S., & Augustyn, M. (2004). *Developmental and behavioral pediatrics* (2nd ed.). Hagerstown, MD: Lippincott Williams & Wilkins.

Partkian, R. (2003). *Before the ABCs: Promoting School Readiness in Infants & Toddlers.* Washington, DC: Zero to Three Press.

Paul, P. (2001). *Language and deafness* (3rd ed.). San Diego, CA: Singular/Thomson Learning.

Paul, R. & Elder, L. (2008). *Critical thinking: Concepts and tools* (5th ed.). Dillon Beach, CA: Foundation for Critical Thinking

Paul, R. (1981). Analyzing complex sentence development. In J. F. Miller (Ed.), *Assessing language production in children: Experimental procedures* (pp. 36–40). Needham Heights, MA: Allyn & Bacon.

Paul, R. (2005). Assessing communication in autism spectrum disorders. In F. R. Volkmar, R. Paul, A. Klin, & D. Cohen (Eds.), *Handbook of autism and pervasive developmental disorders: Vol. 2. Assessment, intervention, and policy* (3rd ed., pp. 799–816). Hoboken, NJ: Wiley.

Paul, R. (2007). *Language disorders from infancy through adolescence: Assessment and intervention* (3rd ed.). St. Louis: Mosby.

Paul, R., & Cascella, P. W. (2006). *Introduction to clinical methods in communication disorders.* Balitimore, MD: Brookes.

Peets, K. F. (2009). The effects of context on the classroom discourse skills of children with language impairment. *Language, Speech, and Hearing Services in Schools, 40,* 5–16.

Pelios, L. V., MacDuff, G. S., & Axelrod, S. (2003). The effects of a treatment package in establishing independent academic work skills in children with autism. *Education and Treatment of Children, 26,* 1–21.

Pellegrini, A. D., McGillicuddy-DeLisi, A. V., Sigel, I. E., & Brody, G. H. (1986). The effects of children's communicative status and task on parents' teaching style. *Contemporary Educational Psychology, 11,* 240–252.

Pena, E., Quinn, R., & Iglesias, A. (1992). The application of dynamic methods to language assessment: A nonbiased procedure. *The Journal of Special Education, 26,* 269–280.

Penagarikano, O., Mulle, J. G., & Warren, S. T. (2007). The pathophysiology of Fragile X syndrome. *Annual Review of Genomics and Human Genetics, 8,* 109–129.

Pence, K. L., Bojczyk, K. E., & Williams, R. S. (2007). Assessing vocabulary knowledge. In K. L. Pence (Ed.), *Assessment in emergent literacy* (pp. 431–480). San Diego, CA: Plural.

Peters-Johnson, C. (1997). Action: School Services. *Language, Speech, and Hearing Services in Schools, 28,* 92.

Phelps-Terasaki, D., & Phelps-Gunn, T. (1992). *Test of Pragmatic Language.* Austin, TX: PRO-ED.

Phillips, N., & Duke, M. (2001). The questioning skills of clinical teachers and preceptors: A comparative study. *Journal of Advanced Nursing, 33,* 523–532.

Piaget, J. (1928). *The child's conception of the world.* London: Routledge and Kegan Paul.

Piaget, J. (1952a). *The child's conception of number.* London: Routledge and Kegan Paul.

Piaget, J. (1952b). *The origins of intelligence in children.* New York: International University Press.

Plante, E., & Vance, R. (1995). Diagnostic accuracy of two tests of preschool language. *American Journal of Speech-Language Pathology, 4,* 70–76.

Pleis, J. R., & Coles, R. (2002). Summary health statistics for U.S. adults: National Health Interview Survey, 1998. National Center for Health Statistics. *Vital Health Stat, 10,* 209.

Population Reference Bureau (2001). *Migration and immigration.* Retrieved from www.prb.org/CPIPR/Topics/MigrationImmigration/Trends.aspx?p=1.

Powell, D. R., Burchinal, M. R., File, N., & Kontos, S. (2008). An eco-behavioral analysis of children's engagement in urban public school preschool classrooms. *Early Childhood Research Quarterly, 23,* 108–123.

Prior, M., & Ozonoff, S. (1998). Psychological factors in autism. In F. R. Volkmar (Ed.), *Autism and pervasive developmental disorders* (pp. 64–108). Cambridge, UK: Cambridge University.

Prizant, B. M., & Rydell, P. J. (1984). Analysis of functions of delayed echolalia in autistic children. *Journal of Speech and Hearing Research, 27,* 183–192.

Prizant, B. M., & Wetherby, A. M. (2006). Critical issues in enhancing communication abilities for persons with autism spectrum disorders. In F. R. Volkmar, R. Paul, A. Klin, & D. Cohen (Eds.), *Handbook of autism and pervasive developmental disorders: Vol. 2. Assessment, interventions, and policy* (3rd ed., pp. 925–945). New York: Wiley.

Prizant, B. M., Wetherby, A. M., & Rydell, P. J. (2000). Communication intervention issues for children with autism spectrum disorders. In A. M. Wetherby & B. M. Prizant, *Autism spectrum disorders: A transactional developmental perspective* (pp. 193–224). Baltimore: Brookes.

Prizant, B. M., Wetherby, A. M., Rubin, E., Laurent, A. C., & Rydell, P. J. (2006). *The SCERTS™ model: A comprehensive educational approach for children with autism spectrum disorders: Vol. 1. Program planning and intervention.* Baltimore, MD: Brookes.

Prizant, B. M., Wetherby, A. M., Rubin, E., Laurent, A. C., & Rydell, P. J. (2006). *The SCERTS™ model: A comprehensive educational approach for children with autism spectrum disorders: Vol. 1. Assessment.* Baltimore, MD: Brookes.

Proctor-Williams, K., Fey, M. E., & Loeb, D. F. (2001). Parental recasts and production of copulas and articles by children with specific language impairment and typical language. *American Journal of Speech-Language Pathology, 10,* 155–168.

Pueschel, S. M. (1990). Clinical aspects of Down syndrome from infancy to adulthood. *American Journal of Medical Genetics [Suppl. 7],* 52–56.

Puranik, C. S., Petscher, Y., Al Otaiba, S., Catts, H. W., & Lonigan, C. J. (2008). Development of oral reading fluency in children with speech or language impairments: A growth curve analysis. *Journal of Learning Disabilities, 41,* 545–560.

Rabidoux, P. C., & MacDonald, J. D. (2000). An interactive taxonomy of mothers and children during storybook interactions. *American Journal of Speech-Language Pathology, 9,* 331–344.

Rafferty, Y., Piscitelli, V., & Boettcher, C. (2003). The impact of inclusion on language development and social competence among preschoolers with disabilities. *Exceptional Children, 69,* 467–479.

Ratner, N. B. (2006). Evidence-based practice: An examination of its ramifications for the practice of speech-language pathology. *Language, Speech, and Hearing Services in Schools, 37,* 257–267.

Ravid, D., Levie, R., & Avivi Ben-zvi, G. (2003). The role of language typology in linguistic development: Implications for the study of language disorders. In Y. Levy & J. Schaeffer (Eds.), *Language competence across populations: Towards a definition of specific language impairment* (pp. 171–196). Mahwah, NJ: Erlbaum.

Redmond, S. M. (2004). Conversational profiles of children with ADHD, SLI, and typical development. *Clinical Linguistics & Phonetics, 18,* 107–125.

Reeve, K. (2005). *Amplification and family factors for children with mild and unilateral hearing impairment.* In National Workshop on Mild and Unilateral Hearing Loss: Workshop Proceedings. Breckenridge, CO: Centers for Disease Control and Prevention 20–21.

Rescorla, L. (2009). Age 17 language and reading outcomes in late-talking toddlers: Support for a dimensional perspective on language delay. *Journal of Speech, Language, and Hearing Research, 52,* 16–30.

Rescorla, L., & Fechnay, T. (1996). Mother-child synchrony and communicative reciprocity in late-talking toddlers. *Journal of Speech and Hearing Research, 39,* 200–208.

Rescorla, L., & Lee, E. (2001). Language impairment in young children. In T. Layton, E. Crais, and L. Watson (Eds.). *Handbook of early language impairments in children: Nature* (pp. 1–55). Albany, NY: Delmar.

Rescorla, L., & Ratner, N. B. (1996). Phonetic profiles of toddlers with severe expressive language impairments (SLI-E). *Journal of Speech and Hearing Research, 39,* 153–165.

Rescorla, L., & Schwartz, E. (1990). Outcome of toddlers with expressive language delay. *Applied Psycholinguistics, 11,* 393–407.

Rey, M., & Rey, H. A. (1985). *Curious George and the Pizza.* Boston, MA: Houghton Mifflin Books for Children.

Reyhner, J. (1992). Policies toward American Indian languages: A historical sketch. In J. Crawford (Ed.), *Language loyalties: A source of the official English controversy* (pp. 41–47). Chicago: University of Chicago Press.

Rhoades, E. A., & Chisolm, T. H. (2000). Global language progress with an auditory-verbal approach. *The Volta Review, 102,* 5–25.

Rhoades, E. A., (2006). Research outcomes of auditory-verbal intervention: Is the approach justified? *Deafness and Education International, 8,* 125–143.

Rice, M. L. (2000). Grammatical symptoms of specific language impairment. In D. V. M. Bishop & L. B. Leonard (Eds.), *Speech and language impairments in children: Causes, characteristics, intervention, and outcome* (pp. 17–34). East Sussex, UK: Psychology Press.

Rice, M. L., & Body, J. (1993). GAPS in the lexicon of children with specific language impairment. *First Language, 13,* 113–132.

Rice, M. L., & Kemper, S. (1984). *Child language and cognition.* Baltimore: University Park.

Rice, M. L., & Oetting, J. (1993). Morphological deficits in children with SLI: Evaluation of number marking and agreement. *Journal of Speech and Hearing Research, 36,* 1249–1257.

Rice, M. L., & Wexler, K. (1995). *Tense over time: the persistence of optional infinitives in English in children with SLI.* Paper presented at the Boston University Conference on Language Development, Boston.

Rice, M. L., Redmond, S. M., & Hoffman, L. (2006). MLU in children with SLI and younger control children shows concurrent validity, stability, and parallel growth trajectories. *Journal of Speech, Language, and Hearing Research, 49,* 793–808.

Rice, M. L., Sell, M. A., & Hadley, P. A. (1991). Social interactions of speech-language impaired children. *Journal of Speech and Hearing Research, 34,* 1299–1307.

Rice, M. L., Warren, S. F., & Betz, S. K. (2005). Language symptoms of developmental language disorders: An overview of autism, Down syndrome, fragile x, specific language impairment, and William syndrome. *Applied Psycholinguistics, 26,* 7–27.

Rice, M. L., Wexler, K., & Cleave, P. (1995). Specific language impairment as a period of optional infinitive. *Journal of Speech and Hearing Research, 38,* 850–863.

Rivera-Gaxiola, M., Klarman, L., Garcia-Sierra, A., & Kuhl, P. K. (2005). Neural patterns to speech and vocabulary growth in American infants. *NeuroReport 16,* 495–98.

Rivers, K., Lombardino, L., & Thompson, C. (1996). Effects of phonological decoding training on children's word recognition of CVC, CV, and VC structures. *American Journal of Speech-Language Pathology, 5,* 113–131.

Roach, A. T., & Elliott, S. N. (2005). Goal attainment scaling: An efficient and effective approach to monitoring student progress. *Teaching Exceptional Children, 37,* 8–17.

Robbins, A. M., Koch, D. B., Osberger, M. J., & Zimmerman-Philips, S. (2004). Effect of age at cochlear implantation on auditory skill development in infants and toddlers. *Archives of Otolaryngology – Head & Neck Surgery, 130,* 570–574.

Roberts, J. E., Mirrett, P. L, & Burchinal, M. (2001). Receptive and expressive communication development of young males with fragile X syndrome. *American Journal on Mental Retardation, 106,* 216–230.

Roberts, J., & Hunter, L. (2002). Otitis media and children's language learning, *American Speech-Language-Hearing Association Leader.* Retrieved May 14, 2007 from www.asha.org/about/publications/leader-online/archives/2002/q4/f021008.htm.

Roberts, J., Rescorla, L., & Borneman, A. (1994). *Morphosyntactic characteristics of early language errors: An examination of specific expressive language delay.* Poster presented at the Symposium on Research in Child Language Disorders, University of Wisconsin, Madison.

Roberts, J. E., Rosenfeld, R. M., & Zeisel, S. A. (2004). Otitis media and speech and language: A meta-analysis of prospective studies. *Journal of Pediatrics, 113,* 238–248.

Robertson, L., & Flexer, C. (1993). Reading development: A parent survey of children with hearing impairment who developed speech and language through the auditory-verbal method. *Volta Review 5,* 253–261.

Robins, D. L., Fein, D., Barton, M. L., & Green, J. A. (2001). The Modified Checklist for Autism in Toddlers: An initial study investigating the early detection of autism and pervasive developmental disorders. *Journal of Autism and Developmental Disorders, 31,* 131–144.

Robinson-Zanartu, C. (1996). Serving Native American children and families: Considering cultural variables. *Language, Speech, and Hearing Services in Schools, 27,* 373–384.

Rogers, C. (1951). *Client centered therapy.* Boston: Houghton Mifflin.

Rogers, S. J. (1999). Intervention for young children with autism: From research to practice. *Infants and Young Children, 12,* 1–16.

Rogers, S. J., & DiLalla, D. (1991). A comparative study of a developmentally based preschool curriculum on young children with autism and young children with other disorders of behavior or development. *Topics in Early Childhood Special Education, 11,* 29–48.

Rogers, S. J., & Lewis, H. (1989). An effective day treatment model for young children with pervasive developmental disorders. *Journal of the American Academy of Child and Adolescent Psychiatry, 28,* 207–214.

Rogers, S. J., Cook, I., & Meryl, A. (2005). Imitation and play in autism. In F. R. Volkmar, R. Paul, A. Klin, & D. Cohen (Eds.), *Handbook of autism and pervasive developmental disorders: Vol. 1. Diagnosis, development, neurobiology, and behavior* (3rd ed., pp. 382–405). Hoboken, NJ: Wiley.

Rogoff, B. (2001). Becoming a cooperative parent in a parent co-operative. In B. Rogoff, C. Turkanis, & L. Bartlett (Eds.), *Learning together: Children and adults in a school community* (pp. 145–155). Oxford: Oxford University Press.

Romski, M. A., & Sevcik, R. A. (1996). Breaking the speech barrier: Language development through augmented means. Baltimore, MD: Brookes.

Romski, M. A., Sevcik, R. A., Adamson, L. B., & Bakeman, R. A. (2005). Communication patterns of individuals with moderate or severe cognitive disabilities: Interactions with unfamiliar partners. *American Association on Mental Retardation, 110* (3), 226–238.

Romski, M. A., Sevcik, R. A., Cheslock, M., & Barton, A. (2006). The system for augmenting language: Augmentative and alternative communication and emerging language intervention. In R. McCauley & M. Fey (Eds.), *Treatment of language disorders in children: Conventional and controversial interventions*. Baltimore: Brookes.

Rondal, J. A. (2004). Intersyndrome and intrasyndrome language differences. In J. A. Rondal, R. M. Hodapp, S. Soresi, E. M. Dykens, & L. Nota (Eds.), *Intellectual disabilities: Genetics, behavior, and inclusion* (pp. 49–113). London: Whurr.

Rondal, J. A., & Comblain, A. (1996). Language in adults with Down syndrome. *Down Syndrome, 8,* 1–9.

Rondal, J. A., & Edwards, S. (1997). *Language in mental retardation.* San Diego, CA: Singular.

Rosalki, J. R., & Karp, S. J. (1999). Guidance on the creation of evidence-linked practice for COIN. *Clinical Oncology, 11,* 28–32.

Rose, S., McAnally, P., & Quigley, S. (2004). *Language learning practices with deaf children* (3rd ed.). Austin, TX: PRO-ED.

Roseberry-McKibben, C., & Hegde, M. N. (2005). *An advanced review of speech-language pathology: Preparation for NESPA and comprehensive examinations* (2nd ed.). Austin, TX: PRO-ED.

Rosemary, C. A., & Roskos, K. A. (2002). Literacy conversations between adults and children at child care: Descriptive observations and hypotheses. *Journal of Research in Childhood Education, 16,* 212–231.

Roseti, S., Tellis, G. M., & Gabel, R. (2001, November). *African-American middle and high school students' perceptions about stuttering.* Seminar presented at ASHA Convention, New Orleans, LA.

Rosin, P. (2006). *Communication skills and challenges of young children with Down syndrome: Bridging research to practice.* Presentation made to The Alberta Early Years Conference, Alberta, Canada.

Rosin, P., & Miolo, G. (2005). *Improving communication skills in children with Down syndrome using performance and literacy-based activities.* Presentation made to 4th International Conference on Developmental Issues in Down Syndrome, Portsmouth, England.

Roth, F., & Paul, R. (2007). Communication intervention: Principles and Procedures. In R. Paul & P. W. Cascella (Eds.), *Introduction to clinical methods in communication disorders* (2nd ed.; pp. 157–178). Baltimore: Brookes.

Rutter, M. (1970). Autistic children: Infancy to adulthood. *Seminars in Psychiatry, 2,* 435–450.

Rutter, M. (2003). Introduction: Autism—the challenges ahead. In G. Bock & J. Goode (Eds.) *Novartis Foundation Symposium on Autism: Neural basis and treatment possibilities* (pp. 1–9). Chichester, UK: Wiley & Sons.

Sabers, D. (1996). By their tests we will know them. *Language, Speech, and Hearing Services in Schools, 27,* 102–108.

Saddler, B., & Graham, S. (2005). The effects of peer-assisted sentence-combining instruction on the writing performance of more and less skilled young writers. *Journal of Educational Psychology, 97,* 43–54.

Salvia, J., & Ysseldyke, J. E. (1995). *Assessment in special and remedial education* (6th ed.). Boston: Houghton Mifflin.

Sandall, S., Giacomini, J., Smith, B. J., & Hemmeter, M. L. (2006). *DEC recommended practices toolkits: Interactive tools to improve practices for young children with special needs and their families* [CDROM]. Missoula, MT: Division for Early Childhood.

Scarborough, H., & Dobrich, W. (1990). Development of children with early language delay. *Journal of Speech and Hearing Research, 33,* 70–83.

Schaaf, R. C., & Miller, L. J. (2005). Occupational therapy using a sensory integrative approach for children with developmental disabilities. *Mental Retardation and Developmental Disabilities Research Reviews, 11,* 143–148.

Schafer, D. S., & Moersch, M. S. (1981). *Developmental programming for infants and young children.* Ann Arbor: University of Michigan Press.

Schalock, R. L. (2004). The emerging disability paradigm and its implications for policy and practice. *Journal of Disability Policy Studies, 14,* 204–215.

Schalock, R. L., & Luckasson, R. (2005). American Association on Mental Retardation's definition, classification, and system of supports and its relation to international trends and issues in the field of intellectual disabilities. *Journal of Policy and Practice in Intellectual Disabilities, 1,* 136–146.

Schalock, R. L., Luckasson, R. A., & Shogren, K. A. (2007). The renaming of "mental retardation": Understanding the change to the term "intellectual disability." *Intellectual and Developmental Disabilities, 45,* 116–124.

Schein, J., & Deck, M. (1974). *The Deaf population of the United States.* Silver Springs, MD: National Association of the Deaf.

Scherer, N. J., & Olswang, L. B. (1989). Using structured discourse as a language intervention technique with autistic children. *Journal of Speech and Hearing Disorders, 54,* 387–396.

Schirmer, B. R. (2000). *Language and literacy development in children who are deaf* (2nd ed.). Boston: Allyn & Bacon.

Schlosser, R. W. (2004). Goal attainment scaling as a clinical measurement technique in communicative disorders: A critical review. *Journal of Communication Disorders, 37,* 217–239.

Schlosser, R. W., & Wendt, O. (2007, November). *Effects of the Picture Exchange Communication System: A systematic review.* Poster session presented at the annual meeting of the American Speech-Language-Hearing Association, Boston, MA.

Schneider, P., & Watkins, R. V. (1996). Applying Vygotskian developmental theory to language intervention. *Language, Speech, and Hearing Services in Schools, 27,* 157–170.

Schopler, E., & Olley, J. (1982). Comprehensive educational services for autistic children: The TEACCH model. In T. B. Gutkin & C. R. Reynolds (Eds.), *Handbook of School Psychology* (3rd ed., pp. 452–475). New York: Wiley.

Schopler, E., Reichler, R. J., & Renner, B. R. (1988). *Childhood Autism Rating Scale (CARS).* Los Angeles, CA: Western Psychological Services.

Schopler, E., Short, A., & Mesibov, G. (1989). Relation of behavioral treatment to "normal functioning": Comment on Lovaas. *Journal of Consulting Clinical Psychology, 57,* 162–164.

Schuele, C. M., & Justice, L. M. (2006, Aug. 15). The importance of effect sizes in the interpretation of research. *The ASHA Leader, 11(10),* 14–15, 26–27.

Schuler, A. L. (1979). Echolalia: Issues and clinical applications. *Journal of Speech and Hearing Disorders, 44,* 411–434.

Scollon, R., & Scollon, S. B. (1980). *Interethnic communication.* Fairbanks, AK: Alaska Native Language Center.

Scott, C. M., & Windsor J. (2000). General language performance measures in spoken and written narrative and expository discourse of school-age children with language learning disabilities. *Journal of Speech, Language, and Hearing Research, 43,* 324–339.

Scott, C. M. (2002). A fork in the road less traveled: Writing intervention based on language profile. In K. G. Butler & E. R. Silliman (Eds.), *Speaking, reading, and writing in children with language learning disabilities* (pp. 219–237). Mahwah, NJ: Erlbaum.

Scott, C. M., & Nelson, N. W. (2009, March). Sentence combining: Assessment and intervention applications. *Perspectives on language learning and education, 16,* 14–20.

Secord, W. (1989). *CELF-R confidence: Understanding confidence intervals, CELF-R Update 2, 2:* 3–4, The Psychological Corporation.

Segal, E. F. (1975). Psycholinguistics discovers the operant: A review of Roger Brown's "A first language: The early stages." *Journal of the experimental analysis of behavior, 23,* 149–158.

Seligman, L. (2004). *Techniques and conceptual skills for mental health professionals.* Upper Saddle River, NJ: Prentice Hall.

Semel, E., Wiig, E. H., & Secord, W. (2003). *Clinical Evaluation of Language Fundamentals – Fourth Edition.* San Antonio, TX: The Psychological Corporation.

Senechal, M., & LeFevre, J. A. (2002). Parental involvement in the development of children's reading skill: A five-year longitudinal study. *Child Development, 73,* 445–460.

Seymour, C. M., & Nober, E. H. (1998). *Introduction to communication disorders: A multicultural approach.* Boston, MA: Butterworth-Heinemann.

Shames, G. H. (2000). *Counseling the communicatively disabled and their families: A manual for clinicians.* Boston: Allyn & Bacon.

Sharma, A. (2007). *Central auditory development and plasticity in infants and children with hearing aids and cochlear implants.* Presented at the AG Bell conference, July 2007, Washington, DC.

Sharma, A., Tobey, E., Dorman, M., Bharadwaj, S., Martin, K., Gilley, P., et al. (2004). Central auditory maturation and babbling development in infants with cochlear implants. *Archives of Otolaryngology – Head & Neck Surgery, 130,* 511–516.

Shattuck, P., Durkin, M., Maenner, M., et al. (2009). Timing of identification of children with Autism Spectrum Disorder: Findings from a population-based surveillance study. *Journal of the American Academy of Child and Adolescent Psychiatry, 48,* 474–483.

Shea, V., & Mesibov, G. B. (2005). Adolescents and adults with autism. In F. R. Volkmar, R. Paul, A. Klin, & D. Cohen (Eds.), *Handbook of autism and pervasive* developmental disorders: Vol. 1. Diagnosis, development, neurobiology, and behavior (3rd ed., pp. 288–311). Hoboken, NJ: Wiley.

Shweder, R. A., Goodnow, J., Hatano, G., LeVine, R. A., Markus, H., & Miller, P. (1998). The cultural psychology of development: One mind, many mentalities. In W. Damon (Ed.), Handbook of child psychology (5th ed., Vol. 1, pp. 865–937). New York: Wiley.

Siegel, B. (1996). Pervasive Developmental Disorders Screening Test. Unpublished manuscript, University of California at San Francisco.

Siegel, B. (1998, June). Early screening and diagnosis in autistic spectrum disorders: The Pervasive Developmental Disorders Screening Test (PDDST). Paper presented at the NIH State of the Science in Autism: Screening and Diagnosis Working Conference, Bethesda, MD.

Siegel, B., & Hayer, C. (1999, April). Detection of autism in the 2nd and 3rd year: the Pervasive Developmental Disorders Screening Test (PDDST). Poster presented at the biennial meeting for the Society for Research in Child Development, Albuquerque, NM.

Sigman, M., & Ungerer, J. (1984). Cognitive and language skills in autistic, mentally retarded, and normal children. Developmental Psychology, 20, 293–302.

Sigman, M., Dissanayake, C., Arabelle, S., & Ruskin, S. (1997). Cognition and emotion in children and adolescents with autism. In C. J. Cohen & F. R. Volkmar (Eds.), Handbook of autism and pervasive developmental disorders (2nd ed., pp. 248–265). New York: Wiley.

Silva-Pereyra, J., Rivera-Gaxiola, M., & Kuhl, P. K. (2005). An event-related brain potential study of sentence comprehension in preschoolers: semantic and morphosyntactic processing. Cognitive Brain Research, 23, 247–285.

Silverman, F. H. (1998). Research design and evaluation in speech-language pathology and audiology (4th ed.). Boston: Allyn & Bacon.

Singer, B. D., & Bashir, A. S. (1999). What are executive functions and self-regulation and what do they have to do with language-learning disorders? Language, Speech, and Hearing Services in Schools, 30, 265–273.

Skinner, B. F. (1957). Verbal behavior. Englewood Cliffs, NJ: Prentice-Hall.

Slobin, D. I. (1973). Cognitive prerequisites for the development of grammar. In C. A. Ferguson & D. I. Slobin (Eds.), Studies of child language development (pp. 175–208). New York: Holt, Rinehart & Winston.

Smedley, A., & Smedley, B. D. (2005). Race as biology is fiction, racism as a social problem is real: Anthropological and historical perspectives on the social construction of race. American Psychologist, 60, 16–26.

Smith, H. L., & Hull, G. A. (1985). Differential effects of sentence combining on college students who use particular structures with high and low frequencies. In D. A. Daiker, A. Kereck, & M. Morenberg (Eds.), Sentence combining: A rhetorical perspective (pp. 17–32). Carbondale, IL: Southern Illinois University Press.

Smith, K. (1992). The acquisition of long-distance wh-questions in normal and specific language-impaired children. Paper presented at the Annual Meeting of the Linguistic Society of America, Philadelphia, PA.

Smith, M. W., & Dickinson, D. K. (1994). Describing oral language opportunities in Head Start and other preschool classrooms. Early Childhood Research Quarterly, 9, 345–366.

Smith, T., Groen, A. D., & Wynn, J. W. (2000). A randomized trial of intensive early intervention for children with pervasive developmental disorder. American Journal of Mental Retardation, 5, 269–285

Snow, C. E., & Ninio, A. (1986). The contracts of literacy: What children learn from learning to read books. In W. H. Teale & E. Sulzby (Eds.), Emergent literacy: Writing and Reading (pp. 116–138). Norwood, NJ: Ablex.

Solomon, R., Necheles, J., Ferch, C., & Bruckman, D. (2007). Pilot study of a parent training program for young children with autism: The PLAY Project Home Consultation program. Autism, 11, 205–224.

Soto, G., & Zangari, C. (Eds.) (2009). Practically speaking: Language, literacy, and academic development for students with AAC needs. Baltimore, MD: Brookes.

Speights Roberts, D., Tingstrom, D. H., Olmi, D. J., & Bellipanni, K. D. (2008). Positive antecedent and consequent components in child compliance training. Behavior Modification, 32, 21–38.

Spencer, L. J., Barker, B. A., & Tomblin, J. B. (2003). Exploring the language and literacy outcomes of pediatric cochlear implant users. Ear and Hearing, 24, 236–247.

Spinelli, M., Rocha, A., Giacheti, C., & Richieri-Costa, A. (1995). Word-finding difficulties, verbal paraphasias, and verbal dyspraxia in ten individuals with fragile X syndrome. American Journal of Medical Genetics, 60, 39–43.

Spiro, M. (1994). Culture and human nature. New Brunswick: Transaction Publishers.

Stahl, S. A. (2004). Vocabulary and the child with learning disabilities. Perspectives: Newsletter of the International Dyslexia Association, 30, 1–4.

Stanovich, K. (2000). Progress in understanding reading: Scientific foundations and new frontiers. New York: Guilford Press.

Stauffer, R. (1970). *The language-experience approach and the teaching of reading.* New York: Harper & Row.

Stein, N., & Glenn, C. (1979). An analysis of story comprehension in elementary school children. In R. Freedle (Ed.), *New directions in discourse processing* (Vol. 2, pp. 53–120). Norwood, NJ: Ablex.

Steppling, M., Quattlebaum, P., & Brady, D. E. (2007). Toward a discussion of issues associated with speech-language pathologists' dismissal practices in public school settings. *Communication Disorders Quarterly, 28,* 179–187.

Sternberg, R. J. (2001). Successful intelligence: Understand what Spearman had rather than what he studied. In J. M. Collis & S. Messick (Eds.), *Intelligence and personality: Bridging the gap in theory and measurement* (pp. 347–373). Mahwah, NJ: Erlbaum.

Sternberg, R. J. (2002). Successful intelligence: A new approach to leadership. In R. E. Riggio, S. E. Murphy, & F. J. Pirozzolo (Eds.), *Multiple intelligences and leadership* (pp. 9–28). Mahwah, NJ: Erlbaum.

Stiggins, R. J. (1997). *Student-centered classroom assessment.* Upper Saddle River, NJ: Prentice Hall.

Stockman, I. J. (1996). The promises and pitfalls of language sample analysis as an assessment tool for linguistic minority children. *Language, Speech, and Hearing Services in Schools, 27,* 355–366.

Stone, W., Ousley, O., Yoder, P., Hogan, K., & Hepburn, S., (1997). Nonverbal communication in 2- and 3-year old children with autism. *Journal of Autism and Developmental Disorders, 20,* 437–453.

Stout, C. E., & Hayes, R. A. (2004). *The evidence-based practice: Methods, models, and tools for mental health professionals.* Hoboken, NJ: Wiley.

Strain, P. S., & Hoyson, M. (2000). The need for longitudinal, intensive social skill intervention: LEAP follow-up outcomes for children with autism. *Topics in Early Childhood Special Education, 20,* 116–122.

Strock, M. (2004). *Autism spectrum disorders (Pervasive developmental disorders).* NIH Publication No. NIH_04–5511, National Institute of Mental Health, National Institutes of Health, U.S. Department of Health and Human Services, Bethesda, MD, 40 pp. www.hnimh.nih.gov/publicat/autism.cfm.

Sudhalter, V., Scarborough, H., & Cohen, I. (1991). Syntactic delay and pragmatic deviance in the language of males with fragile X syndrome. *American Journal of Medical Genetics, 43,* 65–71.

Sulzby, E. S. (1985). Children's emergent reading of favorite storybooks: A developmental study. *Reading Research Quarterly, 20,* 458–481.

Svirsky, M. A. (2000). Language development in children with profound and prelingual hearing loss without cochlear implants. *The Annals of Otology, Rhinology and Laryngology, 109* (12, supplement 2), 99–102.

Svirsky, M. A., Robbins, A. M., Kirk, K. I., Pisoni, D. B., & Miyamoto, R. T. (2000). Language development in profoundly deaf children with cochlear implants. *Psychological Science, 11,* 153–158.

Szatmari, P., & Jones, M. B. (1998). Genetic epidemiology of autism and other pervasive developmental disorders. In F. R. Volkmar (Ed.), *Autism and pervasive developmental disorders,* (pp. 1–9-129). Cambridge, UK: Cambridge University.

Tallal, P. (1988). Developmental language disorders. In J. F. Kavanaugh & T. J. Truss Jr. (Eds.), *Learning disabilities: Proceedings of the national conference* (pp. 181–272). Parkton, MD: York.

Tallal, P., Ross, R., & Curtiss, S. (1989). Familial aggregation in specific language impairment. *Journal of Speech and Hearing Disorders, 54,* 167–173.

Tellis, G., & Tellis, C. (2003). Multicultural issues in school settings. *Seminars in Speech and Language, 24,* 22–26.

Terrell, S. L., & Jackson, R. S. (2002). African Americans in the Americas. In D. E. Battle (Ed.), *Communication disorders in multicultural populations* (3rd ed.). Boston: Butterworth-Heinemann.

Terrell, S. L., Battle, D. E., & Grantham, R. B. (1998). African American cultures. In D. E. Battle (Ed.), *Communication Disorders in Multicultural Populations,* (2nd ed., pp. 31–71). Boston: Andover Medical Publishers.

Tharpe, A. M. (2007). *Assessment and management of minimal, mild, and unilateral hearing loss in children.* Retrieved August 8, 2007 from www.audiologyonline.com/articles/article_detail.asp?article_id=1889.

Thiemann, K. S., & Goldstein, H. (2004). Effects of peer training and written text cuing on social communication of school-age children with pervasive developmental disorder. *Journal of Speech, Language, and Hearing Research, 47,* 126–144.

Thompson, C. K. (2007). Complexity in language learning and treatment. *American Journal of Speech and Language Pathology, 16,* 3–5.

Thompson, R. H., Cotnoir-Bichelman, N. M., McKerchar, P. M., Tate, T. L., & Dancho, K. A., (2007). Enhancing early communication through infant sign training. *Journal of Applied Behavioral Analysis, 40,* 15–23.

Thordardottir, E. T., & Weismer, S. E. (2002). Verb argument structure weakness in specific language impairment in relation to age and utterance length. *Clinical Linguistics and Phonetics, 16,* 233–250.

Timler, G. R., Olswang, L. B., & Coggins, T. E. (2005b). Social communication interventions for preschoolers: Targeting peer interactions during peer group entry and cooperative play. *Seminars in Speech and Language, 26,* 170–180.

Timler, G. R., Olswang, L. B., Coggins, T. E. (2005a). "Do I Know What I Need to Do?" A social communication intervention for children with complex clinical profiles. *Language, Speech, and Hearing Services in Schools, 36,* 73–85.

Tomasello, M. (1988). The role of joint attentional processes in early language development. *Language Sciences, 10,* 69–88.

Tomasello, M., & Bates, E. (2001). General introduction. In M. Tomasello & E. Bates (Eds.), *Language development: The essential readings* (pp. 1–11). Malden, MA: Blackwell.

Tomblin, J. (1996). Genetic and environmental contributions to the risk for specific language impairment. In M. Rice (Ed.), *Toward a genetics of language* (pp. 191–210). Hillsdale: Erlbaum.

Tomblin, J., Records, N., Buckwalter, P., Zhang, X., Smith, E., & O'Brian, M. (1997). Prevalence of specific language impairment in kindergarten children. *Journal of Speech, Language, and Hearing Research, 40,* 1245–1260.

Tomlinson, C. (2003). *Fulfilling the promise of the differentiated classroom: Strategies and tools for responsive teaching.* Alexandria, VA: Association for Supervision and Curriculum Development.

Tonge, B. J., Brereton, A. V., Gray, K. M., & Einfeld, S. L. (1999). Behavioral and emotional disturbance in high-functioning autism and Asperger syndrome. *Autism, 3,* 117–130.

Torgesen, J. K. (1998, Spring/Summer). Catch them before they fall: Identification and assessment to prevent reading failure in young children. *American Educator,* 1–8.

Torgesen, J. K., & Bryant, B. R. (2004) *Test of Phonological Awareness-Second Edition: PLUS.* Austin, TX: PRO-ED.

Torgesen, J. K., Alexander, A. W., Wagner, R. K., Rashotte, C. A., Voeller, K. K. S., & Conway, T. (2001). Intensive remedial instruction for children with severe reading disabilities: Immediate and long-term outcomes from two instructional approaches. *Journal of Learning Disabilities, 34,* 33–58.

Trauner, D., Wulfeck, B., Tallal, P., & Hesselink, J. (2000). Neurological and MRI profiles of children with developmental language impairment. *Developmental Medicine and Child Neurology, 42,* 470–475.

Treiman, R. (1985). The structure of spoken syllables: Evidence from novel word games. *Cognition, 15,* 49–74.

Treiman, R. (1991). Children's spelling errors on syllable-initial consonant clusters. *Journal of Educational Psychology, 83,* 346–360.

Treiman, R., & Bourassa, D. C. (2000). The development of spelling skills. *Topics in Language Disorders, 20,* 1–18.

Tropper, B., & Schwartz, R. G. (2009). Neurobiology of child language disorders. In R. G. Schwartz (Ed.), *Handbook of child language disorders* (pp. 174–200). New York: Psychology Press.

Tsai, L. Y. (2005). Recent neurobiological research in autism. In D. Zager (Ed.), *Autism spectrum disorders: Identification, education, and treatment* (3rd ed., pp. 47–87). Mahwah, NJ: Erlbaum.

Tsatsanis, K. D. (2005). Neuropsychological characteristics in autism and related conditions. In F. R. Volkmar, R. Paul, A. Klin, & D. Cohen (Eds.), *Handbook of autism and pervasive developmental disorders: Vol. 1. Diagnosis, development, neurobiology, and behavior* (3rd ed., pp. 365–381). Hoboken, NJ: Wiley.

Tyler, A., Lewis, K., Haskill, A., & Tolbert, L. (2003). Outcomes of different speech and language goal attack strategies. *Journal of Speech, Language, and Hearing Research, 46,* 1077–1094.

Tymchuk, A. J., Andron, L., & Rahbar, B. (1988). Effective decision-making problem-solving training with mothers who have mental retardation. *American Journal on Mental Retardation, 92,* 510–516.

Ukrainetz, T. (2006). The many ways of exposition: A focus on discourse structure. In T. Ukrainetz (Ed.), *Contextualized language intervention: Scaffolding preK-12 literacy achievement* (pp. 247–288). Eau Claire, WI: Thinking Publications.

Ukrainetz, T. A. (2005). What to work on how: An examination of the practice of school-age language intervention. *Contemporary Issues in Communication Sciences and Disorders, 32,* 108–119.

Ukrainetz, T. A., Harpell, S., Walsh, C., & Coyle, C. (2000). A preliminary investigation of dynamic assessment with Native American kindergarteners. *Language, Speech, and Hearing Services in Schools, 31,* 142–154.

Ukrainetz, T. A., Justice, L. M., Kaderavek, J. N., Eisenberg, S. L., Gillam, R. B., & Harm, H. M. (2005). The development of expressive elaboration in fictional narratives. *Journal of Speech, Language, and Hearing Research, 48,* 1363–1377.

U.S. Department of Education (2002). *Twenty-fourth annual report to congress on the implementation of the Individuals with Disabilities Education Act.* Washington, DC: Government Printing Office.

U.S. Department of Education, Institute of Education Sciences, National Center for Education Statistics, *National Assessment of Educational Progress (NAEP), 2002 Writing Assessment.* Accessed October 7, 2009 at http://nces.ed.gov/nationsreportcard/pdf/stt2002/writing/2003532OH4.PDF.

United States Preventive Services Task Force. (1989). *Appendix A Task Force Ratings [Electronic version].* Retrieved October 13, 2006, from www.ncbi.nlm.nih.gov/books/bv.

Uwer, R., Albrecht, R., & von Suchodoletz, W. (2002). Automatic processing of tones and speech stimuli in children with specific language impairment. *Developmental Medicine and Child Neurology, 44,* 527–532.

Van Acker, R., Loncola, J. A., & Van Acker, E. Y. (2005). Rett syndrome: A pervasive developmental disorder. In F. R. Volkmar, R. Paul, A. Klin, & D. Cohen (Eds.), *Handbook of autism and pervasive developmental disorders: Vol. 1. Diagnosis, development, neurobiology, and behavior* (3rd ed., pp. 126–164). Hoboken, NJ: Wiley.

Van Borsel, J., Maes, E., & Foulon, S. (2001). Stuttering and bilingualism: A review. *Journal of Fluency Disorders, 26,* 179–205.

van Kleeck, A. (1994). Potential cultural bias in training parents as conversational partners with their children who have delays in language development. *American Journal of Speech-Language Pathology, 3,* 67–78.

van Kleeck, A., Schwarz, A. L., Fey, M., Kaiser, A., Miller, J., & Weitzman, E. (2009). Should we use telegraphic or grammatical input with children in the early stages of language development? Evidence from research and experts. *American Journal of Speech-Language Pathology.*

Van Riper, C. (1978). *Speech correction: Principles and methods.* (6th ed.). Englewood Cliffs, NJ: Prentice-Hall.

Vanderas, A. P. (1987). Incidence of cleft lip, cleft palate, and cleft lip and palate among races: A review. *Cleft Palate Journal, 24,* 216–225.

Vigil, D. C., Hodges, J., & Klee, T. (2005). Quantity and quality of parental language input to late-talking toddlers during play. *Child Language Teaching and Therapy, 21,* 107–122.

Vygotsky, L. (1962). *Thought and language.* Cambridge, MA: MIT Press (Originally published 1934).

Vygotsky, L. S. (1978). *Mind in society: The development of higher psychological processes.* Cambridge, MA: Harvard University Press.

Vygotsky, L. S. (1987). *The collected works of L. S. Vygotsky,* Vol. 1. New York: Plenum.

Wacker, D. P., Berg, W. K., Harding, J. W., Anjali, B., Rankin, B., & Ganzer, J. (2005). Treatment effectiveness, stimulus generalization, and acceptability to parents of functional communication training. *Educational Psychology, 25,* 233–256.

Wadman, R., Durkin, K., & Conti-Ramsden, G. (2008). Self-esteem, shyness, and sociability in adolescents with specific language impairment. *Journal of Speech, Language, and Hearing Research, 51,* 938–952.

Wagner, R. K., Torgesen, J. K., & Rashotte, C. A. (1999). *Comprehensive Test of Phonological Processing (CTOPP).* Old Tappan, NJ: Pearson Education.

Wallace, D., & Hammill, D. D. (2002) *Comprehensive Receptive and Expressive Vocabulary Test-Second Edition.* Austin, TX: PRO-ED.

Walpole, S., & McKenna, M. C. (2004). *The literacy coach's handbook: A guide to research-based practice.* New York, Guilford Press.

Warren, S. F., Brady, N. C., & Fey, M. E. (2004). Communication and language: Research design and measurement. In E. Emerson, C. Hatton, T. Thompson, & T. R. Parmenter (Eds.), *The international handbook of applied research in intellectual disabilities* (pp. 385–405). West Sussex, UK: Wiley.

Washington, J. A., & Craig, H. K. (1994). Dialectal forms during discourse of poor, urban, African American preschoolers. *Journal of Speech and Hearing Research, 37,* 816–823.

Wasik, B. A., Bond, M. A., & Hindman, A. (2006). The effects of a language and literacy intervention on Head Start children and teachers. *Journal of Educational Psychology, 98,* 63–74.

Waters, M. (1997). *Transcript of testimony to the U. S. Senate, January 23, 2007, on Ebonics* (pp. 1–3). Retrieved www.pbs.org/newshour/bb/congress/january97/ebonics_1–23.html.

Watkins, R. V., & Rice, M. L. (1991). Verb particle and preposition acquisition in language-impaired preschoolers. *Journal of Speech and Hearing Research, 34,* 1130–1141.

Watkins, R. V., Kelly, D. J., Harbers, H. M., & Hollis, W. (1995). Measuring children's lexical diversity: Differentiating typical and impaired language learners. *Journal of Speech and Hearing Research, 38,* 1349–1355.

Watkins, R., Rice, M. & Moltz, C. (1993). Verb use by language-impaired and normally developing children. *First Language 13,* 133–43.

Watson, J., & Kayser, H. (1994). Assessment of bilingual/bicultural children and adults who stutter. *Seminars in Speech and Language, 15,* 149–164.

Weaver, C. (1996). *Language learning disabilities in school-age children and adolescents.* New York: Pearson/Merrill.

Webb, N. M., Shavelson, R. J., & Haertel, E. H. (2007). Reliability coefficients and generalizability theory. In C. R. Rao & S. Sinharay (Ed.), *Handbook of statistics,* Vol. 26 (pp. 81–124). Radarweg, Amsterdam: Elsevier.

Weir, R. (1962). *Language in the crib.* The Hague, Netherlands: Mouton.

Weismer, S. E., & Robertson, S. (2006). Focused stimulation approach to language intervention. In R. J. McCauley & M. E. Fey (Eds.), *Treatment of language disorders in children* (pp. 267–278). Baltimore, MD: Brookes.

Weismer, S. E., & Thordardottir, E. T. (2002). Cognition and language. In P. J. Accardo, B. T. Rogers, & A. J. Capute (Eds.), *Disorders of language development* (pp. 21–37). Baltimore, MD: York.

Weiss, A. L., (2001). *Preschool language disorders resource guide: Specific language impairment.* San Diego, CA: Singular.

Weitzman, E., & Greenberg, J. (2002). *Learning language and loving it: A guide to promoting children's social, language, and literacy development in early childhood settings* (2nd ed.). Toronto, ON: Hanen Centre.

Wendt, O. (2008, November). *A systematic review of AAC interventions applying graphic symbols for Autism Spectrum Disorders.* Poster session presented at the annual meeting of the American Speech Language-Hearing Association, Chicago, IL.

Werker, J. F., & Tees, R. C. (2005). Speech perception as a window for understanding plasticity and commitment in language systems of the brain. *Developmental Psychobiology, 46,* 233–251.

Westby, C. (1991). Learning to talk, talking to learn: Oral-literate language differences. In C. S. Simon (Ed.), *Communication skills and classroom success* (pp. 334–357). Eau Claire, WI: Thinking Publications.

Westby, C. (1998). Social-emotional bases of communication development. In W. Haynes & B. Shulman (Eds.), *Communication development: Foundations, processes, and clinical applications* (pp. 165–204). Baltimore, MD: Williams & Wilkins.

Westby, C. (2005). Assessing and facilitating text comprehension problems. In H. Catts & A. Kahmi (Eds.), *Language and reading disabilities* (2nd ed., pp. 157–232). Boston: Allyn & Bacon.

Westby, C. (2008). *Language impairments & social-emotional communicative competence.* Accessed via the Web on December 30, 2008 at www.speechpathology.com.

Westby, C. E. (1980). Assessment of cognitive and language abilities through play. *Language, Speech, and Hearing Services in Schools, 11,* 154–168.

Westby, C., & Vining, C. B. (2002). Living in harmony: Providing services to Native American children and families. In D. E. Battle (Ed.), *Communication disorders in multicultural populations* (3rd ed., pp. 135–178). Boston: Butterworth-Heinemann.

Wetherby, A., & Prizant, B. (1989). The expression of communication intent: Assessment guidelines. *Seminars in Speech and Language, 10,* 77–91.

Wetherby, A., & Prizant, B. (1992). Profiling young children's communication competence. In S. Warren & J. Reichle (Eds.), *Causes and effects in communication and language intervention* (pp. 217–251). Baltimore, MD: Brookes.

Wetherby, A., Prizant, B., & Hutchinson, T., (1998). Communicative, social-affective, and symbolic profiles of young children with autism and pervasive developmental disorder. *American Journal of Speech-Language Pathology, 7,* 79–91.

White, J. L. (1984). *The psychology of Blacks: An Afro-American perspective.* New Jersey: Prentice-Hall.

Whitehurst, G. J., & Fischel, J. E. (1994). Early developmental language delay: What, if anything, should the clinician do about it? *Journal of Child Psychology and Psychiatry, 35,* 613–648.

Whitehurst, G. J., & Lonigan, C. J. (1998). Child development and emergent literacy. *Child Development, 69,* 848–872.

Whitmire, K. (2002). The evolution of school-based speech-language services: A half-century of change and a new century of practice. *Communication Disorders Quarterly, 23,* 68–76.

Wiederholt, J. L., & Bryant, B. R. (2001). *Gray Oral Reading Tests–Fourth Edition* (GORT-4). Austin, TX: PRO-ED.

Wiggins, G., & McTighe, J. (1998). *Understanding by design.* Alexandria, VA: Association for Supervision and Curriculum Development.

Wiig, E. H., & Secord, W. A. (2006, Feb. 7). Clinical measurement and assessment: A 25 year retrospective. *The ASHA Leader, 11(2),* 10–11.

Wiig, E. H., Lord Larson, V., & Olson, J. A. (2004). *S-MAPS, Rubrics for Curriculum-Based Assessment and Intervention.* Eau Claire, WI: Thinking Publications.

Wiig, E. H., Secord, W., & Semel, E. (2004). *Clinical Evaluation of Language Fundamentals-Preschool 2.* San Antonio, TX: The Psychological Corporation.

Wilcox, M. J., Kouri, T. A., & Caswell, S. B. (1991). Early language intervention: A comparison of classroom and individual treatment. *American Journal of Speech-Language Pathology, 47,* 49–62.

Wiley, T. G. (1996). Literacy and language diversity in sociocultural contexts. *Literacy and language diversity in the United States.* Washington, DC: Center for Applied Linguistics and Delta Systems.

Wilkerson, D. L. (2000). Documenting clinical service delivery: Writing style and lexical selection. *Contemporary Issues in Communication Science and Disorders, 27,* 6–13.

Wilkes, E. M. & Sunshine Cottage for Deaf Children (1999). *Cottage Acquisition Scales for Listening, Language, and Speech.* San Antonio, TX: Sunshine Cottage School for Deaf Children.

Williams, A. L. (2000). Multiple oppositions: Case studies of variables in phonological intervention. *American Journal of Speech and Language Pathology, 9*, 289–299.

Williams, R. L. (1997). The Ebonics controversy. *Journal of Black Psychology, 23*, 208–214.

Wilson, K., & Chapman, J. (2001). *Bear snores on.* New York: Simon & Schuster Children's Publishing.

Winsler, A. (2003). Introduction to the special issue: Vygotskian perspectives in early childhood education. *Early Education and Development, 14*, 253–269.

Witzig, R. (1996). The medicalization of race: Scientific legitimization of a flawed social construct. *Annuals of Internal Medicine, 125*, 675–679.

Wood, A. J., & Pledger, M. (2001). *In the ocean.* Berkeley, CA: Silver Dolphin Books.

Woodcock, R. W. (1998). *Woodcock reading mastery tests–Revised/normative update (WRMT-R/NU).* Bloomington, MN: Pearson.

World Health Organization (2001). *World Health Report, Mental Retardation.* Retrieved December 4, 2006, from www.who.int/mediacentre/factsheets/fs265/en/.

World Health Organization (2002). *Towards a common language for functioning, disability, and health: The international classification of functioning, disability and health.* Retrieved August, 22, 2007, from www.who.int/classifications/icf/site/beginners/bg.pdf.

Worthy, J. & Rodriguez-Galindo, A. (2006). "Mi hija vale dos personas": Latino immigrant parents' perspectives about their children's bilingualism. *Bilingual Research Journal, 30(2)*, 579–601.

Wray, D., Flexer, C., & Vaccaro, V. (1993). Classroom performance of children who are deaf and hard-of-hearing and who learned spoken communication through the auditory-verbal approach: An evaluation of treatment efficacy. *Volta Review, 99*, 107–119.

Wren, C. (1980). Identifying patterns of syntactic disorder in six-year-old children. *Proceedings from the Symposium on Research in Child Language Disorders 1*, 113–123, Madison: University of Wisconsin, Madison.

Wright, H. H., & Newhoff, M. (2001). Narration abilities of children with language-learning disabilities in response to oral and written stimuli. *American Journal of Speech-Language Pathology, 10*, 308–319.

Xu, H., Kotak, V. C., & Sanes, D. H. (2007). Conductive hearing loss disrupts synaptic and spike adaptation in developing auditory cortex. *Journal of Neuroscience, 27*, 9417–9426.

Yoder, P. J., & Davies, B. (1990). Do parental questions and topic continuations elicit developmentally delayed children's replies: A sequential analysis. *Journal of Speech and Hearing Research, 33*, 563–573.

Yoder, P. J., Kaiser, A. P., & Alpert, C. L. (1991). An exploratory study of the interaction between language teaching methods and child characteristics. *Journal of Speech and Hearing Research, 34*, 155–167.

Yoder, P. J., Kaiser, A. P., Goldstein, H., Alpert, C., Mousetis, L., Kaczmarek, L., & Fischer, R. (1995). An exploratory comparison of milieu teaching and responsive interaction in classroom applications. *Journal of Early Intervention, 19*, 218–242.

Yoder, P. J., Spruytenburg, H., Edwards, A., & Davies, B. (1995). Effect of verbal routine contexts and expansions on gains in the mean length of utterance in children with developmental delays. *Language, Speech, and Hearing Services in Schools, 26*, 21–32.

Yoder, P. J., & Warren, S. F. (2002). Effects of prelinguistic milieu teaching and parent responsivity education on dyads involving children with intellectual disabilities. *Journal of Speech, Language, and Hearing Research, 45*, 1158–1174.

Yoder, P. J., McCathren, R. B., Warren, S. F., & Watson, A.L. (2001). Important distinctions in measuring maternal responses to communication in prelinguistic children with disabilities. *Communication Disorders Quarterly, 22*, 135–147.

Yoshinaga-Itano, C., & de Uzcategui, A. C. (2001). Early identification and social-emotional factors of children with hearing loss and children screened for hearing loss. In E. Kurtzer-White & D. Luterman (Eds.), *Early childhood deafness* (pp. 13–28). Timonium, Maryland: York Press.

Yoshinaga-Itano, C., Sedey, A., Coulter, D., & Mehl, A. (1998). Language of early- and later-identified children with hearing loss. *Pediatrics, 102*, 1161–1171.

Zeidner, M. (2001). Invited forward and introduction. In J. J. W. Andrews, D. H. Saklofske, & H. L. Janzen (Eds.), *Handbook of psychoeducational assessment: Ability, achievement, and behavior in children* (pp. 1–10). San Diego: Academic Press.

Zimmerman, I. L., Steiner, V. G., & Pond, R. E. (2002). *Preschool Language Scale* (4th ed.; PLS-4). San Antonio, TX: Pearson.

Zipoli, R. P. Jr., & Kennedy, M. (2005). Evidence-based practice among speech-language pathologists: Attitudes, utilization, and barriers. *American Journal of Speech-Language Pathology, 14*, 208–22.

Index

AAC devices. *See*
Agumentative/alternative
communication (AAC) system
AAE (African American English).
See African American
English (AAE)
ABA (Applied Behavioral Analysis),
296–298, 303
Abbeduto, L., 248, 249, 261, 262
A-B-C (antecedent-behavior-
consequence) progression, 197,
268–269
ABC (Autism Behavior
Checklist), 291
Abuse, and brain injury, 251
Academic readiness, 322–323
Accents *vs.* dialects, 398
Accommodation, and
communication, 340–341
Acculturation, 393–394
Accuracy, importance of, 99–100, 105
Achenbach, A., 379
Achieving Communication
Independence: A
Comprehensive Guide to
Assessment and Intervention
(ACI), 264–265
Acoustic highlighting, 236, 237, 241
Actions, naming of, 297–298
Activities, 168–169, 195–196,
239, 247
Adams, C., 135, 147, 180, 186
Adamson, L. B., 373
Adaptation, and communication, 341
ADHD (attention-deficit/
hyperactivity disorder),
182–183, 207
Adults. *See also* Parents
behaviors of with children, 8–9,
19, 20, 21
coaching of, 124
African American English (AAE)
in language analysis, 58, 60
morphology of, 179
and obligatory use, 69
and reading, 323
use of in schools, 392–393
variants of, 399
African-based language traditions,
389–390
Age equivalent score, 56

Agumentative/alternative
communication (AAC) system
aids, 359, 360, 361
components of, 358–365
defined, 357
devices, 263
feature match for, 371
myths about, 365
results from, 376
selection sets, 363–364
strategy, 359, 361–363
systems for, 357
team members, 366
technique, 363
Aided language stimulation
(ALS), 372
Albertini, J., 178, 179, 181
Albrecht, R., 236
Alexander Graham Bell Association
(AG Bell), 211, 219
Allen, G., 177
Allen, J., 289
Almond, P. J., 291
Al Otaiba, S., 310
Alpert, C. L., 194, 195, 197, 199, 200
Alphabetic awareness, 311–312
Alt, M., 83
American Association on Mental
Retardation (AAMR), 245,
246, 249, 273
American Psychiatric Association
(APA), 176, 207, 278, 281, 302
American Psychological
Association (APA), 50
American Sign Language (ASL), 215,
218, 224
American Speech-Language Hearing
Association (ASHA), 3, 6, 7,
74, 107, 108, 111, 114, 123,
126, 128, 129, 154, 157, 183,
192, 193, 226, 252, 306, 316,
353, 357, 358, 386, 388, 403
Amplification, use of, 234
Anderson, K., 243
Andrews, R., 206
Andron, L., 255
Angelman syndrome, 251
Antecedent, defined, 8
Antecedent-behavior-consequence
(A-B-C) progression, 197,
268–269

Anthony, J. S., 309
Anthony, S., 227
APD (auditory processing disorder).
See Auditory processing
disorder (APD)
Apel, K., 183, 326, 330, 334
Applebee, A., 330
Applied Behavioral Analysis (ABA),
296–298, 303
Arabella, S., 281
Aram, D., 225
Arick, J. R., 291
Arnold, L. E., 285
ASD (autism spectrum disorder).
See Autism spectrum disorder
(ASD)
Asian nationalities, 391
Asian population
and communication disorders, 400
Asperger, H., 278
Asperger syndrome (AS), 278,
282, 302
See also Autism spectrum disorder
Assertive-responsive communication
scheme, 142–145, 172
Assessments
for AAC, 366–371
for ASD, 290–291
basic components of, 77–79
criterion-referenced, 45, 48,
54, 263
decision making in, 61–62,
104–113, 112–113
dynamic, 402
functional, 263–264
of individual's needs, 369
and intervention goal setting, 48
and minority cultures, 48, 401–403
narrative, 330–331
naturalistic, 188
norm-referenced, 84–87, 263
parent-child, 188–192
participation model, 367, 368
phonological, 78
pretreatment, 203
process of, 74–92
process-oriented measures, 402
psychometric features of, 48–74
reading comprehension, 337
reasons for, 47
reliability of, 50, 54

Assessments (*continued*)
reports of, 89–92
in research studies, 156
speech/articulation, 77–78
spelling, 334
static, 45
static *vs.* dynamic, 108
symbol, 370–371
tools for, 47–48, 230–234, 293
transdisciplinary, 264
writing, 339
Athanasiou, M. S., 191
Atkinson, L., 257
At risk, defined, 111
Attempts, in narratives, 328
Attention, 253, 254
Attention-deficit/hyperactivity
disorder (ADHD), 182–183, 207
Auditory neuropathy/dys-synchrony
(AN/AD), 213–215, 240
Auditory processing disorder (APD),
213–215, 236, 240
Autism. *See also* Autism spectrum
disorder
and FCT, 268
interventions for, 115, 194
and sign language, 223
Autism Behavior Checklist (ABC), 291
Autism Diagnostic Interview-Revised
(ADI-R), 291
Autism Genome Project (AGP)
Consortium, 285
Autism spectrum disorder (ASD)
assessment of, 288–294
criteria for diagnosis, 279
defined, 278
diagnosis of, 278
disorder types within, 281–284
genetic investigations, 285–286
and PECS, 376
prevalence of, 284–285, 302
risk factors for, 285–286
screening tools for, 289
social interaction and
communication, 278–279
Autistic disorder (AD), 281. *See also*
Autism; Autism spectrum
disorder
Avivi Ben-zvi, G., 180
Axelrod, S., 9

Backward design, 118–119
Badian, N. A., 312
Bahr, C. M., 340, 348, 349, 351, 352
Bailey, J., 267
Bain, B., 114
Baird, G., 289
Bakeman, R. A., 373
Baker, L, 182

Baker, S., 217
Baldwin, D., 19
Ball, A. F., 340
Ball, E. W., 319
Bambara, L. M., 269
Baranek, G. T., 281
Barker, B. A., 221
Barker, T. A., 309
Baroff, G. S., 253, 255
Baron-Cohen, S., 281, 289
Baroody, A. J., 20
Barton, A., 373
Barton, M. L., 289
Basal, defined, 56
Baseline, defined, 168
Bashir, A. S., 339, 340
Bates, E., 7, 31, 82, 230
Battle, D. E., 387, 401, 405
Baum, W. M., 137
Bauman, M. L., 285
Bauserman, K. L., 118
Bear, D. R., 153, 314, 333, 336
Beck, I. L., 152, 153, 154
Beckman, A. R., 118
Bedore, L., 177
Beebe, Helen, 220
Behavioral baselines, 269
Behavioral phenotypes, 249
Behavioral theory, influence of,
134–138
Behaviorism, 8, 9, 40, 41
Behaviors
adaptive, 245, 247
and ASD, 280
assessment of play, 190–191
and brain development, 16
challenging, 263–264
entry, 184
and language disorders, 258
linkages between, 11
replacing maladaptive, 266–271
Beirne-Smith, M., 255
Beitchman, J. H., 182
Bellipanni, K. D., 138
Belmont, J. M., 256
Belser, R., 262
Benavides, C., 267
Benigno, J. P., 20
Ben-Shachar, N., 403
Benson, B. J., 339
Berninger, V. W., 313, 335
Berry, J. W., 394
Bettelheim, B., 287–288
Betz, S. K., 260, 262
Beukelman, D. R., 359, 361, 363,
364, 366, 367, 368, 369, 370,
372, 373–374, 379
Bickerton, D., 15, 389
Bilingual-bicultural, 224

Bilingualism, 396–397
Binger, C., 372, 379
Bishop, D., 306
Bishop, D. V. M., 3, 135, 183
Björchk-Åkesson, E., 366
Blachman, B. A., 318, 319
Black, R., 319
Blackstone, S., 365, 371, 379
Blakeley-Smith, A., 267, 268
Blinding, defined, 156
Bliss, L. S., 71, 73, 331
Bloom, L., 24, 258
Bloom, P., 33
Bloom-Pickard, M., 135
Boardman, A. G., 338, 339
Bodfish, J. W., 281
Bodrova, E., 20
Body, J., 178
Body language, 227, 403
Body parts, activities involving, 239
Boehm, A. E., 50, 230
Boehm Test of Basic Concepts,
50, 230
Boettcher, C., 117
Boherty, B. J., 261
Bojczyk, K. E., 82, 83
Bond, M. A., 120
Bondy, A., 376
Bookbinder, L., 57
Books, use of, 237–240
Borneman, A., 181
Bortolini, U., 178
Botting, N., 183
Botwinik-Rotem, I., 15
Bourassa, D. C., 334
Bowen, M., 23
Bowers, L., 86
Boyle, J., 147
Boynton, G. M., 225
Boynton, L., 261
Boyton, S., 238
Bracken, B, 191, 230
Bracken Basic Concept Scale, Third
Edition, (BBCS-3), 230
Brackenbury, T., 81
Bradley, L., 319
Brady, D. E., 128
Brady, N. C., 249
Brain development, 15–18,
251–252, 283, 285
Brain function, 21–22
Bregman, J. D., 280, 282, 283, 284
Brereton, A. V., 282
Bridges, M., 307
Brinton, B., 31, 38, 186
Brody, G. H., 177
Bronfenbrenner, U., 23
Broun, L., 345
Brouwer, C.N., 211

Brown, J., 54, 333
Brown, L., 78
Brown, M. W., 238
Brown, R., 26–27, 38, 59, 140
Brown, S., 402
Brown, V. L., 326
Browne, M. N., 101
Brownell, R., 84, 85
Bruckman, D., 115
Bruner, J., 19, 21,197
Bruno, J., 372
Bryan, M. R., 251, 252
Bryant, B. R., 53, 326
Bryant, P. E., 319
Bucket theory, 332
Buckley, S. J., 261
Buildup/breakdown technique, 141
Buis, K., 339
Burchinal, M., 122, 181, 261
Burgess, S. R., 309
Burns, B. M., 316
Buros Institute of Mental
    Measurements, 53, 87
Bus, A. G., 316
Bush, George W., 324
Butkovsky, L., 200, 204
Butterfield, E. C., 256

Cabell, S. Q., 314
Caesar, L. G., 385, 389
Calandrella, A. M., 28
Camarata, M., 200, 203, 204
Camarata, S. M., 200, 203, 204
Campbell, C., 147
Campbell, T., 74, 402
Cantwell D., 182
Capellini, C., 316, 321
Cardenas-Hagan, E., 322
Carle, E., 238, 239
Carlson, C. D., 322
Carlson, R., 375
Carpenter, A., 67
Carpenter, M., 287
Carpenter, R., 299
Carr, E. G., 267, 268
Carrow-Woolfolk, E., 51, 230, 326
Casadio, P., 31
Casbergue, R. M., 313
Casby, M., 259
Cascella, P. W., 126, 263
Case grammar, 31
Case histories, 76
Caselli, M. C., 31, 178
Caseloads, 306
Case studies
    AAC assessment (Ben), 380–382
    Asperger syndrome (Vijay), 304
    assessment results (Michael),
      95–96

autism (Cameron), 132
cultural differences (Laurimar),
    411–412
Down syndrome (Jonah), 275–276
hearing loss (Katie), 242–243
pragmatic communication (Sachi),
    42–43
reading assessment (Ziquon), 355
scope of intervention (Cole and
    Maria), 174
specific language impairment
    (Zachary), 209
Casey, A. M., 134
CASSLLS (Cottage Acquisition
    Scales for Listening,
    Language, and Speech),
    231–234, 241
Caswell, S. B., 123, 160
Categorical model, 4
Cater, C. M., 295
Cathcart, K., 295
Cat in the Hat, The (Seuss), 317
Catts, H., 118, 183, 306, 307, 309,
    310, 328, 337
Ceiling, in testing, 56
CELF-3 (Clinical Evaluation of
    Language Function–Third
    Edition), 48
CELF-4 (Clinical Evaluation of
    Language Fundamentals–4), 52
CELF-P (Clinical Evaluation of
    Language Function–
    Preschool), 231
CELF-Preschool 2 (Clinical
    Evaluation of Language
    Fundamentals–Preschool 2),
    51, 156
Center for American Progress Task
    Force on Poverty, 388, 389
Centers for Disease Control and
    Prevention, 248, 284, 290
Cepeda, N. J., 125
Chaining, behavioral, 9
Chambers, 393
Chang, F., 316
Chapman, J., 238
Chapman, R. S., 29, 31, 38, 148,
    260, 266
Charman, T., 284
Checklists
    Checklist for Autism in Toddlers
      (CHAT), 289
    early literacy print skills, 46
    play and language, 190–191
Cheng, L., 391, 394, 395, 399, 400,
    401, 403
Cheour, M., 16
Cheslock, M., 373
Chiang, B., 123

Childhood Autism Rating Scale
    (CARS), 291
Childhood disintegrative disorder
    (CDD), 278. See also Autism
    spectrum disorder
Chisolm, T. H., 221
Chomsky, N., 13, 40
Chow, S. M., 316, 321
Chunking, 253, 256
Cirrin, F., 123, 135, 166
Cisar, C., 184
Clancy, B., 16
Clark, J. G., 214
Clarkson, B., 306
Classroom access, 242–243
Classroom-based approach, 123, 163
Cleave, P., 177, 178, 179, 200,
    201, 203
Clegg, M., 182
Clingenpeel, B., 120
Clinical Evaluation of Language
    Function–Preschool
    (CELF-P), 231
Clinical Evaluation of Language
    Function–Third Edition
    (CELF-3), 48
Clinical Evaluation of Language
    Fundamentals–4 (CELF-4), 52
Clinical Evaluation of Language
    Fundamentals–Preschool 2
    (CELF-Preschool 2), 51, 156
Clinical reports, writing of, 91–92
Cloud, N., 322
Cochlear implants, 211, 214, 221
Cochran, P. S., 135
Code switching, 30, 88, 323, 399–400
Coggins, T., 31, 184, 186, 299
Cognitive development, 9–10, 78,
    286–287
Cognitive theory, 9–13, 40, 145–147
Cohen, D., 289, 293, 300
Cohen, I., 261
Cohen, J., 157
Cohen, R., 411
Cohen, W. I., 268
Cole, P. A., 401
Coleman, M., 285
Colton, S., 316, 321
Comblain, A., 258
Communication
    and AS, 282
    achieving independence in,
      264–265
    assertive and responsive, 144
    challenges, 300
    competency in, 4
    cultural differences in, 398, 403
    defined, 2
    display boards for, 360

Communication (*continued*)
 domains of, 113
 effective balance in, 143
 functional, 256
 indirect, 187
 intent, 28
 manual, 222–225
 modalities of, 216, 218–225
 multi-modal, 358
 parent-child, 177
 profiles with ASD, 280
 questions related to, 106
 response to, 148
 SAL users compared with
  others, 373
 social, 184–186, 300
 written, 306–307
Communication Opportunities
  Inventory, 264
Communication probes, 67
Communication Skill Inventory,
  264–265
Communication subdomains
 and form, content, and use, 25
 order of acquisition of, 34
 Subdomain 1 (early pragmatic
  skills), 28–31, 41
 Subdomain 2 (vocabulary
  development), 31–33, 41
 Subdomain 3 (multiple word
  combinations), 33, 41
 Subdomain 4 (morphosyntax
  development), 36–38, 41
 Subdomain 5 (advanced
  pragmatic and discourse
  development), 38–40, 41
Communication system
 levels of, 4–5
Communication temptations,
  use of, 292
Communicative functions, defined,
  291–292
Complex communication needs
  (CCNs), 356, 357, 377
Composite scores, defined, 56
Composition skills, defined, 313
Comprehension
 defined, 336–337
Comprehension, difficulties with, 214
Comprehensive Receptive and
  Expressive Vocabulary Test-
  Second Edition (CRETV-2), 86
Computers, use of, 135, 136,
  348–349
Conboy, B., 402
Condition statements, 165, 173
Conjunctive cohesion, 72
Connectionism, 21–23
Connor, C. M., 323
Consequences, in narratives, 328

Construct validity, 49
Content, with form and use, 149
Content validity, 49
Context
 importance of, 23, 47, 256
 in interventions, 149
 physical, 163
 of stimulus, 134
Contingency, defined, 142
Continuum of naturalness, 162–164,
  167–171, 172
Conti-Ramsden, G., 183, 185
Conversational assertiveness,
  142–145
Conversational discourse, 70, 72
Conversational recast training
  (CRT), 200–204
Conversational repair, 30, 72, 88
Conversational responsiveness,
  142–145
Conversational rules, 30
Cook, I., 281
Coonrod, E. E., 289
Cooperative play, 185, 186
Cormier, S., 228
Corsello, C., 49, 291
Cotnoir-Bichelman, N. M., 222
Cottage Acquisition Scales for
  Listening, Language, and Speech
  (CASSLLS), 231–234, 241
Coulter, D., 217
Counseling, techniques for, 226–227
Cousins, L., 238
Coyle, C., 402
Craig, H., 60, 69, 179, 180, 184, 323
Crain, S., 372, 379
Crain-Thoreson, C., 189
Crais, E. R., 290
Crede, L. A., 333, 335
Creole languages, 15, 389, 398–399
Criteria statements, 165
Criterion-referenced validity, 49
Critical thinking
 decision trees in, 103–104
 parameters of, 99–101, 102–103
 questions in, 101–103, 105
Cross, T., 141, 388
CRT (conversational recast training),
  200–204
Crystal, D., 178
Culatta, B., 160
Cultural conflict, negotiation of, 406
Cultural dialog, 386
Cultural frameworks, defined, 386
Cultural reflection, defined, 386
Cultural sensitivity, 386
Culture
 and ethnicity, 386
 considerations in emergent
  literacy, 322–323

 considerations in reading and
  writing, 340–341
 dominant, 392
 framework of, 397
 individualist *vs.* collectivist,
  395–396
 mainstream, 392–393
C-unit analysis, 60
Curenton, S. M., 321, 331, 383
Curns, A. T., 212
Curriculum-based language
  assessment, 192–193
Curtiss, S., 19, 182
Cuskelly, M., 257
Cyclic strategies, 166–167

Dahlin, M. P., 189
Dale, P. S., 3, 82, 230
Dancho, K. A., 222
Data
 collection of, 168–169, 173
 in EMT, 198–199
 evaluation of quantity of,
  157–158
 keeping of, 167–171
 naturalistic activities, 170–171
 progress monitoring, 126,
  128, 130
 significance of, 156–157
 subjective, 99
Data recording sheet, 169
Davies, B., 200
Dawson, J., 51, 230
Deaf culture, 218, 224
Decibels (dB), 213
Decision making
 in assessment, 104–113
 change/adaptability in, 101, 118
 clinical process, 25–26
 in discourse assessment, 73
 effective, 98–99
Decision trees
 discourse assessment, 73
 dismissal, 129
 for EMT treatment, 198
 for intervention, 164
 spelling intervention, 335
 use of, 103–104
Decoding, 22, 309
Decontextualized information, 71
Deficits, reading and writing, 306
de Kruif, R. E. L. , 122
Delaney, R., 398, 399
DeLoache, J. S., 135
Delprato, D., 195
Demographics, changes in, 384
Denes, P. B., 3
Deno, S. L., 192
Denton, David, 224
Denver model, 295

Descriptive-developmental approach, 3
DesJardin, J., 225
Detection, early
of hearing impairment (EDHI), 216
importance of, 216–217, 220
Detterman, D., 256
de Uzcategui, A. C. , 229
Developmental, Individual Difference, Relationship-based (DOR/Floortime™) approach, 295
Developmental synchrony, defined, 217
Diagnostic and Statistical Manual of Mental Disorders, Fourth Edition, Text Revision (DSM-IV-TR), 278, 302
Diagnostic labels, and assertiveness/responsiveness, 145
Dialects, 3, 179–180, 397–400
Dialogic speech, 320
Dickinson, D. K., 312
Differentiated instruction, defined, 117
DiLalla, D., 295
Dinnebeil, L., 124
Directive language, 177
Disability, defined, 111
Discourse, 30, 39, 73
Discrepancy criterion model, 109–110
Discrete trial therapy (DTT), 297
Discrimination, 253, 254
Displays, fixed vs. dynamic, 363–364
Disruptions in speech, 74. See also Mazing analysis
Dissanayake, C., 281
Distributed practice, defined, 124–125
Diversity, 383–384, 390–400
Dobkins, K. R., 225
Documentation, 156, 203–204
Dodd, B., 176
Dollaghan, C., 63, 72, 74, 134, 278, 402
Donovan, S., 388
Dopamine, and ASD, 285
Dore, J., 79, 80
Dore's Primitive Speech Acts, 80
DOR/Floortime™ (Developmental, Individual Difference, Relationship-based) approach, 295
Dornan, D., 217, 221
Do statements, 165, 173
Dowden, Pat, 365
Downer, J. T., 120
Down syndrome (DS)
and genetic characteristics of, 249, 250

and language skills, 260–261
and reading, 261, 345
Drager, K., 372, 374, 375, 376, 379
Drew, C. J., 253
Drill-and-practice, 9, 162–163, 168
Drill play, 163
D'Silva, K., 375
DSM-IV-TR (Diagnostic and Statistical Manual of Mental Disorders, Fourth Edition, Text Revision), 278, 302
DTT (discrete trial therapy), 297
Dual language programs, 322
Dube, W. V., 253
Duchan, J. F., 159, 160
Duke, M., 101
Dunlap, G., 302
Dunn, D. M., 84, 156
Dunn, L. M., 84, 156
Durand, V. M., 268
Durkin, K., 185
Dykens, E. M., 248, 251
Dynamic assessment, 45–46
Dynamic displays, 364
Dyslexia, 183

Easterbrooks, S., 217
EBP (evidence-based practice), 134, 153–158
Echolalia, 280
Eckstein, K., 16
Ecological approach
and ID, 274
implications of, 23
tenets of, 23, 40
use of, 41, 264
Ecological model of ID, 245, 246, 247, 274
Edmonson, H., 268
Edmunds, K. M., 118
Edwards, A., 200
Edwards, D., 39
Edwards, P. A., 340
Edwards, S., 266
Effectiveness, in interventions, 99
Effect-size estimates, 157
Efficacy studies, for LSL, 220–221
Ehren, B. J., 109, 118, 125
Ehri, L., 309, 333
Einfeld, S. L., 282
Eisenberg, L. S., 221, 225
Eisenberg, S. L., 58, 61, 205, 206
Eitan, T., 403
Elder, L., 99, 101
Elliott, S. N., 170
Ellis, S., 20
Elman, J. L., 21
Embedded-explicit approach, 308, 317–322, 353
Emotions, 226, 227–228

Empathizing, and ASD, 281
EMT (enhanced milieu interventions). See Enhanced milieu interventions (EMT)
Encoding, as AAC strategy, 362–363
Engagement, 122, 140
English, as a second language to ASL, 218
Enhanced milieu interventions (EMT). See also Interventions
discussion of, 194–200
documentation of goals, 200
evidence for, 199–200
goals for, 199
strategies in, 197–199
theoretical foundations of, 197
Environment
in backward design, 118–119
factors of in ASD, 286
importance of home, 120
influence of, 247
and language stimulation, 177
management of, 214–215
modification of, 243
Espin, C. A., 339
Ethnic group, defined, 384–385
Ethnic mismatches, 386–397
Evans, J., 379
Evidence
evaluation of, 100–101, 114–115
external/internal, 134
levels of, 154
Evidence-based practice (EBP), 134, 153–158
Exclusionary criteria, 176
Executive Act on Intellectual Disabilities, 244
Executive functioning, 339
Explicit interventions, defined, 317
Explicit phonological awareness intervention (EPAI), 346–348
Expository narratives, 39
Expressive One-Word Picture Vocabulary Test, 84
Extended optional infinitive theory, 177
Extensions and expansions, 172
Extinction of behaviors, defined, 8
Eye contact, 403
Eyer, J., 51, 177, 230
Ezell, H. K., 320

Fading, 137, 269
Fallon, K., 379
Families
addressing adults in, 405
in ASD treatment, 287–288
child communication norms of, 405

Families (*continued*)
  communication of results to, 89–91
  and culture, 395
  importance of, 226, 366
  input from, 76–77
  involvement of, 216
  and pragmatics, 147–148
  and remediation process, 225–226
  role in interventions, 229, 404–405
  routines of, 121
Family interviews, 76–77
FAPE (free, appropriate public education), 115
Fast mapping, 82, 83
Fechnay, T., 177
Feedback, 137–138, 147, 215, 349
Fein, D., 289
Fenson, L., 79, 81, 230, 240
Ferch, C., 115
Ferguson, B., 182
Fernald, A., 31
Fernald, D., 137
Ferretti, R. P., 256
Fersko, T. M., 58, 61
Feuerstein, R., 403
Fey, M. E., 9, 68, 139, 140, 142, 144, 150, 157, 159, 160, 162, 163, 164, 166, 183, 195, 196, 198, 200, 201, 202, 203, 204, 206, 249, 282, 306, 309, 310, 328, 348
Fidelity, defined, 156
Fiderer, A., 314
Figurative speech, 82
File, N., 122
Filipek, P. A., 290
Fine, I., 225
Finestack, L. H., 150
Fink, N. E., 221
Finlay, B., 16
Finney, E. M., 225
Fischel, J. E., 182
Fisher, S. E., 176
Fisher-Price, 238
Fixed displays, 363–364
Flanigan, K., 316, 321
Fletcher, P., 178, 179
Flexer, C., 217, 221, 229
Flodin, M., 359
Floortime approach, 194
Fluency, analysis of, 79
FM systems (assistive listening devices), 233
Focused stimulation, 160, 161–162, 163, 172
Foils, use of, 370
Fombonne, E., 284
Fonts, information from, 341
Food, as reinforcement, 137

Form, with content and use, 24, 149
Formative assessments, 57
Form-content-use model, 89, 91
Forum on Educational Accountability, 324
Foundation for Child Development, 388
Fowler, A. E., 260, 261
Fox, A. V., 176
Fox, L., 302
Fragile X syndrome, 251, 261–262
Free, appropriate public education (FAPE), 115
Freedle, R., 330
Frequency, defined, 212
Friederici, A. D., 16
Friedmann, M., 15
Friedrich, M., 16
Fristoe, M., 78, 263
Frith, C., 285
Fromkin, V., 19
Frost, L., 376
Fujiki, M., 31, 38, 186
Functional Communication Training (FCT), 266–271

Gabriel, L., 256
Gadaire, D. M., 269
Gallagher, T. M., 266
Gallaudet Research Institute, 212, 213, 224
Ganea, P. A., 135
Garcia-Sierra, A., 16
Gardner, M., 84, 85
Garman, M., 178
Gavin, W. J., 178
Geers, A. E., 216–217, 221, 225
Gelman, R., 260
Gender, 49, 176
Gene duplication, 249
General American English (GAE), 323
Generalization, defined, 124
Generalization probe, 168
Genesee, F., 322
Genetic syndromes, 248–249
Gentner, D., 134
Gentry, J. W., 393
Giacheti, C., 262
Giacomini, J., 225
Giant words, 276
Gillam, R. B., 39, 53, 120, 135, 155, 158, 166, 180, 326, 328, 330, 402
Gillam, S. L., 155, 158
Gillberg, C., 289
Gillette, Y., 264, 265, 274
Gillon, G. T., 22, 309, 310, 318, 333, 346, 347, 348
Gilmore, L., 257

Gleitman, L., 33, 260
Glenn, C., 328, 330
Goal attainment scales (GAS), 170–171
Goals
  attack strategies for, 166–167
  communication, 302
  components of, 173
  flexibility in, 166
  importance of, 164
  intermediate, 150–151
  for IT's Fun approach, 273
  literacy, 342
  for reading and writing, 306–307
  writing of, 165–166
Goffman, E., 386
Goldberg D., 221
Goldman, R., 78, 263
Goldman-Fristoe Test of Articulation, 2nd edition, 263
Goldstein, H., 141, 184, 259, 266, 279
González, N., 341
Gonzalez-Mena, J., 386, 387, 406
Goossens, C., 372, 379
Gopnick, M., 176, 179
Gordon, K. A., 17, 217, 225
Graham, S., 206, 339
Grammatical analysis, 68
Granlund, M., 366
Grantham, R. B., 387, 405
Graphs, 168
Gravel, J. S., 211
Gray, K. M., 282
Gray, S., 152
Green, J. A., 289
Green, L., 39
Greenberg, J., 148
Greenhalgh, K. S., 320
Greenspan, S., 194, 259, 295
Greenwald, C., 261
Grela, B., 177
Gresham, F. M., 298
Grief process, 226, 228–229
Griffin, T., 229
Groen, A. D., 297
Guesses, serious, 402
Gutierrez-Clellan, V. F., 402

Haager, D., 109
Hadley, P., 45, 149, 178, 180, 181
Haertel, E. H., 50, 54
Haggerman, R. J., 261
Hahne, A., 16
Hakuta, K., 397
Hall, E. T., 395
Halle, J. W., 268, 269
Halliday, M. A. K., 79, 80, 377
Halliday's Communication Function, 80

Hamayan, E., 322
Hammill, D. D., 52, 86, 206, 326
Hancock, T. B., 140, 148, 194, 196, 197, 198, 199, 200
Hand cues, 237, 241
Handicap, defined, 111
Hand leading, 278–279
Hand-wringing, 283
Hardman, M. L., 253
Harm, M. W., 22
Harpell, S., 402
Harris, G. A., 395
Harris, J. C., 248, 257
Harris, J. L., 341
Harris, M. D., 372, 379
Harrison, R. V., 17, 217
Harrower, J. K., 295
Harry, B., 400
Hart, B., 33, 120, 197, 225, 312
Hartley, J., 341
Haskill, A., 166
Hauser, R., 409
Hauser-Cram, P., 257
Hayer, C., 289
Hayes, A., 257
Hayes, R. A., 99
Haynes, W. O., 45, 79
Head to Toe (Carle), 239
Health, influence of, 247
Hearing, screening for, 77, 232
Hearing age, 220, 233
Hearing loss
    causes of, 210–211
    co-occurring conditions, 212
    degrees of, 212–213, 214
    early detection of, 216–217
    intervention for, 235–240
    and language development, 215–216
    prevalence of, 211
    types of, 211–212, 240
Hearing threshold, 213
Heath, S. B., 21, 340–341, 403
Hegde, M. N., 30, 56
Hello, symbols for, 359
Hemmeter, M. L., 225, 268, 269
Henderson, E. H., 333
Henry, L. A., 256
Hepburn, S., 280
Herron, S. R., 52
Hesketh, L., 260
Hesselink, J., 181
Hester, P. P., 199
Heubert, J., 409
Hickson, L., 217
Hindman, A., 120
Hodapp, R. M., 248, 251
Hodges, J., 141
Hodson, B. W., 78
Hoff, E., 142

Hoffman, L., 59
Hogan, K., 280
Hood, J., 182
Hopkins, J., 45
Horizontal strategies, 166
Horn, D., 160
Houston, T., 217
Howard, D., 176
Howard, M. R., 11
Howlin, P., 185
Hoyson, M., 296
Hresko, W. P., 52
Hrncir, E. J., 257
Huang, R., 45
Hudson, T., 54
Hughes, D. L., 200, 201, 203
Huisingh, R., 86
Hulit, L. M., 11
Hull, G. A., 206
Hunt, K. W., 11, 64
Hunt Berg, M., 371
Hunter, L., 211
Hutchinson, T., 280
Hwa-Froelich, D., 387, 396, 400, 402, 403, 405, 406
Hyperlexia, defined, 277–278, 345

Iacono, T., 376, 379
IDEA (Individuals with Disabilities Education Act), 225, 307. See Individuals with Disabilities Education Act (IDEA)
Idol, L., 117
Iglesias, A., 391, 396, 397, 402
Ima, K., 400
Imada, T., 16
Image rehearsal, 256
Imitation, defined, 145
Immigrants, generational patterns in, 394
Impairment, defined, 111
Inclusion, 116–117, 223
Incorporation, and communication, 341
Independence, in European cultural tradition, 400
Individualism vs. collectivism, 394–396
Individualized Education Program (IEP), 116, 126
Individuals with Disabilities Education Act (IDEA), 222, 401
    and dismissal from therapy, 128
    eligibility for, 116
    and ethnic minority children, 401
    provisions of, 115–117, 130–131, 288
    role of families in, 396

Infants, screening of, 216
Information
    overlap of, 89
    processing of, 182, 254
    transformation of, 255–256
Information processing theories, 21–23, 40, 41, 350
Informativeness, 72
Ingersoll, B., 287
Ingram, D., 178, 179, 180
Initiating events (IE), narratives, 328
Innis, J., 267, 268
Instructions
    embedded, 299, 301
    in interventions, 148
Intellectual ability, 245
Intellectual disability (ID)
    defined, 244, 245, 273
    dimensions of, 245–247
    frequency of, 274
    prevalence of, 248
    risk factors for, 248–252
    syndromes associated with, 250–251
    theoretical model, 246
Intelligence, nonverbal, 259
Interactions
    balanced, 148
    dyadic, 404
    in interventions, 148
    multi-party language, 405
    with peers for school-age students, 185–186
Interactive-to-independent (I to I) model, 342–346, 353
Interactive to Independent model. See I to I (interactive-to-independent) model
International Classification of Functioning, Disability, and Health (ICF), 358
Interpreters, 224–225, 397
Interrater reliability, 54
Interventions
    AAC approaches, 372–377
    adult-directed, 159
    adult- vs. child-directed, 159–162
    child-directed, 159–160
    for children with ASD, 295–303
    cultural considerations, 403–409
    decision making in, 113–119
    differences in approaches, 115
    direct vs. indirect, 124–125
    early, 17, 114, 215, 264–265
    effective, 98–99, 164–171, 298
    efficiency in, 99
    embedded, 317
    evidence-based strategies, 153–158
    goals for, 114, 150, 348, 351
    hybrid, 160

Interventions (*continued*)
keeping data on, 167–171
LSL, 219
for maladaptive behaviors, 269–270
micro and macro levels of, 407–409
narrative, 331
natural *vs.* unnatural activities, 162–163
oral language, 320–321
peer-mediated strategies, 186–188
performance-based, 271–273
phonological awareness (PA), 346–348
as preventative programs, 308
pronoun, 150
reading, 338–339, 346–352
response to, 110, 130
and significant impairment, 342–346
spelling, 334–336
stimuli for, 134–135
structure of, 158–164
using peer groups, 279
writing, 339–340, 351
Intervention targets
diagnosis and identification of, 75–89
identifying communication subdomains, 79–89
subdomain 1, 79
subdomain 4, 82–87
subdomain 5, 87–89
subdomains 2 and 3, 79–82
Invernizzi, M., 46, 153, 314, 316, 333, 336
IQ levels, and ID placement, 245
I to I (interactive-to-independent) model, 342–346, 353
IT's Fun program, 271–273
Ittenbach, R. F., 255

Jackson, R. S., 399, 405
Jacobsen, L. A., 384
Jamieson, B., 296
Janosky, J., 402
Jerger, J., 212, 213–214
Jerger, S., 212, 216–217
Jick, H., 284
Joanisse, M. E., 22
Johnsen, S., 78
Johnston, F., 153, 314, 333, 336
Johnston, J., 39, 180, 236, 328
Johnston, S., 379
Joint visual attention (JVA), 28–29, 287, 299
Jones, M. B., 285–286
Jones, M. C., 273

Jones, S., 149
Jorde, L. B., 385
Joyce, B., 124
Jun, S., 393
Justice, L. M., 20, 46, 120, 123, 124, 131, 135, 150, 156, 157, 310, 312, 314, 316, 317, 320, 321, 328

Kaczmarek, L., 266
Kaderavek, J. N., 20, 118, 124, 131, 135, 189, 225, 228, 239, 241, 310, 312, 314, 316, 317, 342, 344, 345
Kaiser, A. P., 140, 141, 148, 194, 195, 196, 197, 198, 199, 200
Kalyanpur, M., 400
Kamhi, A., 118, 124, 336
Kaniel, S., 403
Kanner, L., 278
Karchmer, M., 218
Katims, D., 256
Kaye, J. A., 284
Kay-Raining Bird, E., 260
Kayser, H., 397
Kearney, P. M., 229
Keeley, S., 101
Kellogg, S., 238
Kennedy, M., 3
Kids Count, 383, 385
Kim, H., 140
King, J. M., 356
Kinsler, K., 57
Kirk, K. I., 221
Kirn, H., 121, 122
Klarman, L., 16
Klee, T., 141, 178
Klin, A., 281, 282, 289, 293, 300
Klinefelter syndrome, 250
Klingner, J., 109, 340
Knowledge, cultural, 341
Koch, D. B., 217, 225
Koegel, L. K., 295
Koegel, R. L., 295
Koenigsknecht, R., 202
Kontos, S., 122
Kotak, V. C., 211
Kouri, T. A., 123, 160
Kovarsky, D., 159, 160
Kramer Paige, T., 379
Krashen, S., 19
Krug, D. A., 291
Kubler-Ross, E., 228
Kucan, L., 152
Kuhl, P. K., 16, 17, 18, 19
Kumin, L., 260
Kunce, L. J., 288
Kurtzer-White, E., 226
Kushner, M. I., 401

Labov, W., 411
Labovitz, E. M., 400
LAC-3 (Lindamood Auditory Conceptualization Test -3), 53
Lahey, M., 24, 258
Lai, J., 20
Landau, B., 262
Landry, S. H., 21
Language
areas of, 6
challenges in learning, 7
cohesive, 321
concepts of, 375
content of, 7
decontextualized, 321
defined, 2
delays in, 3, 40
delay *vs.* disorder, 258–259
domains of, 24–40, 259
expansions/extensions, 141
figurative, 82
form of, 6
home *vs.* school, 399–400
and ID, 260
impairments, 305–306, 307, 323–340
literate, 320
oral skills, 311–312
qualitative analysis of, 60–61
skills for, 306
stages of acquisition, 34
use of, 7
and Williams syndrome, 262
Language Acquisition Device (LAD), 13, 15
Language-age match, 64, 65
Language Arts State Standards, 338
Language development
Brown's stages of, 27–28
comparison of, 181
and HL, 215–216
and sign language, 235
Language disorders
defined, 2
identification of, 107
numbers of children with, 2
vs. language differences, 46, 47, 107
Language experience books, 237–240
Language facilitation techniques, 138–142
Language learners, 31–32, 195
Language sample analysis (LSA)
beginning language learners, 57–62
clinical decision making in, 62
defined, 44–45
later language learners, 63–64
two-step process, 63–64
use of, 57, 263

Language samples, obtaining, 57–58
Language theory, importance of, 188
Larkin, R. F., 331
Larsen, S. C., 206, 326
Larsson, B., 375
Late talkers, 3, 40, 207
    and SLI classification, 176
Latinos, nationalities of, 390–391
Laurent, A. C., 292, 293, 296, 299, 300, 301, 302
Laux, J. M., 228, 241
Lave, J., 342
Law, J., 147
Layton, T., 345
Leadholm, B., 63
LEAP (Lifeskills and Education for Students with Autism and Other Pervasive Behavioral Challenges), 296
Learning
    bottom up, 253–256
    cultural attitudes toward, 401
    differences with ASD, 281
    mediated, 402
    subskill process needed for, 254
    top-down, 252–253, 256–257
    visual, 223
Learning to listen (LTL) technique, 235–237
Least restrictive environment (LRE), 115–116, 288
LeBlanc, J. M., 288
Le Couteur, A., 291
Lee, E., 175, 177, 178, 179
Lee, L., 202, 400
LeFevre, J. A., 225
Leigh, I., 227
Leonard, L., 36, 160, 176, 177, 178, 179, 261
Leong, D. J., 20
Lepola, J., 118
Levie, R., 180
Lewis, K., 166
Liberman, A. M., 309
Liberman, I. Y., 309
Lidz, C., 46, 402
Light, J., 363, 365, 372, 374, 375, 376, 378, 379
Lindamood, P., 53, 326
Lindamood Auditory Conceptualization Test -3 (LAC-3), 53
Ling, D., 217, 231, 232, 241
Ling Six Sound Test, 231, 232, 241
Linguistic chauvinism, 399
Linguistic events, in interventions, 134
Linguistic isolation, 384–385
Linguistic Society of America, 392–393

Listening, in counseling, 227
Listening and spoken language (LSL) interventions, 220–222
Listening and Spoken Language Specialists (LSLS), 219
Literacy
    artifacts, 343
    checklist for, 315
    cultural considerations in, 322–323
    early skills, 46, 119, 314–316
    emergent, 305, 308–323
    I to I model, 342–345
    orientation, 316
    social, 316
Little, T., 307
Loban, W., 60
Loeb, D. F., 57, 178, 179, 201, 203, 204
LoGiudice, C., 86
Lombardino, L., 331
Loncola, J. A., 283
Long, S. H., 150, 200, 201, 203
Lonigan, C. J., 305, 309, 310
Lord, C., 49, 291
Lord Larson, V., 326
Losardo, A., 188
Lovaas, O. I., 296, 297, 298
Lovaas approach. See Applied behavioral analysis
Lovascz, C., 267
Lovelace, S., 154
LRE (least restrictive environment), 115–116, 288
LSA (language sample analysis). See Language sample analysis (LSA)
LSL (listening and spoken language) interventions, 220–222
LSLS (Listening and Spoken Language Specialists), 219
LTL (learning to listen) technique, 235–237, 237
Lucas, T. D., 331
Luckasson, R., 244, 246, 249
Luckasson, R. A., 23
Lukomski, J., 225
Lundgren, C., 58, 61
Luterman, D., 226

MacArthur-Bates Communicative Development Inventory (CDI-2), 79, 81, 230, 240–241
MacDonald, J. D., 145, 177
MacDonald-Connor, C., 216–217
MacDuff, G. S., 9
Macionis, J. J., 391
MacKall, D. D., 238
MacLean, M., 256
MacMillan, D. L., 298

Macroanalysis, in LSA, 66, 69–74
MacSweeney, M., 225
MacTurk, R. H., 257
Madnick, M. E., 268
Mainstreaming, 117, 225
Management talk, 312
Mand-model sequence, 195, 196, 197
Marazziti, D., 285
Marchman, V. A., 230
Marcus, G. F., 176
Marcus, L. M., 288
Margolis, H., 146
Marschark, M., 225
Martin, B., 238
Martin, J., 213–214
Maryland School for the Deaf (MSD), 223, 224
Mashburn, A. J., 120
Maslow, A. H., 226
Massed practice, 125
Massed trials, 269
Mastergeorge, A., 299
Masterson, J. J., 135, 183, 326, 330, 333, 334, 335
Mather, M., 384
Mattie, H. D., 266
Maul, C. A., 30, 56
Mawhood, L., 185
Mayatit, H., 225
Mayo, L., 288
Mazing analysis, 72, 74
McAnally, P., 217
McCabe, A., 71, 73, 328, 331
McCabe, P. P., 146
McCaleb, P., 71
McCarthy, J., 379
McCathren, R. B., 225
McCauley, R. J., 196, 198, 200, 289, 348
McColl, R., 213–214
McComas, J. J., 267
McConnell, S., 302
McEachin, J. J., 298
McEvoy, M., 302
McFadden, T. U., 402
McGillicuddy-DeLisi, A. V., 177
McGinty, A. S., 123, 124
McGregor, K., 32, 151, 152, 177, 178
McKenna, M. C., 337, 340, 355
McKeown, M. G., 152, 154
McKerchar, P. M., 222
McInerney, W., 124
McNaughton, D., 378
McNerney, E., 295
McPartland, J., 281, 282
McRoberts, G. W., 31
McTighe, J., 118
McTigue, E. M., 118
McWilliam, R. A., 120, 121, 122, 134, 140

Mean, defined, 54
Meanings, hidden, 187
Mean length of utterance (MLU)
  calculation of, 59–60
  and language development,
    26–27, 57
  in morphemes (MLUm), 58
  and run-on sentences, 64
Mediation, 20
Mehl, A., 217
Meier, J., 46, 314, 316
Mellott, S., 379
Membrino, I., 178
Memory, 87, 254, 256
Menken, K., 409
Mercer, C. D., 256
Mercer, N., 39
Meryl, A., 281
Mesibov, G., 285, 288, 298
Meta-analysis, 154–155
Metacognition, 146–147
Metacognitive strategies,
    255–256, 271
Metalinguistics, 146
Metaskills, 255–256, 338–339, 350
Meyer, J., 124
Meyer, M., 19, 225
Microanalysis, in LSA, 65–69
Millar, D., 365, 379
Miller, C. G., 286
Miller, J., 63, 72, 74, 139, 260,
    261, 272
Miller, R., 212
Mills, D. L., 16
Mills, N. H., 228, 241
Minshew, N. J., 285
Mintz, T. H., 33
Miolo, G., 266, 271, 272, 273
Mirenda, P., 359, 361, 363, 364,
    366, 367, 368, 369, 370, 372,
    373–374, 376, 379
Mirrett, P. L, 261
Mitchell, R., 218
Mix, K.S., 20
Miyamoto, R. T., 217, 221
MLU (mean length of utterance).
    See Mean length of utterance
    (MLU)
Moats, L., 326
Modeling
  in EMT, 195
  in interventions, 163
  of language, 138, 139–140
  of skills, 146
  VSD use, 374
Modified Checklist of Autism in
    Toddlers (M-CHAT), 289
Moeller, M. P., 215, 217, 225
Moeller, P., 216–217
Moerk, E., 146, 203

Moersch, M. S., 295
Moll, L. C., 341
Montgomery, J., 109, 125
Moog, J. S., 221
Moran, K., 239
Morehead, D., 178, 180
Morgan, G. A., 257
Morgan, M. H., 392
Morphemes
  beginning use of, 35
  counting of, 58
  free/bound, 37
  missing, 233
  sequence of emergence of, 27–28
  and surface theory, 177
Morphology
  awareness of, 331
  defined, 6, 37
  in interventions, 148–151
  knowledge of, 334
Morphophonology, defined, 37
Morphosyntax
  assessment of development,
    82–87
  deficits in, 150, 177–180
  defined, 36–37
  and Down Syndrome, 260
  immaturity in, 61
  skill assessment of, 60
  tasks, 83, 87
  trickle-down effect of errors, 180
Morris, D., 333
Morrow, L. M., 314, 322
Morrow, R. D., 405
Most, T., 225
Motherese, 19
Motivation, 118, 122, 257
Motor development, 280–281
Mulhern, S., 202
Mulle, J. G., 251
Multicultural environment, 99,
    386–398
Multi-modal, defined, 358
Murdoch, B., 217
Murphy, M. M., 261, 262

Nadel, L., 268
Nagell, K., 287
Nagle, R., 191
Nail-Chiwetalu, B. J., 157
Nair, R., 182
Narrative/narratives
  components of episodes, 328–329
  development of, 330, 352
  macrostructure of, 331
  microstructure/macrostructure
    of, 328, 332
  oral, 353
  and SLI, 180, 182
  visual cues for, 332

National Institute of Child Health
    and Human Development,
    325, 337
National Institute on Deafness and
    Communication Disorders
    (NIDCD), 211
National Institutes on Health, 216
National Reading Panel, 33
National Research Council, 280,
    284, 298, 302
National Scientific Council on the
    Developing Child (NSCDC),
    16, 17
Native Americans, 391
Native languages, 397
Nativist theory (psycholinguistic
    theory), 13–15, 40, 41
Nature vs. nurture debate, 15
NCLB (No Child Left Behind), 323,
    324, 407–409
Necheles, J., 115
Needleman, H., 402
Nelson, K. E., 200, 203, 204
Nelson, N. W., 33, 147, 154, 206,
    340, 348, 349, 351, 352
Nemser, J., 379
Neuman, S. B., 322
Neural maturation, 15–18, 40, 41.
    See also Brain development
Neurobiological research,
    implications of, 17
Neuroimaging, of infants, 18
Neurological soft signs, 182
Neuroplasticity, 217
Newcomer, P. L., 52
Newell, 393
Newhoff, M., 183
Niccols, A., 257
Nicholas, J. G., 221, 225
Niessen, N. L., 183
Ninio, A., 314, 316
Niparko, J. K., 221
Nippold, M. A., 45
Nittrouer, S., 236
No Child Left Behind (NCLB), 323,
    324, 407–409
Norm-referenced assessments
  advantages/disadvantages of,
    47–48
  defined, 45
  examples of, 50–53
  psychometric properties of,
    54–56
  validity/reliablity of, 54
  writing reports on, 91
Notari-Syverson, A., 188, 319
Number of different words (NDW),
    defined, 63
Nurius, P. S., 228
Nusbaum, D., 224, 225

Oberecker, R., 16
Objective data, defined, 99
Obligatory context, defined, 68
Observations
  behaviorist, 192
  of classrooms, 192–193
  parent-child book reading,
    188–189
  of play behaviors, 190–191
Ochs, E., 29
O'Connor, R., 319
Odom, S., 302
Oelwein, P., 261, 345
Oetting, J., 45, 149, 179
Olley, J., 295
Olmi, D. J., 138
Olson, J. A., 326
Olswang, L., 31, 114, 184, 186, 200
O'Neil, R. E., 268
Onset-rime, 319
Open combining, 205
Opportunity barriers, 369, 370
Oral-motor movements, problems
    with, 259
Oral narratives, 39, 328
Organization, 253–255
Orman, J., 86
Oross, S., 253
Orthographic knowledge, 334
Ortiz, A. A., 401
Osberger, M. J., 217, 225
Ostrosky, M. M., 268, 269
Otitis media, 210, 211, 396
Ousley, O., 280
Owens, R. E., 38, 67, 137, 253
Ozonoff, S., 295

Pakulski, L. M., 225, 239
Papsin, B. C., 17, 217
Paradigm shift, defined, 215
Parallel-distributed processing (PDP)
    models, 21
Parallel talk, 139, 172
Parents
  counseling of, 226–228
  and CRT training, 203
  and DTT interventions, 297
  effectiveness of training, 199–200
  and language teaching, 194
  and literacy, 314
  in LTL training, 235–237
  role of, 197
  training of, 197
Parham, L. D., 281
Parrish, C., 379
Parsons, A., 379
Partial reinforcement, 137
Participation, 367, 369
Partkian, R., 412
Pashler, H., 125

Patel, P., 182
Pattern, J. R., 255
Paul, P., 4, 217
Paul, R., 58, 63, 64, 69, 77, 78, 99,
    101, 106, 107, 126, 135, 141,
    145, 160, 165, 166, 167, 281,
    289, 293, 300, 328, 330, 379
Pauses, in counseling, 227
Peabody Picture Vocabulary Test-4
    (PPVT-4), 84, 156
Peak, P. K., 52
Pearson, N. A., 53, 326, 330
Peers
  and communication, 301
  importance of, 120
  peer confederate training, 184
  peer entry, 184, 186
  peer mediation, 186–187, 207
Peets, K. F., 39
Pelios, L. V., 9
Pellegrini, A. D., 177
Pena, E., 46, 402
Penagarikano, O., 251
Pence, K. L., 82, 83
Penner, S., 123
Pepe, P., 212
Pepler, D., 257
Percentages, calculation of, 168–169
Percentile rank, defined, 56
Pervasive developmental disorder—
    not otherwise specified
    (PSS-NOS), 278, 284. See also
    Autism spectrum disorder
Pervasive Developmental Disorders
    Screening Test-Stage I (PDDST-
    Stage I), 289
Peters, J., 179
Peters-Johnson, C., 248
Peterson, C., 328
Peterson, J., 182
Petscher, Y., 310
Phelps-Gunn, T., 50
Phelps-Terasaki, D., 50
Phillips, N., 101
Phonemes, similarity between,
    233–234
Phonics instruction, 309
Phonological Awareness and
    Literacy Screening—Pre-
    Kindergarten (PALS-PreK), 316
Phonological awareness (PA)
  deficits in, 183, 310
  developmental age levels for
    skills, 310
  in early interventions, 317–319
  in emergent literacy programs,
    309–310
  importance of, 352–353
  school-age students, 324–327
  vs. phonics, 309

Phonology, 6, 78, 216, 260
Physical impairments, 357
Piaget, J., 9, 12, 19–20, 40, 286–287
Pianta, R. C., 120
Picture Exchange Communication
    System (PECS), 376–377, 378
Pictures, use of, 134–135, 136,
    269–270, 271
Pidgin languages, 15, 389
Pidgin (sign language), 224
Pindzola, R. H., 45, 79
Pinson, E. N., 3
Pinto, J. P., 31
Piscitelli, V., 117
Pisoni, D. B., 221
Pitch, and hearing loss, 212–213
Pitkin, L., 375
Pivotal response training, 295
Plante, E., 83, 289
Plasticity, 16, 17, 217
Plauché, M. B., 313
Play
  in ASD interventions, 287
  observation of, 12, 14, 41,
    292, 294
  routines, 160
Playgroups, 239
Plomin, R., 3
Plunkett K., 16
Pollack, Doreen, 220
Pollard-Durodola, S. D., 322
Pond, R. E., 187, 230
Population Reference Bureau, 384
Poverty, and ethnic groups, 398–399
Powell, D. R., 122
Powell, T. A., 189
Practice, defined, 145–146
Prader-Willi syndrome, 250
Pragmatically Speaking (Soto &
    Zangari), 372
Pragmatics, 39
  in assessments, 79
  categories of, 80
  defined, 7
  development of, 180
  early development of, 29
  functions of, 261, 263
  and HL, 216
  in interventions, 147–148
  skills for school-age students, 88
Prat C., 16
Prediction and encoding, in AAC
    devices, 361
Predictive validity, 49
Prefixes and suffixes, 152–153
Preschoolers, intervention for, 114
Preschool Language Scale, 4th
    edition (PLS-4), 187, 230, 263
Pretti-Frontczak, K., 124
Prevention approach, 111–112, 252

Price, T. S., 3
Print concepts, 311–312
Print referencing, 320
Private speech, 20
Prizant, B., 71, 290
Prizant, B. M., 138, 280, 292, 293, 296, 299, 300, 301, 302
Problem solving, metaskills for, 255–256
Processing, simultaneous/ successive, 255
Processing differences, accommodation of, 255
Proctor-Williams, K., 201, 204
Progress, monitoring of, 126–128, 128–130, 294
Prompts, 135–136, 152, 269
Pullout models, 123
Punishment, defined, 9
Puranik, C. S., 310
Pye, C., 81

Qualitative data, 126
Qualitative language analysis, 64–65
Quantitative data, 126
Quattlebaum, P., 128
Questions
    in critical thinking, 101–103, 105
    direct, 146
    literal, inferential, critical, 337
    open-ended vs. closed, 228
    related to communication, 106
    in routines-based interviews, 121
    in traditional vs. RTI assessments, 108
Quigley, S., 217
Quinn, R., 402

Rabidoux, P., 177, 342, 344, 345
Race, concept of, 385
Race/ethnic background, and hearing loss, 212, 213
Rafferty, Y., 117
Rahbar, B., 255
Randomization, of research subjects, 155
Rashotte, C. A., 326
Ratner, N. B., 134, 157, 182
Ravid, D., 180
Raw score, defined, 56
Reading
    and African American English, 323
    aloud vs. silently, 345–346
    comprehension, 336–339
    conventional, 305–306
    development of, 183
    and Down syndrome, 261
    emergent, 239
    for oral language learning, 320

pattern of failure, 110
prevention of disabilities in, 308
Receptive language, 2–3
Receptive One-Word Picture Vocabulary Test-2000 Edition (ROWPVT), 85
Receptive vocabulary, 82
Redmond, S. M., 59
Reeve, K., 233
Referencing, defined, 71
Referents, defined, 71
Reflecting feeling, 227–228
Regulatory communication acts, 373
Rehearsal, and memory, 256
Reichle, J., 372, 379
Reichler, R. J., 291
Reinforcement
    continuous, 137
    delay of, 269–270
    in interventions, 159–160
    positive and negative, 8
    social, 137
    use of, 137–138, 147, 269
Reliability, importance of, 100
Remediation, classroom contexts for, 123–125
Renner, B. R., 291
Reports, guidelines for writing, 92
Request, as a pragmatic function, 67
Rescorla, L., 3, 175, 177, 178, 181, 182
Research
    bias in, 155–156
    contamination in, 156
    Level I, 154, 155, 160
    Level II, 155, 157, 160
    Level III, 155, 157, 160
    Level IV, 155, 157
    quality of, 154–157
Resource allocation, 21, 107
Response/responsiveness to intervention (RTI), 107–110
Responses, eliciting, 135–137
Rett syndrome (RS), 278, 283–284, 302. See also Autism spectrum disorder
Rey, H. A, 241
Rey, M., 241
Reyhner, J., 397
Reznick, J. S., 230
Rhoades, E. A., 221
Rhoads, S., 379
Rhyming, 108, 152, 309, 319
Rhyner, P. M., 314
Rice, M. L., 33, 59, 176, 177, 178, 179, 180, 181, 260, 262
Richieri-Costa, A., 262
Rigler, D., 19
Rigler, M., 19
Risley, T., 33, 120, 225, 312

Rivera-Gaxiola, M., 16, 17
Rivers, K., 331, 384
Roach, A. T., 170
Robbins, A. M., 217, 221, 225
Roberts, J., 181, 211, 261
Robertson, L., 221
Robertson, S., 160
Robins, D. L., 289
Robinson-Zanartu, C., 402, 403
Rocha, A., 262
Rochon, J., 182
Rodriguez-Galindo, A., 397
Rogers, C., 226
Rogers, S. J., 281, 286, 287, 295
Rogers-Warren, A. K., 197
Rogoff, B., 342
Rohrer, D., 125
Romski, M. A., 372, 373, 379
Rondal, J. A., 258, 260, 261, 262, 266
Root word, defined, 83
Rose, S., 217
Rosemary, C. A., 312
Rosen, S., 135
Roseti, S., 387
Rosin, P., 266, 271, 272, 273
Roskos, K., 312, 322
Ross, R., 182
Roth, F., 165, 167
Roulstone, S., 147
Routine, defined, 120
Routines-based interviews (RBI), 120–123
Rubin, E., 292, 293, 296, 299, 300, 301, 302
RubiStar, 127
Rubrics
    and data collection, 170
    defined, 126, 128
    for storytelling, 127
Rudebusch, J., 109, 125
Rules and tools, 272
Ruskin, S., 281
Ruthsatz, J., 256
Rutter, M., 185, 285, 291
Rydell, P. J., 138, 280, 292, 293, 296, 299, 300, 301, 302
Rylance, B., 123

Sabbadini, L., 178
Sabers, D., 87
Sabotage, 237
Sacks, B. I., 261
Saddler, B., 206
Salonen, P., 118
Salvia, J., 263
Sandall, S., 225
Sanes, D. H., 211
Scaffolding, 20, 188–190
Scanning, in AAC systems, 363

Scarborough, A. S., 121, 122, 140
Scarborough, H., 261
SCERTS approach (social communication, emotional regulation, and transaction support), 298–302, 303
Schafer, D. S., 295
Schafer, G., 16
Schalock, R. L., 23, 244, 245, 246, 249
Scherer, N. J., 200, 301
Schieffelin, B., 29
Schirmer, B. R., 217, 229
Schlosser, R. W., 273, 365, 376
Schmidt-Robb, B., 217
Schneider, N., 184
Schneider, P., 138
School-age children, 114, 186–187
School success, and discourse development, 38
Schopler, E., 288, 291, 295, 298
Schreibman, L., 287
Schroeder, S. R., 288
Schuele, C. M., 156, 157
Schuler, A. L., 280
Schwartz, R. G., 17
Schwartz, S. E., 260
Scollon, R., 397, 398
Scollon, S. B., 397, 398
Scope of information, 107
Scores, normal distribution of, 54
Scott, C. M., 183, 206, 328
Screening, 74, 288–290
Scripts, 19, 184, 187, 271
Secord, W., 47, 51, 52, 56, 156, 187, 231
Sedey, A., 217, 225
Sedey, A. L., 225
Segal, E. F., 27
Seidenberg, M. S., 22
Self talk, 139, 172
Seligman, L., 228
Sell, M. A., 180
Semantic deficits, 151–153, 216
Semantics, 7
Semantic transparency, defined, 151–152
Semel, E., 51, 52, 156, 187, 231
SEM (Standard Error of Measure), 56
Senechal, M., 225
Sensorimotor skill development, and ASD, 286–287
Sentence combining intervention, 193, 204–207
Sentence expansion, 205
Sentence recasts, 138, 172, 193, 200–201, 202
Sentences
complex, 69, 70, 205

documentation of, 69
modality of, 201
Separatist patterns, 394
Service delivery models, defined, 123
Sevcik, R. A., 372, 373, 379
SGDs (speech generating devices), 359
Shaken baby syndrome (SBS), 251
Shames, G. H., 227
Shankweiler, D., 309
Shaping, 8, 136–137
Sharma, A., 17, 217, 225, 236
Shattuck, P., 290
Shavelson, R. J., 50, 54
Shea, V., 285, 288
Sherbenou, R., 78
Shogren, K. A., 23
Short, A., 298
Shoshan, Y., 295
Showers, B., 124
Shweder, R. A., 404, 405
Siegel, B., 289
Sigel, I. E., 177
Sigman, M., 281, 286
Signing Exact English (SEE), 224
Sign language
arguments for, 225
baby signs, 222
choices in, 224
and language development, 235
use of, 223–224
Silva-Pereyra, J., 16
Silverman, F. H., 156
Simkin, Z., 183
Singer, B. D., 339, 340
Skinner, B.F., 8, 267
Skinner, B.F. (1957), 7
SLI (specific language impairment). See Specific language impairment (SLI)
Slobin, D. I., 149, 331
Smaldino, J., 243
Smedley, A., 385
Smedley, B. D., 385
Smith, B. J., 225
Smith, H. L., 206
Smith, K., 21, 178, 179
Smith, M. W., 312
Smith, T., 297, 298
Snell, M. E., 256
Snow, C. E., 314, 316
Snowling, M. J., 183, 331
Social constructivist theory, 350
Social function, improving, 301
Social interaction theory
in EPAI, 346
implications of, 20–21
influence of, 41
and intervention techniques, 119, 138–145

and language development, 19
principle of, 40
Social intervention, 184
Social Networks (Blackstone & Hunt Berg), 371
Social participation theory, 342
Sociocultural theory, 19–21
Software, for writing lab, 349. See also Computers, use of
Solomon, R., 115
Sommers, R., 217
Soresi, S., 251
Soto, G., 372, 379
Sounds
intensity level of, 213
segmentation/blending, 319
sound sandwiches, 237
Spanish, 396–397
Specific language impairment (SLI)
characteristics of, 177–182
criteria for, 176, 207
defined, 175
genetic basis for, 176–177
interventions for, 194
problems associated with, 182–184
in school-age children, 183
Speech, 2, 140–141
Speech camp, 271
Speech chain model, 3–6
Speech generating devices (SGDs), 359
Speights Roberts, D., 138
Spelling, 331–336
SPELT-3 (Structured Photographic Expressive Language Test-3), 51, 230
Spencer, L. J., 221
Spinelli, M., 262
Spruytenburg, H., 200
Stahl, S. A., 337, 355
Standard deviation, defined, 55
Standard English, 398
Standard Error of Measure (SEM), 56
Standardized testing, 401, 409. See also Norm-referenced assessments
Standard scores, 54
Stanine, defined, 56
Stanovich, K., 311, 321
Statements, do, condition, and criterion, 165
Stauffer, R., 237, 322
Stein, N., 328, 330
Steiner, V. G., 187, 230
Steppling, M., 128
Sternberg, R. J., 253
Stewart, S. R., 154
Stiggins, R. J., 314

Stimuli, choosing for intervention, 134–135
Stimulus overselectivity, defined, 253
Stone, W., 280, 289
Stories/storytelling, 127, 322, 328, 331
Stout, C. E., 51, 99, 230
Strain, P. S., 296
Strock, M., 287
Strong, C. J., 320
Strong, J., 67
Structured Photographic Expressive Language Test-3 (SPELT-3), 51, 230
Studies, 204, 270–271
Sudhalter, V., 261, 262
Suffixes and prefixes, 152–153
Sullivan, A., 316
Sulzby, E., 189, 305, 316, 320
Sunshine Cottage for Deaf Children, 231, 234, 241
Surface theory, 177
Svirsky, M. A., 221
Swank, L., 316
Swank, P. R., 21
Sweeney, J. A., 285
Swingley, D., 31
Syllable recognition, 318
Symbolic recognition, 344–345
Symbols, in AAC, 358–359
Syntactic bootstrapping, 33
Syntax, 6, 38, 216
System for Augmenting Language (SAL), 372–373, 378
Szatmari, P., 285–286

TACL-3 (Test of Auditory Comprehension of Language), 230
Talking diary, 272
Tallal, P., 177, 181, 182
Tangel, D. M., 319
Tansuhaj, P., 393
Tasks, 182, 253, 318–319
Tate, T. L., 222
Taylor, O. L., 401
TBI (traumatic brain injury), 249–250
Teachers, working with, 124, 223, 340
Teaching, 196, 197, 346–347
Teams, transdisciplinary, 254
Technology, use of, 17
Tees, R. C., 225
Tellis, C., 396, 403
Tellis, G., 396, 403
Templeton, S., 153, 314, 333, 336
Terrell, S. L., 387, 399, 405
Testing, high-stakes, 409. *See also* Assessments

Test of Auditory Comprehension of Language (TACL-3), 230
Test of Early Written Language-2 (TEWL-2), 52
Test of Language Development Intermediate 3 (TOLD-I:3), 52
Test of Narrative Language (TNL), 53
Test of Nonverbal Intelligence (Brown, Sherbenou, & Johnson), 78
Test of Phonological Awareness-2nd Edition PLUS (TOPA-2+), 53
Test of Pragmatic Language (TOPL), 50
Test questions, 403, 404
Test-retest reliability, 54
Test-teach-retest approach, 402
TEWL-2 (Test of Early Written Language-2), 52
Thal, D., 82, 230
Therapy, dismissal from, 127, 128, 129
Thiemann, K., 184, 279
Thompson, C., 164, 331
Thompson, R. H., 222
Thordardottir, E. T., 151, 182
Tier 1 instruction, 109
Tier 1 interventions, 108, 126
Tier 2 instruction, 109
Tier 2 interventions, 109, 126
Tier 3 instruction, 109
Time delay, in EMT, 196, 197
Time orientation, 395–396
Timler, G. R., 31, 184, 186
Tingstrom, D. H., 138
TNL (Test of Narrative Language), 53
Tokens. *See* Number of different words (NDW)
Tolbert, L., 166
TOLD-I:3 (Test of Language Development Intermediate 3), 52
Tomasello, M., 7, 287
Tomblin, B., 216–217
Tomblin, J. B., 176, 183, 221, 306, 307, 309, 310, 328
Tomlinson, C., 117
Tonge, B. J., 282
TOPA-2+ (Test of Phonological Awareness-2nd Edition PLUS), 53
Topics, control and maintenance of, 72
TOPL (Test of Pragmatic Language), 50
Torgesen, J. K., 53, 110, 308, 312, 326
Total communication, 218, 224
Touch, sensitivity to, 280

Training sequence, phonological awareness, 347
Transactional model, 203
Transaction support, 299
Transfer
  in learning, 254
  near/far, 255–256
Translocation (genetic mutations), 248–249
Traumatic brain injury (TBI), 249–250
Trauner, D., 181
Treatment and Education of Autistic and Related Communication-Handicapped Children (TEACCH), 295
Treiman, R., 309, 334
Trembath, D., 372
Trent, J. A., 141
Tropper, B., 17
Tsai, L. Y., 285, 286
Tsatsanis, K.D, 281
T-Score, defined, 56
TTR (type-token ratio), 63
T-unit analysis, 57, 63–64, 69, 206
T-units, defined, 63
Turnbull, A., 268
Tyler, A., 166, 167
Tymchuk, A. J., 255
Tzuriel, D., 403

Ukrainetz, T., 39, 115, 321, 402
Ungerer, J., 286
Universal newborn hearing screening (UNHS), 216
U.S. Department of Education, 312, 386
Utterance segments, 57–58
Uwer, R., 236

Vaccaro, V., 221
Vadasy, P. F., 319
Validity, 49, 100
Van Acker, E. Y., 283
Van Acker, R., 283
Vance, R., 289
van IJzendoorn M. H. , 316
van Kleeck, A. , 140, 405
Van Meter, A. M., 33, 154, 340, 348, 349, 351, 352
Van Riper, C., 139
Vasdev, S., 267, 268
Vaughn, S., 109
Vauras, M., 118
Verbal rehearsal, 256
Verbs
  action, 148
  auxiliary, 60, 137–138, 150, 160
  cognitive, 320–321
  difficulty learning, 151

in *do* statements, 165
state, 148
Vertical strategies, 166
Videotaping, use of, 170
Vigil, D. C., 141, 387, 402, 403, 405, 406
Vining, C. B., 391, 396, 397
Visual scene displays (VSDs), 373–376, 378
Visual storage, 334
Vocabulary
checklist for, 81
comprehension of, 233–234
delays in development of, 81
descriptive, 320–321
development of, 31–33, 180, 196–197
effect of socioeconomic levels, 33
expressive, 82
instruction in, 154
interventions in, 33, 152
nuance in, 152
with prefixes and suffixes, 153
Tier 2 *vs.* Tier 3, 153
using pictures for, 135
Volkmar, F. R., 281, 282, 289, 293, 300
von Suchodoletz, W. , 236
Vul, E., 125
Vygotsky, L. S., 19–20, 40, 138, 188, 197, 225, 342

Wacker, D. P., 270, 271
Wadman, R., 185
Wagner, R. K., 326
Wallace, D., 86
Walpole, S., 340
Walsh, C., 402
Ward, M., 379
Warren, S. F., 225, 249, 260, 262, 266, 269
Warren, S. T., 251
Washington, J., 60, 69, 179, 180, 323
Wasik, B. A., 120
Wasowicz, J., 326
Waters, M., 392
Watkins, R. V., 33, 63, 138

Watson, A.L., 225
Weaver, C., 206
Webb, N. M., 50, 54
Webb, S. J., 285
Web sites, 157, 158, 374
Weighting principle, 21–22
Weinberg, A., 31
Weir, R., 141
Weismer, S. E., 151, 160, 182
Weiss, A. L., 176
Weissenburger, J. W., 339
Weitzman, E., 148
Welliver, M., 379
Welsh, J., 200, 204
Wendt, O., 376, 377
Wenger, E., 342
Werker, J. F., 225
Westby, C., 138, 146, 191, 320, 331, 391, 396, 397, 400
Wetherby, A. M., 138, 280, 290, 292, 293, 296, 299, 300, 301, 302
Wexler, K., 177, 178, 181
Whitehurst, G. J., 182, 305
Whiteman, B. C., 199
Whitmire, K., 109, 118, 125
Wieder, S., 194, 295
Wiederholt, J. L., 326
Wiggins, G., 118
Wiig, E. H., 47, 51, 52, 156, 187, 231, 326
Wilcox, M. J., 28, 123, 160
Wilder, J., 366
Wiley, T. G., 340
Wilkerson, D. L., 92
Wilkes, E. M., 231, 234, 241
Williams, A. L., 167
Williams, D. R., 385, 389
Williams, R. L., 383, 393
Williams, R. S., 82, 83
Williams syndrome, 250, 262
Wilson, K., 238
Windsor J., 183, 328
Winsler, A., 20
Witzig, R., 385
Wixted, J., 125
Wood, A. J., 238

Woodcock, R. W., 326
Wooding, S. P., 385
Woods, C. B., 253
Word combinations, 34–36, 67–68
Word prediction, 362
Word sorts, 336
The WORD Test-2, 86–87
Workload analysis, 306
Worksheets, 66
World Health Organization, 248, 358, 367
Worthy, J., 397
Wray, D., 217, 221
Wren, C., 178
Wright, H. H., 183
Writing
development of, 313–314
emergent, 312–314, 322
school-age students, 339–340
Writing lab (WL) approach, 348–353
Writing probes, 193
Writing process, 348
Wulfeck, B., 181
Wynn, J. W., 297

Xu, H., 211

Ylvén, R., 366
Yoder, D. E., 139
Yoder, P., 194, 195, 197, 200, 225, 266, 280
Yoshinaga-Itano, C., 216–217, 225, 229
Ysseldyke, J. E., 263

Zangari, C., 372, 379
Zeidner, M., 49, 89
Zhang, Z., 183, 306, 309, 310, 328
Zimmerman, I. L., 187, 230, 263
Zimmerman-Philips, S., 217, 225
Zipoli, R. P. Jr., 3
Zone of proximal development (ZPD), 20, 188, 225
Z-score, defined, 56
Zukowski, A., 262